Y0-BXX-227

Atherosclerosis and Its Origin

Atherosclerosis and Its Origin

edited by

MAURICE SANDLER

DEPARTMENT OF ANATOMY, DIVISION
OF BASIC HEALTH SCIENCES, EMORY
UNIVERSITY, ATLANTA, GEORGIA

GEOFFREY H. BOURNE

YERKES REGIONAL PRIMATE RESEARCH
CENTER, EMORY UNIVERSITY,
ATLANTA, GEORGIA

1963

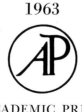

ACADEMIC PRESS

NEW YORK and LONDON

ACADEMIC PRESS INC.
111 Fifth Avenue, New York 3, New York

United Kingdom Edition published by
ACADEMIC PRESS INC. (LONDON) LTD.
Berkeley Square House, London W.1

LIBRARY OF CONGRESS CATALOG CARD NUMBER: 63-21406

PRINTED IN THE UNITED STATES OF AMERICA

Contributors

Numbers in parentheses refer to the page on which the author's contribution begins.

Sv. BERTELSEN, *Institute of Pathological Anatomy, Department of Pharmacology, University of Copenhagen, Frederick d. Femetes, Denmark* (119)

GEOFFREY H. BOURNE, *Yerkes Regional Primate Research Center, Emory University, Atlanta, Georgia* (515)

ROBERT C. BUCK, *Department of Microscopic Anatomy, University of Western Ontario, London, Canada* (1)

I. L. CHAIKOFF, *Department of Physiology, University of California, Berkeley, California* (349)

JACK C. GEER, *Department of Pathology, Louisiana State University School of Medicine, New Orleans, Louisiana* (39)

JOHN W. GOFMAN, *Department of Physics, Division of Medical Physics, The Donner Laboratory, University of California, Berkeley, California* (197)

W. STANLEY HARTROFT, *The Research Institute of the Hospital for Sick Children, University of Toronto, Toronto, Ontario, Canada* (439)

ANCEL KEYS, *Laboratory of Physiological Hygiene, School of Public Health, University of Minnesota, Minneapolis, Minnesota* (263)

JOHN ESBEN KIRK, *Division of Gerontology, Washington University, School of Medicine, St. Louis, Missouri* (67)

S. LINDSAY, *Department of Pathology, University of California School of Medicine, San Francisco, California* (349)

Z. LOJDA, *Laboratory of Angiology, Faculty of Medicine, Caroline University, Prague-Krč, Czechoslovakia* (459)

HENRY C. McGILL, JR., *Department of Pathology, Louisiana State University School of Medicine, New Orleans, Louisiana* (39)

OLGA MRHOVA, *Institute for Cardiovascular Research, Charles University, Prague-Krč, Czechoslovakia* (459)

MAURICE SANDLER, *Department of Anatomy, Division of Basic Health Sciences, Emory University, Atlanta, Georgia* (515)

JEREMIAH STAMLER, *Heart Disease Control Program, Chicago Board of Health, Chicago, Illinois* (231)

JACK P. STRONG, *Department of Pathology, Louisiana State University School of Medicine, New Orleans, Louisiana* (39)

v

LEON SWELL, *Lipid Research Laboratory, Veterans Administration Center, Martinsburg, West Virginia* (301)

MEYER TEXON, *Department of Forensic Medicine, New York University School of Medicine, New York, New York* (167)

WILBUR A. THOMAS, *Department of Pathology, Albany Medical College, Albany, New York* (439)

C. R. TREADWELL, *Department of Biochemistry, George Washington University School of Medicine, Washington, D. C.* (301)

WEI YOUNG, *Division of Medical Physics, University of California, Berkeley, California* (197)

T. ZEMPLÉNYI, *Institute for Cardiovascular Research, Prague-Krč, Czechoslovakia* (459)

Preface

With ever-increasing rapidity the information and literature concerning atherosclerosis is growing. It is impossible at the present time for any one individual to read and assimilate all the available information, especially that derived from disciplines far removed from his own. It would take at once an individual who was a clinician, pathologist, electron microscopist, histochemist, biochemist, and lipid chemist to even stand a chance. This volume is intended to serve as a starting point for the beginner in the field of atherosclerosis research enabling him to ascertain the state of this field at the present time. At the same time, the experienced worker in this field may find the information contained useful in helping him to fit information which he has in with that available from other disciplines. Although not intended for practicing physicians or medical students, they too may be able to see clearer the areas of controversy, especially with regard to diet and its effects on atherosclerosis as well as information as to the diagnostic tools available.

We have attempted to cover the field of atherosclerosis focusing on the human lesion, reverting to information from lower species when the information has not yet been obtained in man. We have included chapters on the histology, pathology, and metabolism of arterial tissue. Believing as do the more sophisticated workers in the field today that there is no one cause of atherosclerosis, we have included chapters on the role of ground substance, hemodynamics, serum lipids, hormones, diet, and the arterial wall metabolism in the development of the lesion.

In view of the importance placed on lipid metabolism in the development of atherosclerosis we felt the need of a chapter on the interrelationship of lipids in blood and tissues, since, for the most part, all that we measure at the present time is blood lipids especially in the clinical situation. Moving on then to experimental atherosclerosis, we felt the need for a description of the naturally occurring lesions in animals, for in order to be certain that the experimental results are due to the manipulation of the experimentor one must be extremely aware of what occurs spontaneously.

We then find discussed methods of inducing the lesion which are in vogue today, followed by a description of the state of metabolism of the aortic wall in the rabbit and then the histochemistry of the lesion in the rat, dog, and man.

We must express our appreciation to all authors for their cooperation and care in preparing this manuscript. The Editors have felt that in a field such as this it was not their place to suggest the removal of a concept because it does not agree with those in vogue today or, in fact, with other authors in this same volume. We feel that any concept which is provoking will generate ideas and will therefore generate further knowledge.

Finally a word of thanks to the staff of Academic Press for their cooperation and care in helping to bring this work to press.

September, 1963

M. SANDLER

G. H. BOURNE

Contents

Histogenesis and Morphology of Arterial Tissue
ROBERT C. BUCK

Natural History of Human Atherosclerotic Lesions
HENRY C. MCGILL, JR., JACK C. GEER, AND JACK P. STRONG

Intermediary Metabolism of Human Arterial Tissue
and Its Changes with Age and Atherosclerosis
JOHN ESBEN KIRK

The Role of Ground Substance, Collagen, and Elastic Fibers
in the Genesis of Atherosclerosis
S. BERTELSEN

The Role of Vascular Dynamics in the Development
of Atherosclerosis
MEYER TEXON

The Filtration Concept of Atherosclerosis and Serum Lipids
in the Diagnosis of Atherosclerosis
JOHN W. GOFMAN AND WEI YOUNG

The Relationship of Sex and Gonadal Hormones
to Atherosclerosis
JEREMIAH STAMLER

The Role of the Diet in Human Atherosclerosis and Its Complications

ANCEL KEYS

Interrelationships of Lipids in Blood and Tissues

LEON SWELL AND C. R. TREADWELL

Naturally Occurring Arteriosclerosis in Animals:
A Comparison with Experimentally Induced Lesions
S. LINDSAY AND I. L. CHAIKOFF

Induction of Experimental Atherosclerosis in Various Animals
W. STANLEY HARTROFT AND WILBUR A. THOMAS

Enzymes of the Vascular Wall in Experimental
Atherosclerosis in the Rabbit

T. Zemplényi, Z. Lojda, and O. Mrhová

Histochemistry of Atherosclerosis in the Rat, Dog, and Man

Maurice Sandler and Geoffrey H. Bourne

—1—

Histogenesis and Morphology of Arterial Tissue

Robert C. Buck

I. Introduction

For a number of reasons, the morphological features of normal arteries cannot be fully described in a single chapter. Consideration must be given to species differences, to differences from one site to another in one species, and to certain changes in these features which occur with the passage of time. Time is a particularly important variable in an analysis of the structure of human arteries, since an understanding of aging effects provides the basis for an intelligent approach to the study of arteriosclerosis.

In this chapter I have tried to survey certain recent work which I consider to be especially significant and, in particular, I have emphasized the electron microscopic studies. Electron microscopy has contributed greatly to the understanding of arterial structure, and although many problems remain, it is true to say that even the most casual observation of properly prepared arteries with the electron microscope provides answers to at least a few of the problems on which investigators of the past spent many futile years. Only part of this gain has been brought about through a higher resolution provided by the electron microscope; much has depended upon better preservation and embedding techniques. Recent improvements in technique, particularly in such electron straining methods as the phosphotungstic acid stain used by Pease and Molinari (1960), have contributed substantially, and further development of such methods will continue to do so.

Since the subject of this book is arteriosclerosis it may not be impertinent to emphasize the importance of regarding the arterial wall as a structure containing living cells having, in greater or lesser degree, such general properties of protoplasm as growth and metabolic activity. The changes observed in arteriosclerosis are, of course, dependent upon many factors, but not the least of these are the living processes of the cells in the vessel wall. It is therefore necessary, in reviewing the morphology and histogenesis of arteries, to include some description of the dynamic properties and potentialities of their component cells. For this reason I have discussed the results of various experimental procedures designed to investigate these properties.

II. Endothelium

A. The Height of Endothelial Cells

The endothelium is a cellular layer which forms a continuous lining throughout the arterial tree. The lining is extremely delicate, and unless gently handled and properly fixed it will be lost or distorted. A good way to fix it in large blood vessels is by perfusion *in situ* under slight pressure for a short time, and follow this by immersion fixation. In smaller arteries of experimental animals the endothelium is fixed well by dribbling fixative for a few minutes over the adventitia while blood continues to flow, and completing fixation by immersion. The vessels should not be cut into small blocks until partially dehydrated.

The height of arterial endothelium may often seem to depend upon the size or type of artery. In small arteries or arterioles the cells are often cuboidal or even columnar, while in the aorta they are usually squamous. However, if the vascular system is perfused with the fixative under slight pressure the endothelium of smaller arteries also appears flattened. Obviously, since the smaller vessels undergo relatively greater post-mortem contraction the height of the endothelium is simply an index of the relative amount of contraction. There is probably no fundamental difference in the height of endothelium in different kinds of arteries.

The high parts of the endothelium of contracted small arteries contain the nuclei which often appear to bulge into the lumen because they come to lie on the "crests" of the folds in the internal elastic lamina (Altschul, 1957). The cytoplasm between the high points may often remain extremely thin. With the electron microscope such thin areas can be observed to represent only the combined thickness of the inner and outer plasma membranes and a fraction of a micron of interposed cytoplasm.

B. Cell Boundaries

The endothelial cells have a long axis paralleling that of the vessel. They are fitted together in a mosaic pattern best appreciated by a study of the surface with whole mounts or with split-off endothelium (Häutchen preparations). Various techniques may be used to make such preparations but probably the simplest is to stain the fresh tissue with silver nitrate. Details of this method are given by Lautch *et al.* (1953) who were largely responsible for reviving the method and applying it to the study of arteriosclerosis. An excellent review of the subject is included in a paper by Poole *et al.* (1958), in which they also describe their modifications of the technique by which the most exquisite rendering of the cell boundaries is accomplished. Sinapius (1956) has also provided a comprehensive review of the literature on the staining of vessels with silver, and from this and his own observations he concluded that chloride ion is responsible for the binding of silver. Chloride may be leached out by soaking in distilled water, but if the tissue is subsequently treated with chloride ion, the endothelium regains its original staining affinity. After studying the distribution of the silver lines in relation to the nuclei, Sinapius (1956) concluded that they did not always represent the intercellular boundaries. Often the nuclei appeared to be located immediately under silver lines. The correctness of this conclusion has been denied by Florey *et al.* (1959).

There are changes in the pattern of silver lines which are related to aging. Cotton and Wartman (1961) studying the aorta, pulmonary artery, and renal artery of man, found that the principal changes were some loss of polarity of the cells (so that the pattern was no longer orderly in relation to the vessel axis) and the appearance of greater

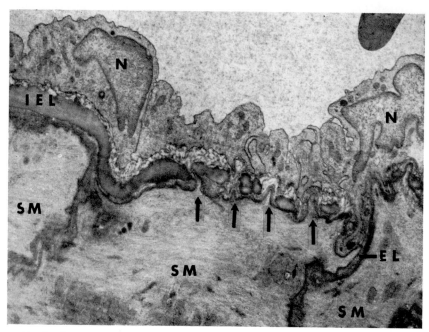

Fig. 1. Low power view of the inner surface of the constricted rat femoral artery showing high endothelium and bulging nuclei (N). The long dark lines in the endothelium indicate points of junction between adjoining cells. The endothelium is separated from the internal elastic lamina by a light space containing the endothelial cell basement membrane and some collagen fibrils. The internal elastic lamina (IEL), which is continuous with elastic lamellae (EL) separating the smooth muscle cells (SM) of the media, shows several fenestrations into which the smooth muscle basement membrane, or sarcolemma, projects (arrows). Vestopal section, stained with phosphotungstic acid. Magnification: × 9700.

variation in the size of cells, with some many times the normal size. In addition, very large cells having up to 9 nuclei in a rosette arrangement were also observed in old age.

With the electron microscope the abutting plasma membranes (Figs. 1 and 2) of adjoining endothelial cells are readily seen. The plasma membrane of one cell is separated from that of its neighbors by a remarkably uniform "gap" of about 100 A. In fact, there is probably no real "gap" at all, for the area of low density may be filled with a part of the membrane not visualized in the electron micrograph. The perfectly parallel course of the two membranes, in spite of convolutions, would suggest that this is the case. The extent and complexity of this interface, as seen in sections cut at right angles to the plane of the endothelium, depends largely upon the heights of the cells. In the high endothelium of small vessels fixed by immersion a long, wavy, often interdigitating boundary exists; in the lower endothelium of perfusion-fixed vessels the interface is usually shorter and straighter. The longer interface is associated with vascular constriction and the shorter one with dilatation. The implication of these observations is that, in some cases at least, the morphological basis of the boundary between the cells need represent nothing more specialized than simply their coming into contact with each other, for its extent can be varied by varying the degree of constriction of the vessel.

On the other hand, in some vessels endothelial cell junctions show special morphological features which suggest a function in holding the cells together. In the rabbit coronary artery certain stretches of plasma membrane along surfaces of mutual contact are occasionally seen to be slightly more dense than other parts (Parker, 1959). True desmosomes are rarely seen in arterial endothelium although they are present in certain types of capillaries (Farquhar, 1961).

Fine intracellular fibrils, sometimes seen in endothelial cells of small vessels may perhaps be associated with desmosomes. Florey and Grant (1961) and Rhodin (1962) stated that fibrils were commonly seen. Fibrils observed in certain endothelial cells of the human dermis and subcutaneous tissue were considered by Hibbs *et al.* (1958) to represent contractile elements. They believed that special blood vessels possessing such contractile endothelium might be important in the regulation of skin temperature by their control over blood flow. In view of the common occurrence of fibrils in endothelial cells (Fig. 2) the existence of special contractile endothelium is questionable. The function of fibrils in endothelium, and in such cells as those of the hepatic parenchyma, is still not understood.

C. Intercellular "Cement"

The question of the existence of intercellular "cement" at endothelial cell junctions has been under study for many years. A review of the evidence for supposing that a cement material exists between endothelial cells and is stained by silver nitrate was given by Chambers and Zweifach (1947) and Zweifach (1959). According to McGovern (1955) the cement substance is a normal secretion of the endothelial cells of veins, although mast cells may produce a film of similar material after injury to the vessel.

By studying the silver lines in thin sections and also in spreads of the surface membrane with the electron microscope, I observed that although the intercellular boundaries were stained the silver appeared to be bound to the abutting plasma membranes and not to any material between them (Buck, 1958a). My interpretation was that the specific distribution of silver was determined by its becoming entrapped in the tiny "gap" between the cells, from which it did not diffuse out during the subsequent rinsing to remove excess silver.

The question has recently been very carefully investigated by Poole *et al.* (1958) and Florey *et al.* (1959). With the light and electron microscopes they also failed to find any evidence supporting the view that silver stains a cement substance. Their conclusion was ". . . that 'cement' in the sense understood by earlier workers, does not exist. This statement must be qualified in two ways. In the first place, although there is no layer of intercellular material of a thickness corresponding to the thickness of silver lines, there appears to be a thin space between endothelial cells which no doubt contains some substance, although this substance is not specifically stained by silver nitrate. In the second place, the fact that there is no cement does not mean that the considerable body of knowledge about the staining properties and reactions of 'cement' is valueless. On the contrary, if, as seems likely, previous workers who have studied the staining properties of 'cement' have really been studying the properties of the endothelial cell surface, the potential interest of their works is increased" (Florey *et al.*, 1959).

Further evidence for the absence of cement was provided by Stehbens (1962) who made autoradiographs of Häutchen preparations of endothelium after administering sulfate-S^{35}. Since one would expect cement to belong to the group of sulfated mucopolysaccharides his failure to observe any significant activity corresponding to the sites of intercellular boundaries argues against the cement concept.

D. Cellular Morphology

The unique structural feature of the endothelial cells is that they line the blood vessels. Otherwise, as seen with the light microscope, they have few remarkable morphological characteristics. Within the cytoplasm, which is usually slightly basophilic, formed structures are difficult to discern. The shape of the nuclei varies with the height of the cells, being flat and oval in low endothelium and spherical or even elongated in the opposite axis in contracted vessels with high endo-thelium. With the exception of occasional binucleated cells and the giant cell masses found in regenerating or otherwise abnormal vessels, the endothelium consists of individual cells, each with a single nucleus. With appropriate techniques one or two small nucleoli can be demon-strated.

Electron micrographs reveal that the usual cytoplasmic organelles are present, namely, mitochondria, Golgi apparatus, endoplasmic reticu-lum, and a pair of centrioles (Fig. 2). The membranes and vesicles of the Golgi apparatus as well as the rough surfaced membranes of the endoplasmic reticulum (those having attached ribosomes) are rather inconspicuous in normal endothelial cells. There are also certain other membranous structures having no attached ribosomes. Some of these which are relatively large and empty can be shown by serial sections to consist of tubular invaginations of the surface plasma membrane (Buck, 1958a). Pockets of this type may extend most of the distance through the cell.

A striking membranous component, and one which has attracted attention for some time (Palade, 1953), is the pinocytic vesicle (some-times called *caveolae intracellulares;* Parker, 1959). These tiny in-vaginations of the surface membrane (Fig. 2) of rather uniform size (50 to 60 mμ) have been observed by many workers. Although particularly numerous in capillaries and arterioles (Palade, 1953; Moore and Ruska, 1957; and many others) and in the aorta (Buck, 1958a; Pease and Paule, 1960), they are found in the endothelium of all kinds of vessels. Great numbers of them may project into a narrow layer of cytoplasm close to the plasma membrane, and in this same layer are often found many tiny spherical vesicles, unattached to the plasma membrane. The free vesicles are identical in size with those whose lumen is open at the plasma membrane. It is a reasonable assumption that they represent a different phase of the activity of a single type of structure, and that this activity is concerned with the transport of materials into or out of the cell.

E. Permeability

The function of pinocytic vesicles in the transport of injected colloidal gold particles has been demonstrated in capillary endothelium by Palade (1961), who observed a higher concentration of particles in the vesicles than in the rest of the cytoplasm. Studying this phenomenon in the aortic endothelium after the injection of colloidal thorium dioxide, I observed particles in larger vacuoles (Fig. 3) but failed to

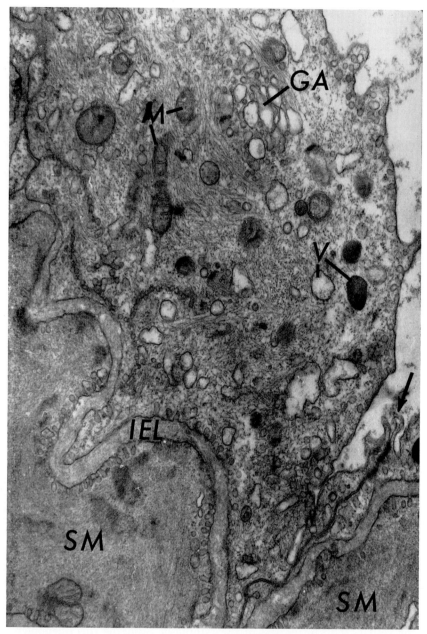

Fig. 2. Most of this figure shows part of a single endothelial cell of a human testicular artery. The plasma membranes of this cell and the abutting endothelial cell are separated from each other by a light, uniform "gap" of about 100 A. The point

demonstrate them in pinocytic vesicles (Buck, 1958a). An explanation for this negative result may be that, although the individual thorium particle is small enough to enter the vesicle, the aggregates of particles which one observes after intravenous injection are probably too large.

Pinocytic vesicles are not confined to the inner surface of the endothelial cells. Many are found at the outer plasma membrane and at the boundary between adjacent cells. They exist also in other types of cells, such as smooth muscle. Bennett (1956) has postulated a mechanism of transport from the inner to outer membranes involving pinocytic vesicles. Moore and Ruska (1957) have suggested that the term "cytopempsis" more appropriately describes the one-way passage through the whole cell. Zweifach (1959) believes that such a form of transport, if it exists, is of limited significance.

The fact that the arterial endothelium is permeable to certain macromolecules has been well established, both by the early work with colloidal dyes (reviewed by Duff, 1932) and by modern isotope techniques using such substances as labeled serum albumen (Duncan *et al.*, 1959) and labeled cholesterol as part of a lipoprotein moiety (Duncan and Buck, 1959). One can only speculate at the present time about which of the cytoplasmic structures is implicated in the transport of specific substances through the endothelium. Pinocytic vesicles may be concerned only with materials in aqueous solution, including probably the colloidal dyes, and certain proteins and lipoproteins. However, diffusion, "active transport," and phagocytosis may all be involved in the passage of other materials. Of these, only the process of phagocytosis is reflected in the morphology of the cell, and it can be recognized by the appearance of certain vacuoles.

Vacuoles, or membrane-bounded spaces, are uncommon in normal endothelium, but they can be induced to appear by various experimental means. They are seen in great numbers (Fig. 4), for example, in arterial endothelium from edematous areas produced by intermittent occlusion of an artery (Buck, unpublished). Probably the content of such clear vacuoles is largely water, which may have entered the cell by pinocytosis. Vacuoles revealed by other experiments are more clearly

---

of junction terminates at the lumen in a fold or "flap" (arrow). The cells rest on the corrugated internal elastic lamina (IEL), outside of which is the smooth muscle (SM) of the media. The endothelial cell cytoplasm contains many fine fibrils everywhere except in the Golgi zone (GA), where vacuoles and vesicles are present. Many pinocytic vesicles exist at the plasma membrane of the inner and outer surfaces. Similar vesicles are seen deep in the cytoplasm, and in this picture they are mainly arranged in rows. Mitochondria (M) and clear and dense vacuoles (V) are present. Lead stained Epon section. Magnification: $\times$ 27,000.

indicative of the phagocytic capacity of arterial endothelium. Lipid vacuoles are seen in aortic endothelium after feeding a diet containing corn oil and cholesterol, but very few are present if only cholesterol is added to the diet (Buck, 1958b). Pease and Paule (1960) observed intracellular elastin in normal rat endothelium, apparently taken up by

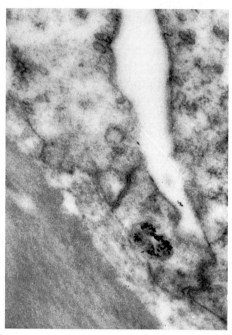

Fig. 3. Endothelium of rabbit aorta 3 hours after intravenous administration of colloidal thorium dioxide. Aggregates of particles are seen in the membrane-bounded inclusion. Methacrylate section. Magnification: 48,000.

phagocytosis. With the electron microscope I have observed vacuoles containing particles of thorium dioxide in the rat and rabbit aortic endothelium (Fig. 3) a few hours after the intravenous injection of Thorotrast (Buck, 1958a). This finding is at variance with the observations of Simonton and Gofman (1951) and Duff *et al.* (1954) who failed to observe phagocytosis under similar conditions using the light microscope. Duff *et al.* (1954) did observe considerable uptake of thorium particles in the rabbit aortic endothelium only after feeding a cholesterol-rich diet. They concluded that the phagocytic capacity of the arterial endothelium was acquired by exposure of the cells to high serum cholesterol. It seems likely that the relatively low phagocytic property of arterial endothelium, often requiring the use of the electron microscope for its demonstration, may be greatly enhanced by cholesterol feeding and also by a number of other experimental procedures or pathological processes, for example, by arterial ligature (Ferrara, 1950). Blood pigments, although taken up by phagocytosis in many other

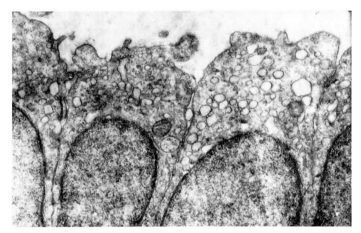

FIG. 4. Endothelium of rat femoral artery showing many clear vacuoles in the cytoplasm. Edema was produced in the leg by intermittent occlusion of the vessels with a cuff. Vestopal section. Magnification: × 18,000.

tissues, are apparently not found in human arterial endothelium (Cappell *et al.,* 1957).

There is also the question of permeation at intercellular boundaries. The morphological studies which formed the basis of the controversy over the existence of "stomata" in normal arteries (reviewed by Altschul, 1954) are now largely of historical interest, since the possibility of detecting the permeation of materials between cells with the light microscope seems, in retrospect, to have been hopeless. Indirect evidence that permeation at these sites does take place in capillaries has been obtained by Chambers and Zweifach (1947). They suggested that certain materials must pass through intercellular boundaries because transport through the cells would involve too great an expenditure of energy. The question has been reviewed recently by Zweifach (1959). My observations are of a negative type. Injected particulate matter, thorium dioxide, was not observed in the intercellular boundaries of rat or rabbit aorta (Buck, 1958a). Obviously the results of this experiment should not be interpreted as excluding the possibility of the passage of other substances of smaller size.

F. Penetration by Cells

Endothelium is also permeable to certain kinds of cells, and, in this case, the entrance is probably effected through intercellular junctions. The classic studies of Clark and Clark (1935) on the endothelium of capillaries of the rabbit ear showed that with mild injury the endothelial surface became sticky, so that circulating leucocytes adhered to it. Also using the transparent chamber in the rabbit ear, Florey and Grant (1961) have reinvestigated the question of cell penetration following injury with ultraviolet light. Their observations were made with the electron microscope. They found that leucocytes, either polymorpho-nuclears or monocytes, first flattened on the side contacting the endo-thelium. The authors were unable to provide definite information on the point of entry through the endothelium, whether between the cells or not. The basement membrane was often pushed ahead of the leuco-cytes which, in some cases, formed a substantial layer between the endothelium and extraendothelial tissue. In an earlier study with the light microscope Poole and Florey (1958) saw macrophages penetrating the aortic endothelium of cholesterol-fed rabbits, and under these conditions the cells entered at the intercellular boundaries. Williams (1961) considered that the rather slight trauma associated with simply freeing a vessel from its bed was sufficient to induce stickiness of the endothelium toward macrophages.

An interesting structural feature of the inner plasma membrane of certain arteries may possibly be related to cellular or molecular pene-tration. Inwardly projecting "flaps" at the intercellular boundaries have been described by Sinapius and Schreil (1956), Pease and Paule (1960), and others. A rather complicated flap of funnel shape is seen in capillaries of the choroid of the eye in fish (Fawcett and Wittenberg, 1962). The inconstancy of "flaps," at least in mammalian arteries, suggests to me that they may represent folds in the inner plasma mem-brane produced by arterial constriction (Fig. 2).

G. Regeneration of Arterial Endothelium

The question of the regenerative capacity of endothelium of arteries is an important one for the problem of arteriosclerosis. It involves such phenomena as the ability of endothelium to grow out and cover fibrin thrombi (Duguid, 1952), the recanalization of vessels, and the growth of collateral arteries following obstruction.

The rate of regeneration of endothelium in injured arteries is usually said to be rather low. Efskind (1941) found that after mechanical trauma to large arteries growth of a covering layer from the surrounding endothelium was slow, and large defects were covered by the transformation of cells of the subendothelial tissue. In a study of the regeneration of rabbit aortic endothelium Poole *et al.* (1958, 1959) found that although the rate of repair was probably rapid for a few days after injury, it was then very much slower, so that more than a year passed before regeneration was complete. They observed migration of endothelial cells from the margins of a scraped area beginning 24 hours after injury and then, from the second to the fifth day, numerous mitoses of these cells. The authors provided convincing photographs of both sectioned material and surface spreads, and there seems to be no possibility that the mitotic cells were of subendothelial origin. The regenerated endothelium had an irregular pattern due to the great variation in the size of the cells and to their somewhat random orientation. Multinucleated giant cells were present from an early date.

Rapid regeneration over a small area may occur. Crawford (1956), studying sections of the human carotid artery from patients who died at various intervals after puncture of the artery for angiograms, noted that the fibrin plug was completely covered by new endothelium in 6 or 8 days. Proliferation of endothelial cells was seen at 18 hours.

A species difference was said by Cotton *et al.* (1961) to account for the more rapid rate of regeneration seen in dog arteries than that observed by Poole *et al.* (1958) in the rabbit. In their experiments a circular patch of endothelium slightly larger than a centimeter was removed by gentle abrasion from the opened dog aorta. Healing took place by the rapid proliferation of pre-existing endothelium at the margins of the denuded area, so that the defect was completely covered in 3 weeks. A growth rate of 0.5 mm per day was calculated. Mitosis of endothelial cells was observed at 8 days and 15 days; no attempt was made to study mitosis in earlier stages. In these experiments the regenerating endothelium grew over a fibrin thrombus which covered the bare area in all but one dog to which heparin had been administered. The authors urged caution in the application to man of the results of animal experiments on vascular healing.

In another experiment, involving the substitution of a knitted "Dacron" graft for part of the aorta of the baboon, Florey *et al.* (1961) observed a high rate of growth of the new endothelium (pseudo-intima). In fact, the rate was almost exactly the same as that determined by Cotton *et al.* (1961) for the dog aorta, namely about 0.5 mm per day.

The question of the life span of endothelial cells and their replacement in the normal artery has been discussed by Altschul (1954, 1961). He considered that during the life of the organism these cells were subjected to potentially damaging influences from pressure, flow, arterial constriction, and turbulence. He therefore supposed that considerable replacement must be constantly in progress. Because of the virtual absence of endothelial cells in mitosis in normal arteries Altschul belived that amitotic division must account for their replacement. On the other hand, he found that mitosis did occur in fetal arteries and ligated arteries.

The nature of the physical forces exerted upon endothelial cells deserves more consideration from morphologists than it has generally received. Altschul (1957) has demonstrated that in prolonged arterial constriction (24 hours) the nuclei change their position and come to be arranged in rows on the "crests" of the folded internal elastic lamina. Such a displacement of the nuclei would suggest that powerful forces are acting on the cells during extreme arterial constriction.

It seems to me less likely that the normal conditions of pressure, flow, and turbulence have any effect on endothelium. If the possible effects of pulsatile flow are disregarded, there is no reason to suppose that endothelium is subjected to greater outwardly directed pressure than cells in other sites. A transmural pressure gradient extends across the wall (Burton, 1954, 1962a) so that, although a considerable pressure difference exists between the outside of the vessel and its lumen, a smaller difference is present between any two points inside the wall. The closer together these points lie, the smaller is the pressure difference. For this reason the very thin endothelial cell must have virtually the same pressure on its outer surface as it has on its luminal surface. Moreover, certain parts of the arterial wall, such as the elastic fibers, have a physical character especially adapted to resist the blood pressure. As a result the pressure gradient is not uniform, but varies from point to point in a manner proportional to the ability of the particular structures to withstand pressure. Thus, the pressure gradient is dissipated largely in structures other than endothelium.

The concept of laminar flow (Burton, 1954; McDonald, 1960) suggests that there is not any appreciable force due to "friction." In theory, the blood in contact with the endothelium does not move, and the highest rate of flow occurs in the axis of the lumen. Turbulent flow, and especially flow associated with a bruit, would seem to be potentially damaging to endothelium since the concept of laminar flow does not apply here. (see also the discussion in Chapter 5 of work reported by Texon). Recently, Dr. Margot Roach, of our Department of Biophysics, allowed me to examine some of her specimens in which turbulent flow, with a bruit, had been present for several months. The specimens consisted of part of the dog femoral artery distal to a partial obstruction. Although the wall of the artery was dilated (poststenotic dilatation) I could find no evidence of abnormality of the endothelium in sections examined with the light microscope or with the electron microscope.

H. Metaplasia

Studies on the metaplastic transformation of other cell types into endothelium have been reviewed by Altschul (1954, 1961). The characteristic feature of the endothelial cell is that it forms the lining of the vessel. Any other kind of cell in this location would be difficult or impossible to distinguish from an endothelial cell. It may be that under certain conditions monocytes can form a vascular lining (Buck, 1961).

The transformation of endothelial cells into other types is generally believed to occur under certain conditions of repair. Altschul (1961) believed that endothelium could dedifferentiate into immature connective tissue cells which had the potential for changing again into endothelium, smooth muscle, or even cartilage and bone. Ferrara (1950) and Schaeffer and Radasch (1924) found that after the application of two ligatures to the rabbit carotid artery, endothelial cells were desquamated; in the lumen of the vessel they became transformed into various types of phagocytic cells and into fibroblasts. The observations of Malyschew (1929) were similar except that he observed hematopoiesis in the doubly litigated segment. According to Williams and Montgomery (1959) the proliferation of endothelium after chemical injury to a segment of artery begins after 1 week, when a layer several cells thick is formed. They stated that this layer, derived from surrounding healthy endothelium, gave rise to fibroblasts and later to smooth muscle cells. An essentially similar view of the potentialities of endothelium in doubly ligated arteries was expressed by Mehrotra (1953).

My observations (Buck, 1961) are not in accord with this view. In fact, with the electron microscope I have not seen the development of more than a single layer of endothelial cells during the repair process following mechanical or thermal injury or after ligature. If the endothelium is destroyed by freezing a length of artery, new endothelium grows from the surrounding healthy endothelium to provide a single cell layer over the surface. Concurrently new smooth muscle cells grow into a subendothelial location. These are derived not from the endothelium but from the media. The origin of these cells will be discussed in connection with the growth of subendothelial tissue.

I. Basement Membrane

In the smaller branches of the arterial tree a basement membrane is usually demonstrated in association with the outer plasma membrane of the endothelial cells. In the aorta a basement membrane is virtually absent (Buck, 1958a; Pease and Paule, 1960). The basement membrane of very small arteries may be shared between the endothelial cell and smooth muscle, and in larger muscular arteries it is part of the general basement membrane system extending throughout the media (Pease and Molinari, 1960). Thus, the basement membrane, composed of acid mucopolysaccharide, may be continuous with deposits of this material in the subendothelial region.

According to Curran (1957) the endothelium of capillaries and other small vessels incorporates injected S^{35}-sulfate, a finding which would imply the capacity of the endothelium for forming basement membranes. However, in his autoradiographic studies, Stehbens (1962) was unable to confirm this work since he found virtually no activity over capillaries, small arteries or veins, or over the endothelium of larger arteries. If the basement membrane is, in fact, composed of sulfated mucopolysaccharide, the question of its origin remains unsettled.

III. Subendothelium

A. Diffuse Intimal Thickening

The subendothelial layer of normal human arteries is extremely variable in thickness, depending principally upon which artery is being considered and upon the age of the subject. In all the arteries of the fetus the endothelium with its basement membrane lies directly against the internal elastic lamina. The latter occasionally shows short lengths of so-called "splitting" or "reduplication." This process, and the associated accumulation of small pools of acid mucopolysaccharide, probably represents the earliest stages in the development of a subendothelial layer. According to Movat *et al.* (1958) most newborn infants show some evidence of this change, and between 6 months and 1 year of age additional elastic but few collagen fibers may form in this layer.

The cells associated with the elaboration of the elastic fibers and mucopolysaccharide, even at this early stage, are smooth muscle cells. In the coronary arteries "splitting" of the internal elastic lamina occurs in the first year of life, followed by the growth of smooth muscle into the "split" (Gross *et al.*, 1934). Discontinuities in the internal elastic lamina allow the passage of cells from the media. In the poplitial and lower brachial arteries similar changes appear in the first and second decades (Robertson, 1960).

Throughout childhood the number of subendothelial smooth muscle cells in the coronary arteries and aorta continues to increase, so that by early adulthood a well developed tunica intima is present. In the coronary arteries a musculoelastic layer having smooth muscle cells longitudinally arranged is supplemented in later decades by one or two distinct inner layers. The elastic-hyperplastic layer of Gross *et al.* (1934), lying immediately inside the musculoelastic layer, consists of elastic fibers and circularly arranged smooth muscle. The innermost layer, the connective tissue layer of Gross *et al.* (1934), contains a high proportion of collagen.

The human aorta shows similar age-related changes (Movat *et al.*, 1958). In the second decade there develops a musculoelastic layer with much smooth muscle and an elastic-hyperplastic layer consisting of irregularly arranged smooth muscle, histiocytis, occasional fibroblasts, delicate elastic fibers, and ground substance. These changes are particularly pronounced in the abdominal aorta. In this region a third, and innermost, layer appears in middle age consisting largely of collagen and elastic fibers, mucopolysaccharide, and a few cells. In old age atrophy and collagen replacement of smooth muscle are found. Movat *et al.* (1958) considered the hyperplastic changes were of great importance, as they corresponded in their location to the sites of future atherosclerotic change. In their opinion the process of diffuse intimal thickening, a normal age-related phenomenon, predisposes to the development of atherosclerosis and constitutes, in fact, a prerequisite for this pathological change. Others regard diffuse intimal thickening as part of the picture of atherosclerosis (Wilens, 1951; Prior and Jones, 1952).

B. Subendothelium at Bifurcations

Aside from the diffuse thickening of the intima there is found a focal growth of subendothelial tissue at the sites of arterial branching. Wagenvoort (1954) observed muscular rings at points of branching from the aorta. According to Conti (1953), cushions of smooth muscle and elastic fibers, often polyploid in shape, may regulate the flow of blood in certain areas. Stehbens (1960) observed intimal pads around the bifurcations of cerebral arteries of fetuses and infants. The pads consisted of longitudinally arranged smooth muscle formed into strata by alternation with elastic lamellae. The endothelium over the pads showed no evidence of proliferation.

Smooth muscle pads developing in fetal life at arterial bifurcations may later give rise to much more extensive subendothelial tissue. Robertson (1960) considered that the longitudinal bands of smooth muscle in the subendothelium of the poplitial and brachial arteries represented a progression of the development of the branch pads, although he stated that cells also entered the longitudinal bands by passing through fenestrations in the internal elastic lamina. This seems to be a point on which more information is needed. A useful study might be made of the spread of smooth muscle cells in relation to age, for example by observing their extension through the aortic subendothelial space from the points of branching of the intercostal arteries.

C. Subendothelium in Experimental Animals

1. NORMAL CONDITIONS

In addition to the growth of subendothelial tissue in diffuse intimal thickening and at arterial bifurcations an essentially similar development appears as a consequence of a variety of experimental procedures. Usually these experiments have been performed on laboratory animals, and it is therefore necessary to realize that, in general, normal experimental animals do not usually show any appreciable degree of diffuse intimal thickening. In the aortas of the rat, rabbit, cat, and ferret only a few unit fibrils of collagen were found in the subendothelial space (Buck, 1958a). Keech (1960) observed an increase in the number of subendothelial collagen fibrils in the rat aorta with aging. Pease and Paule (1960) observed no subendothelial cellular elements in the rat aorta. Parker (1959) found no cells in the subendothelium of the rabbit coronary arteries. On the other hand, Lopes de Faria (1961) observed localized intimal cushions in large and small coronary arteries of older rabbits. At many points of bifurcation of large arteries there were longitudinally oriented smooth muscle cells. In smaller arteries the cushions were frequently unrelated to branchings.

2. EFFECTS OF ARTERIAL LIGATURE

The application of a ligature is one of the simplest and most commonly studied means of provoking the development of a cellular subendothelial layer in experimental animals. A single ligature may be applied or two ligatures may be separated by a short length of artery. In either case the result is a striking growth of new tissue leading eventually to obliteration of the vessel. References are given by Buck (1961) to the many early experiments of this type. According to my observations the cells of the subendothelium seen a few weeks after ligature are virtually all of one kind, namely modified smooth muscle cells. They assume a two-layered arrangement similar to that observed in the human coronary arteries affected by diffuse intimal thickening (Fig. 5). The cells of the inner layer have a circular disposition and those of the outer layer, lying immediately against the internal elastic lamina, are longi-

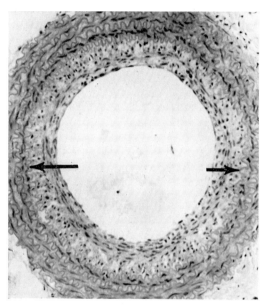

FIG. 5. Internal carotid artery of the rat immediately proximal to the site of ligature 16 weeks previously. The thick intima consists of two layers, an inner circular and an outer longitudinal. The arrows indicate the position of the internal elastic lamina. Paraffin section, hematoxylin and eosin. Magnification: × 115.

tudinally arranged. No fibroblasts can be found. The extracellular material contains many elastic fibers and a little collagen.

My observations on ligated arteries differ in certain respects from those of many who have studied this phenomenon. All agree that a concentric growth of subendothelial cells appears, but some regard these cells as proliferated endothelium (Carden, 1936-1937; Mehrotra, 1953) or as fibroblasts differentiated from endothelium (Schaeffer and Radasch, 1924; Malyschew, 1929; Ferrara, 1950) or as leucocytes (Schaeffer and Radasch, 1924).

The nature of these cells is an important point to establish because the information which can be obtained from this simple experiment is, I think, directly applicable to the much more complicated problem of atherosclerosis. Atherosclerosis represents the morphological response to some kind of arterial injury, although the nature of the injury is not completely understood. Most experimentally induced injuries to arteries, including ligature, show a consistent pattern of repair, and the repair process involves the organization of some of the same cellular elements as those concerned with the repair in the atherogenic process. Moreover, since there is strong evidence that the regions of the arterial tree first and most severely affected by atherosclerosis are sites of pre-existing intimal thickening, it is important to understand the potentialities of the cells of this particular kind of tissue for such properties as phagocytosis, collagen and elastic fiber production, and lipid and mucopolysaccharide synthesis.

Using only the light microscope for studying the cytology of intimal thickening, one is likely to have difficulty in making a positive identification of certain types of cells. As stated, the cells of ligated arteries have been variously described as endothelial cells, leucocytes, fibroblasts, and smooth muscle. Studies with the electron microscope have shown that one reason for the confusion may be that these cells, although all of one type, show certain features which are usually considered to be characteristic of fibroblasts, on the one hand, and macrophages on the other, as well as the features of smooth muscle. That is, the cells of the thickened intima are not ordinary smooth muscle. There could not be so much confusion if this were so.

Altschul (1950, 1954, 1961) has reviewed the earlier literature on these cells, which he termed "intermediate" cells, believing them to have features of endothelium, of mesenchymal cells, and of smooth muscle. He felt that they might be derived from either the smooth muscle of the media or from the endothelium.

When studied in electron micrographs these cells (Fig. 6) show a unique combination of certain features (Buck, 1961). They have a narrow peripheral margin of fibrillated cytoplasm, the individual fibrils being about the same size as those in ordinary smooth muscle. In several other respects the cells differ from smooth muscle of the arterial media: (1) the fibrils, even many months after tying the ligatures, never fill the greater part of the cytoplasm; (2) an extensive, branching ergastoplasm is the principal cytoplasmic organelle; (3) Golgi apparatus and mitochondria are prominent; (4) many dense inclusions are seen, sometimes of such large size that one must consider the likelihood of active phagocytosis in these cells. The extreme development of the ergastoplasm resembles that in active fibroblasts or osteoblasts, so that one thinks of these cells as producers of some extracellular protein material.

I think there can be little doubt that these cells arise from the smooth muscle of the media. They frequently lie partly in the media and partly in the subendothelial space, apparently penetrating the fenestrations of the internal elastic lamina. Small nests of them develop under the endothelium and acquire a coating of elastic tissue, so that the appearance of a "split" in the internal elastic lamina is produced. It is

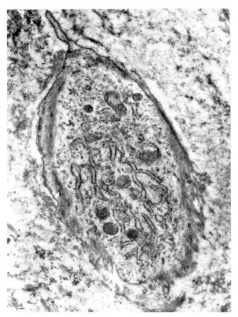

Fig. 6. Oblique section through a modified smooth muscle cell in the subendothelium of a doubly ligated segment of the rat internal carotid artery, 2 weeks after the application of ligatures. Myofilaments are confined to the narrow band of dense cytoplasm immediately under the plasma membrane. The nonfibrillary part of the cytoplasm, much more plentiful here than in the ordinary smooth muscle cell, contains a well developed system of ergastoplasmic membranes, some mitochondria and dense inclusions. Vestopal section, uranyl acetate stain. Magnification: × 8000.

the further growth of these cells over the few weeks or months following ligature that is entirely responsible for the obliteration of the lumen.

3. REPAIR FOLLOWING LOCALIZED FREEZING

Another simple method of producing subendothelial growth is to freeze a short length of artery. Observations on the repair of the rabbit aorta after local freezing were reported by Taylor *et al.* (1950). I have made essentially similar observations with the electron microscope on the repair of the rat internal carotid artery after freezing. Since these experiments have not been published it may perhaps be appropriate to describe them here.

A chrome-plated brass rod, cooled in crushed solid carbon dioxide, was applied for about 1 minute to the exposed artery, the wound closed, and the animals were killed 5, 10, 30, 60, and 120 days later. The frozen

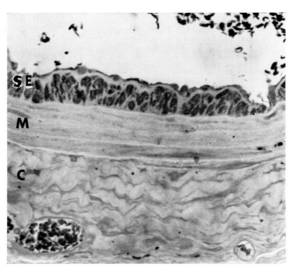

Fig. 7. Transverse section through the rat internal carotid artery showing the repair process 60 days after local freezing. A continuous layer of endothelium covers the surface. The subendothelium (SE) contains 2 or 3 layers of longitudinally oriented smooth muscle cells. The thin media (M) is represented by several pale elastic membranes between which are fine collagen and elastic fibers, but virtually no cells. A thick layer of coarse collagen fibers (C) encloses the vessel. Vestopal section, toluidine blue staining, light micrograph. Magnification: × 320.

part, marked by a suture in adjacent muscle, was treated in the usual way for paraffin or polyester embedding for light or electron microscopy respectively.

Degeneration of endothelium was apparent 5 days after injury, and of smooth muscle of the media, 10 days after injury. A new endothelium was present in the 30-day specimens, and at this time the smooth muscle of the media had completely degenerated. However, by 30 days, but particularly at 60 and 120 days after injury, new modified smooth muscle cells (resembling those in ligated arteries) lay between the old internal elastic lamina and the new endothelium (Fig. 7). In all specimens the new smooth muscle cells were longitudinally oriented in the vessel. In some cases they formed little bundles of a few cells, but later there was a continuous layer of longitudinal smooth muscle under the endothelium. Here also was a new formation of elastic fibers and much mucopolysaccharide. Outside this layer the original elastic lamellae persisted for the whole 120-day period, although the media was extremely thin because it contained virtually no cells.

In interpreting these results one must assume that the cells of both endothelium and media were killed by the freezing procedure. The new growth of these cells was probably from the healthy artery at either end of the frozen part.

There is a resemblance between the repair following freezing and the cyclic changes in ovarian arteries described by Sohma (1908). He found that with each menstrual cycle, and particularly with each pregnancy, regeneration of smooth muscle occurred in the subendothelium, so that eventually a new vessel was formed inside the old. Whether this regeneration is due to endocrine effects or, as seems more likely, to periodic fluctuations in the functional demand has not been established, and this is obviously a fruitful field for research.

D. Significance and Function of Subendothelial Smooth Muscle

It is noteworthy that only one kind of cell was found in the subendothelium of ligated or frozen arteries. This cell, derived from the smooth muscle of the media, must be responsible for the production of the extracellular materials, the identified components of which are elastic fibers and mucopolysaccharide. The property of synthesizing these materials is compatible with their possession of prominent ergastoplasmic membranes, since this is a feature of cells with pronounced protein synthetic activity.

It now seems likely to me that, if we exclude the repair following thrombosis, the process of repair in arteries after many different kinds of injury is essentially the same. A fundamental difference from the repair in many other tissues is that the cells involved are smooth muscle, rather than fibroblasts, and the fibers are mainly elastic, rather than collagen. These generalizations apply only to the simplest kinds of repair, for in certain conditions fibroblasts and collagen fibers may contribute to the development of the intima. This is the case in the lesions of human atherosclerosis or of long-term atherosclerosis in animals. Florey *et al.* (1961) found that collagen fibers were prominent in the pseudointima following grafting, although it is perhaps significant that they did not identify any fibroblasts in the lesions. These are complex situations in which one is perhaps not aware of the effects of such factors as thrombosis, calcification, lipid synthesis, and vascularization. Even so, atherosclerosis does show the same general pattern of repair. The principal cell in the lesions of long-term cholesterol atherosclerosis of rabbits is the modified smooth muscle cell, although a few fibroblasts and macrophages are also present (Buck, 1962). Parker (1960) has shown that the "foam" cell of much earlier lesions in rabbit coronary arteries is, in fact, a lipid-filled smooth muscle cell. Recently Greer *et al.* (1961) have emphasized the phagocytic capacity of smooth muscle cells, stating that practically all the lipid in the early fatty streaks of human arteries is contained in these cells. In avascular granulation tissue of focal elevations of the arterial lining only smooth muscle cells were observed (Haust *et al.,* 1960).

If smooth muscle cells are able to produce mucopolysaccharide and elastic fibers one of the principal functional differences remaining between them and the fibroblasts is their ability to contract. An obvious function of the new muscle cells might seem to be that of restoring the power of the injured vessel to constrict or dilate. However, since the cells are frequently arranged longitudinally it is hard to see how the function of contraction can be effectively used to oppose the dilating force of the blood pressure. Their contractions may, however, provide an important stimulus for the production and orientation of the elastic fibers and, in some cases, collagen fibers also. Virtually nothing is known about the effect of mechanical force on the growth of elastic fibers, although collagen fibrillogenesis has been rather thoroughly studied from this standpoint. It has been shown repeatedly that tension promotes the development of collagen fibers. Thus, a strong pulling force must be present for the complete regeneration of a severed tendon. If the nerve to the muscle associated with the cut tendon is damaged, tendon regeneration is very incomplete (Buck, 1953). In the developing subendothelial layer of arteries one observes that the tapered processes of smooth muscle cells terminate in association with very fine elastic fibers. The elastic tissue forms the framework to which the smooth muscle is harnessed. It seems possible to me that the smooth muscle not only synthesizes the material of the elastic fibers but may also be responsible for spinning out the fibers and causing them to be arranged as a supporting framework.

In summary, the cells of the subendothelium originate from the smooth muscle of the media; they retain a peripheral contractile layer of cytoplasm; they acquire additional synthetic apparatus directed particularly toward elastic fiber production; they are probably ameboid and phagocytic.

IV. Fibers and Ground Substance

A. Elastic and Collagen Fibers

The extent and arrangement of the arterial elastic fiber network provides a basis for the classification into so-called elastic arteries and muscular or distributing arteries. There are, of course, other differences between these types of arteries, such as the ratio of wall thickness to lumen diameter, which becomes progressively higher in smaller arteries (Burton, 1954).

The highest proportion of elastic tissue is found in the aorta where very thick lamellae constitute 30 to 40% of its weight (Hass, 1942b). Each lamella is composed of fibers in one plane. In the aorta the fibers are arranged in clockwise and counterclockwise helices, the direction alternating regularly from one lamella to the next (Kokott, 1929; Hass, 1942a). In muscular arteries the major elastic membranes are reduced to the internal and external elastic laminae, the external being often inconspicuous. In the cerebral arteries of man the external lamina is often absent (Benninghoff, 1930) except in the newborn (Hassler and Larsson, 1962).

The elastic membranes are not solid sheets of elastin, but, as stated above, they are composed of fibers. Fenestrations exist at intervals in the membranes through which cells and materials may pass. The penetration by smooth muscle is particularly obvious in conditions which stimulate the development of the subendothelium, but even in the normal artery the fenestrations often contain extrusions of smooth muscle cytoplasm (Pease and Paule, 1960). In small arteries of the heart (Moore and Ruska, 1957) and in the major coronary arteries (Parker, 1959), part of the endothelial cell cytoplasm may project outward through the gaps. Sometimes the fenestrations are filled with little bundles of collagen fibers (Pease and Paule, 1960). An *in vitro* study of the human external iliac artery perfused with lipid-containing serum showed that lipoproteins passed freely through the fenestrations, but not at other points (Wilens and McCluskey, 1954).

When studied with the light microscope the heavy elastic membranes of the aorta frequently appear to be smooth, dense, wavy bands, alternating with the layers of smooth muscle. In electron micrographs the lamellae have quite irregular surfaces, the irregularity being produced by numerous fine fibers attached to their surfaces. In small arteries (Moore and Ruska, 1957; Parker, 1959) as well as in the aorta (Pease and Paule, 1960) the elastic lamellae form part of a continuous elastic skeleton of much finer fibers in which the smooth muscle cells are embedded. Only in the smallest of arterioles and in arteriovenous anastomoses are elastic fibers absent.

The suggestion of a relationship between elastic fibers and acid mucopolysaccharides dates at least from the studies of Schultz (1922) who considered that the metachromatic substance of the artery contained the building material for elastic fibers. More recently, numerous workers have observed that elastic tissue degeneration is associated with the accumulation of acid mucopolysaccharides (Moon and Rinehart, 1952; Taylor, 1953; Bunting and Bunting, 1953; Movat *et al.*, 1958; Moon, 1957). Gillman (1959) considers that elastic membranes consist of a hyaline core enclosed by an elastic component, with the whole complex embedded in a layer of mucopolysaccharide.

There is now evidence that normal elastic fibers also are not homogeneous, but have at least two components. Moore and Ruska (1957) reported that the internal elastic lamina consisted of materials having different electron densities. Parker (1959) observed many fine fibrils, without periodicity, embedded in a matrix material. Pease and Molinari (1960), studying sections stained with phosphotungstic acid, were able to resolve two components with quite different staining affinities. They observed a finely vesicular pattern in which tiny cavities of a lightly stained component were distributed through a densely stained material. The pale cavities were apparently continuous with the surrounding mucopolysaccharide. Their interpretation was that elastic fibers develop by the deposition of the specific dense material in the pre-existing matrix. According to Moore and Schoenberg (1959) the mucopolysaccharide associated with elastic fibers may be hyaluronic acid, rather than a sulfated mucopolysaccharide. They observed that elastic fibers could be demonstrated in the human umbilical artery at 12 to 13 weeks of fetal life, at which time no sulfated mucopolysaccharide was present. However it is possible that the staining methods used by these authors may have lacked the necessary sensitivity. The problem needs to receive further study, preferably with S^{35}-labeling.

Aging is accompanied by a loss of elasticity of elastic fibers and by their infiltration with mineral salts (Blumenthal *et al.*, 1944). Although the collagen content of the aorta of man (Hass, 1943) and the mouse (Karrer and Cox, 1961) increases with aging, the amount of elastic tissue does not change significantly. In the mouse the number of elastic lamellae remains constant, but they double in thickness in the first 20 days of life, thereafter remaining of constant size (Smith *et al.*, 1951). The age changes in elastic tissue of arteries have recently been reviewed by Lansing (1959).

The collagen content of the media of normal muscular arteries is low. In the larger vessels of this type a few unit fibrils are observed forming scattered small bundles between smooth muscle cells. Fibrils are also found on either side of the internal elastic lamina. In the aorta collagen is much more plentiful, particularly in the human. In the aorta of the rat, unit fibrils are distributed in a random way, having no apparent relationship to the much more plentiful elastic fibers or to the muscle cells (Pease and Paule, 1960).

B. Ground Substance

Metachromasia is apparent even in the human fetal aorta, but the intensity of staining increases greatly soon after birth, particularly in the inner third of the media (Schultz, 1922). The staining continues to increase with age (Taylor, 1953), perhaps in association with the elastic tissue degeneration referred to above.

With the light microscope an extensive distribution of ground substance is not obvious in muscular arteries, where stainable material is largely confined to both surfaces of the internal elastic lamina (Bunting and Bunting, 1953). In electron micrographs, material of a character suggesting mucopolysaccharide extends throughout the media and is continuous with the ground substance in which the internal elastic lamina is embedded (Parker, 1959; Pease and Molinari, 1960). Around each smooth muscle cell a thin layer of mucopolysaccharide forms the basement membrane. It seems unlikely that this material is the same as the much more abundant ground substance of the aorta, for the media of the aorta incorporates S^{35}-sulfate (Odeblad and Boström, 1953; Buck, 1955; Buck and Heagy, 1958; Stehbens, 1962; and others) while the media of muscular arteries shows no significant S^{35} uptake. The extensive chemical studies of Kirk and his colleagues (reviewed by Kirk, 1959) have shown that both nonsulfated mucopolysaccharides and chondroitin sulfate are found in a variety of human arteries. It is possible that the nonsulfated mucopolysaccharides are represented in the basement membrane system.

V. Smooth Muscle of the Media

A. Arrangement

Direct observations on the development of the muscle coat of regenerating arteries were made by Clark and Clark (1940) in transparent chambers of the rabbit ear. Extraendothelial cells contacting the endothelial tube soon increased greatly in number. Thickening of the walls was due to mitosis of existing cells and to the addition of surrounding cells. These flattened, elongated "adventitial" cells lying parallel to the vessel were later observed to round up and then to change their axis to a transverse one, their processes extending around the vessel. They resembled cells in the muscular walls of arteries present in the original ear tissue. Only 6 days, or less, were required to produce a continuous sheet of cells around the endothelial tube, and by the eighth day typical active contractions were seen. The "adventitial" cells were rather undifferentiated at the time of their appearance, and Karrer (1960), studying the development of the chick aorta with the electron microscope, observed the transformation of similar fibroblast-like cells in the early embryo into typical smooth muscle cells of later embryos.

The media of distributing arteries in man and experimental animals, studied by a maceration and dissection technique, shows closely united smooth muscle cells having a helical arrangement (Strong, 1938). This pattern was said to provide for the propagation of a myogenically co-ordinated contracting impulse. According to Rhodin (1962) the angle of the helix in the femoral artery of the mouse is about 30 degrees. Some normal vessels of the rabbit ear, not arteriovenous anastomoses, have additional longitudinal smooth muscle cells (Rossatti, 1956).

In the aorta the presence of heavy elastic lamellae alternating with interlamellar spaces containing the smooth muscle makes the arrangement more complicated. Each muscle cell extends from one lamina to the next. In each interlamellar space the long axes of the cells are parallel to each other, but oblique in relation to the elastic lamellae. Their angle alternates from one layer to the next so that in a cross section of the vessel a zig-zag pattern is seen. The angle depends upon the degree of contraction of the vessel. The alternating angular pattern seen in a section represents alternating clockwise and counterclockwise helices which, on contraction, can cause a rather small decrease in the diameter of the vessel (Burton, 1954; McDonald, 1960) by throwing the elastic lamellae into longitudinal corrugations.

With the exception of capillary endothelial cells in the outer third of the media of the aorta in man and certain other species, smooth muscle is virtually the only type of cell in the arterial media. It must be assumed, therefore, that in the media, as in the subendothelium, the smooth muscle cell forms and maintains the elastic and collagen fibers and the ground substance. This is perhaps to be expected, in view of its origin from fibroblast-like cells of the embryo, but it is, nevertheless, a view which seems only recently to have been emphasized (Pease and Paule, 1960).

The basement membrane system, referred to in Section IV encloses each muscle cell (Policard *et al.,* 1955). It now seems definitely established that in vascular smooth muscle the "intercellular bridges" seen with the light microscope (for early views see McGill, 1909) do not represent pro-

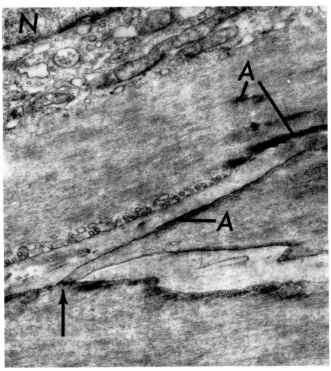

FIG. 8.   Parts of three smooth muscle cells from the media of the human testicular artery. The edge of the nucleus (N) and the sarcoplasmic organelles are in the upper part of the figure. The remainder of the cytoplasm contains fine myofilaments, dense bodies, or attachment devices (A), and pinocytic vesicles. The pinocytic vesicles appear either as invaginations of the plasma membrane or as spherical structures close to it. They are absent over those areas of the plasma membrane fused with the attachment devices. The pale material between the cells is largely elastic fibers. A point of contact is seen between a long process of one cell and the lateral margin of another (arrow). Epon section. Magnification: × 25,100.

toplasmic continuity between cells (Moore and Ruska, 1957; Parker, 1959; Fawcett, 1959; Pease and Paule, 1960; Rhodin, 1962). Although protoplasmic continuity is lacking there are many points of intimate contact between adjoining cells (Figs. 8 and 9). The cellular projections extending to these points of contact give the appearance of bridges when

seen with the light microscope. Similar conclusions have been drawn
from a number of studies of smooth muscle from other sites.

According to Pease and Paule (1960) the smooth muscle cells of the
rat aorta show side-to-side points of contact at which the plasma membranes are separated from each other by about 150 to 200 A. Keech (1960)

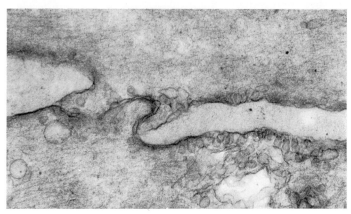

Fig. 9. Part of two smooth muscle cells from the media of the human testicular
artery. Fine myofilaments and pinocytic vesicles are present. The abutting plasma
membranes form a point of contact between the lateral margins of the cells. Epon
section, lead stained. Magnification: × 45,000.

did not observe contact points in the rat aorta. In the mouse femoral
artery the interdigitated ends of the cells, rather than the lateral margins,
show large areas with a light intercellular space of only about 100 A
(Rhodin, 1962). The plasma membrane at these points does not show
any special features, such as desmosomes.

B. Cellular Morphology

Prosser *et al.* (1960) and Rhodin (1962) have indicated how different
the morphology of the vascular smooth muscle is from that of the viscera.
Generalizations in regard to the physiology of vascular smooth muscle,
as well as its structure, are likely to be misleading if they are based on
the study of muscle from intestine, uterus, or other sites (Burton, 1962b).

The smooth muscle cells in arterial media are apparently much
smaller than those of other sites. According to Prosser *et al.* (1960) the
cells of the pig carotid artery measure only 3μ in diameter and only 30μ
in length. Rhodin (1962) observed that in relaxed small arteries of the
mouse the cells had a diameter of about 1.5 to 2.5μ and a length of 60μ.
Under the conditions of his experiments the cells were long cylinders,

showing only occasional branching. In the more commonly observed contracted state the cells are thicker and shorter, and fusiform in shape.

An elongated nucleus near the center of the cell frequently shows a kinked appearance in constricted vessels. This state is represented in electron micrographs by deep folds of the nuclear membrane. At either pole of the nucleus most of the mitochondria and rough surfaced endoplasmic reticulum tend to be concentrated. The cell center is also found in this region. Surrounding this axial core is the major portion of the cytoplasm filled largely with myofilaments embedded in a structureless cytoplasmic matrix. A smooth surfaced component of the endoplasmic reticulum, concentrated immediately under the plasma membrane, consists of numerous pinocytic vesicles and inpocketings, resembling those of the endothelium (Figs. 8 and 9).

The unique morphological feature of the smooth muscle cell is found in the type and arrangement of its myofilaments. The fibrillary material of the cytoplasm in cells in the arteriolar wall, described by Policard *et al.* (1955), was oriented in a general longitudinal direction. Myofilaments were described by Pease and Molinari (1960) as approximately 30 A in diameter, coursing in a general longitudinal direction, but not perfectly oriented, so that a feltwork arrangement existed. Filaments were said to be less well defined and less numerous in the aortic media. Rhodin (1962) found that the filaments averaged about 80 A in diameter and were quite short, perhaps a micron, or that they were longer but twisted about each other. No periodicity has been described in the filaments of arterial smooth muscle.

The question of how the energy of the myofilaments is harnessed has been a puzzle for many years, and, in fact, if the filaments are really as short as 1μ the answer remains obscure. However, the studies of Pease and Molinari (1960) have provided evidence that certain dense bodies, earlier noticed by a number of workers, may act as "attachment devices" for the myofilaments. These elongated bodies, about 0.5μ in length, are particularly numerous and pronounced close to the plasma membrane (Fig. 8). Although well developed in muscular arteries, they are said to be less conspicuous in smooth muscle of the aorta (Pease and Paule, 1960) and in smooth muscle of other tissues, such as the intestine (Rhodin, 1962). Pease and Molinari (1960) have observed the convergence of myofilaments toward the dense bodies, although this appearance is denied by Prosser *et al.* (1960). Keech (1960) considered dense bodies at the plasma membrane to be comparable to desmosomes, and, noting that in the rat aorta they were found only at points of attachment to elastic fibers, considered that they might play a role in the mechanical attachment of the smooth muscle to the elastic skeleton. On the basis of certain extraction procedures applied to the smooth muscle Prosser *et al.* (1960) concluded that the dense bodies were composed of protein, but not the contractile protein of the myofilaments. If, as seems likely, many of these bodies are attached to the plasma membrane they may provide a means for transmitting the contraction of the myofilaments to this surface, and thence to the extracellular fiber system. Rhodin (1962) noted that the dense bodies of intestinal smooth muscle were sometimes absent in the relaxed state, although present in contracted cells. The appearance of folding of the plasma membrane at these sites in contracted arteries, described by Pease and Molinari (1960), provides further support for their hypothesis of the "attachment devices."

C. Walls of Arteriovenous Anastomoses

The arteriovenous anastomosis is a special type of artery in which one might expect to find the ultimate in the constricting mechanism and in nervous control. Although the arteriovenous anastomoses may have no special significance in arteriosclerosis their morphology is worth considering from the standpoint of the basic properties of the structural elements of vascular tissue. In the rabbit ear they are known to be capable of complete closure and wide dilatation in response to environmental temperature changes (Clark and Clark, 1934), and their function in the control of body temperature by this means is very likely, especially in the rabbit, whose temperature control is undoubtedly influenced by the large surface area of the ears. The references to the many tissues and many species in which arteriovenous anastomoses have been discovered are given by Daniel and Prichard (1956) who have contributed greatly to the knowledge of these structures through their studies of the arterio-venous anastomoses in the tongue of the dog and in the human external ear (Prichard and Daniel, 1953, 1956) and the ears of 8 species of animals (Daniel and Prichard, 1956).

The structure of the arteriovenous anastomoses varies from species to species, but, in general, they consist of thick walled vessels of arteriolar size arising from arteries up to 300μ in diameter (Rossatti, 1956). In many species the arteriovenous anastomoses have "epithelioid" cells in the wall, distinguishable from ordinary smooth muscle cells by their larger size, their larger, lighter stained nuclei, and their location close to the lumen (Prichard and Daniel, 1956). The internal elastic lamina is absent, and, according to these authors, the endothelium is probably incomplete. Great numbers of nerve fibers are found in the adventitia, and a few have been observed running between the cells of the media.

In the hope of discovering some special structural character of the muscle cells which would correlate with the functional peculiarities of the arteriovenous anastomoses I recently undertook to examine these vessels with the electron microscope. I was also interested in trying to find some nerve endings in the media, for these have so far eluded electron microscopists studying other kinds of arteries (Parker, 1959; Pease and Molinari, 1960; Rhodin, 1962). Even nerve fibers are not demonstrated between the muscle cells of the media of ordinary arteries by specific histological methods or by electron microscopy. A network of unmyelinated fibers surrounds the medial coat (Woolard, 1926). Some of these end on the surface of the media in small swellings, but the majority end by attrition (Weddell, 1961). In electron micrographs unmyelinated fibers are often seen in the cytoplasm of Schwann cells in the adventitia. Although in this brief study I did not discover any special character of the muscle, or any nerve endings, certain other observations were of interest. Since no electron microscopic study of the arteriovenous anastomoses has been published, my results may warrant brief mention here.

The tissue was obtained on three separate occasions from the ears of 4 young rabbits. The rabbits were killed by a large dose of Nembutal given intraperitoneally. A 22-gauge needle attached to a 20-ml syringe was then inserted into a marginal vein of the ear, the point being directed distally. An injection was given slowly into the vein of 10 to 15 ml of 1% buffered osmium tetroxide. After several minutes a second injection was made through the same needle, this time consisting of Higgins India ink. When the vessels were blackened the distal two-thirds of the ear was cut off. The skin was peeled from the convex surface, and discarded. The other piece of tissue, containing the exposed subcutaneous blood vessels, was immersed for 30 minutes in the fixative. Under a fume hood the preparation was studied with a dissecting microscope. Arteriovenous anastomoses were recognized by their characteristic convoluted course, and their identity was checked by gently compressing the vessels so that some of the India ink was forced from the vein through the arteriovenous anastomosis to the artery. A rectangular piece of tissue containing the cartilage and the arteriovenous anastomosis was cut out with a razor blade. The cartilage was easily peeled away, and a tiny block, just visible to the naked eye, was then carried through the usual steps of the Vestopal embedding procedure. Sections were mounted on "single hole" grids (0.6-mm diameter hole) coated with Formvar. These were found to be necessary in order to see all of the tissue in the section.

After several specimens had been examined it was a simple matter to observe the characteristic morphology of the arteriovenous anastomoses with the electron microscope (Fig 10). They differed from other vessels of comparable size which served as controls for the technique. The striking feature of the media was the total absence of elastic fibers. Instead, the muscle cells were separated by wide and almost empty spaces. No internal elastic lamina was present. The continuous endothelium rested on a basement membrane which it shared at points with the muscle cells. At other points the endothelium was well separated from the muscle. Each muscle cell was invested in a basement membrane that only occasionally joined the basement membrane of neighboring muscle cells. The intervening space was electron lucid. It sometimes contained profiles of sectioned cytoplasm, thought to be mainly processes of other smooth muscle cells. A few unit fibrils of collagen, but no elastic fibers, were contained in the intercellular spaces.

The smooth muscle cell was the only type observed in the media. These cells showed considerable size variation, both apparent and real. They possessed relatively few myofilaments in comparison with the usual arterial smooth muscle cells, and their cytoplasm appeared relatively light. The arrangement of cells was much less regular than that in an artery or arteriole. The outermost cells were usually arranged roughly circularly, but the inner cells were often oblique or even longitudinal.

Except that the adventitia contained a much greater number of unmyelinated nerve fibers than are usually seen in other arteries, the other components of the wall were not remarkable. The endothelium differed in no way from that of other arteries.

It is possible that some of the thin structures traversing the intercellular spaces of the media were nerve fibers, for the fine branches of unmyelinated fibers might be difficult to distinguish from the processes of smooth muscle. However, no nerve endings were recognized.

The failure to observe "epithelioid" cells in the electron micrographs is not surprising, since they are said to be rare in the arteriovenous anastomoses of the rabbit ear (Clara, 1927). More interesting results might have been obtained if the same technique had been applied to the study of the ear arteriovenous anastomoses of other species, such as the sheep, in which "epithelioid" cells are plentiful. The absence of elastic tissue

Fig. 10. Part of the wall of an arteriovenous anastomosis in the rabbit ear. A continuous endothelium is present, and the dense line at the point of contact of two cells may represent a desmosome (arrow). No elastic fibers are present. Wide spaces separate the smooth muscle cells (SM) of the media. In the adventitia the cytoplasm of a Schwann cell (S) contains small unmyelinated nerve fibers. Vestopal section, uranyl acetate stain. Magnification: $\times$ 18,000.

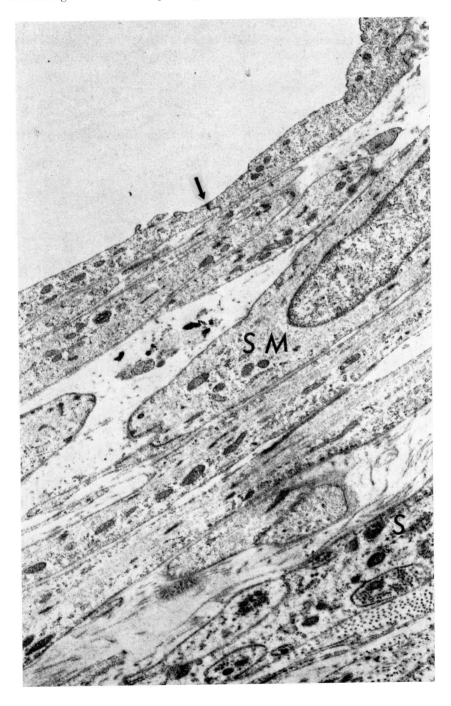

is confirmed, and this finding is in keeping with the concept of the function of elastic fibers in small arteries, namely, that they provide vasomotor stability (Burton, 1954). The significance of the wide spaces between muscle cells is obscure. They do not appear to be artifacts, for small arteries in the same tissue did not show this feature.

Acknowledgment

My own work which has been included in this review has been largely supported by grants from the Life Insurance Medical Research Foundation.

References

Altschul, R. (1950). "Selected Studies on Arteriosclerosis." C. C Thomas, Springfield, Illinois.

Altschul, R. (1954). "Endothelium, Its Development, Morphology, Function and Pathology." Macmillan, New York.

Altschul, R. (1957). *Arch. Pathol. Anat. Physiol. Virchow's* **330**, 357.

Altschul, R. (1961). *In* "Blood Platelets," Henry Ford Hospital Symposium, pp. 23-39. Little, Brown, Boston, Massachusetts.

Bennett, H. S. (1956). *J. Biophys. Biochem. Cytol.* **2** (Suppl.), 99.

Benninghoff, A. (1930). *In* "Handbuch der mikroscopischen Anatomie des Menschen" (W. v. Möllendorff, ed.), Vol. 6, Pt. 1, pp. 1-232. Springer, Berlin.

Blumenthal, H. T., Lansing, A. I., and Wheeler, P. A. (1944). *Am. J. Pathol.* **20**, 665.

Buck, R. C. (1953). *J. Pathol. Bacteriol.* **66**, 1.

Buck, R. C. (1955). *J. Histochem. Cytochem.* **3**, 435.

Buck, R. C. (1958a). *J. Biophys. Biochem. Cytol.* **4**, 187.

Buck, R. C. (1958b). *Am. J. Pathol.* **34**, 897.

Buck, R. C. (1961). *Circulation Res.* **9**, 418.

Buck, R. C. (1962). *Brit. J. Exptl. Pathol.* **43**, 236.

Buck, R. C., and Heagy, F. C. (1958). *Can. J. Biochem. Physiol.* **36**, 63.

Bunting, C. H., and Bunting, H. (1953). *A.M.A. Arch. Pathol.* **55**, 257.

Burton, A. C. (1954). *Physiol. Rev.* **34**, 619.

Burton, A. C. (1962a). *In* "Handbook of Physiology" (W. F. Hamilton, ed.), Vol. I, Sect. 2, pp. 85-106. Am. Physiol. Soc., Washington, D. C.

Burton, A. C. (1962b). *Physiol. Rev.* **42** (Suppl. 5), 1.

Cappell, D. F., Hutchison, H. E., and Jowett, M. (1957). *J. Pathol. Bacteriol.* **74**, 245.

Carden, G. A. (1936-1937). *Yale J. Biol. Med.* **9**, 39.

Chambers, R., and Zweifach, B. (1947). *Physiol. Rev.* **27**, 436.

Clara, M. (1927). Quoted by Daniel and Prichard (1956).

Clark, E. R., and Clark, E. L. (1934). *Am. J. Anat.* **54**, 229.

Clark, E. R., and Clark, E. L. (1935). *Am. J. Anat.* **57**, 385.

Clark, E. R., and Clark, E. L. (1940). *Am. J. Anat.* **66**, 1.

Conti, von G. (1953). *Acta Anat.* **18**, 234.

Cotton, R. E., and Wartman, W. B. (1961). *Arch. Pathol.* **71**, 15.

Cotton, R. E., Harwood, T. R., and Wartman, W. B. (1961). *J. Pathol. Bacteriol.* **81**, 175.

Crawford, T. (1956). *J. Pathol. Bacteriol.* **72**, 547.

Curran, R. C. (1957). *J. Pathol. Bacteriol.* **74**, 347.

Daniel, P. M., and Prichard, M. L. (1956). *Quart. J. Exptl. Physiol.* **41**, 107.

Duff, G. L. (1932). *Am. J. Pathol.* **8**, 219.

Duff, G. L., McMillan, G. C., and Lautsch, E. V. (1954). *Am. J. Pathol.* **30**, 941.

Duguid, J. B. (1952). *Lancet* **ii**, 207.

Duncan, L. E., and Buck, K. (1959). *Circulation Res.* **7**, 765.

Duncan, L. E., Cornfield, J., and Buck, K. (1959). *Circulation Res.* **7**, 390.

Efskind, L. (1941). *Acta Chir. Scand.* **84**, 283.

Farquhar, M. G. (1961). *Angiology* **12**, 270.

Fawcett, D. W. (1959). *In* "The Microcirculation" (S. R. M. Reynolds and B. W. Zweifach, eds.), pp. 1-27. Univ. Illinois Press, Urbana, Illinois.

Fawcett, D. W., and Wittenberg, J. (1962). *Anat. Record* **142**, 231.

Ferrara, A. (1950). *Arch. "De Vecchi" Anat. Pathol. Med. Clin.* **14**, 193.

Florey, H. W., and Grant, L. H. (1961). *J. Pathol. Bacteriol.* **82**, 13.

Florey, H. W., Poole, J. C. F., and Meek, G. A. (1959). *J. Pathol. Bacteriol.* **77**, 623.

Florey, H. W., Greer, S. J., Poole, J. C. F., and Werthessen, N. T. (1961). *Brit. J. Exptl. Pathol.* **42**, 236.

Gillman, T. (1959). *A.M.A. Arch. Pathol.* **67**, 624.

Greer, J. C., McGill, H. C., and Strong, J. P. (1961). *Am. J. Pathol.* **38**, 263.

Gross, L., Epstein, E. Z., and Kugel, M. A. (1934). *Am. J. Pathol.* **10**, 253.

Hass, G. M. (1942a). *A.M.A. Arch. Pathol.* **34**, 807.

Hass, G. M. (1942b). *A.M.A. Arch. Pathol.* **34**, 971.

Hass, G. M. (1943). *A.M.A. Arch. Pathol.* **35**, 29.

Hassler, O., and Larsson, S. E. (1962). *Acta Anat.* **48**, 1.

Haust, M. D., More, R. H., and Movat, H. Z. (1959). *Am. J. Pathol.* **35**, 265.

Hibbs, R. G., Burch, G. E., and Phillips, J. H. (1958). *Am. Heart J.* **56**, 662.

Karrer, H. E. (1960). *J. Ultrastruct. Res.* **4**, 420.

Karrer, H. E., and Cox, J. (1961). *J. Ultrastruct. Res.* **5**, 1.

Keech, M. K. (1960). *J. Biophys. Biochem. Cytol.* **7**, 533.

Kirk, J. E. (1959). *In* "The Arterial Wall" (A. I. Lansing, ed.), pp. 161-191. Williams & Wilkins, Baltimore, Maryland.

Kokott, W. (1929). *Z. Zellforsch. Mikroskop. Anat.* **8**, 772.

Lansing, A. I. (1959). *In* "The Arterial Wall" (A. I. Lansing, ed.), pp. 136-160. Williams & Wilkins, Baltimore, Maryland.

Lautsch, E. V., McMillan, G. C., and Duff, G. L. (1953). *Lab. Invest.* **2**, 397.

Lopes de Faria, J. (1961). *Acta Anat.* **46**, 230.

McDonald, D. A. (1960). "Blood Flow in Arteries." Arnold, London.

McGill, C. (1909). *Am. J. Anat.* **9**, 493.

McGovern, V. J. (1955). *J. Pathol. Bacteriol.* **69**, 283.

Malyschew, B. F. (1929). *Arch. Pathol. Anat. Physiol. Virchow's* **272**, 727.

Mehrotra, R. M. L. (1953). *J. Pathol. Bacteriol.* **65**, 307.

Moon, H. D. (1957). *Circulation* **16**, 263.

Moon, H. D., and Rinehart, J. F. (1952). *Circulation* **6**, 481.

Moore, D. H., and Ruska, H. (1957). *J. Biophys. Biochem. Cytol.* **3**, 457.

Moore, R. D., and Schoenberg, M. D. (1959). *J. Pathol. Bacteriol.* **77**, 163.

Movat, H. Z., More, R. H., and Haust, M. D. (1958). *Am. J. Pathol.* **34**, 1023.

Odeblad, E., and Boström, H. (1953). *Acta Chem. Scand.* **7**, 233.

Palade, G. E. (1953). *J. Appl. Phy.* **24**, 1424.

Palade, G. E. (1961). *Circulation* **24**, 368.

Parker, F. (1959). *Am. J. Anat.* **103**, 247.

Parker, F. (1960). *Am. J. Pathol.* **36**, 19.

Pease, D. C., and Molinari, S. (1960). *J. Ultrastruct. Res.* **3**, 447.

Pease, D. C., and Paule, W. J. (1960). *J. Ultrastruct. Res.* **3**, 469.

Policard, A., Collet, A., and Giltaire-Ralyte, L. (1955). *Bull. Microscop. Appl.* **5**, 3.

Poole, J. C. F., and Florey, H. W. (1958). *J. Pathol. Bacteriol.* **75**, 245.

Poole, J. C. F., Sanders, A. G., and Florey, H. W. (1958). *J. Pathol. Bacteriol.* **75**, 133.

Poole, J. C. F., Sanders, A. G., and Florey, H. W. (1959). *J. Pathol. Bacteriol.* **77**, 637.

Prichard, M. M. L., and Daniel, P. M. (1953). *J. Anat.* **87**, 66.

Prichard, M. M. L., and Daniel, P. M. (1956). *J. Anat.* **90**, 309.

Prior, J. T., and Jones, D. B. (1952). *Am. J. Pathol.* **28**, 937.

Prosser, C. L., Burnstock, G., and Kahn, J. (1960). *Am. J. Physiol.* **199**, 545.

Rhodin, J. A. G. (1962). *Physiol. Rev.* **42** (Suppl. 5), 48.

Robertson, J. H. (1960). *J. Clin. Pathol.* **13**, 199.

Rossatti, B. (1956). *J. Anat.* **90**, 318.

Schaeffer, J. P., and Radasch, H. E. (1924). *Am. J. Anat.* **33**, 219.

Schultz, A. (1922). *Arch. Pathol. Anat. Physiol. Virchow's* **239**, 415.

Simonton, J. H., and Gofman, J. W. (1951). *Circulation* **4**, 557.

Sinapius, D. (1956). *Z. Zellforsch. Mikroskop. Anat.* **44**, 27.

Sinapius, D., and Schreil, W. (1956). *Protoplasma* **47**, 217.

Smith, C., Seitner, M. M., and Wang, H. (1951). *Anat. Record* **109**, 13.

Sohma, M. (1908). *Arch. Gynaekol.* **84**, 377.

Stehbens, W. E. (1960). *Am. J. Pathol.* **36**, 289.

Stehbens, W. E. (1962). *J. Pathol. Bacteriol.* **83**, 337.

Strong, K. C. (1938). *Anat. Record* **72**, 151.

Taylor, C. B., Baldwin, D., and Hass, G. M. (1950). *A.M.A. Arch. Pathol.* **49**, 623.

Taylor, H. E. (1953). *Am. J. Pathol.* **29**, 871.

Wagenvoort, C. A. (1954). *Acta Anat.* **21**, 70.

Weddell, G. (1961). *In* "Advances in Biology of Skin" (W. Montagna and R. A. Ellis, eds.), Vol. II, pp. 71-78. Pergamon, New York.

Wilens, S. L. (1951). *Am. J. Pathol.* **27**, 825.

Wilens, S. L., and McCluskey, R. T. (1954). *Circulation Res.* **2**, 175.

Williams, A. W. (1961). *J. Pathol. Bacteriol.* **81**, 419.

Williams, A. W., and Montgomery, G. L. (1959). *J. Pathol. Bacteriol.* **77**, 63.

Woolard, H. H. (1926). *Heart* **13**, 319.

Zwiefach, B. W. (1959). *In* "The Arterial Wall" (A. I. Lansing, ed.), pp. 15-45. Williams & Wilkins, Baltimore, Maryland.

—2—

Natural History of Human Atherosclerotic Lesions*

Henry C. McGill, Jr., Jack C. Geer,† and Jack P. Strong†

I. Introduction

A. Importance of Natural History

Knowledge of the natural history of human atherosclerosis, including a clear distinction between arterial lesions and morbidity and mortality

* These studies were supported in part by PHS grants HE-6581 and HE-2549 from the National Heart Institute, Public Health Service.

† Dr. Geer and Dr. Strong are recipients of Research Career Development Awards (Dr. Geer, G-M-K3-15333; Dr. Strong, G-M-K3-15150) from the Division of General Medical Sciences, National Institutes of Health, USPHS.

resulting from them, is essential to investigation of the causes and complications of the lesions. Each investigation into or statement concerning atherosclerosis should be directed to a specific stage in the natural history of the process—type of mural arterial lesions, vascular occlusion, or ischemic damage to vital organs.

Atherosclerosis begins in childhood; proceeds rapidly in some arteries during adolescence and in others during early adulthood; undergoes a series of complex changes in subsequent decades; and begins to result in clinically manifest disease during early middle age. It is therefore no wonder that ideas of pathogenesis should be highly variable, depending on the stage of the process studied and the method by which observations are made. Moreover, its long natural history and protean manifestations have caused many difficulties in interpretation of experimental and epidemiological data.

To evaluate the results of animal experimentation, experimental models should be compared with the human counterpart with respect to pathogenesis, tempo of development, and distribution of lesions, as well as morphology. It is inappropriate to make inferences concerning human ischemic heart disease from observations on uncomplicated fatty streaks in animals. Such reasoning not only ignores interspecies variability; it also ignores the process by which human clinical disease develops. The ideal experimental model should duplicate not only the first stage of the lesions but also the intermediate and final stages.

The use of clinical disease as the end point in epidemiological studies may account for not finding strong associations with suspected etiological agents. These difficulties occur more frequently in a population such as that of the United States in which prevalence and severity of arterial lesions are high even in persons who have no clinical manifestations. Measures of extent and severity of arterial lesions may be more useful as disease measures in epidemiological studies, since the agents that cause arterial lipid deposition and progression into fibrous plaques may be quite different from those that precipitate clinical disease years later.

B. The Problem of Necropsy Selection in Reconstructing Natural History

To study preclinical lesions we must reconstruct the pathogenesis of atherosclerosis by multiple observations on necropsied individuals. If such a reconstruction is valid, it must be made from a portion of the necropsy population that reflects the extent and severity of atherosclerotic lesions in the living population, but the necropsy population is not a representative sample of the living population nor even of all deaths.

McMahan (1961) has shown that, in the United States, deaths assigned to cardiovascular disease (the leading category) are least likely to be necropsied; in fact, there is an almost inverse relation between frequency of assigned cause of death and probability of a necropsy being performed.

To minimize the effect of necropsy selection in our studies, we have stratified necropsies from a large general hospital and a medicolegal service not only by age, sex, and race, but also by principal cause of death and the presence of chronic diseases believed to be associated with increased atherosclerosis. Cases with hypertension and diabetes mellitus, and those dying of the complications of atherosclerosis itself, have been removed to eliminate bias; accidental and traumatic deaths have been used as an internal control representing the best available sample of the living population. While accidental death cases are in no sense random samples, they do form a group in which the terminal illness has the least conceivable effect on atherosclerotic lesions. We have found no significant or consistent difference in atherosclerotic lesions between accidental and natural death cases, when deaths due to atherosclerosis, diabetes mellitus, and hypertension are excluded from the natural death series.

C. Grading Atherosclerotic Lesions

Description of a process such as the development of atherosclerotic lesions requires a method of measuring its effects. Only recently have attempts been made to evaluate atherosclerotic lesions more precisely than by grading into three or four categories. A variety of grading methods have been described (Gore and Tejada, 1957; Roberts *et al.*, 1959; Holman *et al.*, 1960; Daoud *et al.*, 1962; Eggen *et al.*, 1962) ranging from visual estimation of the extent of different types of lesions to the application of complex measuring instruments. Each of these methods has advantages and limitations; a method must be selected appropriate to the objective.

The procedure used in our laboratory (Holman, 1958a) has been to preserve longitudinally opened arteries flattened against chipboard. The vessels are stained grossly with Sudan IV and packaged in plastic bags for storage and examination. The percentage of intimal surface covered by lesions and the proportion of diseased surface occupied by each of the four major types of grossly distinguishable lesions are estimated visually. Simple calculations give an average value of the proportion of intimal surface covered by each of the different types of lesions—fatty streaks, fibrous plaques, complicated lesions (ulceration, hemorrhage, or thrombosis), and calcified lesions.

D. Working Concept of Pathogenesis

Figure 1 shows a working hypothesis of the pathogenesis of atherosclerosis. The first structural abnormality that can be classified as "atherosclerosis" is lipid in the intima. Lipid deposition begins in the aorta in the first year of life; in the coronary arteries, in the second decade; in the intracranial arteries, in the third decade. These fatty deposits are

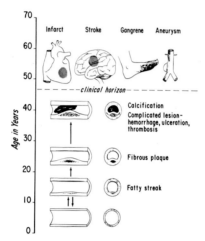

Fig. 1.　Diagrammatic concept of the pathogenesis of atherosclerosis.

seen grossly in the fresh or formalin-fixed vessel as yellow opaque flecks or streaks on the intimal surface.

Connective tissue accumulates about some fatty deposits; and the fatty deposit becomes covered by a cap of fibrous material, which gives the plaque its white, glistening appearance (pearly plaque, fibrous plaque). It is well established that fatty streaks chronologically precede fibrous plaques and more advanced lesions, and many favor the idea that the fatty streak is transformed into the fibrous plaque. Why some fatty streaks undergo this change and others regress is a critical question.

It is the fibrous plaque that sets the stage for clinically manifest disease. Hemorrhage within the plaque and thrombosis over a plaque may reduce the size of the arterial lumen and produce partial or complete ischemia. Ischemia may then result in angina pectoris, myocardial infarction, cerebral infarction, or peripheral gangrene.

This concept of pathogenesis shows that therapy or prophylaxis of diseases due to atherosclerosis may be undertaken at any one of several points. If the terminal complications leading to clinical disease could be prevented, we could prevent crippling and fatal disease though the basic arterial lesions would remain unaltered. A superior approach would seem to be prevention of the lesions which set the stage for occlusion and ischemia.

The entire process from the earliest arterial lesion to ischemic damage is part of the natural history of human atherosclerosis; emphasis in this chapter will be given to the arterial lesions and especially to early and intermediate lesions—the fatty streak and the fibrous plaque.

II. Coronary Artery Lesions

A. Prevalence and Extent of Gross Lesions

Because of the high rates of ischemic heart disease in middle-aged adults in North America and Western Europe, there is no doubt that clinically the coronary artery system is the most significant one affected by atherosclerosis. It has long been recognized that coronary atherosclerotic lesions occur in young people, but only recently has the extent and severity of these lesions in young adults been appreciated (Yater *et al.*, 1948; Enos *et al.*, 1955; Rigal *et al.*, 1960).

Our study of the coronary arteries of 548 patients from New Orleans (Strong and McGill, 1962) confirmed the early onset of coronary lesions in this population. Gross lesions before the age of 10 years were rare (one in 22); but fatty streaks were present in many cases in the second decade (22 of 44). Thereafter, practically all cases had coronary lesions. Fibrous plaques began to appear in the white males in the second decade, in the Negro in the third decade, and in the females of both races in the fourth decade.

Figure 2 shows the average extent (per cent of intimal surface involved) of grossly visible coronary lesions in each of the four sex and race groups in New Orleans by age. This quantitative assessment of lesions demonstrates the early onset of coronary lesions in young white males, in whom fatty streaks and fibrous plaques occupy a considerable portion of the intimal surface in the second decade, and in whom a marked increase in fibrous plaques occurs in the third and fourth decades.

Complicated and calcified lesions are first found in white males in the fourth decade, at least a decade earlier than in the other sex-race groups. White males have more extensive lesions of all types up to age 40 years; they remain ahead but by a smaller margin for the next two decades; by the seventh decade, there is little difference among the sex-race groups.

B. Relation of Coronary Artery Lesions to Clinical Disease

Some observers attribute geographic, racial, and sex differences in the incidence of myocardial infarction to differences in the severity of atherosclerosis (Blache and Handler, 1950; Stamler, 1958; Wainwright, 1961) others suggest that the modern epidemic of ischemic heart disease may be due primarily to an increased tendency to thrombosis (Bronte-Stewart, 1961; Hartroft, 1961; Morris and Crawford, 1961). The problem

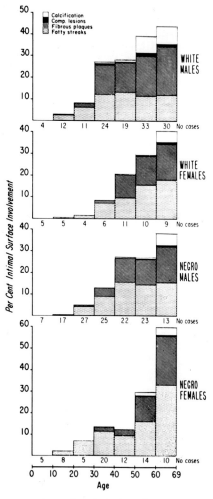

Fig. 2. Coronary artery atherosclerotic lesions by age, race, and sex in New Orleans; ages 1-69 years. Key to graph: Clear area, Calcification; Solid black area, Complicated lesions; Hatched area, Fibrous plaques; Dotted area, Fatty streaks.

is accentuated by finding many persons with severe and extensive coronary artery lesions who have died of causes other than ischemic heart disease, and an occasional case with coronary lesions of limited extent dying of myocardial infarction.

To test for correlation between coronary artery lesions and ischemic

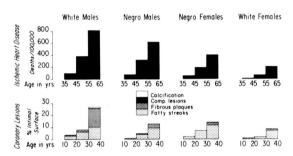

FIG. 3. Comparison of mortality rates from ischemic heart disease (420.0 and 420.1), ages 35-64 in Louisiana; and coronary artery lesions, ages 10-39 years in New Orleans by race and sex.

heart disease, mortality rates for four sex-race groups in Louisiana have been compared with coronary artery lesions (Strong and McGill, 1962). In the second, third, and fourth decades quantitative measurement of coronary lesions rank white males highest, white females lowest, and Negroes intermediate—the same order as mortality rates from ischemic heart disease in the 30-year age span from 35 to 64 years (Fig. 3). Thus, coronary artery lesions in groups of young individuals accurately predict the group's relative frequency of ischemic heart disease 25 years later. These data support the hypothesis that extent and severity of coronary atherosclerosis determine the risk of ischemic heart disease in a population. Other reports (Higginson and Pepler, 1954; McGill *et al.*, 1959; Gore *et al.*, 1960; Hirst *et al.*, 1960, 1962; Mathur *et al.*, 1961; Scott *et al.*, 1961) comparing coronary lesions between different populations have shown a similar correspondence between extent of coronary lesions (particularly fibrous plaques and more advanced lesions in young adults) with estimates of ischemic heart disease mortality in these areas. More data concerning lesions in different populations will be forthcoming from a cooperative study in which our laboratory and others are participating (e.g., Standard Operating Protocol, 1962).

We have found that cases dying with myocardial infarction have on the average more coronary lesions than those dying without myocardial infarction (Fig. 4). The difference between cases with and cases without infarction is not as great as one might expect, however; and these data illustrate the magnitude of the clinically silent lesions in a high risk group—the underwater portion of the iceberg, as it has been called (Morris, 1957).

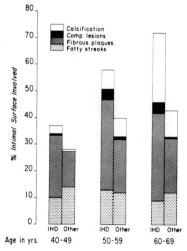

Fig. 4. Comparison of coronary artery lesions in 40 to 69-year old white males dying of ischemic heart disease with those in white males dying of other causes.

C. Histology and Electron Microscopy of Coronary Artery Lesions

1. Methods

Despite many studies of the morphological and histochemical characteristics of human atherosclerotic lesions, disagreement continues regarding their pathogenesis. It has been said that any theory of atherosclerosis can be proved by proper selection of histological sections. Our studies have been directed toward determining the origin of the fatty streak and its transformation into the fibrous plaque, and for this purpose we have examined the coronary arteries of young individuals, principally those between 10 and 40 years of age, by light and electron microscopy.

Tissues for electron microscopy were chosen according to gross type of lesion—fatty streaks, fibrous plaques, and complicated lesions. When only small, scarcely visible fatty streaks were present in a young individual, it was assumed that these represented the earliest lesion identifiable as atherosclerosis (Geer *et al.*, 1961).

To study the transition of fatty streaks into fibrous plaques, a separate study was performed; standard longitudinal blocks from 82 North American and Colombian cases were taken from the first portion of the anterior descending branch of the left coronary artery immediately distal to the origin of the left circumflex artery (Robertson *et al.*, 1963).

This site, prone to early and frequent development of fatty streaks and fibrous plaques in North American white males, can be predicted to have lesions with a high probability of progressing from fatty streaks to more advanced lesions. In groups that are much less likely to develop severe lesions (such as females), there is a lower probability of progressing. Eighty-two cases ranging in age from 10 to 39 years were examined by light microscopy with stains for lipid and connective tissues.

The following description of the origin and progression of coronary lesions is derived from these two studies.

2. MUSCULOELASTIC INTIMAL THICKENING

Gross and associates (1934), Fangman and Hellwig (1947), and Dock (1946) have described progressive thickening, with age, of the coronary intima composed of musculoelastic, elastic-hyperplastic, and collagenous layers extending in that order from media to endothelium. In the electron microscope, the musculoelastic and elastic-hyperplastic layers were composed of smooth muscle, elastic tissue, collagen, and intervening space presumably filled with ground substance. The smooth muscle cells in the elastic-hyperplastic layer were round, in contrast to their fusiform shape in the musculoelastic layer.

The collagenous layer in young persons appeared to contain little collagen when observed by light microscopy; there were scattered collagen fibers in electron micrographs. Collagen was increased in this layer in older persons. The collagenous layer also contained many round cells, some with and some without the cytoplasmic myofilaments typical of smooth muscle. Their similarity and juxtaposition to smooth muscle have suggested that they may all be the same basic cell type, but in different stages of differentiation.

The role of intimal thickening in the development of atherosclerosis has long been a subject of debate. Those arteries that have the most marked intimal thickening are the most prone to develop severe atherosclerosis (Sappington and Cook, 1936), but intimal thickening does not inevitably progress to atherosclerosis. For example, in the 82 cases, there was no difference in coronary intimal thickening (excluding lipid-containing lesions) between Colombians and North Americans nor between males and females. It appears that other changes must take place before atherosclerosis develops. The many unanswered questions about intimal thickening are subjects for future investigation—the nature of the stimulus that causes the intima to thicken; the source of the smooth muscle cells; and the reason for the change from musculoelastic to elastic-hyperplastic to collagenous with age.

3. Fatty Streaks

The histological counterpart of the coronary fatty streak in young persons is shown in Fig. 5. Stainable lipid occurred in any of the three layers of the coronary intima, usually in the elastic-hyperplastic or

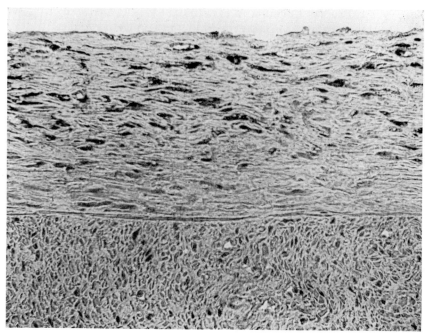

Fig. 5. Coronary artery, male, Colombia, South America, age 25 years. Intimal thickening with numerous cells containing stainable lipid (black in photograph). Oil red O-hematoxylin. Magnification: $\times$ 275.

collagenous layers. When such lesions were examined by electron microscopy the lipid was found in smooth muscle cells (Fig. 6).

4. Transition of Fatty Streaks to Fibrous Plaques

It is likely that the intracellular lipid accumulations in early coronary fatty streaks are reversible, just as similar changes in liver, kidney, and heart are reversible. In some fatty streaks, however, the cells became engorged with lipid and resembled foam cells. The stimulus to fibrosis—the transition from fatty streak to fibrous plaque—appeared to be the release of intracellular lipid into the extracellular space because of cellular degeneration and death. The extracellular lipid incited an inflammatory reaction—a reaction to injury, evidenced by infiltration with small round cells and occasional neutrophilic leucocytes (Fig. 7). Such inflammatory lesions occurred in 12 of 39 cases 30 to 39 years of age; 9 of the 12 cases were white males. Inflammatory lesions also occurred in 2 of 5 white males in the 20 to 29-year age group and were found only in white males in this decade of life. The high incidence of

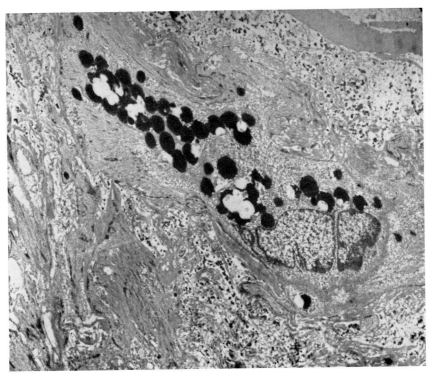

FIG. 6. Coronary artery, white male, age 23 years. Smooth muscle cell in the intima from a lesion that grossly appeared as a fatty streak. Numerous dense lipid inclusions in the cytoplasm; the center of some of the inclusions is clear, probably due to incomplete penetration of osmium fixative. Myofilaments in the cytoplasm identify the cell. Magnification: × 4000.

inflammatory lesions in white males is consistent with their propensity to severe, extensive, and progressive gross coronary lesions and to ischemic heart disease in later life.

The inflammatory stage of coronary atherosclerosis was accompanied by ingrowth of capillaries at the base of the lesion from the vasa vasorum (Figs. 8 and 9). Collagen increased until the typical fibrous plaque was formed, with a fibrous cap covering a core of lipid material (Fig. 9).

Thus, gradual transition from a fatty streak to a fibrous plaque was demonstrated.

5. Fibrous Plaques

The typical fibrous plaque is shown in Fig. 9. In electron micrographs (Fig. 10), the fibrous cap was composed of fusiform cells, collagen, and

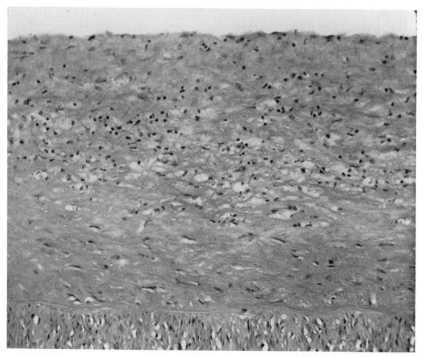

Fig. 7. Coronary artery, white male, age 39 years. Thickened intima with foam cells and numerous small round cells, some of which are polymorphonuclear leucocytes. Hematoxylin and eosin. Magnification: × 3000.

scattered small elastic fibers. Some of the fusiform cells were smooth muscle; others that could not be identified may have been fibroblasts or fibrocytes. Many contained intracytoplasmic lipid particles. Collagen was tightly clustered about the fusiform cells and dispersed between them, along with small elastic fibers and unidentified small dense bodies (Fig. 10). In the lipid core of the fibrous plaque there were extracellular clefts representing crystals of cholesterol ester, dense crystalline bodies that were probably calcium, and extracellular lipid particles.

Fibrin incrustation on the intimal surface was found in 3 of the 82 cases studied by light microscopy; all 3 cases were females. The incorporation of such fibrin incrustations could produce further intimal thickening, but the infrequency with which they occurred and the group in which they occurred cast doubt on their playing a primary role in intimal thickening or atherosclerosis.

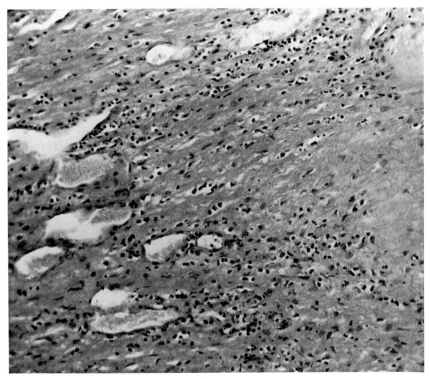

FIG. 8. Coronary artery, white male, age 31 years. Vascular channels at the margin of fibrous plaque with round cells. Hematoxylin and eosin. Magnification: × 300.

Many questions remain concerning the origin and composition of the fibrous plaque. Some of the cells within the fibrous cap are smooth muscle cells, but many others cannot be identified. The role of fibrin in the genesis of the fibrous plaque has not been determined; we have found fibrin in electron micrographs of such lesions in only one instance—a coronary plaque with overlying thrombosis and hemorrhage into its base. Fibrin may be present with greater frequency but in a form not readily identifiable by electron microscopy.

D. The Occlusive Event in the Coronary Arteries

There is much evidence indicating that coronary artery lesions, especially fibrous plaques, set the stage for coronary occlusion. It is doubtful from examination of ischemic heart disease deaths, however, that fatty streaks, fibrous plaques, and calcified lesions alone or in

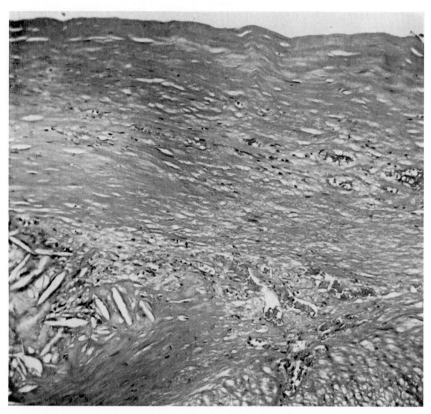

Fig. 9. Coronary artery, white male, age 36 years. Fibrous plaque with core of lipid material and cap of fibrous tissue. Vascularization of the plaque by extension of vessels from vasa vasorum at margin of lipid core. Hematoxylin and eosin. Magnification: × 100.

combination produce the occlusive event that precipitates clinical disease. Another event must be superimposed on the pre-existing arterial lesion.

The event, or sequence of events, that causes occlusion of a coronary artery and thereby clinical disease has been the subject of numerous investigations, but there remains considerable difference of opinion regarding the nature of the event itself and the mechanism by which it occurs (see the review by Crawford, 1961). The event most widely regarded as responsible for coronary occlusion is thrombosis, but thrombosis is found in most studies only in about half of the cases. The variations in the incidence of thrombotic occlusion reported are con-

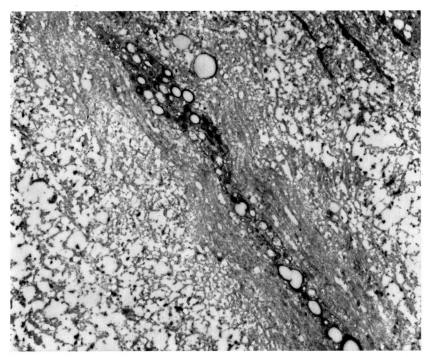

FIG. 10. Coronary artery, white male, age 56 years. Electron micrograph of fusiform cell from cap of fibrous plaque. Cell is filled with lipid inclusions and identification of cell type is not possible. Collagen fibers are clustered about the cell and small dense bodies are present in the interstitial tissue away from the cell. Magnification: $\times$ 4730.

siderable and no doubt depend on the method of detecting thrombi and the ages of the subjects. Intimal hemorrhage with rapid expansion of an intimal lesion has been suggested as a cause of coronary occlusion, but the relative frequency and importance of this as a cause of coronary occlusion is subject to debate. Atheromatous embolism, multiple atherosclerotic plaques in all major coronary branches, and vasospasm also have been considered as causes of coronary occlusion. It is evident that no single event or sequence of events is common to all cases of coronary occlusion. Whatever the sequence of events is that produces acute coronary occlusion, mural atherosclerotic lesions are prerequisite for occlusion; but other changes must be superimposed on the mural lesion for acute occlusion to occur.

III. Aortic Atherosclerosis

A. Natural History of Gross Lesions

Aortic atherosclerosis is a less frequent cause of morbidity and mortality than coronary or cerebral atherosclerosis, but its clinical manifestations are assuming increasing importance with the increasing average age of the population. The aorta is the largest, most accessible, and most convenient artery to examine; its usefulness as an indicator of atherosclerosis in other arterial systems, however, depends on the degree to which it can predict the extent and severity of atherosclerotic lesions in other arteries.

Efforts in our laboratory were first concentrated on the natural history of aortic atherosclerosis in young individuals (Holman *et al.*, 1958b). Intimal fatty streaks occurred in every case 3 years of age or older. The prevalence and extent of fatty streaks were not affected by the terminal illness; accidental death cases did not differ significantly from natural death cases, adolescent Negroes had more extensive aortic fatty streaks than whites.

Fibrous plaques were detected first in the second decade but were insignificant quantitatively until the fourth decade. Despite the greater surface involvement with fatty streaks in the adolescent Negro, there were more fibrous plaques in the white cases in the fourth decade.

Particular attention was given to the topographical distribution of aortic lesions. The aortic ring was the first area involved by fatty streaks in the first decade of life. The aortic valve leaflets themselves were not affected; the anterior leaflet of the mitral valve was usually involved. In the aortic arch fatty streaks were small and discrete, usually occurring about the orifices of the carotid and subclavian arteries. In the descending thoracic aorta, in the second and third decades, fatty streaks developed in a distinctive pattern as longitudinal streaks on the posterior aorta between and immediately lateral to the intercostal vessels. In the abdominal aorta fatty streaks occurred as larger irregular areas with no consistent pattern.

The study was later extended to 1348 cases of all ages (Strong and McGill, 1963). The average extent (per cent of intimal surface) of lesions by age in white and Negro cases of both sexes is shown in Fig. 11. The previous finding of more extensive aortic fatty streaks in Negroes than in whites in the second decade of life was confirmed. Fibrous plaques and calcified and complicated lesions were more extensive in whites than in Negroes in older age groups. Within each race, there was little sex difference in aortic lesions; white males 30–59 years of age had only slightly

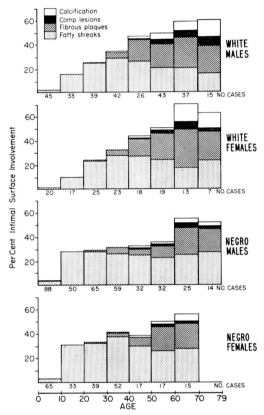

Fig. 11. Aortic atherosclerotic lesions by age, race, and sex in New Orleans; ages 1–79 years.

more fibrous plaques, complicated lesions, and calcified lesions than white females. Negroes showed no consistent sex differences in aortic atherosclerotic lesions. These findings were in contrast with those regarding the coronary arteries, where there was significant sex difference.

A severity index that was developed to relate extent of lesions to rank order of severity was calculated for each abdominal aorta (Holman et al., 1960). In Fig. 12, the averages of these indices for each sex and race are compared. After age 40, white cases had higher average indices than the Negro cases, but sex differences were not consistent nor were they of any appreciable magnitude. Thus, it does not appear that a single index calculated from measures of the different lesions show relationships not apparent from measures of the extent of the lesions themselves.

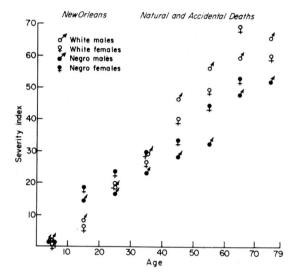

Fig. 12. Aortic atherosclerosis severity index for the abdominal aorta by age, race, and sex in New Orleans: ages 1–79 years.

B. Correlation between Aortic and Coronary Artery Lesions

If only the presence of lesions were considered, there would be a high correlation between lesions in coronary arteries and those in aortas, but correlation calculated from the extent of each type of lesion was low. Six measures of atherosclerosis in the aorta were tested for correlation with five measures of atherosclerosis in corresponding coronary arteries in 517 cases. There was a statistically significant but low correlation between the extent of most of these lesions with lesions in the other arterial segment. Total intimal surface involvement, extent of fibrous plaques, and aortic severity index (Section III, C) were correlated best between the two arteries, with coefficients from 0.5 to 0.6. Aortic fatty streaks correlated very poorly with all coronary lesions, and in some instances there was a small negative correlation. Although most positive coefficients of correlation were statistically significant, correlation coefficients of the order of 0.5 and 0.6 are not strong and indicate that one lesion measure predicts only a small proportion of the lesion measure in the other artery.

When populations differ greatly in incidence of ischemic heart disease and severity of coronary atherosclerosis, aortic atherosclerotic lesions in these same populations show the same trend of differences as do coronary lesions, especially fibrous plaques and more advanced atherosclerotic lesions (Tejada and Gore, 1957; Tejada *et al.*, 1958; Strong *et al.*, 1958, Restrepo and McGill, 1959; Gore *et al.*, 1960; Hirst *et al.*, 1962). It is doubtful, however, that examinations of aortic lesions alone could distinguish clearly between populations with small or moderate differences in coronary lesions and ischemic heart disease.

C. Histology and Electron Microscopy of Aortic Lesions

1. MUSCULOELASTIC INTIMAL THICKENING

Intimal thickening is present in the aorta and progresses with age (Wilens, 1951; Prior and Jones, 1952; Movat *et al.*, 1958). We observed the thickened intima to be composed predominantly of smooth muscle cells and elastic tissue, with collagen and considerable tissue space in which no structures were visible in electron micrographs. There were cells in this layer that did not contain cytoplasmic myofilaments, but the many transitional forms between smooth muscle and the cells without myofilaments suggested that they were all the same basic cell type. The significance of intimal thickening has been discussed in regard to the coronary arteries, and there is no reason to believe the situation is different in the aorta.

2. FATTY STREAKS

The aortic fatty streak in the light microscope showed an intima of varying thickness (usually thicker in the abdominal portion) containing stainable lipid. In some lesions the lipid was in fine droplets and intimately associated with elastic plates; in others, there were collections of foam cells (Fig. 13); and in still others, there were small aggregates of lipid droplets that appeared intracellular. The more advanced lesions had localized collections of lipid with cholesterol clefts; and such lesions frequently were infiltrated with small round cells and occasional segmented neutrophils, resembling the inflammatory lesions in coronary arteries.

Fatty streaks from young individuals—that is, those in the second decade of life—that showed no necrosis, cholesterol clefts, or calcification were presumed to represent the early stage in the formation of a fatty streak. In the electron microscope the lipid was within smooth muscle cells (Fig. 14) just as in the coronary arteries. Smooth muscle cells with

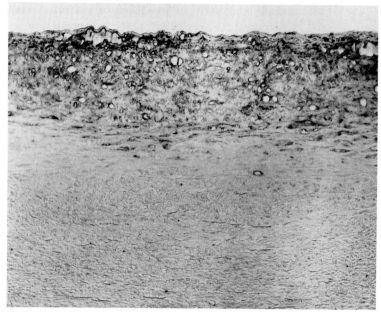

Fig. 13. Descending thoracic aorta, Negro female, age 18 years. Thickened intima with numerous cells containing lipid in their cytoplasm. This lesion grossly was a fatty streak. Oil red O-hematoxylin. Magnification: × 100.

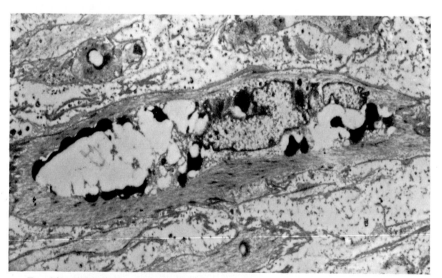

Fig. 14. Abdominal aorta, white male, age 35 years. Lipid inclusions in the cytoplasm of a smooth muscle cell from an intimal lesion that grossly was a fatty streak. Magnification: × 5900.

numerous lipid inclusions were interpreted as transitional forms to foam cells.

Three morphologically different intracellular lipid inclusions were found in aortic lesions. In the small and presumably early lesions in young individuals, the lipid inclusions in the smooth muscle cells typi-

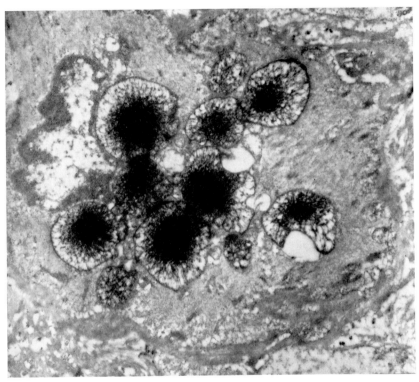

Fig. 15. Descending thoracic aorta, white female, age 31 years. Smooth muscle cell with cytoplasmic lipid inclusions. The lipid inclusions have a central dense zone with radiating filaments of dense material. Magnification: × 10,200.

cally had a dense center from which fine strands of dense material radiated to the periphery of the inclusion (Fig. 15). These inclusions were limited by a double membrane. In lesions with a large amount of lipid, lipid inclusions in smooth muscle cells were either dense and homogeneous or appeared as clear spaces in the cytoplasm. We suspect that the first type of inclusion is lipoprotein, and that the latter two types of inclusion are lipids of varying degrees of saturation. If a lipid is unsaturated it will deposit osmium during fixation and will, in effect, become denatured, no longer possessing the properties of a lipid. Since the plastics used for processing the tissue are lipid solvents, a lipid that retains the properties of a lipid (a saturated lipid in this case) would be dissolved away. Thus, the site of a saturated lipid in the tissue would appear as clear space in electron micrographs, and unsaturated lipid would appear as an area of greater density.

The lipid in the early aortic fatty streak was predominantly of the type that appeared as an inclusion in smooth muscle cytoplasm with a dense center and radiating filaments. In contrast, the lipid inclusions in the coronary fatty streaks were usually dense and homogeneous. This morphological difference is probably a reflection of a chemical difference in the lipid, such as had been demonstrated by Böttcher and associates (1959).

3. Fibrous Plaques

Inflammatory lesions have been seen frequently in the aorta, but have not been studied by electron microscopy. More advanced lesions in the electron microscope show increased collagen, smooth muscle cells with and without lipid, extracellular cholesterol clefts, aggregates of dense crystalline material (probably calcium), foam cells, and small dense bodies. These features are identical to those in coronary artery lesions. There is no single site in the aorta where lesions having a high probability of progressing from fatty streaks to fibrous plaques and complicated lesions occur; therefore, it is more difficult to document histologically the transition from fatty streak to fibrous plaque. Transitional lesions do occur, however, and there is no reason to believe that the pathogenesis of aortic and that of coronary lesions are significantly different except that regression of aortic fatty streaks may be more likely to occur, especially in Negroes (Section III, A).

IV.　Cerebral Artery Lesions

A.　Method of Study

The cerebral arteries have not been studied as extensively as the aorta and coronary arteries owing to the difficulty with which they are dissected. There are two large anatomical divisions of the cerebral vasculature, intracranial and extracranial; any study designed to correlate clinical disease with arterial lesions should include examination of both divisions. The statements reported here are based on studies by Moossy (1959, 1962). The vessels were opened longitudinally and processed in the same manner as the coronary arteries and aortas (Section I, C).

B. Natural History of Gross Lesions

Atherosclerosis was first detected in the second decade of life in extra-cranial cerebral arteries as scattered intimal fatty streaks. In the third decade the carotid sinus portion of the internal carotid artery was regularly involved by fatty streaks and fibrous plaques. The involvement of the carotid sinus increased in the fourth and fifth decades; the cavernous portion of the internal carotid was nearly always involved; and occasionally there were lesions in the petrous portion of the internal carotid. In these same decades the cervical portion of the internal carotid sometimes had a few fatty streaks and fibrous plaques, and fatty streaks and fibrous plaques were found in the vertebral arteries principally about their origins. In the sixth, seventh, and eighth decades lesions increased in extent and severity in the sites described, and the portion of the vertebral arteries between their origin and their entrance into the cranium became more extensively involved. The lesions in this portion of the vertebral arteries were in some cases distributed like rungs in a ladder, located at the level of the foramina of the transverse processes of the cervical vertebrae (C2–C6), and may have been related to cervical spine osteoarthritis.

Atherosclerosis was first detected grossly in the intracranial cerebral arteries in the third decade, in contrast to the onset of lesions in the coronary arteries in the second and in the aorta in the first decade. The initial lesions were found in the internal carotid and vertebral arteries at the points these vessels entered the cranial cavity. In the fourth and fifth decades intimal involvement with atherosclerosis increased; lesions appeared at the origins of the middle and posterior cerebral arteries and in the rostral one-third and caudal one-third of the basilar artery. In the sixth, seventh, and eighth decades there was involvement of any or all portions of the intracranial arteries, but typically the most advanced lesions were found at the sites where they occurred in the fourth and fifth decades. The variation in percentage of intimal surface involvement was considerable in each decade, and the number of cases was too small to stratify each decade by sex and race.

The lesions in the extracranial cerebral arteries occurred approximately a decade later than those in the aorta, but thereafter their tempo of development and gross appearance were similar. Lesions in the intracranial arteries were detected two decades later than those in the aorta, and most of the lesions had the gross appearance of fibrous plaques. The clear chronological antecedence of fatty streaks was not as demonstrable in the intracranial arteries as it was in the aorta and coronary arteries.

C. Histology of Cerebral Artery Lesions

Fibromuscular and fibroelastic intimal thickening has not been studied in the intracranial or extracranial arteries as extensively as in the aorta or coronary arteries. Intimal fatty streaks in the cerebral arteries always showed a thickened intima, but whether they were always

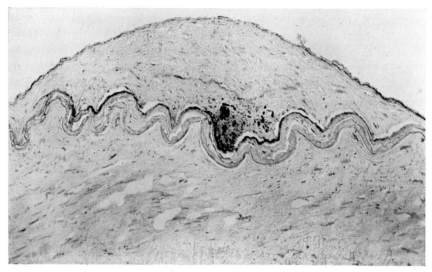

Fig. 16. Middle cerebral artery, white male, age 84 years. Intimal fibrous plaque with stainable lipid in the core of the lesion (black in photograph). Oil red O-hematoxylin. Magnification: × 160.

preceded by intimal thickening without lipid has not been definitely demonstrated. Histologically, the lesions in the extracranial cerebral arteries were similar to those in the aorta.

The intracranial cerebral arteries differed from the aorta and coronary arteries by the absence of an external elastic membrane. The media of the intracranial arteries was thin compared to the lumen diameter and contained only small and scattered elastic fibers. The intima of the normal artery was composed of endothelium lying on the internal elastic membrane except at sites of branching, where the intima was thickened in a cushion-like fashion near the orifice of the branching vessel. The relationship of these intimal "cushions" to fibromuscular intimal thickening such as was seen in the coronary arteries remains to be determined.

The histological appearance of most of the lesions in the intracranial arteries corresponded to their gross appearance as fibrous plaques, with considerable collagen associated with the lipid (Fig. 16). The fibrous plaques always contained stainable lipid, which was located in the core of the lesion and was often inconspicuous in contrast to the thick cap of fibrous tissue. The histogenesis of this lesion has yet to be determined. Making a study of a single site in the cerebral arteries, as was done with the coronary arteries (Section II, C), would do much to enhance our knowledge of the pathogenesis of cerebral atherosclerotic lesions.

V. Summary and Conclusions

Human atherosclerosis begins in childhood, many years before it precipitates clinical manifestations—indeed, most lesions never produce clinical disease. The first alteration recognizable as atherosclerosis is the intimal fatty streak, which appears grossly in the aorta in the first decade of life; in the coronary arteries, in the second decade; and in the intracranial arteries, in the third decade. The histological counterpart of the fatty streak is an intracellular accumulation of particulate lipid in smooth muscle cells. This lipid deposition is probably reversible, but some of these seemingly innocuous intimal fatty streaks progress to fibrous plaques and other more advanced, potentially clinically significant lesions.

Some fibrous plaques may undergo further change—internal hemorrhage from their intrinsic blood vessels, necrosis and sloughing, or formation of an overlying thrombus. The significant result of these processes is reduction in the size of the arterial lumen and ischemia of the tissue supplied by that artery. Only when ischemia becomes sufficiently severe to produce clinical symptoms and signs does clinical disease become apparent.

The risk of developing clinical disease is determined in large part by the extent and severity of advanced atherosclerotic lesions in the individual or in the group. However, other factors, such as coagulability of the blood or adequacy of collateral circulation, would be expected to affect the risk of clinical disease in groups that have arterial atherosclerotic lesions to an identical degree and extent.

Our studies have suggested that a critical step in the pathogenesis of atherosclerosis is the transformation of the fatty streak to the fibrous plaque. The hypothesis is suggested that so long as lipid remains within the cells in which it originates, the lesion is reversible; when these cells become disrupted by excessive lipid accumulation, or when they die and release their lipid into the interstitial spaces, an inflammatory and reparative reaction occurs that leads to the formation of the fibrous plaque.

Recognition of the stepwise sequential development of atherosclerosis is essential to fruitful investigation of the process. The agent that initiates the fatty streak may be (and probably is) different from the agent that influences the formation of a thrombus over a fibrous plaque. Experimental models and epidemiological studies should be related to specific stages of the process in humans. Prophylaxis of the human disease may be attempted at any one of several different stages in the process; a promising opportunity would seem to be at the stage of conversion of fatty streak to fibrous plaque.

Future investigation of atherosclerosis can be profitably directed along the following lines:

(1) The origin and nature of the coronary musculoelastic intimal thickening, in which atherosclerotic lesions begin—whether this is a "normal" anatomical structure, or whether it forms in response to an injurious stimulus.

(2) The stimulus responsible for accumulation of fat in the smooth muscle cell—whether this results from an internal metabolic derangement, hormonal imbalance, nutritional imbalance, phagocytosis of lipid, or other.

(3) Identification of the conditions that determine the fate of the fatty streak—whether this is determined by amount of lipid, nature of the lipid, or reactivity of the individual tissues.

(4) Shifting emphasis in epidemiological studies from clinical disease to arterial lesions, with the hope of relating specific environmental factors to specific stages of the process of atherosclerosis.

REFERENCES

Blache, J. O., and Handler, F. P. (1950). *A.M.A. Arch. Pathol.* 50, 189.
Böttcher, C. J. F., Woodford, F. P., Ter Haar Romeny, C. C., Boelsma, E., and van Gent, C. M. (1959). *Nature* 183, 48.
Bronte-Stewart, B. (1961). *Federation Proc.* 20 (Pt. III), 127.
Crawford, T. (1961). *J. Atherosclerosis Res.* 1, 3.
Daoud, A. S., Goodale, F., Florentin, R., and Beadenkopf, W. G. (1962). *Arch. Pathol.* 73, 74.
Dock, W. (1946). *J. Am. Med. Assoc.* 131, 875.
Eggen, D. A., Strong, J. P., and McGill, H. C., Jr. (1962). *Lab. Invest.* 11, 732.
Enos, W. F., Jr., Beyer, J. C., and Holmes, R. H. (1955) *J. Am. Med. Assoc.* 158, 912.
Fangman, R. J., and Hellwig, C. A. (1947). *Am. J. Pathol.* 23, 901 (Abstr.).
Geer, J. C., McGill, H. C., Jr., and Strong, J. P. (1961). *Am. J. Pathol.* 38, 263.
Gore, I., and Tejada, C. (1957). *Am. J. Pathol.* 33, 875.
Gore, I., Robertson, W. B., Hirst, A. E., Hadley, G. G., and Koseki, Y. (1960). *Am. J. Pathol.* 36, 559.
Gross, L., Epstein, E. Z., and Kugel, M. A. (1934). *Am. J. Pathol.* 10, 253.
Hartroft, W. S. (1961). *Federation Proc.* 20 (Pt. III), 135.

Higginson, J., and Pepler, W. J. (1954). *J. Clin. Invest.* **33**, 1366.

Hirst, A. E., Jr., Gore, I., Hadley, G. G., and Gault, E. W. (1960). *A.M.A. Arch. Pathol.* **69**, 578.

Hirst, A. E., Jr., Piyaratn, P., and Gore, I. (1962). *Am. J. Clin. Pathol.* **38**, 162.

Holman, R. L., McGill, H. C., Jr., Strong, J. P., and Geer, J. C. (1958a). *Lab. Invest.* **7**, 42.

Holman, R. L., McGill, H. C., Jr., Strong, J. P., and Geer, J. C. (1958b). *Am. J. Pathol.* **34**, 209.

Holman, R. L., Brown, B. W., Gore, I., McMillan, G. C., Paterson, J. C., Pollak, O. J., Roberts, J. C., and Wissler, R. W. (1960). *Circulation* **22**, 1137.

McGill, H. C., Jr., Strong, J. P., Holman, R. L., McMahan, C. A., Tejada, C., Restrepo, C., Lichtenberger, E., and Galindo, L. (1959). *Circulation* **20**, 974 (Abstr.).

McMahan, C. A. (1961). Paper presented at the International Population Conference, New York University, New York, September 11-16, 1961.

Mathur, K. S., Patney, N. P., and Kumar, V. (1961). *Circulation* **24**, 68.

Moossy, J. (1959). *Neurology* **9**, 569.

Moossy, J. (1962). *Res. Publ. Assoc. Res. Nervous Mental Diseases* (in press).

Morris, J. N. (1957). "Uses of Epidemiology," p. 44. Livingstone, Edinburg and London.

Morris, J. N., and Crawford, M. D. (1961). *Lancet* **i**, 47 (Letter to the editor).

Movat, H. Z., More, R. H., and Haust, M. D. (1958). *Am. J. Pathol.* **34**, 1023.

Prior, J. T., and Jones, D. B. (1952). *Am. J. Pathol.* **28**, 937.

Restrepo, C., and McGill, H. C., Jr. (1959). *A.M.A. Arch. Pathol.* **67**, 618.

Rigal, R. D., Lovell, F. W., and Townsend, F. M. (1960). *Am. J. Cardiol.* **6**, 19.

Roberts, J. C., Jr., Moses, C., and Wilkins, R. (1959). *Circulation* **20**, 511.

Robertson, W. B., Geer, J. C., Strong, J. P., and McGill, H. C., Jr. (1963). *J. Exptl. Mol. Pathol.* (in press).

Sappington, S. W., and Cook, H. S. (1936). *Am. J. Med. Sci.* **192**, 822.

Scott, R. F., Daoud, A. S., Florentin, R. A., Davies, J. N. P., and Coles, R. M. (1961). *Am. J. Cardiol.* **8**, 165.

Stamler, J. (1958). *J. Am. Dietet.* **A34**, 701.

Standard Operating Protocol of the International Atherosclerosis Project. (1962). Joint publication of the Department of Pathology, Louisiana State University School of Medicine, New Orleans and the Institute of Nutrition of Central America and Panama, Guatemala.

Strong, J. P., and McGill, H. C., Jr. (1962). *Am. J. Pathol.* **40**, 37.

Strong, J. P., and McGill, H. C., Jr. (1963). *J. Exptl. Mol. Pathol.* (in press).

Strong, J. P., McGill, H. C., Jr., Tejada, C., and Holman, R. L. (1958). *Am. J. Pathol.* **34**, 731.

Tejada, C., and Gore, I. (1957). *Am. J. Pathol.* **33**, 887.

Tejada, C., Gore, I., Strong, J. P., and McGill, H. C., Jr. (1958). *Circulation* **18**, 92.

Wainwright, J. (1961). *Lancet* **i**, 366.

Wilens, S. L. (1951). *Am. J. Pathol.* **27**, 825.

Yater, W. M., Traum, A. H., Brown, W. G., Fitzgerald, R. P., Geisler, M. A., and Wilcox, B. B. (1948). *Am. Heart J.* **36**, 334, 481.

—3—

Intermediary Metabolism of Human Arterial Tissue and Its Changes with Age and Atherosclerosis*

JOHN ESBEN KIRK

I. Introduction

In view of the significance of arteriosclerosis as a disease entity, the acquisition of information about the metabolism of human arterial tissue is of definite importance. This subject has received less attention than several other factors in connection with the theories about the pathogenesis of arteriosclerosis. On the basis of biochemical enzyme studies made in the reviewer's department during the last 15 years, the main metabolic aspects of human arteries have been established. These inves-

* The studies performed in the author's department were supported by a grant from the National Institutes of Health, Public Health Service (PHS-891).

tigations have revealed that the vascular wall contains enzymes of the glycolytic pathway, hexosemonophosphate shunt, tricarboxylic acid cycle, malate shunt, and oxidative chain; in addition, the activities of several special enzymes have been assayed. Because of the numerous enzymes present in tissues, the available information must, however, still be considered as being somewhat incomplete.

A great disparity exists in the histological structure of large, elastic and medium-sized, muscular-walled arteries. Although such arteries show many metabolic similarities, the differences in tissue structure are to some extent reflected in the enzyme activities of these blood vessels. For this reason, observations made on one type of arteries are not necessarily applicable to other arteries. Biochemical studies on separate types of blood vessels are therefore desirable, and in the present review the available data about the human aorta, pulmonary artery, and coronary artery will be reported. The fact that the pulmonary artery rarely is the site of severe arteriosclerotic changes justifies a special consideration of the metabolic pattern of that blood vessel.

The investigations on the enzymes of human arterial tissue have in many instances shown significant changes in activities with age. These observations may be of some importance because of a possible relationship between certain aging metabolic changes in the vascular wall and increased susceptibility to arteriosclerosis. The comparatively greater longevity of humans than of most other animal species makes systematic studies of the correlation between age and enzymic concentrations of human blood vessels of particular significance.

In the case of several enzymes, notable differences have been recorded between the activities of normal and arteriosclerotic tissue portions. Although it is difficult to evaluate whether the observed enzymic changes are the cause or the result of arteriosclerosis (Kirk, 1959b), this type of research work constitutes a necessary approach to the subject of atherogenesis. It may be expected that comprehensive investigations in this field will disclose whether the limiting enzymes in the main metabolic pathways are affected by the presence of arteriosclerosis (Kirk, 1959b).

The enzymic patterns of the vessels of animals have been studied to a certain extent by various investigators. The reported observations include enzymic assays of both normal arteries and blood vessels with induced atherosclerosis. The arteries of animals in general distinguish themselves by being less susceptible to spontaneous arteriosclerosis than human arteries, and for that reason comparative metabolic studies on animal and human tissue samples may provide valuable information about the factors involved in the pathogenesis of arteriosclerosis. In this chapter, however, the references to metabolic observations on animal blood vessels will be limited to a brief description of those enzymes and cofactors which have not yet been investigated in human arterial samples. It is believed that such supplementary information may be of a certain value.

In addition to biochemical studies on arterial tissue, histochemical investigations on the presence and activity rates of enzymes in the human arterial wall have been reported. Although histochemical studies often provide valuable information about the localization of enzymes in the tissue, the histological preparatory procedures are generally associated with a loss in enzyme activities. In the present review, only quantitative biochemical studies and investigations performed with isotopically labeled compounds will be considered.

II. Total Metabolism

Determinations of the total metabolism of human aortic tissue (Kirk *et al.*, 1953b, c, 1954a) have shown a rather low respiratory rate (Table I), the mean Q_{O_2} value of intima-media sections of samples obtained

TABLE I

TOTAL METABOLIC RATES OF NORMAL HUMAN AORTIC TISSUE

Process	Rate
Respiration (Q_{O_2})	0.26
Anaerobic glycolysis ($Q_G^{N_2}$)	0.90
Aerobic glycolysis ($Q_G^{O_2}$)	0.66

within 2 to 4 hours after death being 0.26 (range 0.22 to 0.36); this respiratory rate is only about 2% of that exhibited by liver tissue. It should be noted that the assays of the arterial samples were made under sterile conditions with a special procedure developed by Kirk and his associates (1954b; Kirk and Hansen, 1951, 1952a). In this method both the oxygen consumption and carbon dioxide production are measured, and the technique is so accurate and sensitive that it is applicable to tissues with Q_{O_2} rates as low as 0.01. In the assays of the respiratory rate of the aortic samples a modified Krebs phosphate buffer (pH 7.1) with a 0.2% glucose concentration was used as incubation medium.

The respiratory quotient of the aortic samples showed an average value of 0.91, this finding being in accordance with the concept of a predominantly carbohydrate metabolism by the tissue.

The respiratory rates of endothelial cells derived from human aortic specimens have been determined by Lazzarini-Robertson (1962a). The average oxygen consumption observed for the intima cells from normal samples was 0.094 μmoles/10^7 cells per hour, whereas a higher respiratory rate of 0.148 μmoles/10^7 cells per hour was recorded for atherosclerotic endothelial aortic cells.

An extensive investigation (Kirk *et al.*, 1953b, c, 1954a) on the rate of glycolysis by human aortic tissue (intima-media samples) revealed a rather high glycolytic activity, the mean $Q_G^{N_2}$ value being 0.90 (Table I). It was further demonstrated that the glycolysis rate is relatively independent of the oxygen tension, the aerobic glycolysis rate ($Q_G^{O_2}$) being only 30% lower than the anaerobic value. This observation of a low Pasteur effect in arterial tissue has received much attention. Because aerobic glycolysis is functioning in the tissue, lactic acid must steadily be formed in the arterial wall. This formation of acid from the neutral compounds of glucose and glycogen could result in a low pH of the tissue which may be of importance in controlling the activities of some enzyme functions and may play a role in the prevention of calcification (Lehninger, 1959).

In the studies conducted by Kirk *et al.*, both the lactic acid formation and glucose utilization by the tissue samples were measured. These assays generally showed good agreement, although slightly more glucose disappeared than could be accounted for as lactate and by oxidation. It was suggested by the investigators that the small amount of extra glucose disappearing may have been converted to glycogen. The subsequent demonstration of enzymes of the glycogen pathway in the human aortic wall (Kirk, 1962a) would tend to support this assumption.

Investigations recently reported by Fontaine *et al.* (1960a) on the rates of respiration and glycolysis exhibited by human peripheral artery samples showed a metabolic pattern essentially similar to that observed by Kirk *et al.* for the human aorta. Both the normal and the pathological arterial specimens were obtained at surgery from patients suffering from obstructive vascular diseases. The results of these studies are presented in Table II. For comparative purposes, values recorded by Kirk *et al.* for 10 human aortic samples assayed within 2 to 8 hours after death have been included in the table. The reported data reveal a moderately lower glycolysis rate in the peripheral arteries than in the aorta. It is of interest to note that the pathological artery specimens studied by Fontaine *et al.* showed a lower respiratory rate and a higher rate of glycolysis than the normal tissue portions.

The predominance of glycolysis observed for both the aorta and peripheral arteries is a factor of significance with regard to the energy formation in the tissue by the metabolic processes. A calculation was

TABLE II

COMPARISON OF RESPIRATORY AND GLYCOLYSIS RATES BY HUMAN PERIPHERAL ARTERY
TISSUE AND AORTIC TISSUE

Tissue and reference	Number of samples	Micromoles oxygen consumed/gm wet tissue/ hour	Micromoles lactic acid produced/gm wet tissue/ hour
Normal peripheral artery tissue (Fontaine *et al.*, 1960a)	3	3.26	2.20
Pathological peripheral artery tissue (Fontaine *et al.*, 1960a)	12	1.27	3.88
Aortic tissue assayed 2–8 hours after death (Kirk *et al.*, 1954a)	10	1.93	6.93

made (Kirk *et al.*, 1954a) of the energy production by glycolysis and by oxidation in experiments on 43 aortic intima-media samples. It was found that the tissue glycolysis contributed an average of 51% and the respiration 49% of the total energy production by the tissue. Essentially similar conclusions were reached by Fontaine *et al.* (1960a) on the basis of their studies on peripheral human arteries.

If the results derived from the *in vitro* experiments are applicable to the tissue *in vivo,* this may, according to Zemplényi (1962) indicate a rather unfavorable energy metabolism in the arterial wall. This assumption is based on the fact that 1 mole of glucose through glycolysis supplies only 2 moles of ATP, whereas 39 moles of ATP are provided by complete oxidation of glucose via the tricarboxylic acid cycle. The rate of aerobic glycolysis exhibited by the arterial tissue is somewhat unusual from a biological point of view and, as stated by Lehninger (1959), this type of metabolism needs a proportionally greater supply of glucose for energy production than that required by tissues in which the glucose is oxidized to a greater extent. Attention should, however, also be directed to the fact that the total metabolic rate of the arterial tissue is rather low as compared with more active tissues, and this aspect may constitute a favorable feature with regard to the maintenance and survival of the arterial wall.

Since human arterial samples are used for grafting, a study was made of the effect of prolonged storage of the specimens at $1°C$ on the tissue respiration and glycolysis (Kirk *et al.*, 1954a); the maintenance of sterility of the samples was ascertained by bacterial cultures. A marked tendency was noted for the Q_{O_2} value to decrease with time of storage (Fig. 1), but it should be pointed out that in several of the aortic specimens a detectable oxygen consumption was found even after storage for 25 to 30 days. Histological examinations of the stored samples showed that the intima remained relatively intact and that the nuclei of the smooth muscle cells were still discernible although their number was reduced.

In accordance with the observations made on the respiratory rate of

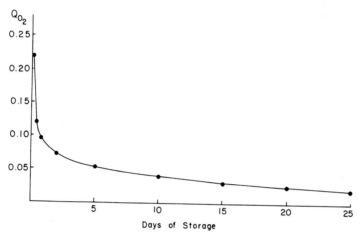

Fig. 1. Effect of storage on rate of respiration (Q_{O_2}) of human aortic tissue. $N = 12$. The curve was constructed on the basis of data observed by Kirk *et al.* (1954a).

the aortic samples, the glycolysis of the tissue declined markedly when the specimens were stored over long periods at 4°C (Fig. 2). A certain glycolytic activity was, however, still exhibited by the tissue after several weeks of storage and by some samples for even more than 100 days.

These findings suggest a high degree of stability in the elementary metabolic machinery of the arterial wall and indicate some favorable features of the metabolic pattern.

One anatomical aspect of the human aorta requires consideration in connection with the evaluation of the metabolic condition of the tissue. The internal one-half to two-thirds of the aortic wall is not supplied with capillaries (Woerner, 1951) and is therefore dependent on diffusion from the aortic lumen and from the vasa vasorum for its supply of oxygen and nutrients; a review of the literature pertaining to this subject has been given by Kirk and Hansen (1952b). The average thickness of the avascular layer ranges from 0.84 mm in young adults to 1.10 mm in middle-aged persons (Wellman and Edwards, 1950). It is as yet unknown whether other mechanisms besides diffusion are of importance for the supply of the arterial wall. It does not seem unlikely, as suggested by various investigators, that the passage *in vivo* of a filtrate through the wall as the result of mechanical forces may contribute to the supply of oxygen and nutrients. In spite of this uncertainty, measurements of the diffusion coefficient values for various significant metabolic compounds would seem warranted.

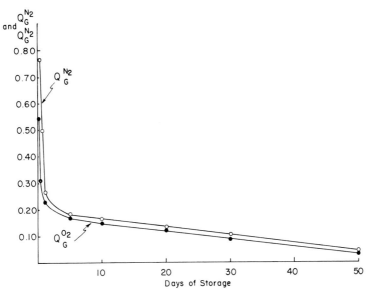

Fig. 2. Effect of storage on rates of anaerobic $(Q_G N_2)$ and aerobic $(Q_G O_2)$ glycolysis of human aortic tissue. $N = 12$. The curve was constructed on the basis of data observed by Kirk *et. al.* (1954a).

Determinations of the diffusion coefficients of several solutes (at $37°C$) for membranes of the intima-subintima and media layers of the human aorta have been made by Kirk and Laursen (1954a, d, e, 1955b; Kirk *et al.,* 1953a) using the procedure described by Kirk and Johnsen (1951; Johnsen and Kirk, 1955). Assays were made separately of the diffusion coefficients of nitrogen, oxygen, carbon dioxide, lactate, iodide, and glucose. The diffusion coefficient was defined in the classic way (Hill, 1928-1929) as the number of units of a substance which diffuses through 1 sq cm of the membrane in 1 minute at a concentration gradient of 1 unit per milliliter per centimeter. Expressed in this way, the coefficient for gases and for nongaseous solutes can be directly compared.

The average diffusion coefficient of oxygen for human aortic tissue from young adults was 0.000505. When compared with the respiratory rate of the tissue, calculations reveal that the layer thickness which can be supplied with oxygen through diffusion is 0.91 mm. The corresponding value for middle-aged and old individuals (diffusion coefficient = 0.000606) is 1.00 mm. These estimated depths to which oxygen can penetrate through diffusion indicate a low margin of reserve for the oxygen supply of the normal aortic wall.

One important finding in the study by Kirk and Laursen was an increase with age in the diffusion coefficient values for the various compounds studied (Table III). The increased permeability of the aortic tissue with age is illustrated in Fig. 3 in which the diffusion coefficient values for glucose have been plotted against the age of the subjects. An analysis of the data reported in Table III indicates that the diffusion

TABLE III

MEAN DIFFUSION COEFFICIENTS FOR AORTIC TISSUE OBSERVED FOR VARIOUS AGE GROUPS[a]

Age group years	Number of samples	Nitrogen	Oxygen	Carbon dioxide	Lactate	Iodide	Glucose
			Intima-Subintima Layer				
10–39	13	0.000393	0.000439	0.000359	0.000098	0.000253	0.000074
40–59	20	0.000500	0.000550	0.000400	0.000098	0.000318	0.000101
60–80	18	0.000492	0.000501	0.000442	0.000166	0.000363	0.000128
			Media Layer				
10–39	13	0.000499	0.000505	0.000329	0.000064	0.000230	0.000061
40–59	20	0.000548	0.000607	0.000367	0.000076	0.000244	0.000075
60–80	17	0.000597	0.000605	0.000419	0.000107	0.000289	0.000091

[a] The diffusion coefficient is defined according to Hill (1928-1929) as the number of units of a substance diffusing through 1 sq cm of the membrane in 1 minute at a concentration gradient of 1 unit per milliliter per centimeter.

coefficients of the compounds with molecular weights ranging from 90 to 180 (lactate, iodide, glucose) increased to a greater extent with age than the coefficient values for the substances with lower molecular weights (nitrogen, oxygen, carbon dioxide). If the concept of a membrane pore theory is accepted, these findings would suggest an increase with age particularly in the number of larger sized pores in the aortic tissue. In this connection it should be mentioned that investigations made on a connective tissue membrane (human tentorium cerebelli) which rarely exhibits pathological changes failed to show any significant variation in permeability with age (Laursen and Kirk, 1955b).

Comparisons were further made of the diffusion coefficients for normal and arteriosclerotic tissue portions of the same aortas. In these studies, the coefficient values for the arteriosclerotic samples were found to be about 70% higher than those observed for the normal aortic specimens.

It has recently been suggested by Lehninger (1959) that the increase with age in the permeability of the aorta demonstrated by Kirk and Laursen may cause a faster removal of lactic acid from the tissue. Ac-

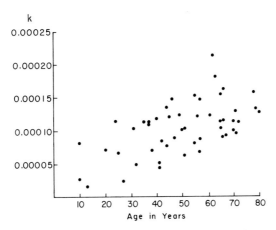

Fig. 3. Variation with age in the diffusion coefficient of glucose for membrane preparation of human aortic intima (with attached subintimal tissue). k = Diffusion coefficient, defined according to Hill (1928-1929) as the number of units of a substance diffusing through 1 sq cm of a membrane in 1 minute at a concentration gradient of 1 unit per milliliter per centimeter. From Kirk and Laursen (1955b).

cording to Lehninger, this might result in a higher pH of the media layer in the aged arterial wall and could be a factor of importance in the process of calcification by facilitating the formation of insoluble calcium phosphate compounds in the tissue.

Studies on the permeability of human arterial tissue to serum lipids (Wilens and McCluskey, 1954) and to albumin, globulin, and hemoglobin (Hirst and Gore, 1962) have also been reported, but these investigations do not provide quantitative measurements. Since the diffusion of these high-molecular compounds is not directly related to the metabolism of the arterial wall or comparable with the permeability rates of the metabolites studied by Kirk and Laursen, the available information derived from these and similar studies will not be reviewed in the present chapter.

III. Enzymes of Human Arterial Tissue

The acquisition of information about the intermediary metabolism of the arterial wall includes measurements of the concentrations of enzymes and cofactors present in the tissue. The application of isotope techniques to arterial samples also constitutes an important approach to the elucidation of the various metabolic functions exhibited by the tissue.

The enzyme studies performed by the reviewer have been carried out on homogenates of arterial tissue obtained fresh at autopsy. The measurements were made on intima-media samples of the aorta, pulmonary artery, and coronary artery. Approximately 100 specimens of the aorta and pulmonary artery have been included in each investigation to permit an evaluation of the relation of enzyme activity to age. In the case of the aortic and coronary artery samples, the enzyme determinations were conducted separately on normal and arteriosclerotic tissue portions from the same arteries. The mean activity values observed for the arteriosclerotic samples have been expressed in percentages of the activities recorded for the normal segments of the arteries.

The measurements of the enzyme activities of homogenates of the arterial tissue samples represent the contributions of the different cell types present in the vascular wall. It seems a reasonable approach first to obtain information about the metabolism exhibited by homogenates of the intima-media layers. At a later stage, observations on individual cell types in the arterial tissue would be advisable because the various cells assumedly have special physiological functions and metabolic properties.

Most of the enzymes have been assayed by procedures utilizing spectrophotometric analyses, but in many instances the high connective tissue content of the vascular wall has made it necessary to modify the available methods or to develop new techniques. The procedures as applied to crude tissue extracts must also eliminate interference by other enzymes. The activity measurements were made at optimal pH, in the presence of the required cofactors, and usually at a substrate concentration permitting a zero order reaction. It is generally agreed that determinations of enzyme activities under such conditions afford a reliable measurement of the enzyme concentrations present in the tissue and thus provide a useful basis for comparison of such values. It should be pointed out in this connection that enzyme values determined under these optimal conditions do not necessarily correspond to the activities exhibited by the tissue *in vivo* because the concentrations of substrates and cofactors are usually lower in the intact tissue. The actual quantities of substrates available *in vivo* for various enzymes are, however, difficult to evaluate since there is little likelihood that intermediate products will accumulate when enzymes of a metabolic chain are operating normally.

The enzyme systems reported in the present survey will be grouped according to the metabolic pathways and subdivisions to which they belong. In order to avoid arbitrary units, the activity values will, when possible, be expressed as millimoles of substrate metabolized per gram wet tissue per hour. Average activities observed for nonpathological tissue portions derived from young adults have been chosen for expression of the normal tissue enzyme values. A brief review will further be made of the metabolic activities of arterial tissue determined by the quantitative tetrazolium technique (Kirk and Laursen, 1955b). Because 2, 3, 5-triphenyltetrazolium chloride has a rather high diffusion coefficient for human arterial tissue, this method can be applied both to tissue slices and homogenates. Comparative studies made in the reviewer's department (Laursen and Laursen, 1958) of the rates of formazan formation and oxygen consumption of human arterial tissue have revealed that metabolic activities measured by the tetrazolium technique are only 3-5% of those observed by manometric determination of oxygen consumption by the tissue; these comparisons were performed by recalculation of the values to the common denominator of oxidation-reduction microequivalents moved per milligram of dry tissue per hour. In spite of this discrepancy for which no cause has been revealed, quantitative tetrazolium studies are of a certain significance because the formation of formazan (compound extracted with acetone and determined spectrophotometrically) usually is proportional to the metabolic tissue activity (Laursen and Laursen, 1958). These observations on arterial tissue are in accordance with those reported for other human tissues (Laursen and Laursen, 1958) and for animal tissues (Barker and Schwartz, 1954; Barker, 1955).

The general description of arterial enzyme activities will be based on the observations made on samples derived from adult subjects. Statistically significant age changes ($p < 0.05$) recorded for normal aortic and pulmonary artery samples will be presented graphically. For comparative purposes, the mean enzyme values for arteriosclerotic tissue portions are listed in percentages of the activities exhibited by the normal segments of the same blood vessels. Since values recorded for arteriosclerotic samples may be partly influenced by a replacement of the arterial tissue with inert non-nitrogenous material, the enzyme activities of the pathological tissue will be expressed both on the basis of wet tissue weight and tissue nitrogen content.

Separate surveys will be made of enzyme values observed for children and of differences between activities of arterial specimens from sexually mature male and female persons.

A. Enzymes of Carbohydrate Metabolism

1. Glycolytic Pathway

Of the eleven enzymes in this metabolic subdivision, only five have been studied in detail in human arterial tissue (Table IV). Investigations on two additional enzymes (phosphoglyceric kinase and phosphoglyceromutase) are currently in progress in the reviewer's department.

TABLE IV

Mean Enzyme Activities of Normal Human Arterial Tissue Glycolytic and Glycogen Pathways

Enzyme	Aorta	Pul-monary artery	Cor-onary artery	Unit
Glycolytic pathway				
Hexokinase	0.013	0.011	—	mM of substrate metabolized/ gm wet tissue/hour
Phosphoglucoisomerase	1.85	1.62	2.05	Same as above
Aldolase	0.056	0.073	0.099	Same as above
Enolase	0.24	0.27	0.24	Same as above
Lactic dehydrogenase	1.06	0.86	0.68	Same as above
Glycogen pathway				
Glycogen phosphorylase	0.100	0.138	0.103	Same as above

The reported activity values for the various enzymes in the glycolytic pathway show great differences. It will be noted for instance that the average hexokinase activity was found to be less than 1% of the mean activity of phosphoglucoisomerase. This finding supports the contention that investigations aimed at identifying the limiting enzyme systems within each metabolic subdivision may prove rewarding.

Through catalysis by hexokinase, glucose undergoes an obligatory phosphorylation as the initial step in its metabolism. An energy-rich phosphate bond is used in the reaction, and this endergonic metabolic process is considered to be essentially irreversible. The resulting compound, glucose-6-phosphate, is not only the sequential metabolite in the glycolytic chain of reactions but constitutes also the initial substrate for the enzymes of the oxidative shunt pathway.

In the investigation performed in the reviewer's department (Brandstrup *et al.*, 1957) the hexokinase activity was assayed by measurement of the rate of disappearance of glucose. In the previous study by Kirk *et al.* (1954a) in which the respiration of intact aortic tissue was determined in the presence of glucose, a mean glucose utilization of 0.43 mg per gram wet tissue per hour was observed. A higher glucose utilization (1.80 mg per gram wet tissue per hour) was recorded in the hexokinase assays which were performed on tissue homogenates with the use of a glucose substrate solution supplemented with ATP, but this activity rate must still be considered as being remarkably low.

The second enzyme of the glycolytic pathway, phosphoglucoisomerase distinguishes itself by having a very high concentration in human aortic and pulmonary artery tissue (Brandstrup *et al.*, 1957). A special investigation conducted on coronary artery samples (Kirk *et al.*, 1958) revealed an even higher phosphoglucoisomerase activity in this medium-sized blood vessel.

The observations made on the aldolase enzyme in human aortic tissue (Kirk and Sørensen, 1956a, b) are of particular interest because these studies have shown a notable increase in the aldolase concentration of that tissue with age (Fig. 4), whereas lower values were found for arteriosclerotic than for normal tissue portions (Table XI). The average activity of the arteriosclerotic tissue was only 29% of that of the normal aorta sections, and this difference between arteriosclerotic and normal tissue portions is the greatest recorded for the many enzymes studied in the reviewer's department.

The presence of a rather high enolase activity in human arterial tissue (Wang and Kirk, 1959) may be of some importance because the reaction catalyzed by enolase provides the generation of a high-energy phosphate bond through the conversion of 2-phosphoglyceric acid to phosphoenolpyruvic acid. In view of the predominance of glycolysis in the arterial tissue, this enzyme may play a significant role in the exergonic aspect of the arterial wall.

The last enzyme in the glycolytic pathway, lactic dehydrogenase, also exhibits a comparatively high activity in the arterial tissue (Matzke *et al.*, 1957; Kirk *et al.*, 1958). In analogy with the observations made on aldolase, the aortic tissue level of lactic dehydrogenase increases with age until 50-59 years and then shows a decrease in subsequent decades (Fig. 4). A similar but less pronounced variation with age was observed for the pulmonary artery (Fig. 5) whereas the lactic dehydrogenase concentration remained essentially unchanged throughout life in the coronary artery.

In human arterial tissue, a notable activity of an enzyme adjunct to the glycolytic pathway, phosphomannoseisomerase has recently been demonstrated by Kirk, using the assay method described by Bruns *et al.* (1958a). This enzyme converts mannose-6-phosphate to fructose-6-phosphate and thus provides the arterial tissue with the opportunity to utilize mannose-containing carbohydrate compounds.

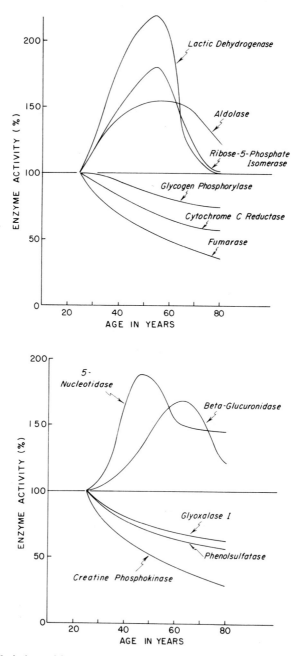

Fɪɢ. 4. Variation with age in enzyme activities of normal human aortic tissue.

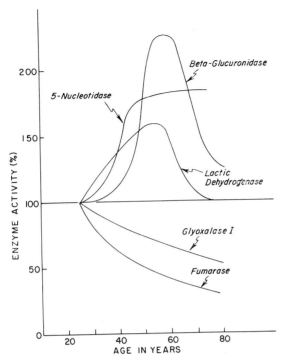

FIG. 5. Variation with age in enzyme activities of human pulmonary artery tissue.

2. GLYCOGEN PATHWAY

The first step in the synthesis of glycogen consists in the conversion of glucose-6-phosphate to glucose-1-phosphate through the action of phosphoglucomutase. According to current concepts, the synthesis of glycogen from glucose-1-phosphate takes place mainly through the functioning of the uridyl transferase enzyme. Although glycogen phosphorylase may operate in both the synthetic and degrading directions, this enzyme in the tissue is believed to act principally in the process of the breakdown of glycogen (Stetten and Stetten, 1960).

The presence of phosphoglucomutase in human aortic, pulmonary artery, and coronary artery tissue has been demonstrated by Kirk using the assay method described by Noltmann and Bruns (1958). In the application of this procedure to arterial tissue, addition of the glucose-1,6-diphosphate coenzyme to the substrate is required.

Measurements of the glycogen phosphorylase activity of human arterial tissue (Table IV) were made (Kirk, 1962a) with a modification of the method of Buell *et al.* (1958). In this assay procedure, glucose-1-

phosphate is used as substrate for the enzyme and the amount of ortho-phosphate liberated is determined colorimetrically. The addition of adenylic acid to the incubation mixture assures the measurement of both the active and inactive form of the phosphorylase.

The studies on the glycogen phosphorylase in aortas and coronary arteries showed a significant decrease in the activity of this enzyme with age (Fig. 4), and markedly lower values were found for arteriosclerotic than for normal tissue portions (Tables XI and XII). The reductions in the glycogen phosphorylase activities associated with aging and arterio-sclerosis are probably due to atrophic changes in the smooth muscular tissue of the vessel wall. In the pulmonary artery, which is not suscep-tible to arteriosclerosis, higher glycogen phosphorylase concentrations were recorded and no variation with age was observed. With regard to this enzyme, a notorious difference has thus been demonstrated between the aorta and coronary artery on one side and the pulmonary artery on the other side.

In connection with the glycogen phosphorylase it should be noted that rather high concentrations of glycogen have been reported (Schmidt and Hillenbrand, 1953) for samples of human peripheral arteries (Table V). The lower values observed for arteriosclerotic specimens were associ-ated with histologically demonstrable atrophy of the muscular tissue; in samples from patients suffering from endarteritis obliterans, the re-corded moderately higher glycogen concentrations were related to mus-cular hypertrophy in the vascular wall.

TABLE V

GLYCOGEN CONCENTRATION OF HUMAN FEMORAL ARTERY[a]

Condition of artery	Per cent of wet weight
Normal	0.070
Arteriosclerosis	0.030
Endarteritis obliterans	0.092

[a] The values were calculated on the basis of data reported by Schmidt and Hillenbrand (1953).

3. HEXOSEMONOPHOSPHATE SHUNT

In human arterial tissue, the presence of enzymes of the hexosemono-phosphate shunt was first demonstrated by Kirk (1958, 1959e; Kirk *et al.*, 1959). Studies have been completed on three of the enzymes in this meta-bolic pathway (Table VI) and work on the transketolase activity of the arterial tissue is in progress.

The direct oxidative pathway of glucose-6-phosphate metabolism pro-

TABLE VI

Mean Enzyme Activities of Normal Human Arterial Tissue
Hexosemonophosphate Shunt

Enzyme	Aorta	Pulmonary artery	Coronary artery	Unit
Glucose-6-phosphate dehydrogenase	0.115	0.092	0.102	mM of substrate metabolized/gm wet tissue/hour
6-Phosphogluconate dehydrogenase	0.010	0.013	0.019	Same as above
Ribose-5-phosphate isomerase	0.0034	0.0045	0.0045	Same as above

ceeds in a cycle via 6-phosphogluconate, ribulose-5-phosphate, and sedoheptulose-7-phosphate to hexosemonophosphate. This shunt is of particular interest because it provides an alternate pathway for the metabolism of carbohydrates. No lactic acid is formed in the oxidative shunt, and as previously pointed out by the reviewer (Kirk, 1958), the use of this pathway may be of importance for a tissue like the arterial wall which is chiefly dependent on diffusion for the removal of lactic acid. The fact that two of the enzymes (glucose-6-phosphate dehydrogenase and 6-phosphogluconate dehydrogenase) supply TPNH through their functioning is also an important feature because TPNH is required for the synthesis of fatty acids and cholesterol. In view of the assumed significance of lipid metabolism in the arterial wall in connection with atherogenesis, the operation of the hexosemonophosphate shunt in human arterial tissue may therefore be a subject which requires special consideration. This pathway also provides a mechanism for generating the pentose phosphate compounds required in the formation of nucleic acids and nucleotides.

The extent to which the intact tissue uses this shunt as compared with the glycolytic pathway cannot be evaluated with certainty on the basis of the enzyme measurements performed on homogenized tissue samples. Information about this subject may be obtained through comparative investigations with glucose-1-C^{14} and glucose-6-C^{14} as described by Bloom and Stetten (1953, 1955). By following such a procedure, a notable functioning of this pathway in the guinea pig aorta has recently been demonstrated by Sbarra *et al.* (1960).

The completed investigations on the enzymes in human arterial tissue (Table VI) have shown marked differences in the enzyme concentrations of this pathway. The activity of glucose-6-phosphate dehydrogenase, the first enzyme in the hexosemonophosphate shunt is approximately 10 times as great as that of the subsequent enzyme, 6-phosphogluconate dehydrogenase. These two TPN-dependent enzymes also differ with regard to the relationship between arteriosclerotic changes and enzymic activities. Distinctly lower concentrations of glucose-6-phosphate dehydrogenase were observed in arteriosclerotic than in normal tissue portions, whereas no significant differences were recorded for the 6-phosphogluconate dehydrogenase enzyme (Tables XI and XII).

The ribose-5-phosphate isomerase of the aortic tissue distinguishes itself by showing an increase in concentration with age (Fig. 4) whereas no significant variation was observed for the pulmonary artery. A rather remarkable finding with regard to this enzyme is that higher values were recorded for arteriosclerotic than for normal aortic tissue portions (Table XI). Since it has been shown that the ribose-5-phosphate isomerase activity of human red blood cells is about 1000 times as high as that of the arterial tissue, the possibility exists that the higher enzyme values observed for the arteriosclerotic tissue portions may be due, at least to some extent, to the presence of capillaries which were not detectable by macroscopic inspection of the samples.

The procedure for transketolase determination recently developed by Bruns *et al.* (1958b) has been applied by the reviewer to human arterial tissue, and such assays have shown the presence of notable concentrations of this enzyme in aortic, pulmonary artery, and coronary artery tissue.

4. TRICARBOXYLIC ACID CYCLE

A main phase of glucose metabolism starts with the conversion of pyruvic acid to the acetyl-CoA compound. The complete oxidation of the acetyl moiety of acetyl-CoA is subsequently effected by means of the cyclic mechanism known as the tricarboxylic acid cycle. Of the seven enzymes included in this metabolic subdivision, the activities of five have been studied in the reviewer's department (Table VII). Investigations on succinic dehydrogenase have further been reported by Maier and Haimovici (1957, 1958).

The presence in human aortic tissue of a moderate activity of aconitase was first reported by Laursen and Kirk (1955a). In a subsequent study (Kirk, 1961a) a large number of aortic and pulmonary artery samples was assayed for the tissue concentration of this enzyme. The aconitase measurements were made by determination of the quantity of citric acid formed through incubation of the tissue with cis-aconitic acid.

TABLE VII

Enzyme	Aorta	Pulmonary artery	Coronary artery	Unit
Tricarboxylic acid cycle				
Aconitase	0.021	0.027	—	mM of substrate metabolized/gm wet tissue/hour
Isocitric dehydrogenase	0.063	0.071	0.082	Same as above
Succinic dehydrogenase	0.035	—	—	Same as above
Fumarase	0.178	0.328	—	Same as above
Malic dehydrogenase	0.57	0.71	0.98	Same as above
Malate shunt				
TPN-malic enzyme	0.011	0.010	0.012	Same as above

As compared with other enzymes in the tricarboxylic acid cycle, the aconitase activity of human arterial tissue is rather low; this aspect makes investigations on the enzyme of particular interest. A marked tendency was found for the aconitase level of the pulmonary artery to exceed that of the aorta; the mean values observed for the pulmonary artery samples were 136% (wet tissue) and 140% (tissue nitrogen) of those of the aortic samples derived from the same subjects, the t values of the differences being, respectively, 6.90 and 6.05. Significantly lower enzyme concentrations were recorded for arteriosclerotic than for normal tissue specimens (Table XI).

The TPN-linked isocitric dehydrogenase enzyme operates in the tricarboxylic acid cycle by catalyzing the transformation of D-isocitric acid to oxalosuccinic acid; a decarboxylation of this compound subsequently takes place with the formation of α-ketoglutaric acid. The isocitric dehydrogenase enzyme is further of importance through its production of TPNH, the compound which is required for the synthesis of fatty acids and cholesterol.

The isocitric dehydrogenase activity observed for human arterial tissue (Kirk and Kirk, 1959a; Kirk 1960c) is about 300 times as high as that found for human serum. In both the aorta and coronary artery, essentially similar activity values were recorded for the arteriosclerotic and normal tissue portions of the same blood vessels (Tables XI and XII).

The investigations on the activity of succinic dehydrogenase in human arterial tissue were initiated in the reviewer's department (Kirk and Laursen, 1954b, c; 1955a) by quantitative measurement of the formazan formation resulting from incubation of intima-media tissue segments in a succinate-phosphate buffer medium to which triphenyltetrazolium had been added. A notable succinic dehydrogenase activity was observed for human aortic tissue, the formazan formation averaging 0.107 mg per gram of wet tissue following a 40-minute incubation at 39°C; this value is 8 times as high as that observed for samples incubated in buffered glucose solution. This conspicuous difference is illustrated in Fig. 6.

In subsequent investigations (Kirk *et al.*, 1955) a comparison was made of the rates of respiration of aortic tissue in succinate-phosphate and glucose-phosphate buffer media. The oxygen consumption by the arterial tissue was found to be 4.4 times as high in the succinate-containing medium as in the control experiments. A marked depression of the respiration was attained through addition of malonate to the incubation mixture, this finding confirming the existence of the succinic dehydrogenase activity in the human arterial wall.

Approximately equal activities of succinic dehydrogenase were reported by Kirk *et al.* (1955) and by Maier and Haimovici (1957, 1958) for the human aorta. Comparative assays were made by the latter authors of the activities of this enzyme in the aortic arch, descending thoracic aorta, and abdominal aorta. The mean Q_{O_2} values recorded for the three aortic segments in samples derived from 0- to 17-year-old subjects were, respectively, 1.00, 1.17, and 0.72 indicating a lower succinic dehydrogenase activity in the abdominal aorta than in the arch and thoracic aorta in this age group. Assays of samples obtained from 21- to 73-year-old individuals revealed a notable decrease with age in the enzymic activities of all three segments, the average values for these aortic specimens being 0.44 (arch), 0.50 (thoracic descending aorta), and 0.53 (abdominal aorta).

Investigations on the fumarase enzyme (Laursen and Kirk, 1955a; Sørensen and Kirk, 1955, 1956) showed a marked and consistent decrease in activity with age in both the aorta (Figs. 4 and 7) and the pulmonary artery (Fig. 5). In contrast to this, no significant variation with age in the malic dehydrogenase activity was recorded (Matzke *et al.*, 1957). This DPN-dependent enzyme exhibits an appreciable activity in the aorta, pulmonary artery, and coronary artery (Kirk *et al.*, 1958).

Studies are currently in progress by Kirk on an adjunct enzyme, glutamic dehydrogenase. This enzyme catalyzes the interconversion of ketoglutarate and glutamate and thus establishes an interrelationship between the tricarboxylic acid cycle and amino acid metabolism.

Fig. 6. Photograph of samples from a normal thoracic aorta incubated for 40 minutes with triphenyl tetrazolium chloride in buffered glucose solution (1), citrate medium (2), and succinate medium (3). From Kirk and Laursen (1955a).

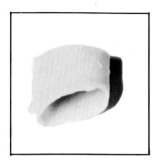

1

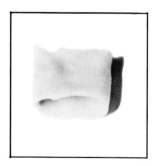

2

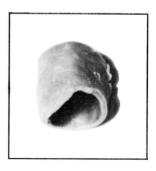

3

PLATE I

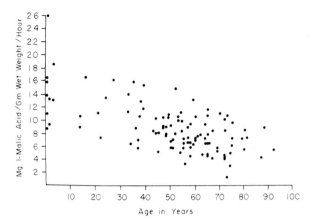

FIG. 7. Scattergram showing variation with age in fumarase activity of human aortic (thoracic) tissue. The figure was constructed on the basis of data recorded by Sørensen and Kirk (1956).

5. MALATE SHUNT

The TPN-malic enzyme is most unusual since it seems to catalyze simultaneous dehydrogenation and decarboxylation of malic acid without going through the step of oxalic acid:

$$\text{L-Malate} + \text{TPN} \rightleftharpoons \text{pyruvate} + CO_2 + \text{TPNH}$$

In studies conducted in the reviewer's department (Kirk and Kirk, 1959a; Kirk, 1960c) the activity of this enzyme in human arterial tissue (Table VII) was found to be only 2% of that recorded for the DPN-malic dehydrogenase in the tricarboxylic acid cycle (Matzke *et al.*, 1957; Kirk *et al.*, 1958). The demonstration of a definite activity of the TPN-malic enzyme in the arterial tissue may nevertheless be of metabolic importance since this finding indicates that the malate shunt is operating in the human arterial wall.

6. OXIDATIVE CHAIN

In this stepwise process, the tissue makes use of electron carrier systems which are intermediates in redox potential between the dehydrogenase substrates and oxygen. The final product of this reaction is water which is formed when the negatively charged oxygen combines with hydrogen released at an earlier stage. The three enzymes associated with the oxidative chain (Table VIII) have been studied in human arterial tissue (Maier and Haimovici, 1957, 1958; Kirk, 1962c).

The determinations of the diaphorase activity in the arterial samples

TABLE VIII

MEAN ENZYME ACTIVITIES OF NORMAL HUMAN ARTERIAL TISSUE
OXIDATIVE CHAIN

Enzyme	Aorta	Pulmonary artery	Coronary artery	Unit
Diaphorase	0.110	0.103	0.109	mM of substrate metabolized/gm wet tissue/hour
Cytochrome c reductase	0.030	0.032	0.027	Same as above
Cytochrome c oxidase	0.060	—	—	Same as above

were made with the use of a quantitative procedure (Kirk, to be published) in which the decolorization time of 2,6-dichlorophenolindophenol is measured visually in the presence of DPNH and NaCN. This method permits an accurate assay of the diaphorase activity in specimens with a high connective tissue content. The diaphorase enzyme is closely related in function to cytochrome c reductase; both enzymes mediate the transfer of electrons from DPNH to electron acceptors, but diaphorase distinguishes itself from cytochrome c reductase by being inert with cytochrome c. In the evaluation of tissue diaphorase activities the fact must be considered that cytochrome c reductase is capable of catalyzing the reduction of 2,6-dichlorophenolindophenol in the presence of DPNH. In contrast to this, diaphorase does not interfere with the measurement of the cytochrome c reductase activity, because cytochrome does not serve as an electron acceptor in the functioning of diaphorase. On the basis of these facts, the determination of the activities of both enzymes in the same tissue samples is advisable.

The mean diaphorase and cytochrome c reductase activities were found to be definitely lower in the arteriosclerotic tissue (Tables XI and XII). The cytochrome c reductase activity decreased significantly with age in the aorta (Fig. 4) whereas no certain change was observed for the pulmonary artery or coronary artery.

In the investigation by Maier and Haimovici (1957) the cytochrome c oxidase activity of aortic samples from 21- to 73-year-old persons was found to be only 50% of that recorded for specimens from 0- to 17-year-old subjects. Essentially similar values were observed for the aortic arch, thoracic aorta, and abdominal aorta (Maier and Haimovici, 1957, 1958).

B. Enzymes of Protein Metabolism

Various groups of enzymes are involved in the metabolism of proteins. The only enzymes of this category which have been studied in

TABLE IX

MEAN ENZYME ACTIVITIES OF NORMAL HUMAN ARTERIAL TISSUE
PROTEOLYTIC ENZYMES

Enzyme	Aorta	Pulmonary artery	Coronary artery	Unit
Leucine aminopeptidase	1.37	1.49	1.60	Milligrams of naphthylamine formed/gm wet tissue/hour
Autolysis	0.95	1.25	1.77	Milligrams of tyrosine released/gm wet tissue/hour
Cathepsin	2.18	1.18	1.38	Same
Total proteolysis	3.13	2.43	3.15	Same

human arterial tissue (Table IX) are leucine aminopeptidase (Green *et al.*, 1955; Kirk, 1960a) and cathepsin (Kirk, 1962b).

The presence of leucine aminopeptidase in the human aorta was first reported by Green *et al.* in 1955, but only three samples were included in the study. In a subsequent investigation by Kirk (1960a) on this exopeptidase, enzyme measurements were made on a large number of aortic, pulmonary artery, and coronary artery specimens. The enzyme activities observed for the aorta and pulmonary artery were ten times as high as that of normal human serum, and even greater values were recorded for the coronary artery.

It is generally assumed that the breakdown of proteins in tissues is catalyzed by cathepsin, but the actual function of this proteolytic enzyme in living cells has not yet been established. In contrast to this, the participation of cathepsin in autolysis of animal cells has been demonstrated by several investigators (Eder *et al.*, 1939; Belfer *et al.*, 1943) indicating that this enzyme serves to cleave the proteins of the cells after death.

The studies on cathepsin in arterial tissue are of particular interest because it was shown by Bavina and Kritsman in 1953 that notably higher proteolytic activities were exhibited by arteriosclerotic than by normal tissue in rabbits. These findings were later confirmed by Kirk (1962b) in investigations on human aortic and coronary artery samples. A special denatured hemoglobin preparation was used as substrate for the enzyme and the extent of enzymic cleavage was expressed in terms of tyrosine released from the substrate. Separate measurements were made in the presence and in the absence of the substrate. The former values were classified as total proteolysis and those observed in the control tests as autolysis. In accordance with the conventional terminology, the difference between the two proteolytic assays was designated as cathepsin activity.

The mean values observed for arteriosclerotic aortic tissue portions were 122% (autolysis), 145% (cathepsin), and 131% (total proteolysis) of those recorded for the normal tissue. The corresponding percentage figures for the coronary artery samples were 115, 178, and 145. These results emphasize the possible significance of this proteolytic enzyme in connection with the process of arteriosclerosis and may reflect the presence of a higher proportion of dead cells in the arteriosclerotic tissue.

In a study by Kritsman and Bavina (1954) the rate of incorporation of radioactive-labeled amino acids into the proteins of the aorta was found to be lower in rabbits with induced atherosclerosis than in normal animals. A distinctly lower incorporation of methionine-S^{35} into the aortas of old oxen than into the arterial samples of young cattle was subsequently reported by Fontaine *et al.* (1960a, b).

C. Enzymes of Lipid Metabolism

In view of the great volume of research work on atherogenesis, it would seem logical to place special emphasis on the lipid metabolism of the arterial wall (Kask, 1962). Several histochemical investigations (Müller and Neumann, 1959; Tischendorf and Curri, 1959) have been reported on the functioning of a lipase in human arteries, but quantitative biochemical determinations have not yet been conducted on that esterase. The reason enzyme studies are lacking in this important metabolic subdivision is that information has only recently become available about the intermediary reactions involved in lipid synthesis and catabolism. The knowledge is not yet complete with regard to this subject (Bloch, 1960), and because of the many technical difficulties associated with the assay of enzymes catalyzing the processes of lipogenesis and fatty acid oxidation, it may be expected that progress in this field will be somewhat delayed. However, important data about the total enzymic function in the arterial tissue in connection with lipid metabolism have been supplied through isotopic investigations.

The *in vitro* synthesis by aortic tissue of fatty acids and steroids from C^{14}-labeled acetate has been observed for several animal species. Special studies on the ability of human fetal aortic samples to synthesize these compounds were reported by Paoletti *et al.* in 1958. The formation of fatty acids and of cholesterol from C^{14}-labeled acetate was, respectively, 31 and 40% of the values encountered for hepatic tissue, whereas the biosynthesis results recorded with the use of C^{14}-labeled mevalonic acid were only 3 and 7% of the hepatic activity. In a subsequent investigation by Azarnoff (1958) on human aortas from adults, the *in vitro* synthesis of digitonine-precipitable steroids was also observed, but incorporation of acetate into cholesterol purified as a dibromide compound was not established. Lipid synthesis by human intimal cells isolated from normal

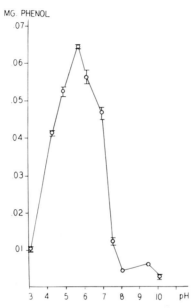

Fig. 8. Phosphomonoesterase activities of human aortic tissue at various pH levels. Assays performed with the use of disodium phenylphosphate as substrate. From Kirk and Praetorius (1950a).

and from arteriosclerotic tissue areas has recently been described by Lazzarini-Robertson (1962a, b).

D. Phosphatases and Phosphorylases

In human arterial tissue the presence of a nonspecific phosphomono-esterase with a pH optimum at 5.75 was first discovered by Kirk and Praetorius (1949, 1950a, b) through assays of aortic homogenates. Disodium phenylphosphate was used as substrate for the enzyme. A plot of the enzyme activity against the pH showed two peaks (Fig. 8); a major one appeared at pH 5.75 (acid phosphatase) and a minor one at pH 9.5. It was deduced that the smaller peak expressed traces of alkaline phosphatase since the enzyme function was enhanced by addition of magnesium chloride to the incubation medium.

The previously assumed absence of a phosphatase in the arterial wall had for many years been a subject of importance in the discussion of the pathogenesis of arterial calcification. The failure by earlier investigators to demonstrate the presence of this enzyme in the arterial tissue could be ascribed to the fact that previous phosphatase studies had been conducted only at an alkaline reaction.

In a subsequent investigation by Kirk (1959a) the acid phosphatase activities of the human aorta, pulmonary artery, and coronary artery were assayed with the use of *p*-nitrophenylphosphate as substrate (Table X). The presence in human arteries of both acid and alkaline phosphomonoesterases has been confirmed by Antonini and Weber (1951).

A remarkable feature of human arterial tissue is its high concentration of adenosinetriphosphatase (Baló *et al.*, 1948-1949; Banga and Nowotny, 1951a, b). The studies by these authors indicate that both elastic and muscular-walled vessels contain two different adenosinetriphosphatases. One of these is myosin-bound and has a pH optimum at 7.0, whereas the other is water-soluble and exhibits maximal activity at pH 9.0. The latter enzyme which splits off both the terminal and the central phosphate groups of ATP and inosine triphosphate has been found only in arterial tissue and was designated as adenylpyrophosphatase by Baló *et al.* As might be expected, the muscular-walled arteries, like the femoral artery were found to contain greater quantities of myosin-bound enzyme than the aorta. In both muscular and elastic arteries, however, the special arterial adenosinetriphosphatase (adenylpyrophosphatase) was present in the highest concentration.

Studies of the adenosinetriphosphatase of the human aorta, coronary artery, and peripheral arteries have further been reported by Antonini and Weber (1951). It was subsequently demonstrated by Kirk (1959a) that the arterial tissue contains both an adenylpyrophosphatase and an inorganic pyrophosphatase. In the inorganic pyrophosphatase determinations, sodium pyrophosphate instead of ATP was used as substrate. The adenylpyrophosphatase was found to have its highest activity at pH 8.1 and in the presence of a magnesium concentration of 1 mM; in contrast to this, the optimal activity of the inorganic pyrophosphatase was exhibited at pH 7.2 and at a magnesium level of 15 mM. These observations on the pH and magnesium dependency suggest the functioning of two different enzymes in the arterial wall.

Assays of the arterial samples revealed that the tissue concentrations of adenylpyrophosphatase and inorganic pyrophosphatase are approximately equal (Table X). The adenylpyrophosphatase values observed in Kirk's study are about twice as high as those reported by the previous

TABLE X

MEAN ENZYME ACTIVITIES OF NORMAL HUMAN ARTERIAL TISSUE
PHOSPHATASES AND PHOSPHORYLASES

Enzymes	Aorta	Pulmonary artery	Coronary artery	Unit
Phosphomonoesterase (pH 5.75)	0.050	0.034	0.034	mM PO_4 liberated/gm wet tissue/hour
Adenylpyrophosphatase	0.24	0.26	0.44	Same as above
Inorganic pyrophosphatase	0.20	0.24	0.38	Same as above
5-Nucleotidase	0.16	0.07	0.10	Same as above
Purine nucleoside phosphorylase	0.009	0.013	0.020	mM of substrate metabolized/gm wet tissue/hour
Creatine phosphokinase	0.128	0.260	0.330	Same as above

investigators; this discrepancy may be due to the small number of samples assayed by the other authors. It is of interest to note that the arterial enzyme level is of similar magnitude to that found for striated muscles (Banga and Nowotny, 1951a). Although the exact nature of the enzymes responsible for the adenosinetriphosphatase activity of the arterial tissue has not yet been established, their metabolic functions are assumedly related to the physiological processes of the smooth muscular component in the vessel wall. In this connection it should be pointed out that the biological role of the inorganic pyrophosphatase is obscure at present.

The presence of another specific phosphatase, 5-nucleotidase in human aortic tissue was first reported by Reis in 1950, who in subsequent publications (Reis, 1951; Ahmed and Reis, 1958) provided further details concerning the properties of the enzyme. This phosphatase which has a pH optimum at 7.8 acts only on adenosine-5-monophosphate (AMP) and inosine-5-monophosphate. The concentration of 5-nucleotidase in the arterial wall is unusual since it has been found by Reis (1950) to be of the same magnitude as that observed for ossifying cartilage and about 15 times as high as the activity in skeletal muscle. These findings by Reis were confirmed by Antonini and Weber (1951). In a later study by Kirk (1959d) which included a large number of arterial samples, an even higher concentration of this phosphatase was recorded for human aortic tissue and a considerable increase with age in the enzyme level was demonstrated in both the aorta (Fig. 4) and the pulmonary artery (Fig. 5). The high content of 5-nucleotidase in the arterial tissue and the fact that it exhibits maximal activity near the physiological pH deserve attention because it has been suggested by Reis (1950, 1951) that it may play a role in the process of tissue calcification.

In connection with this review of the dephosphorylating enzymes of the arterial tissue it should be mentioned that Carr *et al.* (1954, 1955) have found a notable myokinase activity in the coronary artery of cattle. The myokinase enzyme catalyzes the conversion of ADP to ATP and AMP and is therefore closely connected with the functioning of both the adenylpyrophosphatase and the 5-nucleotidase. So far no studies have been conducted with the purpose of demonstrating the presence of myokinase in human arterial tissue.

An appreciable concentration of creatine phosphokinase in human arterial tissue has further been established by Kirk (1961d, 1962d). This enzyme participates in both the generation and utilization of energy-rich compounds. In the dephosphorylation of creatine phosphate, ADP is required as phosphate acceptor; the replenishment of ATP through the action of this transphosphorylase is of great metabolic significance especially with regard to the physiological function of the muscular tissue in the arterial wall. The assumption that creatine phosphokinase is associated mainly with the smooth muscle component of the vascular wall is supported by the finding of a 10 times higher activity of the enzyme in the brachial artery than in the aorta.

A marked tendency was noted for the aortic enzyme level to decrease with age (Fig. 4) and in all the assayed samples, the arteriosclerotic portions exhibited a distinctly lower creatine phosphokinase activity than the normal tissue (Table XI). These enzymic changes may be related to atrophic processes in the muscular tissue of the aortic wall and probably represent findings of definite pathophysiological significance.

In contrast to the observations on creatine phosphokinase, a study

TABLE XI

Mean Enzyme Activities of Arteriosclerotic Aortic Tissue Expressed in Percentages of Activities of Normal Tissue Portions[a]

Enzymes	Wet tissue (%)		Tissue nitrogen (%)	
Hexokinase	81	$p < 0.01$	91	ns
Phosphoglucoisomerase	91	$p < 0.05$	99	ns
Aldolase	29	$p < 0.001$	—	
Enolase	99	ns	—	
Lactic dehydrogenase	82	$p < 0.01$	96	ns
Glycogen phosphorylase	58	$p < 0.001$	63	$p < 0.001$
Glucose-6-phosphate dehydrogenase	65	$p < 0.01$	67	$p < 0.01$
6-Phosphogluconate dehydrogenase	105	ns	104	ns
Ribose-5-phosphate isomerase	120	$p < 0.05$	144	$p < 0.001$
Aconitase	87	$p < 0.001$	89	$p = 0.02$
Isocitric dehydrogenase	97	ns	101	ns
Fumarase	55	$p < 0.01$	—	
Malic dehydrogenase	81	$p < 0.01$	103	ns
TPN-malic enzyme	94	ns	97	ns
Diaphorase	79	$p < 0.001$	85	$p < 0.001$
Cytochrome c reductase	79	$p < 0.001$	84	$p < 0.001$
Leucine aminopeptidase	100		110	$p < 0.1$
Autolysis	114	ns	122	ns
Cathepsin	118	$p < 0.05$	145	$p < 0.001$
Total proteolysis	115	$p < 0.02$	131	$p < 0.001$
Phosphomonoesterase (pH 5.75)	95	ns	98	ns
Adenylpyrophosphatase	85	$p < 0.01$	86	$p < 0.01$
Inorganic pyrophosphatase	88	$p < 0.01$	91	$p < 0.05$
5-Nucleotidase	89	$p < 0.02$	95	ns
Purine nucleoside phosphorylase	127	$p < 0.001$	142	$p < 0.001$
Creatine phosphokinase	54	$p < 0.001$	58	$p < 0.001$
Glyoxalase I	79	$p < 0.001$	—	

[a] The statistical evaluation of differences is presented in the third and fifth columns.

TABLE XII

MEAN ENZYME ACTIVITIES OF ARTERIOSCLEROTIC CORONARY ARTERY TISSUE EXPRESSED IN PERCENTAGES OF ACTIVITIES OF NORMAL TISSUE PORTIONS[a]

Enzymes	Wet tissue (%)		Tissue nitrogen (%)	
Phosphoglucoisomerase	76	$p < 0.01$	—	
Enolase	90	$p < 0.1$	—	
Lactic dehydrogenase	81	$p < 0.01$	—	
Glycogen phosphorylase	35	$p < 0.01$	34	$p < 0.01$
Glucose-6-phosphate dehydrogenase	74	$p < 0.01$	77	$p < 0.01$
6-Phosphogluconate dehydrogenase	84	ns	91	ns
Ribose-5-phosphate isomerase	107	ns	115	ns
Isocitric dehydrogenase	104	ns	103	ns
Malic dehydrogenase	66	$p < 0.01$	—	
TPN-malic enzyme	97	ns	97	ns
Diaphorase	84	$p < 0.01$	87	$p < 0.02$
Cytochrome c reductase	85	$p < 0.05$	88	$p < 0.1$
Leucine aminopeptidase	113	ns	109	ns
Autolysis	106		115	
Cathepsin	164		178	
Total proteolysis	132		145	
Phosphomonoesterase (pH 5.75)	127	$p < 0.01$	135	$p < 0.05$
Adenylpyrophosphatase	80	$p < 0.01$	93	ns
Inorganic pyrophosphatase	81	$p < 0.01$	89	ns
5-Nucleotidase	111	ns	111	ns
Purine nucleoside phosphorylase	127	$p < 0.1$	120	$p < 0.05$
Glyoxalase I	77	$p < 0.001$	—	

[a] The statistical evaluation of differences is presented in the third and fifth columns.

on the purine nucleoside phosphorylase enzyme (Kirk, 1961b) demonstrated a significantly higher activity of this phosphorylase in arteriosclerotic than in normal arterial tissue (Tables XI and XII). The increased enzyme concentration in the pathological tissue is somewhat unusual and should be considered in connection with the pathogenesis of arteriosclerosis.

E. Other Enzymes

Investigations have been completed on several other enzymes in human arteries (Table XIII). One of these enzymes, β-glucuronidase (Dyrbye and Kirk, 1955, 1956) which hydrolyzes glucuronides has recently received some attention because of its possible role in mucopolysaccharide catabolism and in tissue regeneration. In comparison with the glucuronidase activities of human parenchymatous organs, the arterial enzyme levels observed by Dyrbye and Kirk were quite low, namely only about 0.5% of those reported for liver tissue. A tendency was noted for the enzyme concentration in the aorta and pulmonary artery to increase until the age of 50-69 years after which a decrease occurred (Figs. 4 and 5). In the same investigation, higher β-glucuronidase activities were observed for arteriosclerotic than for normal aortic tissue portions, whereas lower values for arteriosclerotic intima samples subsequently were reported by Kayahan (1960).

TABLE XIII

MEAN ENZYME ACTIVITIES OF NORMAL HUMAN ARTERIAL TISSUE
OTHER ENZYMES

Enzyme	Aorta	Pulmonary artery	Coronary artery	Unit
β-Glucuronidase	0.00017	0.00015	0.00015	mM of substrate metabolized/gm wet tissue/ hour
Phenolsulfatase	0.000023	0.000025	0.000020	Same as above
Glyoxalase I	1.23	1.70	1.00	Same as above
Carbonic anhydrase	0.01	—	—	E.U./mg wet tissue

In a study by Branwood and Carr (1960) which included a large number of coronary artery samples, the β-glucuronidase activities recorded for the intima layer of that blood vessel were similar to those observed by Dyrbye and Kirk for the human aorta; higher enzymic values were likewise encountered by Branwood and Carr for the arteriosclerotic tissue specimens.

A low, but definite phenolsulfatase activity (Dyrbye and Kirk, 1955; Kirk and Dyrbye, 1956) was also demonstrated in human arterial tissue. The level of this enzyme in the aorta showed a notable decrease with age (Fig. 4) and with progressive arteriosclerosis. The change with age in the enzyme activity of the pulmonary artery samples was less conclusive. Phenolsulfatase catalyzes the hydrolysis of sulfuric acid esters, but the physiological significance of this factor in the vascular tissue has not been established.

One unusual finding in the arterial enzyme research studies is a very high concentration of a special enzyme, glyoxalase I (Kirk and Kirk, 1959b; Kirk, 1960b) which catalyzes the condensation of methylglyoxal and glutathione. There is apparently no natural substrate (methylglyoxal) for this enzyme in the tissue, and it is therefore not possible to draw any conclusions regarding the physiological function of glyoxalase I. In both the aorta and the pulmonary artery, the enzyme level was found to decline significantly with age (Figs. 4 and 5).

Of other enzymes studied, carbonic anhydrase is of special interest since this enzyme may be indirectly associated with both the glycolytic and oxidative metabolism of the tissue. Assays made by Kirk and Hansen (1950, 1953) on homogenates prepared from the media layer of human aortic samples showed a measurable activity of this enzyme in all the samples analyzed; the recorded values were corrected for the minute amounts of red blood cells present in the homogenates. The observed mean enzyme concentration of 0.01 enzyme units (E.U.) per milligram of wet tissue is only about 1% of that found in red blood cells, but is nevertheless noteworthy. Whether the significant function of carbonic anhydrase in the arterial tissue is a catalysis of the hydration of carbon dioxide or of the dehydration of carbonic acid is not known. If, however, carbonic acid is formed in large amounts in the arterial wall as a metabolic end product or through neutralization of lactic acid by bicarbonate, a catalysis of the dehydration of carbonic acid might serve a useful purpose by facilitating the removal of this compound from the tissue since the diffusion rate of carbon dioxide is higher than that of carbonic acid.

Determinations of the thromboplastin activity of human vascular tissue have been made by several investigators during the last few years (Astrup and Claassen, 1957; Witte and Bressel, 1958; Astrup *et al.*, 1959; Kirk, 1960d, 1961c, e, 1962e; Coccheri and Astrup, 1960, 1961; Perlick, 1961; Astrup and Coccheri, 1962; Donner, 1962). The presence of this enzyme in the arterial wall has received some attention in connection with Duguid's (1948) theory about the pathogenesis of arteriosclerosis. It is generally believed that the arterial thromboplastin is a factor of importance in the process of blood clotting when the vascular wall is damaged, but the role of this enzyme in the formation of a thrombus in the vascular lumen when the tissue is intact remains uncertain. It has been suggested by Emmrich (1961) that tissue thromboplastin may be released from desquamated endothelial cells, and recent experiments (Shimamoto, 1962; Shimamoto *et al.*, 1962) have revealed that isolated rabbit aortas perfused with saline solution release thromboplastin directly into the vessel lumen when epinephrine in physiological doses is added to the perfusion solution.

The findings reported by the various investigators on the thromboplastin of human blood vessels in general show good agreement. The average thromboplastin values observed by Kirk for different layers of the aorta and pulmonary artery are presented in Table XIV. In this study, the thromboplastin activities exhibited by the tissue were calculated quantitatively with the use of the conventional double logarithmic plot (Fig. 9); a thromboplastin preparation and homogenates of the gray matter of human brain tissue were used as standards.

The results listed in Table XIV indicate that lower thromboplastin activities usually were recorded for fibrous-lipid arteriosclerotic portions of the aortas than for the normal tissue specimens. A lower thromboplastin activity of fibrous arteriosclerotic tissue has also been observed by Perlick (1961) who ascribes the difference to the presence of a higher

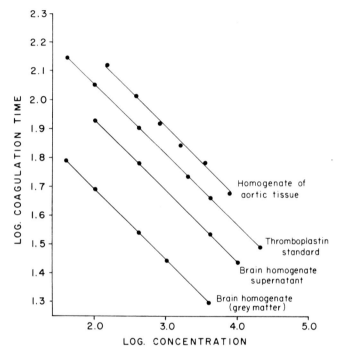

Fig. 9. Double logarithmic plot for calculation of thromboplastin activities of human vascular tissue samples. Tissue concentrations are expressed in micrograms of wet weight and thromboplastin standard in micrograms of solution employed (properly prepared Simplastin suspension). Coagulation times expressed in seconds. From Kirk (1962e).

concentration of antithromboplastin factors in the arteriosclerotic tissue. One interesting finding in the reviewer's study is the extremely low thromboplastin concentration of the ulcerated arteriosclerotic areas, which is only about one-tenth of that encountered for the fibrous-lipid portions.

A calculation was made of the correlation between age and arterial thromboplastin activities. A significant decrease with age was observed in the thromboplastin content of the arteriosclerotic (fibrous-lipid) aortic intima tissue ($r = -0.55$, $t = 2.87$, $p < 0.01$). This decrease may be

TABLE XIV

THROMBOPLASTIN ACTIVITIES OF BLOOD VESSELS EXPRESSED IN PERCENTAGE OF ACTIVITY
OF HUMAN BRAIN TISSUE (GRAY MATTER)

Blood vessel and tissue	Percentage of activity
Normal aorta	
Intima	3.4
Media	2.8
Adventitia	1.8
Arteriosclerotic aorta	
Lipid-fibrous intima	2.0
Lipid-fibrous media	2.3
Ulcerated tissue	0.2
Pulmonary artery	
Intima	1.2
Media	1.4

related to an increased formation of hard fibrous tissue in connection
with the progressive development of arteriosclerotic changes with advancing age. In contrast to the decline in the thromboplastin activity of
the aortic arteriosclerotic tissue with age, the thromboplastin values of
the nonarteriosclerotic intima layer of the pulmonary artery showed a
tendency to increase with age $(r = +0.38,\ t = 2.05,\ p < 0.05)$. This is
illustrated in Fig. 10 in which the individual pulmonary thromboplastin
values have been plotted.

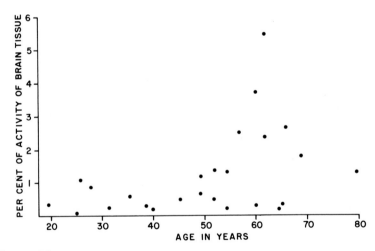

FIG. 10. Effect of age on thromboplastin activity of human pulmonary artery intima
layer. From Kirk (1961e).

In human arterial tissue the presence of monoamine oxidase (Thompson and Tickner, 1951) and cholinesterase (Thompson and Tickner, 1953) has further been established, but too few samples were included in these studies to permit an evaluation of the normal vascular enzyme tissue levels. In the monoamine oxidase experiments, tyramine hydrochloride was used as substrate for the enzyme; evidence that oxidative deamination was effected by a monoamine oxidase was obtained through demonstration of the resulting aldehyde in the incubation mixture by use of the 2,4-dinitrophenylhydrazine reaction. The investigations on the cholinesterase indicate that this enzyme in the human aorta is chiefly, but not entirely a pseudo-cholinesterase.

Assays have been made by Mandel and Kempf (1960) on the glutamic oxalacetic transaminase activity in bovine aortas. Essentially similar values were observed for old and for young animals, the mean activities being, respectively, 0.0213 and 0.0224 mM of substrate transformed per gram wet tissue per hour (at 25°C). Information about the concentration of this enzyme in human vascular tissue is lacking.

F. Metabolism of Arterial Mucopolysaccharides

Studies on the activities in human arterial tissue of enzymes involved in the synthesis of mucopolysaccharides have not as yet been reported. Valuable information concerning the rate of turnover of the sulfated mucopolysaccharides in arterial tissue has, however, recently been obtained through the use of radioactive-labeled sulfate.

Several *in vivo* and *in vitro* investigations on various animal specimens have revealed high rates of sulfate incorporation into the arterial wall (Fig. 11). A review of the literature pertaining to this subject has been made by Kirk (1959c). The reported high incorporation rates suggest that the arterial tissue cannot be considered as inert with regard to this metabolic aspect.

An *in vitro* study performed by Dyrbye (1959a, b) on human aortic samples is of particular interest. In this investigation sterile intima-media tissue portions were incubated for 45 hours at 38°C in Tyrode's solution containing S^{35}-labeled sodium sulfate. The acid mucopolysaccharides were subsequently isolated from the tissue as described by Dyrbye and Kirk (1957) and the radioactivity of the material was determined. As seen from Table XV, a definite decrease with age in the rate of sulfate incorporation by the aortic tissue was found. This observation was later confirmed by Hauss *et al.* (1962).

G. Cofactors and Coenzymes

Many of the enzymes in the arterial wall are dependent on cofactors and coenzymes for their functioning. Several of the enzyme systems are

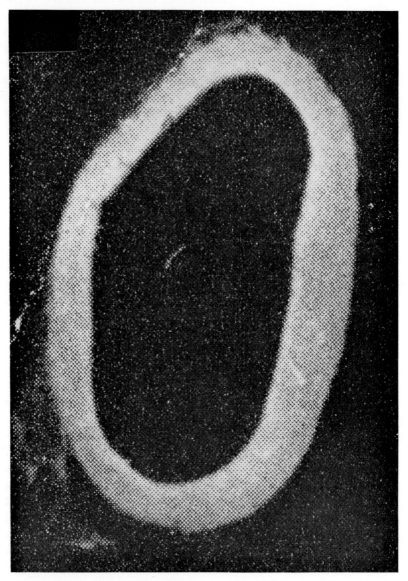

FIG. 11. Incorporation of radioactive-labeled sulfate by aorta of rabbit fetus. From Boström and Odeblad (1953).

TABLE XV

INCORPORATION *in Vitro* OF RADIOACTIVE-LABELED SULFATE BY SULFATED
MUCOPOLYSACCHARIDES OF HUMAN ARTERIAL SAMPLES[a]

Age	Number of samples	Cpm/mg hexosamine/ hour of incubation
Fetus	1	182
25–47 years	9	33
57–80 years	8	8

[a] The values were calculated on the basis of data reported by Dyrbye (1959a, b).

activated by the divalent metallic magnesium ion. Information about the
concentration of this cofactor in human arterial tissue is therefore of
definite importance. A significant increase in the magnesium content of
normal aortic tissue from 0.010% at the age of 30 years to 0.041% at
60 years was observed by Buck (1951), whereas Rechenberger and Hevelke
(1955) over the same age range found a decrease in the tissue magnesium
level from 0.011 to 0.003%. In both studies, however, increased magnesium concentrations were recorded for arteriosclerotic tissue portions.
In view of the controversial observations on normal aortic tissue, further
investigations on the arterial content of this mineral compound would
be desirable.

Studies on the coenzyme concentrations in human aortic tissue (Table
XVI) have shown comparatively high values for both nicotinic acid

TABLE XVI

COENZYME CONCENTRATIONS OF HUMAN AORTIC TISSUE

Coenzyme	Micrograms/ gm wet tissue
Nicotinic acid	20.0
Free riboflavin + flavin mononucleotide	0.40
Flavin adenine dinucleotide	0.98
Total riboflavin	1.38
Glutathione	220.0

(Chang *et al.,* 1955) and riboflavin (Schaus *et al.,* 1955), the determination of the nicotinic acid compound serving as a reliable measurement
of the tissue level of phosphopyridine nucleotides. The nicotinic acid
and total riboflavin values listed in the table are about 20% and 10%
of the corresponding contents observed for human liver tissue. In view
of the low respiratory rate of the aortic tissue, the concentrations of
these compounds in the vascular wall must be considered as being rather
high.

A tendency was noted for the nicotinic acid (Fig. 12) and total riboflavin (Fig. 13) contents of the human aorta to decrease with age. The reduction in the riboflavin concentration seemed to affect the free riboflavin + flavin mononucleotide and the flavin adenine dinucleotide fractions to approximately the same extent.

In order to investigate the rate of breakdown of the pyridine nucleo-

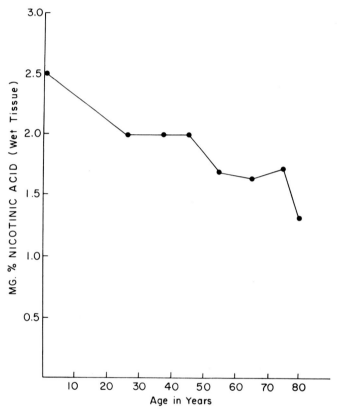

Fɪɢ. 12. Effect of age on nicotinic acid concentration of human aortic tissue. N = 65. The curve was constructed on the basis of data reported by Chang *et al.* (1955).

tides in the aortic tissue during storage of the samples, experiments were conducted (Chang *et al.*, 1955) in which the coenzyme content was determined by the fluorometric procedure of Burch (1952). A rapid destruction of DPN was found to occur at 37°C (Fig. 14), but no decrease in the total nicotinic acid concentration of the tissue was observed. These findings indicate the presence of an appreciable activity of the DPNase enzyme in the human arterial wall. A decrease in the flavin adenine dinucleotide content of the stored aortic samples was similarly noted

(Schaus *et al.*, 1955); this reduction in the FAD content was associated with an increase in the free riboflavin + flavin mononucleotide fraction.

Investigations on the concentrations of free nucleotides, adenosine nucleotides, and uridine nucleotides in samples of bovine aortas have recently been reported by Kempf *et al.* (1961). In these studies lower

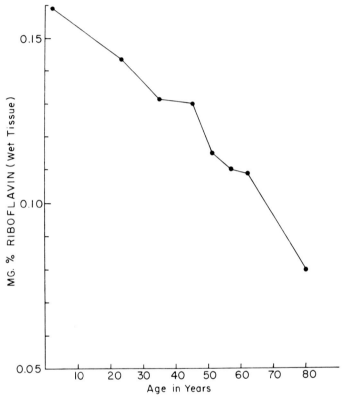

Fig. 13. Effect of age on total riboflavin concentration of human aortic tissue. N = 100. The curve was constructed on the basis of data reported by Schaus *et al.* (1955).

coenzyme values were recorded for aortas from old oxen than from young animals.

The presence of cytochrome c in human aortic tissue has been demonstrated by Kirk (1959b), but because of the low concentration of this compound in the tissue, exact determinations of the cytochrome c level in the arterial wall have not been possible. The isolation of cytochrome c was performed by a modification of the method described by Carruthers (1947).

TABLE XVII

Enzyme Activities and Coenzyme Concentrations of Arterial Samples from Children (0–10 Years) Expressed in Percentages of Values Observed for Adults (18–35 Years)[a]

Enzymes and coenzymes	Aorta				Pulmonary artery			
	%	t of diff.	D.f.[b]		%	t of diff.	D.f.[b]	
Hexokinase	70	1.47	14	ns	64	2.05	14	p < 0.1
Phosphoglucoisomerase	77	1.47	14	ns	54	3.26	14	p < 0.01
Aldolase	90	0.54	20	ns	100	0.00	16	—
Enolase	59	3.26	19	p < 0.01	29	7.50	19	p < 0.001
Lactic dehydrogenase	50	2.52	20	p = 0.02	70	1.70	15	ns
Glycogen phosphorylase	93	0.43	16	ns	—	—	—	—
Glucose-6-phosphate dehydrogenase	32	3.55	24	p < 0.01	—	—	—	—
6-Phosphogluconate dehydrogenase	119	0.79	18	ns	95	0.40	15	ns
Ribose-5-phosphate isomerase	64	2.07	19	p < 0.1	—	—	—	—
Aconitase	148	2.75	25	p < 0.02	68	1.52	15	ns
Isocitric dehydrogenase	106	0.42	20	ns	100	0.00	13	—
Fumarase	121	1.25	16	ns	82	1.13	16	ns
Malic dehydrogenase	100	0.00	20	—	78	1.38	16	ns
TPN-malic enzyme	91	0.27	18	ns	88	0.98	18	ns
Diaphorase	65	2.83	18	p < 0.02	—	—	—	—
Cytochrome c reductase	91	0.79	18	ns	—	—	—	—
Leucine aminopeptidase	100	0.00	21	ns	—	—	—	—
Autolysis	66	1.35	14	ns				
Cathepsin	100	0.00	14					
Total proteolysis	87	0.44	14	ns				
Phosphomonoesterase	51	5.80	24	p < 0.001	55	4.74	21	p < 0.001
Adenylpyrophosphatase	93	0.50	24	ns	90	0.61	20	ns
Inorganic pyrophosphatase	71	1.82	22	p < 0.1	49	3.15	20	p < 0.01
5-Nucleotidase	40	6.38	26	p < 0.001	75	1.24	23	ns
Purine nucleoside phosphorylase	95	0.29	24	ns	112	0.90	12	ns

TABLE XVII (*continued*)

Enzymes and coenzymes	Aorta			Pulmonary artery		
	%	*t* of diff.	D.f.[b]	%	*t* of diff.	D.f.[b]
Creatine phosphokinase	96	0.15	19	ns	—	—	—
Phenolsulfatase	115	0.15	20	ns	—	—	—
Glyoxalase I	116	1.00	21	ns	100	0.00	17
Nicotinic acid	132	1.60	12	ns	—	—	—
Riboflavin	116	0.88	13	ns	—	—	—
Glutathione	128	1.02	15	ns	—	—	—

[a] The percentage values were calculated on the basis of wet tissue weight.
[b] D.f. = degrees of freedom.

Glutathione is a coenzyme of glyoxalase I and a prosthetic group of the glyceraldehyde-3-phosphate dehydrogenase enzyme. Measurements by Wang and Kirk (1960) of the total glutathione level in human aortic samples (Table XVI) showed a tendency for the tissue content of this compound to increase with age; essentially similar values were recorded for normal and arteriosclerotic tissue portions.

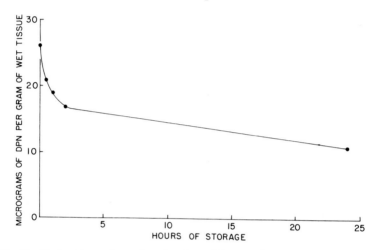

FIG. 14. Destruction of aortic phosphopyridine nucleotides through action of DPNase in arterial tissue. The curve was constructed on the basis of data observed by Chang *et al.* (1955).

The presence of notable concentrations of coenzyme A in aortic tissue has been reported by Paoletti *et al.* (1959) and Kim *et al.* (1960) for various animal species. This coenzyme is of great importance in many metabolic functions, including the synthesis of lipids and the channeling of metabolic components of carbohydrates, lipids, and proteins into the tricarboxylic acid cycle. In these investigations, aortic tissues of the species which are most susceptible to atherosclerosis showed the greatest levels of this coenzyme and also the highest rates of biosynthesis of lipids from C^{14}-labeled acetate. No determinations of coenzyme A in human arterial tissue have been recorded.

H. Comparison of Enzyme Activities in Arterial Samples from Children and Young Adults

The studies conducted on arterial enzyme systems have shown that vascular samples obtained from children frequently exhibit different activity levels than those derived from adults. For evaluation of the enzymic pattern in the aorta and pulmonary artery of children, a comparison was made of the values observed for samples (wet weight) from 0- to 10-year-old children and 18- to 35-year-old subjects. The comparative statistical data are presented in Table XVII.

The recorded percentage values indicate the presence of a significantly higher aconitase activity in the aortic tissue of children and distinctly lower concentrations of the following eight enzymes: enolase, lactic dehydrogenase, glucose-6-phosphate dehydrogenase, ribose-5-phosphate isomerase, diaphorase, phosphomonoesterase, inorganic pyrophosphatase, and 5-nucleotidase. Essentially similar differences between young and adult tissue values were observed for the pulmonary artery.

When more extended studies have been made on vascular specimens from children it is expected that additional significant differences in enzyme activities between children and adults will be disclosed.

I. Comparison of Enzyme Activities in Arterial Samples from Sexually Mature Men and Women

The correlation between hormone activities and atherogenesis has received much attention in the last decade mainly through the work on sex hormone effects conducted by Stamler, Pick, and Katz. Several reviews of this subject have been reported which include surveys of both animal experiments and clinical studies (Katz and Stamler, 1953; Pick *et al.,* 1959; Stamler *et al.,* 1959; Katz and Pick, 1961; Schettler, 1961; Kask, 1962). In view of the significance of this subject it seemed desirable to make a comparison of enzyme activities in human arterial samples derived from sexually mature men and women. On the basis of a suggestion made by Malinow (1962), the statistical evaluation was made on enzyme values recorded for 18- to 54-year-old individuals.

The calculated data are presented in Table XVIII in which the enzyme activities of arterial samples from women are expressed in percentages of those observed for male subjects. These percentage values and statistical calculations indicate that more pronounced sex differences in enzyme concentrations are exhibited by the aorta than by the pulmonary artery. In spite of the limited number of coronary artery samples (16-28) available for comparisons, the trend recorded for that blood vessel is somewhat similar to that observed for the aorta.

The results show that distinctly lower activities of glucose-6-phosphate dehydrogenase, 6-phosphogluconate dehydrogenase, isocitric dehydrogenase, and TPN-malic enzyme were found in the aortic wall of female than of male subjects. Since these four enzymes provide TPNH through

TABLE XVIII

ENZYME ACTIVITIES AND COENZYME CONCENTRATIONS OF ARTERIAL SAMPLES FROM FEMALE SUBJECTS EXPRESSED IN PERCENTAGES OF VALUES OBSERVED FOR MALE INDIVIDUALS (18–54 YEARS)[a]

Enzymes and coenzymes	Aorta %	t of diff.	D.f.[b]		Pulmonary artery %	t of diff.	D.f.[b]		Coronary artery %	t of diff.	D.f.[b]	
Hexokinase	115	1.31	24	ns	120	1.09	21	ns	—	—	—	
Phosphoglucoisomerase	106	0.76	24	ns	118	1.35	23	ns	100	0.00	16	
Aldolase	99	0.09	49	ns	96	0.42	42	ns	—	—	—	
Enolase	91	0.84	38	ns	87	1.50	33	ns	71	1.84	20	$p < 0.1$
Lactic dehydrogenase	109	0.34	30	ns	88	0.80	28	ns	100	0.00	19	ns
Glycogen phosphorylase	111	0.80	49	ns	93	0.45	35	ns	88	0.58	14	ns
Glucose-6-phosphate dehydrogenase	64	3.15	36	$p < 0.01$	80	1.52	35	ns	76	1.94	16	$p < 0.1$
6-Phosphogluconate dehydrogenase	76	1.80	28	$p < 0.1$	80	1.46	29	ns	82	1.08	16	ns
Ribose-5-phosphate isomerase	107	0.37	33	ns	88	0.70	27	ns	—	—	—	
Aconitase	95	0.64	60	ns	108	0.76	36	ns	94	0.54	19	ns
Isocitric dehydrogenase	84	2.75	31	$p = 0.01$	120	0.93	27	ns	—	—	—	
Fumarase	96	0.26	39	ns	107	0.30	35	ns	111	0.50	19	ns
Malic dehydrogenase	98	0.20	30	ns	118	0.90	27	ns	63	1.82	17	$p < 0.1$
TPN-malic enzyme	73	2.34	24	$p < 0.05$	89	0.54	20	ns	89	0.93	21	ns
Diaphorase	91	0.83	59	ns	86	1.63	59	ns	86	0.90	21	ns
Cytochrome c reductase	100	0.00	59		100	0.00	59		98	0.24	24	ns
Leucine aminopeptidase	98	0.45	38	ns	89	1.45	36	ns	—	—	—	
Autolysis	65	1.89	43	$p < 0.1$	98	0.06	31	ns	—	—	—	
Cathepsin	143	1.88	43	$p < 0.1$	135	0.65	31	ns	—	—	—	
Total proteolysis	128	1.95	43	$p < 0.1$	107	0.24	31	ns	—	—	—	
Phosphomonoesterase	100	0.00	35	ns	87	1.68	36	ns	89	0.83	24	ns
Adenylpyrophosphatase	84	1.78	36	$p < 0.1$	95	0.58	36	ns	104	0.19	20	ns
Inorganic pyrophosphatase	86	1.28	34	ns	75	2.22	35	$p < 0.05$	103	0.22	21	ns
5-Nucleotidase	129	2.30	41	$p < 0.05$	105	1.43	39	ns	134	1.98	22	$p < 0.1$

TABLE XVIII (*continued*)

Enzymes and coenzymes	Aorta				Pulmonary artery				Coronary artery			
	%	t of diff.	D.f.[b]		%	t of diff.	D.f.[b]		%	t of diff.	D.f.[b]	
Purine nucleoside phosphorylase	78	2.15	55	p < 0.05	102	0.16	43	ns	95	0.35	14	ns
Creatine phosphokinase	98	0.08	46	ns	—	—	—		—	—	—	
Glyoxalase I	95	0.60	43	ns	100	0.00	39		100	0.00	26	
Riboflavin	100	0.00	31		—	—	—		—	—	—	
Glutathione	92	0.34	31	ns	105	0.21	10	ns	—	—	—	

[a] The percentage values were calculated on the basis of wet tissue weight.

[b] D.f. = degrees of freedom.

their functioning, this recorded sex difference ought to be considered in connection with the problem of atherogenesis.

Moderately higher activities of 5-nucleotidase were found in both the aortic and coronary artery specimens from women. It has been reported by Blankenhorn (1962) that with increasing age the calcium deposition in the human aorta is more variable in women than in men, but evidence of higher aortic calcium values for the 18- to 54-year age group has not been presented. A calculation by the reviewer of individual analytical data published by Hevelke (1954) showed essentially similar calcium concentrations in the femoral artery of men and women for various age groups between 18 and 54 years. The higher 5-nucleotidase values observed for female arteries apparently do not indicate that the sex difference in this enzymic activity is associated with increased arterial calcification.

IV. Discussion and Conclusions

The extensive literature dealing with research studies on the pathogenesis of arteriosclerosis has provided rather conclusive evidence that several etiological factors are involved in the development of this disease entity. With regard to the intermediary metabolism of arterial tissue, it may be assumed that investigations in this field will prove to be of both direct and indirect value in supplying important answers to the many-sided problem of atherogenesis.

The completed enzyme studies reported in the present survey have revealed the presence in the human arterial wall of metabolic subdivisions which are similar to those observed for other tissues. Some remarkable findings have, however, been disclosed with regard to the metabolism of the arterial tissue. The low Pasteur effect exhibited by the human aorta is noticeable, and the demonstration of appreciable activities of adenylpyrophosphatase and 5-nucleotidase in the arterial tissue adds a further interesting aspect to the metabolic pattern. Although the human aorta has a low respiratory rate, the observed high incorporation of sulfate into the arterial mucopolysaccharides indicates that the arterial wall cannot be considered as being metabolically inert.

Because of the many unexpected findings, the studies on the arterial intermediary metabolism in the reviewer's opinion should be extended to include comprehensive investigations of all the enzymes present in the tissue for which appropriate assay procedures can be made available.

There is no adequate interpretation of the reported variations in enzyme activities in connection with aging. In the case of some enzymes, the effect of age on the activity values may to some extent be the result of changes in the tissue composition of the arterial wall. As an example, the decrease with age in the glycogen phosphorylase and creatine phosphokinase activities of the aorta is probably associated with atrophic changes in the muscular component of the vessel wall. The occurrence of pre-arteriosclerotic changes in macroscopically normal tissue portions may similarly account for some of the aging changes; this applies to those arteries in which the observed variation with age proceeds in the same direction as the changes recorded for the arteriosclerotic tissue samples.

Assays of human arteriosclerotic tissue portions have shown that the various enzymes are differently affected by the pathological changes. This dissimilar response of the enzymes to the development of arteriosclerosis is of particular interest. The fact that many enzymes remain unchanged and that some even exhibit higher activities in the arteriosclerotic tissue indicates that the variations in enzymic activities associated with atherogenesis are not due merely to a replacement of the vascular tissue with the deposit of inert material. These findings suggest that further comprehensive studies in this field of pathology may prove rewarding, and in such investigations special emphasis should be placed on those enzymes which exhibit higher activities in the arteriosclerotic tissue areas. Since considerable differences in enzyme activities occasionally were displayed by various arteriosclerotic portions of the same blood vessels (Kirk, 1962a, e), the expression of enzymic values on the basis of the type of arteriosclerosis present in the assayed tissue portions will probably yield additional valuable information.

The marked differences in the quantities of substrate metabolized by various enzymes per unit of arterial tissue is also a fact deserving special notice. As previously remarked, the low activities exhibited by some enzymes in the arterial wall may make it possible to identify the limiting enzyme systems within each metabolic pathway; through separate studies on arteriosclerotic tissue portions it will further be disclosed whether these particular enzymes are affected by the pathological tissue changes. Since the failure of the functioning of a single enzyme frequently will obstruct the activity of a whole metabolic pathway, such findings may be of definite pathophysiological significance.

One promising feature with regard to future work on arterial intermediary metabolism is that comparative biochemical studies may provide an opportunity for identification of some of the factors involved in the pathogenesis of arteriosclerosis (Kirk, 1962f). Although most human arteries are susceptible to arteriosclerosis to an appreciable extent, certain types of arteries rarely exhibit visible pathological changes. This lack of susceptibility to arteriosclerosis applies to the diaphragmatic arteries (Wartman, 1933) and the internal mammary arteries (Duff and McMillan, 1951). Comparative investigations on selected types of human and animal arteries may similarly be advisable. As an example, it has been pointed out by Bürger (1954) that whereas cerebrovascular hemorrhage constitutes an important disease in human subjects, such condition is practically unknown in animals. For this reason, determinations of the chemical composition and metabolic pattern of both human and animal cerebral arteries may be expected to afford some explanation concerning the factors associated with the development of severe pathological changes in the human brain arteries.

Continued studies on the enzyme systems in normal and pathological sections of the arterial wall are undoubtedly of primary significance. The enzymes are compounds which are essential for the biological functioning of tissues, and because of the importance of arteriosclerosis as a disease entity, it is anticipated that in the future special emphasis will be placed on the intermediary metabolism of human arterial tissue.

REFERENCES

Ahmed, Z., and Reis, J. L. (1958). *Biochem. J.* **69**, 386.
Antonini, F. M., and Weber, G. (1951). *Arch. "De Vecchi" Anat. Patol. Med. Clin.* **16**, 985.
Astrup, T., and Claassen, M. (1957). *Proc. 6th European Congr. Haematol. Copenhagen, 1957* p. 455.
Astrup, T., and Coccheri, S. (1962). *Nature* **193**, 182.
Astrup, T., Albrechtsen, C. K., Claassen, M., and Rasmussen, J. (1959). *Circulation Res.* **7**, 969.
Azarnoff, D. C. (1958). *Proc. Soc. Exptl. Biol. Med.* **98**, 680.
Baló, J., Banga, I., and Josepovits, G. (1948-1949). *Z. Vitamin- Hormon- Fermentforsch* **2**, 1.
Banga, I., and Nowotny, A. (1951a). *Acta Physiol. Acad. Sci. Hung.* **2**, 317.
Banga, I., and Nowotny, A. (1951b). *Acta Physiol. Acad. Sci. Hung.* **2**, 327.
Barker, S. B. (1955). *Endocrinology* **57**, 414.
Barker, S. B., and Schwartz, H. S. (1954). *J. Alabama Acad. Sci.* **26**, 81.
Bavina, M. V., and Kritsman, M. G. (1953). *Biokhimiya* **18**, 548.
Belfer, S., Koran, P., Eder, H., and Bradley, H. C. (1943). *J. Biol. Chem.* **147**, 345.
Blankenhorn, D. H. (1962). *Circulation* **26**, 646 (abstr.).
Bloch, K. (1960). "Lipide Metabolism." Wiley, New York.
Bloom, B., and Stetten, D. (1953). *J. Am. Chem. Soc.* **75**, 5446.
Bloom, B., and Stetten, D. (1955). *J. Biol. Chem.* **212**, 555.
Boström, H., and Odeblad, E. (1953). *Anat. Record* **115**, 505.
Brandstrup, N., Kirk, J. E., and Bruni, C. (1957). *J. Gerontol.* **12**, 166.
Branwood, A. W., and Carr, C. J. (1960). *Lancet* **ii**, 1254.
Bruns, F. H., Noltmann, E., and Willemsen, A. (1958a). *Biochem. Z.* **330**, 411.
Bruns, F. H., Dünwald, E., and Noltmann, E. (1958b). *Biochem. Z.* **330**, 497.

Buck, R. C. (1951). *A.M.A. Arch. Pathol.* **51**, 319.

Buell M. V., Lowry, O. H., Roberts, N. R., Chang, M. V., and Kapphahn, J. I. (1958). *J. Biol. Chem.* **232**, 979.

Bürger, M. (1954). "Altern und Krankheit," 2nd ed. Thieme, Leipzig.

Burch, H. B. (1952). *Federation Proc.* **11**, 192 (abstr.).

Carr, C. J., Bell, F. K., Hurst, J. N., and Krantz, J. C. (1954). *Circulation Res.* **2**, 516.

Carr, C. J., Bell, F. K., Rehak, M. J., and Krantz, J. C. (1955). *Proc. Soc. Exptl. Biol. Med.* **89**, 184.

Carruthers, C. (1947). *J. Biol. Chem.* **171**, 641.

Chang, Y. O., Laursen, T. J. S., and Kirk, J. E. (1955). *J. Gerontol.* **10**, 165.

Coccheri, S., and Astrup, T. (1960). *Proc. 3rd European Congr. Cardiol. Rome, 1960* p. 1127.

Coccheri, S., and Astrup, T. (1961). *Proc. Soc. Exptl. Biol. Med.* **108**, 369.

Donner, L. (1962). *J. Atherosclerosis Res.* **2**, 88.

Duff, G. L., and McMillan, G. C. (1951). *Am. J. Med.* **11**, 92.

Duguid, J. B. (1948). *J. Pathol. Bacteriol.* **60**, 57.

Dyrbye, M. O. (1959a). *J. Gerontol.* **14**, 32.

Dyrbye, M. O. (1959b). "Ageing of Human Arterial Tissue." Munksgaard, Copenhagen.

Dyrbye, M., and Kirk, J. E. (1955). *Circulation* **12**, 504 (abstr.).

Dyrbye, M., and Kirk, J. E. (1956). *J. Gerontol.* **11**, 33.

Dyrbye, M., and Kirk, J. E. (1957). *J. Gerontol.* **12**, 20.

Eder, H., Bradley, H. C., and Belfer, S. (1939). *J. Biol. Chem.* **128**, 551.

Emmrich, R. (1961). *In* "Gefässwand und Blutplasma" (R. Emmrich and E. Perlick, eds.), pp. 15-35. Fischer, Jena.

Fontaine, R., Mandel, P., Pantesco, V., and Kempf, E. (1960a). *Strasbourg Med.* **9**, 605.

Fontaine, R., Mandel, P., Pantesco, V., and Kempf, E. (1960b). *J. Cardiovascular Surg.* **1**, 236.

Green, M. N., Tsou, K., Bressler, R., and Seligman, A. M. (1955). *Arch. Biochem. Biophys.* **57**, 458.

Hauss, W. H., Junge-Hülsing, G., and Holländer, H. J. (1962). *J. Atherosclerosis Res.* **2**, 50.

Hevelke, G. (1954). *Z. Alternsforsch.* **8**, 130.

Hill, A. V. (1928-1929). *Proc. Roy. Soc.* **B104**, 39.

Hirst, A. E., and Gore, I. (1962) *Circulation* **26**, 657 (abstr.).

Johnsen, S. G., and Kirk, J. E. (1955). *Anal. Chem.* **27**, 838.

Kask, E. (1962). *Angiology* **13**, 35.

Katz, L. N., and Pick, R. (1961). *J. Atherosclerosis Res.* **1**, 93.

Katz, L. N., and Stamler, J. (1953). "Experimental Atherosclerosis." C. C Thomas, Springfield, Illinois.

Kayahan, S. (1960). *Lancet* ii, 667.

Kempf, E., Fontaine, R., and Mandel, P. (1961). *Compt. Rend. Soc. Biol.* **155**, 623.

Kim, J. J., Paoletti, R., and Vertua, R. (1960). *Atompraxis* **6**, 55.

Kirk, J. E. (1958). *Circulation* **18**, 487 (abstr.).

Kirk, J. E. (1959a). *J. Gerontol.* **14**, 181.

Kirk, J. E. (1959b). *Ann. N. Y. Acad. Sci.* **72**, 1006.

Kirk, J. E. (1959c). *In* "The Arterial Wall" (A. I. Lansing, ed.), pp. 161-191. Williams & Wilkins, Baltimore, Maryland.

Kirk, J. E. (1959d). *J. Gerontol.* **14**, 288.

Kirk, J. E. (1959e). *J. Gerontol.* **14**, 447.

Kirk, J. E. (1960a). *J. Gerontol.* **15**, 136.

Kirk, J. E. (1960b). *J. Gerontol.* **15**, 139.

Kirk, J. E. (1960c). *J. Gerontol.* **15**, 262.

Kirk, J. E. (1961a). *J. Gerontol.* **16**, 25.

Kirk, J. E. (1961b). *J. Gerontol.* **16**, 243.

Kirk, J. E. (1961c). *Federation Proc.* **20**, 90 (abstr.).

Kirk, J. E. (1961d). *J. Lab. Clin. Med.* **58**, 933 (abstr.).

Kirk, J. E. (1961e). *Proc. 13th Intern. Symp. Biol. Med. Sci. Henry Ford Hosp. Detroit, 1961.* "Etiology of Myocardial Infarction" (T. N. James and J. W. Keyes, eds.), pp. 273-284. Little, Brown, Boston, Massachusetts, 1963.

Kirk, J. E. (1962a). *J. Gerontol.* **17**, 154.

Kirk, J. E. (1962b). *J. Gerontol.* **17**, 158.

Kirk, J. E. (1962c). *J. Gerontol.* **17**, 276.

Kirk, J. E. (1962d). *J. Gerontol.* **17**, 369.

Kirk, J. E. (1962e). *Proc. Soc. Exptl. Biol. Med.* **109**, 890.

Kirk, J. E. (1962f). *Proc. 51st Ann. Meeting Intern. Acad. Pathol. Montreal 1962* p. 45.

Kirk, J. E., and Dyrbye, M. (1956). *J. Gerontol.* **11**, 129.

Kirk, J. E., and Hansen, P. F. (1950). *J. Lab. Clin. Med.* **36**, 844 (abstr.).

Kirk, J. E., and Hansen, P. F. (1951). *Federation Proc.* **10**, 208 (abstr.).

Kirk, J. E., and Hansen, P. F. (1952a). *J. Biol. Chem.* **199**, 675.

Kirk, J. E., and Hansen, P. F. (1952b). *In* "Cowdry's Problems of Ageing" (A. I. Lansing, ed.), 3rd ed., pp. 730-763. Williams & Wilkins, Baltimore, Maryland.

Kirk, J. E., and Hansen, P. F. (1953). *J. Gerontol.* **8**, 150.

Kirk, J. E., and Johnsen, S. G. (1951). *Circulation* **4**, 478 (abstr.).

Kirk, J. E., and Kirk, T. E. (1959a). *Federation Proc.* **18**, 261 (abstr.).

Kirk, J. E., and Kirk, T. E. (1959b). *J. Lab. Clin. Med.* **52**, 828 (abstr.).

Kirk, J. E., and Laursen, T. J. S. (1954a). *J. Gerontol.* **9**, 361 (abstr.).

Kirk, J. E., and Laursen, T. J. S. (1954b). *J. Gerontol.* **9**, 362 (abstr.).

Kirk, J. E., and Laursen, T. J. S. (1954c). *Circulation* **10**, 607 (abstr.).

Kirk, J. E., and Laursen, T. J. S. (1954d). *Circulation* **10**, 607 (abstr.).

Kirk, J. E., and Laursen, T. J. S. (1954e). *Ciba Found. Colloq. Aging* **1**, p. 69-79.

Kirk, J. E., and Laursen, T. J. S. (1955a). *J. Gerontol.* **10**, 18.

Kirk, J. E., and Laursen, T. J. S. (1955b). *J. Gerontol.* **10**, 288.

Kirk, E., and Praetorius, E. (1949). *J. Lab. Clin. Med.* **34**, 1617 (abstr.).

Kirk, E., and Praetorius, E. (1950a). *Science* **111**, 334.

Kirk, J. E., and Praetorius, E. (1950b). *Circulation* **2**, 477 (abstr.).

Kirk, J. E., and Sørensen, L. B. (1956a). *J. Gerontol.* **11**, 438 (abstr.).

Kirk, J. E., and Sørensen, L. B. (1956b). *J. Gerontol.* **11**, 373.

Kirk, J. E., Chiang, S. P., and Laursen, T. S. (1953a). *Circulation* **8**, 451 (abstr.).

Kirk, J. E., Effersøe, P. G., and Chiang, S. (1953b). *Federation Proc.* **12**, 231 (abstr.).

Kirk, J. E., Effersøe, P. G., and Chiang, S. P. (1953c). *J. Gerontol.* **8**, 382 (abstr.).

Kirk, J. E., Effersøe, P. G., and Chiang, S. P. (1954a). *J. Gerontol.* **9**, 10 (abstr.).

Kirk, J. E., Hansen, P. F., Effersøe, P. G., and Iversen, K. (1954b). *J. Biol. Chem.* **208**, 17.

Kirk, J. E., Laursen, T. J. S., and Schaus, R. (1955). *J. Gerontol.* **10**, 178.

Kirk, J. E., Matzke, J. R., Brandstrup, N., and Wang, I. (1958). *J. Gerontol.* **13**, 24.

Kirk, J. E., Wang, I., and Brandstrup, N. (1959). *J. Gerontol.* **14**, 25.

Kritsman, M. G., and Bavina, M. V. (1954). *Dokl. Akad. Nauk SSSR* **94**, 721.

Laursen, T. J. S., and Kirk, J. E. (1955a). *J. Gerontol.* **10**, 26.

Laursen, T. J. S., and Kirk, J. E. (1955b). *J. Gerontol.* **10**, 303.

Laursen, T. J. S., and Laursen, R. S. (1958). *Am. J. Clin. Pathol.* **30**, 237.

Lazzarini-Robertson, A. (1962a). National Conference on Fundamentals of Vascular Grafting, Brooklyn, New York (in press).

Lazzarini-Robertson, A. (1962b). *Circulation* **26**, 660 (abstr.).

Lehninger, A. L. (1959). *In* "The Arterial Wall" (A. I. Lansing, ed.), pp. 220-246. Williams & Wilkins, Baltimore, Maryland.

Maier, N., and Haimovici, H. (1957). *Proc. Soc. Exptl. Biol. Med.* **95**, 425.

Maier, N., and Haimovici, H. (1958). *Am. J. Physiol.* **195**, 476.

Malinow, M. R. (1962). Personal communication.

Mandel, P., and Kempf, E. (1960). *Compt. Rend. Soc. Biol.* **154**, 791.

Matzke, J. R., Kirk, J. E., Brandstrup, N., and Wang, I. (1957). *J. Gerontol.* **12**, 279.

Müller, E., and Neumann, W. (1959). *Frankfurter Z. Pathol.* **70**, 174.

Noltmann, E., and Bruns, F. H. (1958). *Z. Physiol. Chem.* **313**, 194.

Paoletti, P., Paoletti, R., and Savi, C. (1958). *Boll. Soc. Ital. Biol. Sper.* **34**, 1416.

Paoletti, P., Tessari, L., and Vertua, R. (1959). *Ric. Sci.* **29**, 2382.

Perlick, E. (1961). *In* "Gefässwand und Blutplasma" (R. Emmrich and E. Perlick, eds.), pp. 211-227. Fischer, Jena.

Pick, R., Stamler, J., and Katz, L. N. (1959). *In* "Hormones and Atherosclerosis" (G. Pincus, ed.), pp. 229-240. Academic Press, New York.

Rechenberger, J., and Hevelke, G. (1955). *Z. Alternsforsch.* **9**, 309.

Reis, J. L. (1950). *Biochem. J.* **46**, 21 (abstr.).

Reis, J. L. (1951). *Biochem. J.* **48**, 548.

Sbarra, A. J., Gilfallan, R. F., and Bardawil, W. A. (1960). *Biochem. Biophys. Res. Commun.* **3**, 311.

Schaus, R., Kirk, J. E., and Laursen, T. J. S. (1955). *J. Gerontol.* **10**, 170.

Schettler, G. (1961). "Arteriosklerose." Thieme, Stuttgart.

Schmidt, C. G., and Hillenbrand, H. J. (1953). *Z. Ges. Exptl. Med.* **120**, 685.

Shimamoto, T. (1962). *Trans. 2nd European Congr. Microcirc. Pavia Italy* p. 23.

Shimamoto, T., Takeuchi, K., and Ishioka, T. (1962). *Circulation* **26**, 672 (abstr.).

Sørensen, L. B., and Kirk, J. E. (1955). *J. Gerontol.* **10**, 470 (abstr.).

Sørensen, L. B., and Kirk, J. E. (1956). *J. Gerontol.* **11**, 28.

Stamler, J., Pick, R., Katz, L. N., Pick, A., and Kaplan, B. M. (1959). *In* "Hormones and Atherosclerosis" (G. Pincus, ed.), pp. 423-442. Academic Press, New York.

Stetten, D., and Stetten, M. R. (1960). *Physiol. Rev.* **40**, 505.

Thompson, R. H. S., and Tickner, A. (1951). *J. Physiol. (London)* **115**, 34.

Thompson, R. H. S., and Tickner, A. (1953). *J. Physiol. (London)* **121**, 623.

Tischendorf, F., and Curri, S. B. (1959). *Acta Histochem.* **8**, 158.

Wang, I., and Kirk, J. E. (1959). *J. Gerontol.* **14**, 444.

Wang, I., and Kirk, J. E. (1960). *J. Gerontol.* **15**, 35.

Wartman, W. B. (1933). *Am. J. Med. Sci.* **186**, 27.

Wellman, W. E., and Edwards, J. E. (1950). *A.M.A. Arch. Pathol.* **50**, 183.

Wilens, S. L., and McCluskey, R. T. (1954). *Circulation Res.* **2**, 175.

Witte, S., and Bressel, D. (1958). *Folia Haematol. (Frankfurt)* [N. S.] **2**, 236.

Woerner, C. A. (1951). *J. Gerontol.* **6**, 165.

Zemplényi, T. (1962). *J. Atherosclerosis Res.* **2**, 2.

—4—

The Role of Ground Substance, Collagen, and Elastic Fibers in the Genesis of Atherosclerosis

S. BERTELSEN

I. Introduction

As early as 1856, Virchow referred to an accumulation of a mucous intimal substance in which lipid from the invading plasma was gradually deposited. He considered the deposition of mucous substance in the intima as an exudative inflammatory process, combined with the fatty deposits, which constitute the earliest atherosclerotic change, to gradually produce a fibrosis in the intima.

Virchow's views have been supported by numerous investigators, and the intimal lipidosis has been the subject of intensive studies. Consequently, local changes in the vascular wall have not been considered very important to the development of atherosclerosis. Only during the last few decades has interest been attached to the age changes in the vascular wall and to their possible importance with regard to the atherosclerotic process. Duff and McMillan (1951) strongly emphasized the importance of the local factors in the aortic wall for the formation of plaques, and the object of the present investigations is solely to determine the morphological and biochemical changes that occur in the elastic type of vessels prior to and simultaneously with the atherosclerotic process.

In the aortic wall and in the pulmonary artery three layers can be distinguished, the tunica intima, the tunica media, and the tunica adventitia (see Chapter 1 by Buck).

The *tunica intima,* whose thickness increases with age, is built up of a few thin elastic fibrils, collagenous fibers, a number of fibroblasts, and an abundance of ground substance.

The *tunica media* consists mainly of concentric elastic membranes. In the space between the membranes is an appreciable amount of basophilic amorphous ground substance containing a great many collagen fibers and cells (fibroblasts and muscle cells). (For a description of cell types see Chapter 1 by Buck and Chapter 2 by McGill *et al.*) The ground substance as well as the collagen fibers are increasing with age, so that the elastic membranes will become separated.

The *tunica adventitia* is relatively thin. It cannot be sharply distinguished from the surrounding connective tissue. Numerous elastic fibers project from the external elastic membrane, and there is a gradual transition from the tunica adventitia to the surrounding loose connective tissue.

In working with vascular tissue, the investigator is soon faced with two important problems: the definition of atherosclerosis and grading of the atherosclerotic lesion in a given aorta. Diverging conceptions of these two factors have made many investigators arrive at widely differing results, and it is not possible to make an immediate comparison between these results.

The former pathological-anatomical definition of atherosclerosis (Boyd, 1950) as an intimal, spotted lipoidal degeneration, with a secondary thickening and sclerosing of the superficial intima, originates directly from Virchow's (1856) conception and description of the pathogenesis of atherosclerosis, namely, that the fat, secondary to the intimal degeneration, is the essential factor in the development of atherosclerosis.

This conception of the nature of atherosclerosis has made many investigators of both experimental and human pathology describe the intimal accumulation of lipid as atherosclerosis, without having ascertained that an actual intimal sclerotic change has occurred.

Intensive studies of atherosclerosis during recent years, and particularly the investigations carried out during the last 10-15 years on the ground substance of the aortic wall have induced investigators in the United States to set up a *study group* under WHO (1958); this study group has suggested an adequate definition of the atherosclerosis concept and has also attempted to lay down general lines for a uniform evaluation of the degree of atherosclerosis of a vessel.

In hardly any other area of pathological anatomy is there so much confusion of ideas as in the investigation of atherosclerosis. The terms arteriosclerosis, atherosclerosis, and atheromatosis are mentioned indiscriminately; and it often happens that authors fail to define the different terms and use them indiscriminately in one and the same publication.

It is often possible by macroscopic examination of an atherosclerotic aorta to distinguish between two different forms of plaques: (a) lipoidal plaques, and (b) fibrous plaques. The term *lipoidal plaque* is applied to superficial yellow and yellowish-gray intimal lesions which are stained selectively by fat stains, and the term *fibrous plaque* is applied to a circumscribed, elevated intimal thickening which is firm and gray or pearly white. Both plaque forms may be complicated by ulceration and calcareous deposits, so that a definite macroscopic evaluation cannot be made. A microscopic examination must therefore be made in order to ascertain the nature of the changes.

In the present study the following terms have been employed:

Intimal lipidosis, meaning an accumulation of lipid in the intima. The lipid is accumulated in lumps with increasing age, and these lumps gradually become macroscopically visible as the so-called *lipoidal plaques.* Pathologists often use the term "atheromatosis" for the lipid accumulation with formation of lipoidal plaques.

Intimal fibrosis, denoting accumulation of collagenous or collagenlike fibrils in the intima. In localized areas the fibrils run a parallel course, with the result that the intima is changed into a *fibrous plaque.* The individual fibrils in a fibrous plaque may swell, the fibrillar structure is gradually obliterated, and the fibrous plaque becomes an *atheroma.*

The definitions of lipoidal and fibrous plaques just mentioned are closely related to the definition prepared by the WHO Study Group (1958).

In evaluating the degree of atherosclerosis, the present investigator has employed a macroscopic surface-evaluation combined with microscopic examinations in order to distinguish between lipoidal and fibrous plaques. Thus the degree of atherosclerosis is expressed by the percentage area of each individual plaque form in relation to the total vascular surface.

A. Chemistry of the Ground Substance

The ground substance in connective tissue consists of mucopolysaccharides together with large amounts of protein. The mucopolysaccharides are present in the form of mucoproteins, mucoids, and glycoproteins. The mucoproteins consist of complexes of acid mucopolysaccharides in polar union with protein, whereas the mucoids and glycoproteins contain carbohydrate groups in covalent bonds with protein. The carbohydrate groups of the mucoids and glycoproteins consist of hexosamine and neutral sugars; and the carbohydrate groups in the mucoproteins are built up of equimolar amounts of hexosamine, hexuronic acid, acetic acid, and possibly sulfuric acid. The mucoproteins and mucoids possess a hexosamine content of more than 4%, and the glycoproteins a lower hexosamine concentration.

Of acid mucopolysaccharides alone there are already at least eight well defined examples (Table I); with the exception of synovial fluid and vitreous humor, both of which contain only hyaluronic acid, all tissues contain more than one of these substances.

Table I shows the acid mucopolysaccharides which have been isolated from connective tissue.

Hyaluronic acid is an unbranched polymer of the disaccharides consisting of N-acetylglucosamine and glucuronic acid united in glu-

TABLE I
ACID MUCOPOLYSACCHARIDES OF CONNECTIVE TISSUE

Acid mucopolysaccharide	Tissue from which isolated
Nonsulfated	
Hyaluronic acid	Aorta, rheumatic nodules, synovial fluid, vitreous humor
Chondroitin	Cornea
Sulfated	
Chondroitin sulfuric acid A	Aorta, bone, cartilage, cornea, ligamentum nuchae
Chondroitin sulfuric acid B	Aorta, heart valves, ligamentum nuchae, skin, tendon
Chondroitin sulfuric acid C	Aorta(?), cartilage, nucleus pulposus, tendon
Heparins	Amyloid, aorta, liver, lungs
Keratosulfate	Bone, cornea, nucleus pulposus
Mucoitin sulfuric acid	Aorta, amyloid, gastric mucosa

cosaminide bonds. Hyaluronic acid is soluble in water, and the solutions are highly viscous. Hyaluronic acid is depolymerized by bacterial as well as testicular hyaluronidase.

Chondroitin is isomeric with hyaluronic acid, the glucosamine being replaced by galactosamine. Like hyaluronic acid it forms viscous solutions, and is depolymerized by testicular and bacterial hyaluronidases. It has been demonstrated with certainty only in the cornea.

Chondroitin sulfuric acids A and C resemble each other closely in composition as well as in their mode of reaction. They are polymers, made up of dissaccharides composed of N-acetylgalactosamine and glucuronic acid. Both carbohydrates are hydrolyzed by testicular, but not by bacterial hyaluronidase. In contrast to chondroitin sulfuric acids A and C, chondroitin sulfuric acid B contains iduronic acid, and it is resistant to testicular as well as to bacterial hyaluronidase. Chondroitin sulfuric acids A, B, and C contain a sulfate ester group in the galactosamine.

Heparins are mixtures of various mucopolysaccharides, built up of glucosamine and glucuronic acid in equimolar quantities, and of variable quantities of ester sulfate. The actual heparin contains three sulfate groups per repeating disaccharide, one of which is N-sulfate. Other heparins are heparitin sulfuric acid and heparin monosulfuric acid. The heparins have various anticoagulant properties, and they are not susceptible to any form of hyaluronidase.

Keratosulfate consists of N-acetylglucosamine, galactose, and sulfate; it is thus the only acid mucopolysaccharide which does not contain uronic acid. It is not susceptible to testicular or bacterial hyaluronidase.

Mucoitin sulfuric acid consists of N-acetylglucosamine, glucuronic acid, and sulfate in equimolar concentrations. It is not depolymerized by any form of hyaluronidase.

Neutral mucopolysaccharides form the carbohydrate groups in mucoids and glycoproteins. In contrast to acid mucopolysaccharides, neutral mucopolysaccharides from connective tissue have not as yet been adequately analyzed. During recent years several authors have shown that mucoids and glycoproteins may constitute important components of the ground substance. The neutral mucopolysaccharides contain hexosamine and neutral sugars (glucose, galactose, mannose, fucose), but they are free from uronic acid and sulfuric acid. Furthermore, some of the neutral mucopolysaccharides prepared of many mucous epithelial secretions, contain a good deal of sialic acid, and these mucoids have been termed sialo-mucins in contrast to fuco-mucins, which contain small amounts of sialic acid.

For further details about mucoproteins, mucoids, and glycoproteins see Meyer (1945, 1953a, b, 1956, 1957), Stacey (1946), Kent and White-house (1955), Bettelheim-Jevons (1958), Meyer *et al.* (1959), Stacey and Barker (1962).

B. Materials and Methods

The material in this investigation is comprised of human aortas and pulmonary arteries obtained fresh from autopsies performed at the Copenhagen County Hospital, Copenhagen University Hospital, and Copenhagen Municipal Hospital.

Numerous experiments have shown that the qualitative and quantitative composition of the connective tissue is subject to the influence of various factors, such as the influence of different hormones (see Chapter 7 by Stamler) on the ground substance. Owing to the special function of the elastic vascular walls, the connective tissue of these walls is further subjected to the variations of blood pressure (see Chapter 5 by Texon) throughout life. It is quite possible that to a certain extent it is these factors which cause many of the demonstrable changes that occur in the vascular wall with age. The human material for this investigation was therefore collected on the basis of the following criteria:

1. No history of hormonal, mesenchymal or hypertensive diseases. No hormone treatment within the last 5 years.

2. No clinical indication of the above mentioned diseases.

3. During autopsy special importance was attached to normal findings in the heart, lungs, and kidneys.

In addition to the above mentioned material, aortas and pulmonary arteries were collected from seven patients with hypertension in the pulmonary circulation.

The histochemical, physiochemical and chemical investigations of the author and collaborators performed on these vessels are presented below.

In the histochemical investigations the tissue specimens were fixed partly in 4% formaldehyde solution and partly in 4% basic lead acetate solution. The tissue specimens were embedded in paraffin. The acid mucopolysaccharides were stained with toluidine blue, alcian blue, and Hale's colloidal iron stain. The neutral mucopolysaccharides were stained with periodic acid-Schiff (PAS), and both forms of mucopolysaccharides were stained with combined PAS-alcian blue and PAS-Hale's stain. The elastic and collagen fibers were shown with Eskelund's elastin staining and van Gieson-Hansen's staining. Lipid was demonstrated with Sudan III, and calcium with alizarin-red S staining.

Proteolytic digestion of disintegrated, dry, defatted tissue was employed in the extraction of acid mucopolysaccharides. The mucopolysaccharides were precipitated with alcohol after previous purification of the extracts (Bertelson and Jensen, 1960b; Bertelsen and Marcker, 1961a, b). The extracted acid mucopolysaccharides were characterized by means of viscometry, paper electrophoresis, chromatography, molecular weight determinations, and biological heparin-activity determinations.

Both acid and neutral mucopolysaccharides were extracted by alkaline extraction for 4 days. The acid and the neutral fraction were then precipitated at an alcohol percentage of 60 and 84 respectively (Meyer and Chaffee, 1941; Meyer, 1945; Glegg *et al.,* 1954; Larsen, 1957).

Furthermore, the precipitated fractions were characterized by means of hexosamine, sulfate, and nitrogen analyses; and for qualitative estimation of uronic acid in the tissue, the carbazole reaction of Dische (1947) was carried out upon the hydrochloric acid hydrolyzates of the tissue samples.

The elastin content in the tissues was determined by the method of Lowry *et al.* (1941), and the results were corrected for the calcium salt content.

The chemical analyses were comprised partly of hexosamine and calcium analyses, and partly of hydroxyproline analyses directly on tissue from the aorta and the pulmonary artery. The analyses were performed on dry, defatted tissue from the intima and the media respectively.

Hexosamine: Blix's (1948) modification of Elson and Morgan's (1933) method.
Calcium: Patton and Reeder (1956), the mineral being solely calculated as $CaCO_3$.
Hydroxyproline: Martin and Axelrod (1953); conversion to collagen was made by the use of 7.46 factor.

The lipid content was determined by ether extraction of the dry tissue. The hexosamine and hydroxyproline contents were corrected for calcium salts in the tissue. The calcium analyses were made on dry, defatted tissue.

II. Histochemical Studies on Arteries of the Elastic Type

In 1911, Björling demonstrated the presence, in human aortic wall, of connective tissue having staining reactions similar to those of mucin. He termed this connective tissue "mucoid connective tissue," and presumed that it was primarily localized in the elastic vascular walls. Later, Schultz (1922, 1923) and Ssolowjew (1923, 1924) confirmed Björling's findings. They showed that the aortic connective tissue reacted strongly metachromatically with cresyl violet, and they were of the opinion that the metachromatic reaction was caused by a considerable content of chondroitin sulfate. The above mentioned studies on the metachromasia of the vascular wall were later repeated by several investigators (Wolkoff, 1924; Holzinger, 1934; Jorpes et al., 1937; Holmgren, 1940; Wislocki et al., 1947; Bunting, 1950; Bunting and Bunting, 1953).

Besides examining the metachromatic reaction, several authors have lately examined the ground substance of the vascular wall by the help of colloidal iron staining, alcian blue staining, and Schiff's reaction (Moon and Rinehart, 1952; Taylor, 1953; Rinehart, 1954; Zugibe et al., 1959; Zugibe and Brown, 1960; Braunstein, 1960). According to the concurrent works of the above mentioned investigators, acid mucopolysaccharides are accumulated in elastic vascular walls with age. Taylor's (1953) investigation further showed that PAS-positive material gradually becomes visible along the elastic fibrils with age.

Faber (1912) was one of the first investigators to mention an appreciable depositing of calcium salts in the aortic tunica media. Some years previously, Mönckeberg (1903) had described the depositing of calcareous salts in the arteries of the muscular type, whereas he found no calcium in the tunica media of aorta. Faber showed that the aortic depositing of calcium began earlier and was considerably more vigorous in the aorta than in the vessels of the limbs. Few authors have devoted their time to the study of the fairly unexplored aortic medial mineralization (Ravault, 1928; Farkas and Fasal, 1929; Haythorn and Taylor, 1936; Haythorn et al., 1936).

Only as late as 1944 did Blumenthal et al. by microincineration on 540 human aortas, demonstrate a uniformly increasing deposition of calcareous salts in the tunica media after the age of 20. They further demonstrated that the intensity of the medial calcification was greater in the abdominal part than in the thoracic part of the aorta, and that the calcification of the media precedes the formation of intimal plaques.

During the last decades, numerous histological works have been published on the lipid in the aortic wall (see Chapter 2 by McGill et al.); the present author does not intend to give a full account of these publications, but wants to mention the interesting finding that completely normal aortic tissue contains considerable amounts of lipid, and that this lipoidal depositing commences even during infancy (Langhaas, 1866; Ribbert, 1918; Aschoff, 1925; Holman et al., 1957; Zugibe and Brown, 1960; Bertelsen, 1961a).

In a number of previous histochemical studies the present author has attempted to elucidate the quantitative and qualitative changes occurring in the connective tissue in the aorta and the pulmonary artery, age changes as well as atherosclerotic changes (Bertelsen and Jensen, 1960a; Bertelsen, 1961a, b; Jensen and Bertelsen, 1961). A brief report on these investigations will be given here, and to facilitate a survey, medial and intimal changes will be mentioned separately.

The histochemical investigations were made on 163 aortas and 32 pulmonary arteries in the age groups 0–90 years; furthermore, 27 fetal aortas were examined.

A. Connective Tissue

1. AORTA

a. *Media.* In the course of the third fetal month, spots of metachromasia become distinctly visible among the elastic fibers in the fetal aorta. The metachromasia is often localized to a zone round the fibroblast-like cells, and it expands with fetal aging, so that the interfibrillar ground substance in the newborn is uniformly metachomatic. Simultaneously, the metachromasia has become more intensified, and the faint color of the β-metachromasia gradually becomes more red-violet. During the course of the first years of life, the metachromatic substance will increase further, and the vigorous γ-metachromasia gradually dominates the picture.

A constant, uniform increase in the amount of ground substance will occur with aging (Figs. 1, 2). The accumulation, largest in the luminal half of the media, takes place primarily from the second to the fourth decade; but after the age of 50, it is impossible to decide whether a further increase in the amount of metachromatic substance occurs.

The alcian blue and colloidal iron stainings are in conformity with the metachromatic staining.

The elastic membranes in the aorta have a regular, undulating course in the fetus after the third or fourth fetal months, in newborn infants, and in children (Fig. 1), but they are gradually pressed apart by the increasing amount of ground substance, and during the latter half of the second decade it is observed that the elastic membranes begin to become ruptured. This is first visible in the membrana elastica interna; its course becomes irregular, and numerous elastic fibrils begin to invade the intima. The fragmentation of the elastic membranes throughout the entire media continues during the third decade. Each single elastic fiber is gradually straightened out, and at the same time fragmentated. The course becomes irregular, often duplicated, with numerous communications visible between the individual fibers (Fig. 2).

During the last part of fetal life a few collagenous fibrils become visible in the ground substance between the elastic membranes. With increasing age the collagenous fibrils become more distinct as they grow thicker and more numerous. The collagenous fibrils are faintly PAS-positive.

The smooth musculature in the aortic wall is rather scanty; it is best

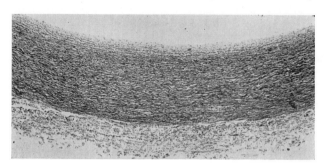

Fig. 1. Aorta from a 2-year-old child. The elastic fibers in the tunica media have a regular, undulating course. The ground substance is scanty. Magnification: 30.

seen with van Gieson-Hansen's staining. The smooth muscle cells are but faintly observable in PAS-staining; they are of a reddish brown color, and easy to distinguish from the usual, red PAS-positive color. Incidentally, treatment with amylase will make the muscle cells less PAS-positive.

During fetal life and during the first years of life the elastic fibers are distinctly PAS-positive, but in the latter half of the first decade they will no longer take stain from Schiff's reagent. Even from fetal life a very thin peripheral argyrophil zone along the elastic fibrils may be seen in Foot's silver staining. This zone will gradually become thicker and finally form a thick mantle round the elastic fibrils. During the third decade the PAS-positive substance will spread through the interfibrillar ground substance, and the PAS-positive reaction is—like the metachromatic reaction—most vigorous in the luminal part of the media.

A moderate proliferation of the fibroblasts occurs with age, but the relationship between cells and ground substance is considerably decreased in aging.

The condition of the media is primarily independent of the degree of atherosclerosis of the superficial intima; large fibrous or lipoidal plaques may, however, be pressed into the luminal part of the media, resulting in a secondary compression and destruction of the elastic fibrils.

b. *The Macroscopically Normal Intima.* During fetal life and the beginning of the first year of life the endothelial cells are located directly on the internal elastic membrane (Fig. 1). From the first or second year after birth an accumulation of metachromatic substance may be observed subendothelially. The metachromasia is a vigorous γ-metachromasia, increasing uniformly with age. Simultaneously a considerable proliferation of fibroblasts occurs (Fig. 2). As previously mentioned, the internal elas-

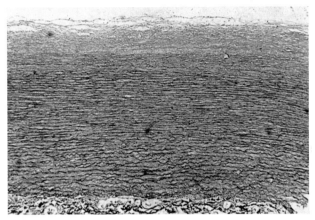

FIG. 2. Aorta from a 40-year-old person. The elastic fibers are pressed apart by the increasing ground substance. The fibers are ruptured and fragmented. The internal elastic membrane is split up. The cells both in the tunica intima and media are mostly fibroblasts. Magnification: 30.

tic membrane will become irregular, ruptured, and fragmented in the course of the second decade, and numerous fragments will be seen invading the intima. Silver staining shows a fine network of filiform argyrophile fibrils. To facilitate a survey, this stage will be termed *the stage of proliferation*; it lasts approximately until the beginning of the third decade, and the depositing of PAS-positive substances or fibrils is negligible during this period.

In the course of the third and fourth decades the intimal thickening changes its character; gradually a PAS-positive substance can be detected in the intima simultaneously with a constant accumulation of metachromatic ground substance. A vigorous proliferation of cells occurs in the intima, and fibroblasts with PAS-positive cytoplasm are often visible surrounded by an extracellular PAS-positive zone. Concurrently with the expansion of the PAS-positive ground substance, fragments of PAS-positive fibrils make their appearance, and the latter become more vigorous with increasing age. In the old intima their course is often undulated, running in dense streaks, surrounded partly by metachromatic

substance, and partly by PAS-positive substance. This stage is termed
the stage of fibrosis.

It should be stressed that intimal changes in aortas with normal gross
appearance are identical with intimal changes in normal parts of atherosclerotic aortas. But in one and the same aorta these changes are often
more advanced in the abdominal aorta than in the thoracic aorta.

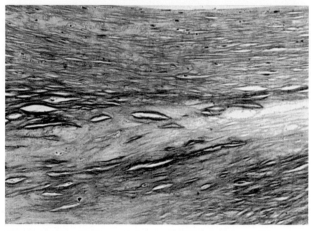

Fɪɢ. 3. Fibrous plaque. The thick collagenous fibrils are running in parallel
bunches. The fibroblasts are visible in the scanty ground substance. Some of the
fibrils are increased in thickness and do not take color; the normal fibrillar structure
is obliterated and an atheroma is formed. Magnification: 120.

c. *The Atherosclerotic Intima.* In the intima a microscopic distinction may be made between *primary fibrous plaques,* i.e., a fibrosis without major amounts of lipid (Fig. 3), and *secondary fibrous plaques,* i.e.,
an area of fibrosis found located luminally to the fairly large *lipoidal
plaques* which often contain cholesterol crystals (Fig. 4).

In connection with a fibrous plaque the thickening of the intima is
markedly increased, and serial sections various distances from the actual
plaque show a distinct increase in the PAS-positive fibrils and a decrease
in the interfibrillar ground substance. Sections made through the actual
fibrous plaques reveal a very scanty ground substance between the thick,
PAS-positive fibrils. The fibrils are accumulated in parallel bunches and
react like collagenous fibrils in van Gieson-Hansen's staining. Only a
few fibroblasts are visible in the scanty interfibrillar metachromatic
ground substance. The fibrils placed centrally in a fibrous plaque may
become swollen, and as a result of this swelling the central part of the

individual fibril does not take color from either Schiff's reagent or van Gieson-Hansen's staining. Gradually, the fibrillar structure is completely obliterated, and a homogeneous substance—an atheroma*—may be formed. The intima above an atheroma may be involved in the necrotizing process; the result will be a defect through the epithelial stratum, and the atheroma is drained into the vascular lumen. It should

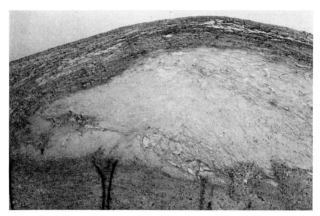

Fig. 4. Lipoidal plaque with sclerosis of the luminal intima, i.e., a secondary fibrous plaque. In the lipoidal accumulation a precipitation of cholesterol crystals is visible. Magnification: 30.

be noted that the intima localized round a primary fibrous plaque contains no more lipid than other intimal parts, and frequently there is no lipid at all, or only negligible amounts of lipid in the actual fibrous part.

A considerable thickening of the intima can often be demonstrated, corresponding to secondary fibrous intimal plaques, for, as indicated above, these plaques are situated luminally in relation to the lipoidal plaques. The structure of this fibrous part is identical with the primary fibrous plaque. Here, too, an atheroma may be formed, which may expand laterally in the direction of the lipoidal plaque or luminally toward the surface of the vessel.

The author would like to emphasize that he has never observed fibrous plaques in the intima without simultaneous and considerable changes in the media, such as accumulation of ground substance, fragmentation of elastic fibrils, and depositing of calcareous salts.

---

* Editors' note: This author's use of the term "atheroma" should be noted since it differs from the general concept of atheroma.

2. The Pulmonary Artery

The structure of the pulmonary artery and the structure of the aorta
are identical, and the age changes in the connective tissue of the
pulmonary artery are similar to—but less pronounced than—those of
the aorta. The elastic fibers in the media have a regular, undulating

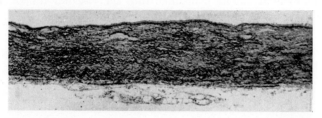

Fig. 5. The pulmonary artery from a 65-year-old person with normal tension in
the pulmonary circulation. The elastic fibers are closely packed and show a regular
course. The ground substance is scanty. The intima is not proliferated. Magnification:
30.

course even in very old individuals, and the interfibrillar ground
substance, consisting mainly of acid mucopolysaccharides, is very scanty.
The intimal proliferation is negligible, and the accumulation of ground
substance here, even in elderly persons, is extremely scanty (Fig. 5).

Enzymic incubations of sections of the aorta and pulmonary artery
gave the following result: incubation with bacterial hyaluronidase in
fetal and infantile aortas will considerably decrease the amount of
metachromatic substance. In aging the metachromatic substance will
soon become resistant to bacterial hyaluronidase, and in the course of
the second or third year it will be impossible to observe any decrease in
the amount of metachromasia after incubation with bacterial hyaluronidase.

It is, however, possible by incubation with testicular hyaluronidase
to remove the metachromasia except from a very narrow subendothelial
zone—and this applies to all ages.

The metachromasia cannot be weakened or removed by ribonuclease.

The PAS-positive parts of the ground substance are resistant to
amylase and testicular hyaluronidase.

B. Calcium Salts

The calcareous depositing in the media starts during the third decade,
increasing uniformly with age. The calcium salts are deposited diffusely
in the ground substance without any observable relation to the elastic
fibers (Fig. 6). There is no indication of major amounts of calcium

below lipoidal or fibrous plaques, and nothing seems to indicate that the calcareous concentrations are larger in the abdominal than in the thoracic aorta, although the medial calcification seems to start earlier in the abdominal portion. It is not possible to distinguish between even appreciable concentration differences, if the amount of calcium in a

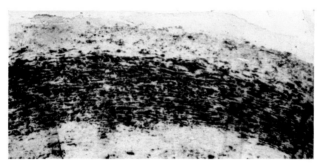

Fig. 6. Medial aortic calcification in a 52-year-old person. Magnification: 30.

section exceeds a certain expansion and quantity, but later biochemical observations have supported the histological supposition.

In intimal parts with normal gross appearance calcareous deposits are never visible, whereas in fibrous plaques calcareous crystals may be demonstrated in close relation to the fibrils (Fig. 7). It is obvious that calcareous deposits in fibrous intimal parts seem to be perfectly accidental. It is not unusual to find a vigorous fibrosis without the least trace of calcium, so that the calcareous precipitation in a plaque must be considered as a complication rather than as a late stage in the atherosclerotic process.

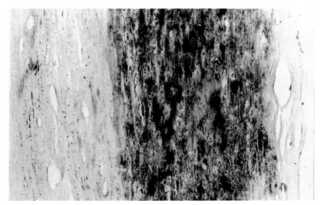

Fig. 7. Fibrous plaque with calcification. The calcium salts are deposited in the ground substance in close relation to the collagenous fibrils. Magnification: 120.

TABLE II

The Patients with Hypertension in the Pulmonary Circulation

No.	Age	Diagnosis	Microscopic findings		Calcium content in % of dry, defatted tissue weight
			Tunica intima	Tunica media	
1	3 months	Coarctation of the aorta	Slight proliferation	Slight thickening	0.4
2	24 years	Mitral stenosis	Vigorous proliferation	Considerable thickening. Mineralization starting in the ground substance	0.7
3	26 years	Interventricular septal defect	Vigorous proliferation	Considerable thickening	0.5
4	31 years	Essential pulmonary hyper-tension	Vigorous proliferation	Considerable thickening	0.5
5	37 years	Aortic valvular stenosis	Vigorous proliferation	Considerable thickening	0.4
6	41 years	Mitral stenosis	Vigorous proliferation	Considerable thickening	0.4
7	68 years	Aortic valvular stenosis	Vigorous proliferation	Considerable thickening. Mineralization starting	0.75

It is noteworthy that fibrous plaques are never visible in the intima except in connection with an appreciable calcareous depositing in the media; this phenomenon is in accordance with the findings of Blumenthal *et al.* (1944) and Lansing (1952).

The histological picture seems to indicate that the calcareous salts are deposited in the intimal and medial ground substance. It is obvious that the intimal depositing occurs in the scanty ground substance in close relation to the collagen-like fibrils. It is impossible, using the light microscope to determine whether there is any relation between the collagenous fibrils and the calcareous crystals in the media.

Calcareous deposits are never found in the media of the pulmonary artery under normal conditions. The present author has made histochemical investigations on pulmonary arteries from seven patients with hypertension in the pulmonary circulation; in two of the seven cases incipient crystalline precipitations were detected in the media, which was markedly thickened in all patients. No calcareous deposits in the intima could be demonstrated in any of the cases (Table II).

C. Lipid

Even during the first years of life a sudanophil substance is visible in the intimal aorta, and both in the stage of proliferation and in the stage of fibrosis there is a uniform increase in the amount of lipid. During the proliferating stage the lipid is diffusely distributed throughout the intima, partly intracellularly (the so-called "foam cells"), and partly extracellularly. In the course of the stage of fibrosis, the lipid is accumulating in large or small extracellular lumps, often surrounded by "foam cells." No cellular or fibrillar reactions around the lipid accumulations are visible in intimal tissue of normal gross appearance (Fig. 8).

Gradually as the size of the lipid lumps increases they can be observed macroscopically as yellowish streaks or spots on the intimal surface, the so-called lipoidal plaques. Only when the lipoidal plaques have grown to a certain size, and if there is a simultaneous appreciable medial alteration, can cholesterol crystals be deposited in the deepest part of the plaques. At this stage a fibrillar reaction is often visible in the superficially covering intima, where a secondary fibrous plaque is formed. As indicated above, the formation of an atheroma in the secondary fibrous plaque may entail an intimal defect through which both the atheromatous material and the more deeply located lipid may drain into the vascular lumen.

The amount of lipid in the media is very scanty in macroscopically

normal, as well as in atherosclerotic vascular tissue, and the lipid is
localized to the most luminal part.

In the pulmonary artery from individuals with normal tension in
the pulmonary circulation, only a minimal diffuse lipidosis is visible
in the scanty intimal ground substance, and there is no indication of
lipid lumps or smallish lipoidal plaques.

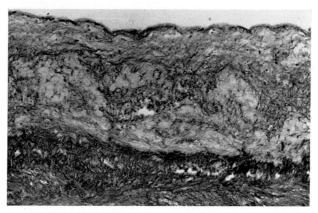

Fɪɢ. 8. Accumulation of lipid in the tunica intima in a 24-year-old person. Intima
is in the stage of proliferation. There is no reaction in the connective tissue. Magnification: 30.

The author has, as mentioned, examined seven patients with hypertension in the pulmonary circulation with a view to elucidating the
relation between the luminal tension in the elastic vessels and the
changes in the vascular wall.

It appears from Table II that all patients were suffering from a
cardiac or a vascular disease, which raised the blood pressure in the
pulmonary circulation. In three of the patients measurements of the
tension in the pulmonary artery were available (Numbers 2, 4, and 5),
and they all showed a marked hypertension (systolic pressure, 80-130 mm
of mercury; diastolic pressure, 40-70 mm).

Autopsy showed in all patients an appreciable thickening of the
wall of the right ventricle, besides a marked hypertrophy of the wall
of the pulmonary artery.

In two of the patients (Numbers 2 and 4) small lipoidal plaques
were visible in the truncus and the principal branches, but there was
no macroscopic sign of fibrous plaques or calcification in any of the
cases.

Microscopy of the sections showed a considerable thickening of the media on account of an accumulation of ground substance, which pressed the elastic fibers apart. There was also an appreciable intimal thickening with a vigorous proliferation of fibroblasts (Fig. 9).

The elastic fibers in the media showed a considerable fragmentation, and numerous elastic fragments were invading the proliferating intima from the internal elastic membrane.

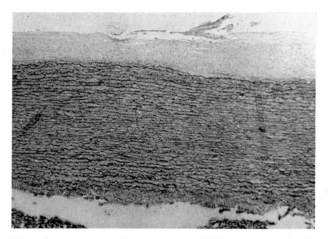

FIG. 9. The pulmonary artery from a person with hypertension in the pulmonary circulation. In the tunica media the ground substance separates the elastic membranes and the intima is vigorously proliferated. Magnification: 30.

There was thus a striking resemblance between the microscopic picture of the seven pulmonary arteries and that of normal aortic walls, and it appeared indeed from histochemical investigations, that the ground substance contained the same chemical components, i.e., acid and neutral mucopolysaccharides. It was of special interest to note that many PAS-positive fibroblasts were located deeply in the intima.

In all patients, there was a diffuse intimal lipidosis with intra- as well as extracellular lipid. In several patients there was a tendency to the formation of lumps in the intima, and this formation of lumps was particularly pronounced in patients with macroscopically lipoidal plaques. No tendency to fibrillar formation in superficial intima was observable.

In two cases (Numbers 2 and 7) staining with alizarin red S showed an incipient depositing of calcareous salts in the media, and calcium analyses showed that the pulmonary artery contained approximately 0.4-0.7% calcium (in relation to dry, defatted tissue weight), which is a distinct rise in proportion to the calcium content in normal pulmonary arteries in individuals from a corresponding age group.

Stainings with toluidine blue, alcian blue, and colloidal iron show that the ground substance in fetal aortas, and aortas and pulmonary arteries from newborn infants contains large amounts of acid muco-polysaccharides, and the nature of the metachromatic reaction as well as incubation experiments give evidence of a fairly appreciable content of hyaluronic acid in the above vessels. With increasing age, the β-meta-chromasia will, however, rapidly become masked, as the accumulation chiefly consists of a γ-metachromatic material, i.e., sulfated mucopoly-saccharides.

Incubation with testicular hyaluronidase further indicates that the accumulated ground substance mostly contains chondroitin sulfates A and/or C, while chondroitin sulfate B or heparins are localized in the subendothelial zone.

Fetal or infantile vessels show—in close relation to the elastic fibrils —a PAS-positive substance, often of a faintly fibrillar structure, and Foot's silver staining distinctly demonstrates that these are reticular threads, localized along the elastic fibrils. A close relationship between the elastic tissue and the argyrophile fibrils in vessels has been demon-strated in both human aortas (Gillman *et al.*, 1957; Bertelsen, 1961a; Jensen and Bertelsen, 1961) and animal aortas (Gillman *et al.*, 1957, 1960; Bertelsen, 1961d).

Reticular fibrils are, in contrast to collagenous fibers, strongly PAS-positive (Lillie, 1947; Wislocki and Dempsey, 1948; Kramer and Wind-rum, 1953). Lhotka and Davenport (1950) found a good similarity be-tween the PAS-reaction and Foot's silver staining of reticular fibrils; they therefore concluded that both color reactions were due to the fact that the reticular threads contain substances with free 1:2 glycol groups. Kramer and Windrum (1953), Windrum (1958), and Pearse (1960) fur-ther demonstrated that, in contrast to collagenous fibers, reticular fibers give a metachromatic reaction after sulfation.

In experiments utilizing reticulin-rich tissue, Glegg *et al.* (1953) found by paper chromatography, that the extracted reticulin contained large amounts of carbohydrates, particularly galactose, glucose, mannose and fucose, whereas tissue rich in collagen, showed a very scanty con-tent of carbohydrate. In agreement with this finding, Windrum *et al.* (1955) discovered that reticulin from kidney cortex contained approxi-mately 4.2% carbohydrate (galactose, mannose, fucose), while the hex-osamine content was very low (0.17%). Collagenous tissue contained a similarly low amount of hexosamine, but a considerably lower amount of galactose, mannose, and fucose; the composition of amino acids was, however, almost identical in reticulin and in collagen.

As indicated above, a homogeneous PAS-positive substance is observable in the media as well as in the intima with aging. This substance is presumably made up of mucoids and glycoproteins, and biochemical investigations show that with advancing years it is possible to isolate from human aortas an increasing amount of neutral carbohydrates containing aldo- and ketohexoses, besides hexosamine (see below).

PAS-staining gives but a very faint picture of the collagenous fibrils in the media, whereas numerous vigorously PAS-positive fragments of a collagenous nature are observable in the intima, and particularly in studying a fibrous plaque, thick, PAS-positive fibrils are seen running in parallel. It has not yet been established whether these fibrils are composed of ordinary collagen, or whether they have a different composition, but they take stain as collagenous fibrils do in van Gieson-Hansen's staining.

As will be mentioned below, biochemical investigations show that fibrous intimal plaques contain appreciable amounts of hydroxyproline, hexosamine, and hexose, whereas the uronic acid reaction is very faint or negative. In contrast to this, histological investigations indicate that fibrous plaques contain only a very scanty amount of ground substance among the fibrils, so that the majority of the hexosamine content in the fibrous plaques may form a constituent part of the fibrils.

The intimal and medial accumulations of acid mucopolysaccharides occur simultaneously, but the most vigorous medial accumulation occurs by far during the two first decades. No vigorous intimal proliferation is visible until a pronounced medial thickening has occurred; and no PAS-positive substance or fibrils appear in the intima until the mineralization has commenced in the media.

Today it is generally held that the mucopolysaccharides are formed in the fibroblasts of the tissue and secreted into the ground substance, and that the collagen molecule is formed within the fibroblast, possibly on or within the endoplasmic reticulum, and then extruded into the surrounding extracellular space (Boucek *et al.*, 1959; Slack, 1959).

It is well known that mucopolysaccharides tend to accumulate in tissue with a low oxygen tension, and that this applies particularly to sulfate-containing mucopolysaccharides (Altshuler and Angevine, 1954), and Wislocki *et al.* (1947), Bunting (1950), and Bunting and Bunting (1953) indicated a certain relation between the accumulation of acid mucopolysaccharides in the vessels and the oxygen tension in the walls.

The distribution of the mucopolysaccharides in the aortic wall seems to indicate that parts with the lowest oxygen tension are exposed to the largest accumulation of mucopolysaccharides. The intima and the luminal part of the media contain by far the largest amount of ground substance, which corresponds to the part of the vascular wall that does not contain vasa vasorum. A comparison between the aorta and the pulmonary artery shows that the aortic wall contains by far the largest amount of ground substance, which is possibly due to the fact that an increased pressure in a vessel will decrease the blood flow of vasa vasorum in the wall, and consequently also decrease the oxygen tension.

The intimal proliferation and later fibrosis, which increases more rapidly after medial calcification has started, may thus easily be explained as a consequence of the ischemic condition which prevails in the aortic wall, and which is probably further aggravated by a depositing of calcium in the media.

The histological picture seems to indicate that the calcareous salts are deposited in the intimal and medial ground substance. The present author interprets the calcareous depositing as a simple mineralization process and advances the theory, based on histochemical investigations, that the medial calcareous crystals are precipitated in the ground substance in close relation to the collagenous fibrils. This theory is not in accordance with that of Blumenthal et al. (1944) and Lansing et al. (1950a, b, c), who interpreted the medial calcareous deposits as a calcium precipitation in and on the elastic membranes, and they call the process an "elastocalcinosis."

To prove this, they used partly microincineration and partly biochemical methods. By basic hydrolysis they isolated and produced elastin in pure form. The fact that this elastin contains large quantities of calcium—increasing greatly with age—is not, as the authors hold, due to a deposit of calcium in the elastic fibrils, but to the fact that calcium is insoluble in basic surroundings. The calcium, deposited in the ground substance between the elastic fibrils, will thus by alkaline hydrolysis be precipitated together with the elastin, and it is therefore present as an impurity and not as a component of the fibrils.

It is the contention of the present author that the intimal calcareous depositing occurs in the scanty ground substance in close relation to the collagen-like fibrils. It is impossible, using the light microscope, to determine with certainty whether there is a relationship between the collagen fibrils and the calcium crystals in the media. The fact that an increasing mineralization may result in a picture which suggests a deposit of calcium outside the elastic fibrils, is probably a quantitative phenomenon. It should be possible by electron microscopic examinations to determine where the crystalline precipitation occurs (see Chapter 2 by McGill *et al.*). As previously mentioned the author interprets the calcification of the media as a typical mineralization, which is understood to mean a depositing of inorganic crystals in or on an organic matrix. More recent investigations into normal calcium deposits in certain organic tissues (bone, dentine, and enamel) show that the process takes place in an organic matrix, consisting partly of ground substance and partly of collagen fibrils (Rubin and Howard, 1950; Glimcher, 1959, 1961). Electron microscopic examinations show that the mineralization starts on the surface of or in the collagen fibrils, all the crystals being orientated with their axes longitudinally along the fibrils (Robinson and Watson, 1952; Rouiller *et al.*, 1952).

How important a role the chondroitin sulfate in the ground substance plays for the mineralization process is still to a certain degree an open question, but several experiments (Boyd and Neuman, 1951; Glimcher *et al.*, 1957; Strates *et al.*, 1957) seem to indicate that besides collagen fibrils, chondroitin sulfate and inorganic materials (Ca^{++}, PO_4^{--}, CO_3^{--}), a still unknown "local factor(s)" is necessary for the start of the mineralization. Einbinder and Schubert (1951) have demonstrated that protein collagen and chondroitin sulfate have great affinity for each other and form complex compounds, and Sobel (1955) in *in vitro* experiments shows that the collagen-chondroitin sulfate complex may be part of a "local factor."

There are several indications that the pressure in the vascular lumen will influence the carbohydrate content as well as the calcium concentration in the vascular wall. This may best be illustrated by considering the pulmonary artery from patients with normal tension in the pulmonary circulation, where only a scanty amount of interfibrillar ground substance is observable, and calcium salts are never deposited in the media. In patients with hypertension in the pulmonary circulation a pronounced accumulation of ground substance is seen in both the media and the intima, and in such cases a depositing of calcium salts may occur (Lansing, 1952).

III. Physiochemical and Chemical Studies of the Ground Substance and Collagen in the Aorta and Pulmonary Artery

A. Isolation and Characterization of the Mucopolysaccharides of Aortic Tissue

Mörner (1895) was the first scientist to isolate acid mucopolysaccharides from vascular tissue, and several investigators have since attempted to isolate and characterize mucopolysaccharides from the aortic wall. For many years isolation was performed by alkaline extraction, but in recent years proteolytic digestion has been used. It is interesting to note that hyaluronic acid was only isolated with certainty from aortic tissue after the latter extraction method had begun to be used.

Krawkow (1898) and Neuberg (1904) isolated "aortaamyloid," a rather impure product, containing chondroitin sulfate. But Levene and López-Suárez (1918) extracted a pure chondroitin sulfate product from calf aortas; and experimenting with isolation of chondroitin sulfate from horse aortas, Stallmann (1937) found a different composition of the mucopolysaccharides in young and old animals.

Hiruma (1923) extracted a substance with antithrombin activity from animal aortas, but gave no further characterization of the substance. Some years later, Jorpes *et al.* (1937), isolated chondroitin sulfate from animal aortas and found a very high sulfur content in acid mucopolysaccharides extracted from calf aortas, while mucopolysaccharides, isolated from pig aortas, contained smaller amounts of sulfur. Heparin was isolated by electrodialysis and precipitation with brucine. While conducting these experiments, Jorpes *et al.* found a correlation between the number of mast cells in the vascular walls and the heparin activity of the extracted mucopolysaccharides, whereas the amount of extracted mucopolysaccharides was independent of the number of mast cells.

Bassiouni (1954) isolated chondroitin sulfate from two human aortas and found that the extracted substance had an anticoagulant effect. During the last decade, Meyer and his associates (Meyer, 1951; Meyer and Rapport, 1951; Meyer *et al.*, 1956, 1957; Linker *et al.*, 1958) have been studying the connective tissue in animal as well as human aortic tissue. Proteolytic enzymic incubation was employed in several of the investigations (Meyer *et al.*, 1956, 1957), and the total quantity of acid mucopolysaccharides was found to constitute approximately 1% of the dry weight of the tissue. Qualitatively, hyaluronic acid composed approximately 15-23% of the mucopolysaccharides, and chondroitin sulfate A 30-45%, chondroitin sulfate B and heparitin sulfate made up the remaining percentage. A later investigation (Kaplan and Meyer, 1960) demonstrates a very similar composition of the acid mucopolysaccharides in human aortic tissue. Hyaluronic acid constituted approximately one-seventh of the extracted substances, decreasing markedly with age. Chondroitin sulfate C composed more than 50% of the mucopolysaccharides, showing a similar tendency to decrease with age, whereas chondroitin sulfate B and heparitin sulfate made up approximately 10% and increased slightly with age. Furthermore, Kaplan and Meyer found no variation in the ratio galactosamine:glucosamine.

Dyrbye and Kirk (1957), Kirk and Dyrbye (1957), and Kirk *et al.* (1958) gave a characterization of acid mucopolysaccharides from 30 human aortas in the age groups 1 to 76 years. No hyaluronic acid, or only insignificant amounts, were isolated, and chromatographic examinations showed that the ratio galactosamine:glucosamine was constant until the age of 60, after which time there was a slight rise.

Bollet *et al.* (1958) identified hyaluronic acid, chondroitin sulfate A and heparin in 5 human aortas, while Yu and Blumenthal (1958) showed that the mucoproteins from bovine aortas had an anticoagulant activity. Detailed studies on the acid mucopolysaccharidal compounds of bovine aortas were published by Berenson (1958, 1959). He identified hyaluronic acid and chondroitin sulfates A and B; chondroitin sulfate A was found to compose approximately 75% of the sulfated mucopolysaccharides. The concentration of acid mucopolysaccharides was highest in the luminal part of the vascular wall.

Buddecke (1960) extracted the acid and neutral mucopolysaccharides of the aortic wall. The acid fraction was identified as: hyaluronic acid, which composed 15%, and chondroitin sulfates A and B, which composed 50%; the remaining percentage was made up of heparin and keratosulfate. The ratio galactosamine:glucosamine increased slightly with age. An analysis of the neutral fraction showed that it was composed of galactose, mannose, and 1-fucose, besides hexosamine.

Gore and Larkey (1960), experimenting recently on human aortas, isolated a fraction which was resistant to testicular hyaluronidase. It was established that the fraction, which was identified as chondroitin sulfate B, had an anticoagulant effect.

Extensive investigations of the mucopolysaccharides in human aortic tissue have been carried out by Bertelsen and his associates during recent years.

Bertelsen and Jensen (1960b), extracting acid mucopolysaccharides from 17 human aortas from individuals in the age group 2 to 84 years, found that the viscosity of the extracted substances was fairly low, but there was a marked tendency toward a higher viscosity in the acid mucopolysaccharides extracted from young aortas. It was presumed that this phenomenon indicated a relative decrease in the content of hyaluronic acid in proportion to sulfated mucopolysaccharides. By enzymic incubation with bacterial hyaluronidase it was established that all vessels, irrespective of age and degree of atherosclerosis, contained hyaluronic acid. Further incubation with testicular hyaluronidase after hydrolysis of the hyaluronic acid showed that the vascular walls contained chondroitin sulfates A and/or C.

The lower viscosity in mucopolysaccharidal mixtures extracted from aortas of the elderly should be interpreted with some caution, since several factors influence the viscosity. It is, therefore, not possible to ascertain definite quantitative conclusions from these measurements alone. The relatively low viscosities must indicate that the hyaluronic acid extracted was low molecular, or that it was present only in a weak concentration.

The relative relationship between hyaluronic acid and sulfated mucopolysaccharides and its variation with age was determined in a later study by Bertelsen and Marcker (1961a). The age of the individuals from whom the samples were obtained ranged from 0 to 80 years. The hyaluronic acid fraction constituted approximately 40-50% in the age group under 20 years, approximately 30-35% in the age group 20-60 years, and between 10 and 20% after the age of 60.

In the last two investigations the quantities of acid mucopolysaccharide material obtained from aortas of various ages decreased with age. In younger age groups the yield was about 1.5-1.8% of dry, defatted tissue weight, whereas the amount of mucopolysaccharides from older aortas composed about 0.4-0.6%.

For further identification of the acid mucopolysaccharide material in the above mentioned investigations each of the aortic samples was subjected to paper electrophoresis and paper chromatography. By electrophoresis it was found that all the acid mucopolysaccharide samples contained two components: a faster moving one exhibiting a mobility similar to that of chondroitin sulfate, and a slower moving one with a mobility similar to that of hyaluronate. The spots indicating the hyaluronate were highly diffuse, which showed that these substances were polymolecular.

The hydrolyzate from the acid mucopolysaccharide samples were seen by chromatography to be mixtures of glucosamine and galactosamine.

Bertelsen and Marcker (1961b) further isolated hyaluronic acid from 12 aortic samples by the method of Simmons (1955). They characterized the hyaluronate with the aid of molecular weight determinations, viscometric measurements, paper electrophoresis, paper chromatography, sulfur analysis, and nitrogen analysis.

Table III shows that the molecular weight of the aortic hyaluronate is very low (average molecular weight, 44,000), and as expected it was not possible to demonstrate any variation in the molecular weight with age.

TABLE III

MOLECULAR WEIGHTS (M) OF HYALURONATE ISOLATED FROM HUMAN AORTAS,
CALCULATED FROM MEASUREMENTS OF THE OSMOTIC PRESSURES[a]

Age (years)	$M \times 10^3$	Nitrogen[c] (%)	Sulfur[c] (%)	Gross appearance
0	44			No plaques
0	43	3.62	0.69	No plaques
0	35			No plaques
$\frac{1}{2}$–2[b]	51	3.59	—	No plaques
6	30	3.18	0.63	No plaques
11	48	—	0.61	No plaques
35	48	4.29	—	Lipoidal plaques
50	43	3.52	0.76	Slight sclerosis
60	47	3.62	—	Slight sclerosis
63	40	—	0.73	Pronounced sclerosis
72	42	3.44	1.30	Pronounced sclerosis
84	60	3.80	0.81	Pronounced sclerosis

[a] After Bertelsen and Marcker, 1961b.

[b] This group consists of three aortas.

[c] Owing to the small amounts of substance at our disposal, only some of the results with nitrogen and sulfur have been determined.

The molecular weights were calculated from colloid osmotic pressure measurements performed by a micro-osmometric method.

Bertelsen and Jensen (1960b) found that the isolated mucopolysac-charidal mixtures had a marked heparin effect, and Bertelsen and Marcker (1961a) showed that the isolated sulfated fraction had an anti-coagulant activity (antithrombin and antithromboplastin activity).

These findings seem to indicate that the aortic wall contains heparin or a heparin-like substance; this is in accordance with the histological investigations which demonstrated a vigorous γ-metachromatic, hya-luronidase-resistant zone subendothelially.

The present author has attempted to give an indication of the dis-tribution of acid and neutral mucopolysaccharides in the aortic wall. The material consisted of 10 human aortas in the age groups 7 to 70 years; only nonsclerotic tissue was employed. The extraction was per-formed with alkali.

Table IV states the amount of extracted fractions in relation to dry, defatted tissue weight.

A considerable rise in the acid fraction and a slighter rise in the neutral fraction are observed with increasing age.

No attempt was made to remove the large amounts of protein im-purities in the two fractions. The hexosamine concentration in the acid fraction fluctuated from 3.3 to 7.9%, and in the neutral fraction from

TABLE IV
FRACTIONS EXPRESSED IN PERCENTAGES OF DRY, DEFATTED TISSUE WEIGHT

Age	Acid Fraction (%)	Neutral fraction (%)
7 months	3.3	3.1
2 years	5.3	4.2
13 years	11.3	4.2
21 years	10.0	6.1
30 years	13.6	4.3
37 years	14.7	4.1
45 years	11.4	4.9
58 years	14.1	5.4
60 years	14.6	6.2
70 years	15.1	6.6

2.9 to 4.1%, and the corresponding sulfate concentration in the acid and the neutral fraction was 1.9 to 3.1% and less than 0.2% respectively.

The acid fraction gave, with Dische's (1947) carbazole reaction, a vigorous positive reaction as an indication of a large content of uronic acid, whereas the neutral fraction only contained traces of, or no, uronic acid. The neutral fraction further contained aldo- and ketohexoses, as it gave characteristic color reactions with cysteine, carbazole, and sulfuric acid (Dische, 1955), besides being vigorously PAS-positive (McManus and Hoch-Ligeti, 1952).

It may be inferred from the hexosamine concentrations in the neutral fraction that the fraction is likely to contain a number of mucoids, which of course does not prevent glycoprotein from forming a constituent part of the fraction.

It is of special interest to see how the hexosamine content of the aortic wall is distributed between the acid and the neutral fractions respectively, for, as mentioned below, the total hexosamine content is found by hexosamine determinations directly on the aortic tissue. Table V shows the hexosamine content of the acid and neutral fractions respectively, and the sulfate content of the acid fraction converted to 100 gm dry, defatted tissue.

The total hexosamine concentration rises markedly with advancing years. The values are in perfect accordance with the concentrations found by Buddecke (1958a, b). Furthermore, it appears that with increasing age the content of hexosamine of the neutral fraction constitutes a decreasing percentage of the total hexosamine.

The rise in the sulfate content of the aortic wall with age is obviously due to an actual rise in the content of sulfated mucopolysaccharides. The ratio sulfate:hexosamine will rise further, which may

TABLE V

HEXOSAMINE AND SULFATE CONTENTS (MG PER 100 GM DRIED, DEFATTED TISSUE)

Age	Acid mucopolysaccharides		Neutral mucopolysaccharides	Total hexosamine content
	Hexosamine	Sulfate	Hexosamine	
7 months	0.26	0.10	0.13	0.39
2 years	0.36	0.15	0.14	0.40
13 years	0.42	0.25	0.15	0.57
21 years	0.49	0.24	0.16	0.65
30 years	0.46	0.28	0.15	0.61
37 years	0.48	0.28	0.17	0.65
45 years	0.55	0.31	0.16	0.71
58 years	—	0.32	—	—
60 years	0.63	0.38	0.18	0.81
70 years	0.68	0.41	0.18	0.86

partly be due to an increase in the amount of sulfated mucopolysaccharides in proportion to nonsulfated mucopolysaccharides, and partly an increased degree of sulfation of the chondroitin sulfates.

A comparison between the above results and the hexosamine content found by direct determination on aortic tissue (Bertelsen, 1961c, 1962) will show that the former constitute approximately 40 to 50% of the directly determined values. This fact is a clear demonstration of the ineffectiveness of the alkaline extraction method.

B. Hexosamine, Estersulfate, and Hydroxyproline Contents in Arteries of the Elastic Type

Jorpes *et al.* (1937) performed sulfate analyses on different animal aortas and found that they contained 2-3% chondroitin sulfate in relation to dry tissue weight.

Faber (1949) found in aortic tissue an increasing content of total sulfate with advancing years. The percentage of sulfate concentration was at least as high in aortas of the senile as in those of younger persons, but he concluded that "the active part" of the vessel showed a rising percentage of sulfate with aging.

Hexosamine analyses on human aortic tissue were performed by Kuzin and Gladyshev (1950). They analyzed 4 samples derived from persons 16 to 58 years of age. The average hexosamine concentrations in intima and media were 1.34 and 1.23% of dry tissue weight respectively.

Kirk and Dyrbye (1956) found in human aortas and pulmonary arteries no changes in the hexosamine content with age. The investigation included 124 samples of the aorta and 91 samples of the pulmonary artery. The analyses were performed on wet homogenates prepared from the intima and media of the vessels, and the results were expressed in relation to nondefatted, wet tissue weight. The mean hexosamine concentration in the aorta was 0.30% calculated on the basis of wet tissue weight; expressed on the basis of dry tissue weight the mean hexosamine concentration for the samples was 1.07%. No significant change in the hexosamine concentration was observed with age. In the samples of the pulmonary arteries the average hexosamine concentration was 0.27% calculated on the basis of wet weight, and 1.12% expressed on the basis of dry tissue weight.

Furthermore, Kirk and Dyrbye (1956) measured the acid-hydrolyzable sulfate content in aorta and pulmonary artery. In the aorta the average concentration was 0.270% of dry tissue weight, and no significant variation in the tissue concentration of sulfate with age was noted. In the pulmonary artery the average concentration of sulfate was 0.291% expressed on the basis of dry tissue weight, and the values were found to be higher for the 50-79 years age group than for younger persons.

Buddecke (1958a, b), in chemical analyses of extracts from sections of thoracic aorta with normal gross appearance, found an increase in the hexosamine content with age, whereas Kaplan and Meyer (1960) found no variation in the relative hexosamine concentrations with age on 33 human aortic extracts.

The first collagen analyses on aortic tissue date back to 1941, when Lowry *et al.* found an average content of 28% of dry, defatted tissue weight. Later analyses, performed by Myers and Lang (1946), showed a rise in the content of collagen in aortic tissue after the fourth decade. The material was comprised of 93 human aortas. Up to the age of 45 there was a constant content of collagen (15.5% of dry tissue weight); after the age of 45, a slight rise to approximately 18-19% was observable. Buddecke (1958a, b) found, however, no change in the collagen content of aortic tissue with age (20-24% of dry, defatted tissue weight).

In a chemical analysis of atheroma-free sections (intima-media) from human aortas, Kanabrocki *et al.* (1960) showed that the collagen levels remained comparatively constant with advancing years (about 20% of dry tissue weight).

All the analyses so far mentioned were carried out on intimal-medial tissue, with the exception of the investigations made by Kuzin and Gladyshev (1950), who analyzed the intima and the media separately. Very few further reports of isolated intimal and medial analyses are available. Pernis and Clerici (1957) determined the chemical composition of hyaline plaques from atherosclerotic aortas and compared the values with those of normal aortic tissue. They found a great decrease of the hexosamine and sulfate content, and a complete disappearance of uronic acid in the plaques in relation to the normal aortic wall. Noble *et al.* (1957) extracted intimal tissue from 60 human aortas, and found in fibrous plaques an increase in the concentration of collagen and an increase in the binding of hexosamine with scleroprotein (collagen and elastin). The total hexosamine concentration, however, remained unchanged with the development of atherosclerosis. In normal intimal tissue the hydroxyproline and hexosamine contents did not increase with age.

The author has in two investigations analyzed the tunica intima and tunica media separately (Bertelsen, 1961c, 1962). The medial analyses were performed on 102 samples of thoracic aorta and 86 samples of pulmonary artery. All the aortic samples were drawn from parts with normal gross appearance, and the pulmonary samples from the pulmonary trunk. The intimal analyses were performed on 20 aortas; 12 of the vessels showed atherosclerosis with distinct fibrous plaques. The analyses were performed on normal intimal tissue as well as plaques.

All the analyses were analyzed for their statistical significance.

Figure 10 shows the hexosamine concentrations in medial and intimal aortic tissue in terms of dry, defatted, and calcium-free weight. During the first four decades there is a significant increase in the hexosamine concentrations; from the fifth decade a small, but regular increase takes place. No significant variation is noted in the older age groups. The average hexosamine contents in medial tissue from an atherosclerotic and a nonatherosclerotic group are identical.

In intimal tissue with normal gross appearance there is a significant increase in the hexosamine content until about the fifth or sixth decades, after this age a slight decrease sets in. The hexosamine content varies irregularly in the fibrous plaques of the individual aortas and shows no correlation with the degree of atherosclerosis. The mean total concentration of hexosamine is on the same level in the fibrous plaques as in the intimal tissue with normal gross appearance.

Table VI demonstrates the hexosamine concentrations in medial tissue from pulmonary arteries at different ages. There is a significant increase in the concentrations with age. The hexosamine concentrations are lower in the pulmonary than in the aortic tissue (grand mean in aorta: 1400 mg per 100 gm dry, defatted, decalcified tissue; in pulmonary artery: 1166 mg).

Figure 11 shows the hydroxyproline concentrations in intimal and medial aortic tissue in terms of dry, defatted, and calcium-free weight.

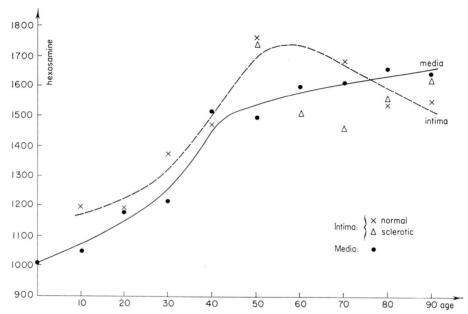

FIG. 10. The hexosamine content in intimal and medial aortic tissue with age and intimal fibrosis (mg per 100 gm dry, defatted, decalcified tissue weight).

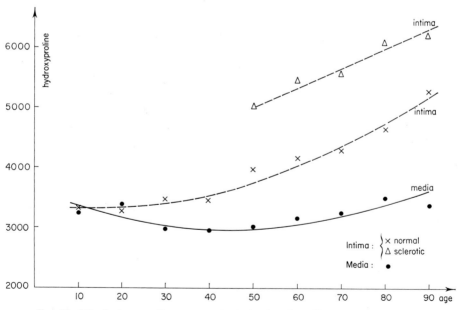

FIG. 11. The hydroxyproline content in intimal and medial aortic tissue with age and intimal fibrosis (mg per 100 gm dry, defatted, decalcified tissue weight).

TABLE VI

HEXOSAMINE AND CALCIUM IN MEDIAL TISSUE FROM PULMONARY ARTERIES AT DIFFERENT AGES[a]

Age groups (years)	Number of samples	Hexosamine content in mg per 100 gm dry, defatted, decalcified tissue[b]	Calcium content in mg per 100 gm dry, defatted tissue
0–1	1	1098	194
1–10	4	973	188
11–20	7	924	152
21–30	7	1046	172
31–40	14	1229	243
41–50	12	1128	255
51–60	10	1170	242
61–70	10	1293	317
71–80	9	1400	557
>80	12	1401	538

[a] After Bertelsen, 1961c.
[b] Grand mean 1166.

In the medial tissue the content remains remarkably constant through life, with a slight decrease in the second to fourth decades.

In normal intimal tissue there is a significant increase of hydroxy-proline with age. In each individual an increased hydroxyproline concentration is observed in the fibrous plaques in relation to normal intimal tissue; and the mean total concentration of hydroxyproline in the sclerotic tissue samples is significantly increased in relation to the concentration in the groups of normal intimal samples.

The author has examined the hydroxyproline concentration in medial tissue from 20 pulmonary arteries; the values were of the same order as those in the aortic tissue.

It appears from present investigations that the physiochemical and chemical analyses of the aortic tissue confirm the morphological picture of the vessel wall.

According to the above results the ground substance of the aortic wall contains mucoproteins, mucoids, and glycoproteins. During the first years after birth, the acid mucopolysaccharides compose approximately 50% of the polysaccharides of the ground substance. The content of both acid and neutral mucopolysaccharides increases with advancing years, but the increase is relatively largest in the acid fraction, so that in the adult aorta it constitutes approximately 75% of the polysaccharides. The demonstrated rise in the hexosamine content by analyses on aortic tissue is therefore primarily attributable to an increase in the acid carbohydrate fraction.

On extracting acid mucopolysaccharides from the aortic wall by proteolytic enzyme incubation, several authors find a decreasing content with advancing years (Dyrbye and Kirk, 1957; Bertelsen and Jensen, 1960b; Bertelsen and Marcker, 1961a), whereas in the present investigation alkaline extraction shows an increase in the acid fraction with age. The latter result is in agreement with the findings of Buddecke (1960), whereas Kaplan and Meyer (1960) did not with certainty demonstrate variations in the extracted amounts with age. It seems established that in comparison with the fairly pronounced increase in the amount of hexosamine, which is visible by direct analyses on the aortic wall, there is a relative rise in the amount of acid mucopolysaccharides in the aortic wall with age. The fall in the extracted acid fraction observed by enzymic digestion can be accounted for as a stronger binding between the mucopolysaccharidal part and protein. This strong binding may be due to the qualitative changes occurring in the acid mucopolysaccharides of the aortic wall in aging, for as Meyer (1953a) and Grossfeld et al. (1957) found, the chondroitin sulfates are appreciably closer bound to protein than hyaluronic acid.

The acid fraction contains both sulfated and nonsulfated mucopolysaccharides, and a marked rise in the ratio of sulfated mucopolysaccharides:nonsulfated mucopolysaccharides is observable with age. This finding is in agreement with Berenson (1958, 1959), Kaplan and Meyer (1960), and Buddecke (1960).

During a long period it was considered questionable whether human aortic tissue contained any hyaluronic acid at all (Meyer et al., 1957). As late as 1959 Meyer and his collaborators (1959) stated that young aortas did contain small amounts of hyaluronic acid, but that the amount would decrease or possibly be obliterated with increasing age and atherosclerosis. Simultaneously Kaplan and Meyer (1960) and the present author succeeded in demonstrating fairly significant amounts of hyaluronic acid in human aortic tissue irrespective of age and atherosclerosis.

The enzymic studies on the qualitative composition of chondroitin sulfate in aortic tissue, reveal the presence of a fraction that is sensible to testicular hyaluronidase, i.e. chondroitin sulfates A and/or C. Kaplan and Meyer (1960) did not find chondroitin sulfate A, but significant quantities of chondroitin sulfate C, which is in agreement with the work of Buddecke and Schubert (1961). Kaplan and Meyer (1960), Buddecke (1960), and Gore and Larkey (1960) further identified chondroitin sulfate B in the aortic wall.

In contrast to Berenson (1958, 1959) and the present author, who found a heparin activity of the extracted substances, Kaplan and Meyer failed to demonstrate heparin in the aortic mucopolysaccharides.

Several investigators have examined the ratio of galactosamine: glucosamine in aortic tissue. On analyzing isolated acid mucopolysaccharides, Kirk and Dyrbye (1957) and Kaplan and Meyer (1960) found the ratio unaltered with age; the former authors found, however, a slight increase in the galactosamine content after the age of 60. On examination of extracted mucopolysaccharides, Buddecke (1960) demonstrated a comparative rise in the galactosamine content in aging, but when he performed fractionated hexosamine analyses directly on aortic tissue, he found a slight increase in the glucosamine content in relation to the galactosamine quantity. Kirk and Dyrbye as well as Kaplan and Meyer employed paper chromatographic methods, whereas Buddecke (1960) used a column chromatographic method. A direct determination of the hexosamine components, carried out on hydrolyzed tissue, should be the very best method, as the distribution of the components in the extracted mucopolysaccharides is not necessarily similar to the distribution in the tissue.

The fact that there is a strong decrease in the hyaluronic acid content with age, and a simultaneous very slight change in the ratio of galactosamine:glucosamine, must signify that increasing age will entail a rise in the content of heparins in the vascular wall. This conclusion is in agreement with Kaplan and Meyer's (1960) results.

The molecular weight of the aortic hyaluronate is very low, but the above finding is in accordance with the low viscosities of the extracted mucopolysaccharides and the diffuse distribution of the hyaluronic acid fraction in electrophoresis.

Buddecke's (1960) investigations of the neutral mucopolysaccharides in the aortic wall are in agreement with the results in the present investigation.

As mentioned above, a number of intimal and medial age changes occur in macroscopically normal aortic tissue. It appears from the present investigations that these changes are quantitatively different in the two layers and that it is necessary to analyze each layer separately in order to obtain any valuable information at all.

A comparison between the present chemical investigations and previous studies will demonstrate that in order to reveal a rise in the hexosamine concentration with age in the intima as well as in the media, it is necessary to make allowance for the large amounts of lipid and calcium that are being deposited in the aorta with increasing years.

Comparisons between the biochemical findings in the media and in the intima show that the hexosamine contents in the two layers are almost identical, whereas there are large deviations in the contents of hydroxyproline, calcium salts, and lipids.

In the normal intima a rise occurs in the hexosamine as well as the hydroxyproline content with age; but the media displays a rise only in the hexosamine content, whereas the amount of hydroxyproline remains more or less constant. The biochemical investigations of intimal tissue are in accordance with the histochemical findings; with advancing years an accumulation of metachromatic substance and a simultaneously increasing amount of collagenous fragments become visible in the intima, whereas in the media only a minor, relative increase in the collagenous elements is observable, besides the vigorous accumulation of metachromatic substances.

Interesting to note is the change that occurs in the intima during the formation of fibrous plaques. Biochemical investigations made by Pernis and Clerici (1957), Noble et al. (1957), and Bertelsen (1962) demonstrated a vigorous increase in the amount of collagen, whereas the content of hexosamine remained more or less unchanged (Noble et al., 1957; Bertelsen, 1962). A further marked fall in the uronic acid concentration was established (Pernis and Clerici, 1957; Bertelsen, 1962) and a simultaneous rise in the content of hexose (Pernis and Clerici, 1957).

As previously mentioned, these changes seem to indicate that the formation of a plaque will involve a vigorous increase in the content of neutral carbohydrates, besides an accumulation of hydroxyproline fibrils. As mentioned the histochemical investigations show that the fibrils in a fibrous plaque are vigorously colored by Schiff's reagent after oxidation with periodic acid, whereas the reaction of the very scanty interfibrillar ground substance is metachromatic. The fact that the fibrils are PAS-positive must indicate either that they are collagenous fibrils that have bound large quantities of neutral carbohydrates to the surface, or that they represent a special kind of fibril, which contains neutral carbohydrates besides large amounts of hydroxyproline.

Experimenting on human skin, Sobel et al. (1958) demonstrated a rise in the content of collagen and a fall in the amount of hexosamine with age, so that a marked decrease occurred in the ratio of hexosamine: collagen. The authors were of the opinion that this ratio indicated the age of the connective tissue. Conditions are somewhat different in the aortic tissue: in the media, the collagen content is relatively constant, whereas the amount of hexosamine is markedly increasing, resulting in a slight rise in the ratio of hexosamine:collagen with age. In normal intimal tissue the ratio is fairly constant until the age of 50 or 60, when a decrease sets in, whereas the ratio in fibrous plaques is decreasing markedly in proportion to normal intimal tissue. The intimal age changes, and particularly the formation of fibrous plaques, may therefore display a certain similarity to the changes occurring in skin as previously pointed out by Yu and Blumenthal (1958).

The local age changes in the aortic wall, described in the present study, no doubt greatly influence the development of atherosclerosis, i.e., the formation of fibrous and lipoidal plaques, as well as complicating calcareous deposits, if any. But it has not yet been fully elucidated to which extent the atherosclerotic process is dependent on medial changes (Blumenthal *et al.*, 1944; Bertelsen, 1961a).

C. Calcium and Lipid Contents in Arteries of the Elastic Type

While analyzing the ground substance in aortic tissue, the investigator should not overlook the fact that large amounts of lipid and calcium are contained in the intima as well as in the media.

Most calcium analyses are carried out on the total aortic wall, and investigators have therefore failed to establish which part of the wall contains the largest amount of calcium (Haythorn *et al.*, 1936; Björnsson, 1941; Kirk and Kvorning, 1949; Faber and Lund, 1949; Buck, 1951). Only very few authors have performed separate analyses on the tunica intima and the tunica media, which gave considerably more regular values and also showed a medial calcium content, uniformly increasing with age (Weinhouse and Hirsch, 1940; Lansing *et al.*, 1950a, b, c, 1951; Lansing, 1959).

The present author has examined the calcium and lipid contents in the tunica media and tunica intima of 102 aortic samples with normal gross appearance, besides the calcium content in fibrous plaques from 12 atherosclerotic aortas. Furthermore, the calcium content in medial tissue from 86 pulmonary arteries was determined.

Figure 12 shows the calcium and lipid concentrations in aortic medial tissue. The calcium content shows a distinct increase with age, whereas the lipid content is low and shows only a slight increase.

Figure 13 demonstrates the calcium and lipid contents in tunica intima of aorta. The calcium concentration is low and without any observable increase, whereas the lipid content increases notably with age.

In fibrous plaques without gross calcium salts the concentrations of calcium range from 400 to 3700 mg per 100 gm dry, defatted tissue weight.

Table VI shows the calcium content of the media of pulmonary

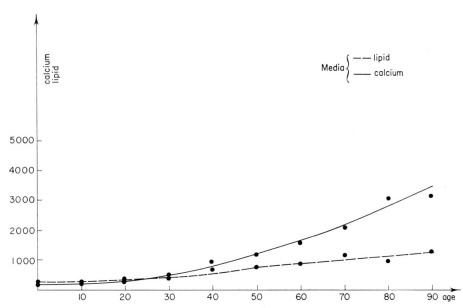

Fig. 12. Age variations in the calcium and lipid concentrations in medial aortic tissue (mg per 100 gm dry, defatted tissue weight).

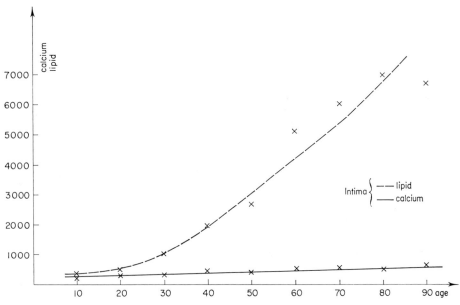

Fig. 13. Age variations in the calcium and lipid concentrations in intima of aortas with normal gross appearance (mg per 100 gm dry, defatted tissue weight).

arteries at different ages; the values are low, and only after the sixth decade do they increase slightly.

The calcium analyses confirm the histochemical findings. In the tunica media there is a uniform increase in the amount of calcium salts with age, independent of the degree of sclerosis in the superficial intima. There is only a scanty calcium content in macroscopically normal intimal tissue, and the calcium concentration varies greatly in fibrous plaques, because the calcareous deposits here represent a more or less incidental complication of the fibrosis.

The diffuse intimal lipidosis starts in early childhood, and in individuals with normal serum cholesterol it is presumably developed concurrently with the increasing thickening of the intima. But in certain cases, such as hypercholesterolemia, a pronounced lipidosis becomes visible without any concurrent accumulation of ground substance (Bertelsen, 1961a).

Lipid and calcium analyses have previously been employed in chemical gradings of aortic atherosclerosis. Since the atherosclerotic process occurs primarily in the intima, it should be imperative that such analyses are made solely on intimal tissue. As the amount of lipid is noticeably increasing in the normal intima, and as fibrous plaques are formed without any relation to the lipid, it is not very likely that the lipid concentration is an expression of the degree of vascular atherosclerosis.* Wells (1933) and Björnsson (1941) demonstrated an appreciable difference between the lipid content in the aorta and its macroscopic status. To sum up, it may be said that the lipid concentration in the intima will express the intimal lipidosis, but it will not throw any light on the distribution of the lipid.

Calcium salts are present as random deposits in the fibrous plaques, and the major part of the calcium content of the vascular wall is found in the tunica media; it is therefore obvious that the calcium concentration is completely unsuitable for grading the degree of atherosclerosis, even if the analyses are performed on isolated intimal tissue. In 1941, Björnsson demonstrated this statistically on large human section material.

As mentioned before, no satisfactory method for graduating the degree of vascular atherosclerosis is yet available (classification of the degree of vascular atherosclerosis is discussed in Chapter 2 by McGill *et al.*). According to the present investigations the atherosclerotic proc-

---

* Editors' note: This is not in agreement with current concepts of the term atherosclerosis and the reader should view this statement with special regard to the definitions given by the author at the beginning of this chapter.

ess occurs primarily solely in the intima, and a determination of the
intimal collagenous content will give a definite indication of the degree
of fibrosis.

Until further investigations are published, the best method for grading the atherosclerosis of the aortic wall is a combined macroscopic and
microscopic evaluation, in which a distinction is made between lipoidal
plaques and primary and secondary fibrous plaques. Each individual
plaque type is placed in relation to the total intimal surface. A further
analysis of the hydroxyproline and lipid concentration in the intima
will give an indication of the amount of collagen and of the lipidosis
present, and the calcium concentration will indicate a possible complicating calcification in the intima.

As previously mentioned, normal intimal tissue contains considerable
amounts of collagen; so the content of hydroxyproline will not directly
indicate the degree of fibrous plaque formation. The uronic acid content
in fibrous plaques is decreasing markedly or becoming completely obliterated; it should therefore be possible from the ratio of hydroxyproline:
uronic acid to obtain a numerical expression of the degree of atherosclerosis in an intimal part.

IV. Elastin Content in Arteries of the Elastic Type

Lowry *et al.* (1941) found the average elastin content in human aortas
to be about 30% of dry, defatted tissue weight, whereas Hass (1942)
demonstrated the content as ranging from 28 to 40% with no correlation
with age. Myers and Lang (1946) found the quantity of elastin to vary
between 37% in the age group 15-29 years, falling to about 27% in
the older age groups.

Lansing (1959) reported on 110 cases, the ages ranging from birth
to 103 years. The elastin was determined as the residue by extraction
of desiccated medial tissue in alkali. The content was found remarkably
constant through life with a mean value of about 42% of the dry tissue
weight. Using alkali extractions Kraemer and Miller (1953) did not find
any change with age in the percentage of aortic elastin, whereas Faber
and Møller-Hou (1952) reported human aortic elastin as being highest
in early life and gradually declining in the last decades of life.

Buddecke (1958a, b) using the method of Lowry *et al.* (1941) found
a significant decrease of the elastin content with age, and recently Scarselli (1961) has shown a highly significant increase in the elastin content
of the human aorta with age between 0 and 20 years. He used a photo-
metric method and expressed the elastin content in relation to dry tissue
weight.

The present author has prepared elastin from medial aortic tissue by the method of Lowry *et al.* (1941). The material consists of 89 aortas and the analyses were made on 1-2 gm dry, defatted medial tissue, and the results were corrected for the content of calcium salts in the tissue.

Table VII shows the average elastin contents in varying age groups. The elastin content of the media remained constant throughout life

TABLE VII
THE ELASTIN CONTENT IN PERCENTAGE OF DRY, DEFATTED, DECALCIFIED TISSUE WEIGHT

Age groups (years)	Number of samples	Elastin (%)
<20	11	42.5
21–30	7	46.3
31–40	9	43.7
41–50	17	41.8
51–60	15	46.5
61–70	16	42.1
>70	14	45.7

with a mean concentration of about 44% of dry, defatted, decalcified tissue.

By qualitative studies Lansing *et al.* (1950a, 1951) determined the amino acid composition of elastin from young and old aortas. The elastin from old aortas was found to contain more aspartic and glutamic acid, and from this result the authors explained the calcification of elastin with age. Thus, the calcification of the elastic tissue in the media occurred as a function of age, and Blumenthal *et al.* (1944) mentioned that the medial "elastocalcinosis" preceded the formation of intimal plaques, that medial calcification occurred more frequently than intimal plaques, and that intimal plaques did not occur without calcification of the elastic tissue of the media.

Furthermore, Lansing *et al.* (1950b) showed that the elastin content of the pulmonary artery was significantly lower than that of the aorta, and pulmonary elastin did not show amino acid age changes.

As mentioned Lansing and collaborators prepared the elastin by alkali extraction. The elastin thus prepared contains minerals, including calcium salts, which have not been dissolved; the minerals are therefore present as an impurity, and not as a component of the fibrils.

V. Factors in the Development of Atherosclerosis

There can hardly be any doubt that the atherosclerotic process in the intima is dependent on both local and general factors. Some hypothetical comments on a number of these theoretical factors will be advancing in the following.

Age changes in the aortic walls denote changes of a uniform nature and appearance which occur both in normal and in atherosclerotic vessels. As will appear from the above, it may be difficult to distinguish between age changes and atherosclerotic changes. Among age changes are all the above changes in the media, i.e., proliferation of cells, accumulation of ground substance, increase in the number of collagen fibrils, and splitting of the elastic membranes, besides the depositing of calcium salts. In the intima the proliferation of fibroblasts, the accumulation of ground substance, and diffuse lipidosis are among the age changes, whereas the formation of lipoidal lumps, lipoidal plaques, with or without secondary fibrosis, and formation of primary fibrous plaques are specific atherosclerotic changes in the vascular wall.

The medial and intimal age changes seem largely dependent on the vascular tension. This is clearly demonstrated by the difference in structure of the aorta and the pulmonary artery, and the change in the pulmonary artery in the case of hypertension in the pulmonary circulation.

Several authors consider the intimal thickening an integrating part of atherosclerosis (Moschcowitz, 1950; Wilens, 1951); the former postulated that the development of intimal thickening was due primarily to the intravascular tension.

There is a relatively uniform intimal thickening throughout the aorta, whereas the atherosclerotic process is distinctly localized to patches, therefore other factors must necessarily influence the development of atherosclerosis. This conception is in agreement with that of Duff and McMillan (1951), who pointed out that the sporadic distribution of the atherosclerotic process proved that an important local factor in the vascular wall is involved in the development of atherosclerosis.

The temporal relationship between the intimal and medial age changes should be observed. The accumulation of acid mucopolysaccharides is greatest in the media during the first years of life, but the intimal thickening gradually increases, and after the mineralization has started in the media the intimal proliferation will increase greatly, and there is a simultaneous accumulation of both acid and neutral mucopolysaccharides. Furthermore, PAS-positive fibrillar fragments will appear in the intima only after the medial mineralization has commenced.

Whether there is an actual correlation between the condition of the media and the intimal fibrosis, has not yet been elucidated, but the present author has never observed fibrous plaques without simultaneous pronounced changes in the tunica media. This observation is in accordance with the results of Blumenthal *et al.* (1944) and Lansing (1952), who found that a medial mineralization preceded the formation of plaques. Faber (1912) pursued the same line of thought.

As the age changes in the media are uniform throughout the total length of the vessel these changes are insufficient in themselves to form fibrous plaques, but must be considered solely as a fundamental factor in the development of atherosclerosis. The local factors that induce the formation of fibrous plaques are not known, but it is very likely that a further localized decrease of the already low oxygen tension in the intima may result in a fibrosis.

The presence of lipid has been a subject of discussion during the last 50-75 years. It is widely held today that lipoproteins are filtered through the intima and resorbed by the vasa vasorum in the luminal part of the media. It is very likely that this filtration is influenced by numerous factors, and the amount of lipid in the intima will probably be dependent on the speed of the filtration, the thickness of the intima, the resorption, etc. Besides the filtration of lipid, a synthesis of both cholesterol and phospholipid occurs in the intima, but it is not ascertained to what extent the lipidosis is due to this synthesis.

It is the experience of the present author that simple lipoidal plaques are often present in the aorta without any marked medial changes, and particularly without any sign of calcareous deposits in the media. As a rule, these lipoidal plaques will, however, be only moderate in size, and precipitations of cholesterol crystals are never seen. Secondary fibrosis of the superficial covering intima above a lipoidal plaque is observed only when the lipoidal accumulation has reached such a size that the intima, superficial to the plaque, has become separated from the media located below; and when the lipoidal accumulation contains precipitations of cholesterol crystals. A secondary intimal fibrosis is never visible without a pronounced medial mineralization.

It is not possible to determine whether the secondary intimal fibrosis is a reaction to the cholesterol crystals in the tissue, or whether it is attributable to the decreased oxygenation in the superficial part of the intima, which has become separated from the media below by the lipoidal plaques. It is probable that both crystalline precipitation and poor oxygenation of the intima will influence the process of fibrosis occurring above a lipoidal plaque.

REFERENCES

Altshuler, C. H., and Angevine, D. M. (1954). *In* "Connective Tissue in Health and Disease" (G. Asboe-Hansen, ed.), pp. 178-195. Munksgaard, Copenhagen.

Aschoff, L. (1925). *In* "Vorträge über Pathologie," pp. 62-84. Fischer, Jena.

Bassiouni, M. (1954). *J. Clin. Pathol.* **7**, 330.

Berenson, G. S. (1958). *Biochim. Biophys. Acta* **28**, 176.

Berenson, G. S. (1959). *Circulation Res.* **7**, 889.

Bertelsen, S. (1961a). *Acta Pathol. Microbiol. Scand.* **51**, 206.

Bertelsen, S. (1961b). *Acta Pathol. Microbiol. Scand.* **51**, 229.

Bertelsen, S. (1961c). *Acta Phamacol. Toxicol.* **18**, 359.

Bertelsen, S. (1961d). *Acta Pathol. Microbiol. Scand.* **53**, 335.

Bertelsen, S. (1962). *J. Geront.* **17**, 24.

Bertelsen, S., and Jensen, C. E. (1960a). *Acta Pathol. Microbiol. Scand.* **48**, 305.

Bertelsen, S., and Jensen, C. E. (1960b). *Acta Pharmacol. Toxicol.* **16**, 250.

Bertelsen, S., and Marcker, K. (1961a). *Acta Pharmacol. Toxicol.* **18**, 1.

Bertelsen, S., and Marcker, K. (1961b). *Nature* **191**, 386.

Bettelheim-Jevons, F. R. (1958). *Advan. Protein Chem.* **13**, 35.

Björling, E. (1911). *Arch. Pathol. Anat. Physiol. Virchow's* **205**, 71.

Björnsson, J. (1941). Arteriosclerosis: a Chemical and Statistical Study. Thesis. Munksgaard, Copenhagen.

Blix, G. (1948). *Acta Chem. Scand.* **2**, 467.

Blumenthal, H. T., Lansing, A. I., and Wheeler, P. A. (1944). *Am. J. Pathol.* **20**, 665.

Bollet, A. J., Anderson, D. V., and Simpson, W. F. (1958). *J. Clin. Invest.* **37**, 858.

Boucek, R. J., Noble, N. L., and Woessner, J. F. (1959). *In* "Connective Tissue, Thrombosis, and Atherosclerosis" (I. H. Page, ed.), pp. 193-211. Academic Press, New York.

Boyd, E. S., and Neuman, W. F. (1951). *J. Biol. Chem.* **193**, 243.

Boyd, W. (1950). "A Text-Book of Pathology." Lea & Febiger, Philadelphia, Pennsylvania.

Braunstein, H. (1960). *A.M.A. Arch. Pathol.* **69**, 617.

Buck, R. C. (1951). *A.M.A. Arch. Pathol.* **51**, 319.

Buddecke, E. (1958a). *Z. Physiol. Chem.* **310**, 182.

Buddecke, E. (1958b). *Verhandl. Deut. Ges. Kreislaufforsch* **24**, 143.

Buddecke, E. (1960). *Z. Physiol. Chem.* **318**, 33.

Buddecke, E., and Schubert, M. (1961). *Z. Physiol. Chem.* **325**, 189.

Bunting, H. (1950). *Ann. N.Y. Acad. Sci.* **52**, 977.

Bunting, C. H., and Bunting, H. (1953). *A.M.A. Arch. Pathol.* **55**, 257.

Dische, Z. (1947). *J. Biol. Chem.* **167**, 189.

Dische, Z. (1955). *Methods Biochem. Anal.* **2**, 313.

Duff, G. L., and McMillan, G. C. (1951). *Am. J. Med.* **11**, 92.

Dyrbye, M., and Kirk, J. E. (1957). *J. Geront.* **12**, 20.

Einbinder, J., and Schubert, M. (1951). *J. Biol. Chem.* **188**, 335.

Elson, L. A., and Morgan, W. T. J. (1933). *Biochem. J.* **27**, 1824.

Faber, A. (1912). "Die Arteriosklerose. Ihre Pathologische Anatomie, ihre Pathogenese und Ätiologie." Fischer, Jena.

Faber, M. (1949). *A.M.A. Arch. Pathol.* **48**, 342.

Faber, M., and Lund, F. (1949). *A.M.A. Arch. Pathol.* **48**, 351.

Faber, M., and Møller-Hou, G. (1952). *Acta Pathol. Microbiol. Scand.* **31**, 377.

Farkas, E., and Fasal, P. (1929). *Beitr. Pathol. Anat. Allgem. Pathol.* **82**, 102.

Gillman, T., Hathorn, M., and Penn, J. (1957). *In* "Connective Tissue. A Symposium" (R. E. Tunbridge, ed.), pp. 120-135. Scientic Public., Oxford.

Gillman, T., Grant, R. A., and Hathorn, M. (1960). *Brit. J. Exptl. Pathol.* **41**, 1.

Glegg, R. E., Eidinger, D., and Leblond, C. P. (1953). *Science* **118**, 614.

Glegg, R. E., Eidinger, D., and Leblond, C. P. (1954). *Science* **120**, 839.

Glimcher, M. J. (1959). *In* "Connective Tissue, Thrombosis, and Atherosclerosis" (I. H. Page, ed.), pp. 97-141. Academic Press, New York.

Glimcher, M. J. (1961). *In* "Macromolecular Complexes" (M. V. Edds, ed.), pp. 53-84. Ronald, New York.

Glimcher, M. J., Hodge, A. J., and Schmitt, F. O. (1957). *Proc. Natl. Acad. Sci. U.S.* **43**, 860.

Gore, I., and Larkey, B. J. (1960). *J. Lab. Clin. Med.* **56**, 839.

Grossfeld, H., Meyer, K., Godman, G., and Linker, A. (1957). *J. Biophys. Biochem. Cytol.* **3**, 391.

Hass, G. M. (1942). *A.M.A. Arch. Pathol.* **34**, 971.

Haythorn, S. R., and Taylor, F. A. (1936). *Am. J. Pathol.* **12**, 303.

Haythorn, S. R., Taylor, F. A., Whitehill, H., Crago, B. S., and Burrier, A. Z. (1936). *Am. J. Pathol.* **12**, 283.

Hiruma, K. (1923). *Biochem. Z.* **139**, 152.

Holman, R. L., McGill, H. C., Strong, J. P., and Geer, J. C. (1957). *Circulation* **16**, 483.

Holmgren, H. (1940). *Z. Mikroskop. Anat. Forsch.* **47**, 489.

Holzinger, J. (1934). *Beitr. Pathol. Anat. Allgem. Pathol.* **94**, 227.

Jensen, C. E., and Bertelsen, S. (1961). *Acta Pathol. Microbiol. Scand.* **51**, 241.

Jorpes, E., Holmgren, H., and Wilander, O. (1937). *Z. Mikroskop. Anat. Forsch.* **42**, 279.

Kanabrocki, E. L., Fels, I. G., and Kaplan, E. (1960). *J. Geront.* **15**, 383.

Kaplan, D., and Meyer, K. (1960). *Proc. Soc. Exptl. Biol. Med.* **105**, 78.

Kent, P. W., and Whitehouse, M. W. (1955). "Biochemistry of the Aminosugars." Butterworths, London.

Kirk, J. E., and Dyrbye, M. (1956). *J. Geront.* **11**, 273.

Kirk, J. E., and Dyrbye, M. (1957). *J. Geront.* **12**, 23.

Kirk, E., and Kvorning, S. A. (1949). *Am. Heart J.* **38**, 476.

Kirk, J. E., Wang, I., and Dyrbye, M. (1958). *J. Geront.* **13**, 362.

Kraemer, D. M., and Miller, H. (1953). *A.M.A. Arch. Pathol.* **55**, 70.

Kramer, H., and Windrum, G. M. (1953). *J. Clin. Pathol.* **6**, 239.

Krawkow, N. P. (1898). *Arch. Exptl. Pathol. Pharmakol. Naunyn-Schmiedeberg's* **40**, 195.

Kuzin, A. M., and Gladyshev, B. H. (1950). *Biokhimiya* **15**, 316.

Langhaas, T. (1866). *Arch. Pathol. Anat. Physiol. Virchow's* **36**, 187.

Lansing, A. I. (1952). *Ann. Internal. Med.* **36**, 39.

Lansing, A. I. (1959). *In* "The Arterial Wall. Aging, Structure, and Chemistry" (A. I. Lansing, ed.), pp. 136-160. Williams & Wilkins, Baltimore, Maryland.

Lansing, A. I., Alex, M., and Rosenthal, T. B. (1950a). *J. Geront.* **5**, 112.

Lansing, A. I., Rosenthal, T. B., and Alex, M. (1950b). *J. Geront.* **5**, 211.

Lansing, A. I., Alex, M., and Rosenthal, T. B. (1950c). *J. Geront.* **5**, 314.

Lansing, A. I., Roberts, E., Ramasarma, G. B., Rosenthal, T. B., and Alex, M. (1951). *Proc. Soc. Exptl. Biol. Med.* **76**, 714.

Larsen, B. (1957). *Acta Rheumatol. Scand.* **3**, 30.

Levene, P. A., and López-Suárez, J. (1918). *J. Biol. Chem.* **36**, 105.

Lhotka, J. F., and Davenport, H. A. (1950). *Stain Technol.* **25**, 129.

Lillie, R. D. (1947). *J. Lab. Clin. Med.* **32**, 910.

Linker, A., Hoffman, P., Sampson, P., and Meyer, K. (1958). *Biochim. Biophys. Acta* **29**, 443.

Lowry, O. H., Gilligan, D. R., and Katersky, E. M. (1941). *J. Biol. Chem.* **139**, 795.

McManus, J. F. A., and Hoch-Ligeti, C. (1952). *Lab. Invest.* **1**, 19.

Martin, C. J., and Axelrod, A. E. (1953). *Proc. Soc. Exptl. Biol. Med.* **83**, 461.

Meyer, K. (1945). *Advan. Protein Chem.* **2**, 249.

Meyer, K. (1951). *Conf. Connective Tissues Trans. 1st Conf. New York 1950* pp. 88-100.

Meyer, K. (1953a). *Discussions Faraday Soc.* **13**, 271.

Meyer, K. (1953b). *In* "Some Conjugated Proteins. A Symposium" (W. H. Cole, ed.), pp. 64-73. Rutgers Univ. Press, Brunswick, New Jersey.

Meyer, K. (1956). *Conf. Polysaccharides Biol. Trans. 1st Conf. Princeton, New Jersey 1955* pp. 31-51.

Meyer, K. (1957). *Harvey Lectures* **51**, 88.

Meyer, K., and Chaffee, E. (1941). *J. Biol. Chem.* **138**, 491.

Meyer, K., and Rapport, M. M. (1951). *Science* **113**, 596.

Meyer, K., Davidson, E., Linker, A., and Hoffman, P. (1956). *Biochim. Biophys. Acta* **21**, 506.

Meyer, K., Hoffman, P., and Linker, A. (1957). *In* "Connective Tissue, A Symposium" (R. E. Tunbridge, ed.), pp. 86-96. Blackwell, Oxford, England.

Meyer, K., Hoffman, P., and Linker, A. (1959). *In* "Connective Tissue, Thrombosis and Atherosclerosis" (I. H. Page, ed.), pp. 181-191. Academic Press, New York.

Mönckeberg, J. G. (1903). *Arch. Pathol. Anat. Physiol. Virchow's* **171**, 141.

Mörner, C. T. (1895). *Z. Physiol. Chem.* **20**, 357.

Moon, H. D., and Rinehart, J. F. (1952). *Circulation* **6**, 481.

Moschcowitz, E. (1950). *J. Am. Med. Assoc.* **143**, 861.

Myers, V. C., and Lang, W. W. (1946). *J. Geront.* **1**, 441.

Neuberg. (1904). *Verhandl. Deut. Pathol. Ges.* **1**, 19.

Noble, N. L., Boucek, R. J., and Kao, K. T. (1957). *Circulation* **15**, 366.

Patton, J., and Reeder, W. (1956). *Anal. Chem.* **28**, 1026.

Pearse, A. G. E. (1960). "Histochemistry. Theoretical and Applied," 2nd ed. Churchill, London.

Pernis, B., and Clerici, E. (1957). *Experientia* **13**, 351.

Ravault, P. P. (1928). *Bull. Histol. Appl. Physiol. Pathol. Tech. Microscop.* **5**, 40.

Ribbert, H. (1918). *Deut. Med. Wochschr.* **44**, 953.

Rinehart, J. F. (1954). *In* "Connective Tissues in Health and Disease" (G. Asboe-Hansen, ed.), pp. 239-250. Munksgaard, Copenhagen.

Robinson, R. A., and Watson, M. L. (1952). *Anat. Record* **114**, 383.

Rouiller, C., Huber, L., Kellenberger, E., and Rutishauser, E. (1952). *Acta Anat.* **14**, 9.

Rubin, P. S., and Howard, J. E. (1950). *Conf. Metab. Interrelations Trans. 2nd Conf. New York* pp. 155-166.

Scarselli, V. (1961). *Nature* **191**, 710.

Schultz, A. (1922). *Arch. Pathol. Anat. Physiol. Virchow's* **239**, 415.

Schultz, A. (1923). *Zentr. Allgem. Pathol. Pathol. Anat.* **33**, 469.

Simmons, N. S. (1955). Atomic Energy Project U.C.L.A. Report 353.

Slack, H. G. B. (1959). *Am. J. Med.* **26**, 113.

Sobel, A. E. (1955). *Ann. N. Y. Acad. Sci.* **60**, 713.

Sobel, H., Gabay, S., Wright, E. T., Lichtenstein, I., and Nelson, N. H. (1958). *J. Geront.* **13**, 128.

Ssolowjew, A. (1923). *Arch. Pathol. Anat. Physiol. Virchow's* **241**, 1.

Ssolowjew, A. (1924). *Arch. Pathol. Anat. Physiol. Virchow's* **250**, 359.

Stacey, M. (1946). *Advan. Carbohydrate Chem.* **2**, 161.

Stacey, M., and Barker, S. A. (1962). "Carbohydrates of Living Tissues." Van Nostrand, Princeton, New Jersey.

Stallmann, B. (1937). *Z. Ges. Exptl. Med.* **101**, 175.

Strates, B. S., Neuman, W. F., and Levinskas, G. J. (1957). *J. Phys. Chem.* **61**, 279.

Taylor, H. E. (1953). *Am. J. Pathol.* **29**, 871.

Virchow, R. (1856). *In* "Gesammelte Abhandlungen zur wissenschaftlichen Medicin," pp. 458-636. Meidinger Frankfurt.

Weinhouse, S., and Hirsch, E. F. (1940). *A.M.A. Arch. Pathol.* **29**, 31.

Wells, H. G. (1933). *In* "Arteriosclerose, A Survey of the Problem" (E. V. Cowdry, ed.), pp. 323-353. Josiah Macy, Jr. Foundation, New York.

WHO-Study Group (1958). *World Health Organ. Tech. Rept. Ser.* **143**, 1.

Wilens, S. L. (1951). *Am. J. Pathol.* **27**, 825.

Windrum, G. M. (1958). *Lab. Invest.* **7**, 9.

Windrum, G. M., Kent, P. W., and Eastoe, J. E. (1955). *Brit. J. Exptl. Pathol.* **36**, 49.

Wislocki, G. B., and Dempsey, E. W. (1948). *Am. J. Anat.* **83**, 1.

Wislocki, G. B., Bunting, H., and Dempsey, E. W. (1947). *Am. J. Anat.* **81**, 1.

Wolkoff, K. (1924). *Arch. Pathol. Anat. Physiol. Virchow's* **252**, 208.

Yu, S. Y., and Blumenthal, H. T. (1958). *J. Geront.* **13**, 366.

Zugibe, F. T., and Brown, K. D. (1960). *Circulation Res.* **8**, 287.

Zugibe, F. T., Brown, K. D., and Last, J. H. (1959). *J. Histochem. Cytochem.* **7**, 101.

—5—

The Role of Vascular Dynamics
in the Development of Atherosclerosis

Meyer Texon

I. Introduction

Vascular hemodynamics integrates the laws of fluid mechanics with the biological response of the blood vessels. The hemodynamic concept of atherosclerosis considers the role of vascular hemodynamics as the primary factor in the development of atherosclerosis. The application of the laws of fluid mechanics to the natural conditions in the circulatory system can account for the localization of atherosclerotic lesions at specific areas of predilection in the arterial tree as well as for its absence in apparently identical adjacent areas of intima. Continuous blood flow governed by the laws of fluid mechanics is prerequisite and conducive to progressive pathological changes. Local effects based upon the laws of hydrodynamics can account for the inception of atherosclerosis and its varied pathological appearance in the aorta and coronary arteries as well as in the arteries of the viscera and extremities. The absence or lesser degree of sclerosis in the pulmonary arteries and in veins is also accounted for on the basis of hemodynamics.

The variations in the severity of atherosclerosis found among individual patients appear to be due principally to individual differences in their hydraulic characteristics. The composite effect of velocity of blood flow, caliber of the lumen, and anatomical geometry are of importance. A biological factor, namely, the capacity for reparative response by the intima to the local hydraulic forces must also be considered. It is here that genetic and species differences in tissue or fabric structure and differences in biological response to injury may determine the nature and degree of atherosclerotic change.

The roles of contributing atherogenic factors such as age, sex, race, diet, nutritional status, habitus, lipid metabolism, drugs, hormones, associated diseases, enzyme systems, hypertension, and stress require reevaluation as secondary or modifying influences. No one of these factors is always present nor is any particular combination present as a common denominator or as a primary factor responsible in a causative sense for atherosclerosis. Atherosclerosis is found in both men and women, in the relatively young as well as in the aged, in hypertensive persons as well as in normotensives and in lean as well as in obese individuals. Notwithstanding available studies of the statistical association of atherosclerosis with lipids, diet, sex, habitus, and ethnic groups, proof of the causal relation of these factors to atherosclerosis is not thereby demonstrated or proved. Statistical associations *per se* cannot be considered scientific proof of causal relation.

On the basis of the constancy of the correlated data obtained from human autopsy specimens and the demonstration of the applicable laws of fluid mechanics in models and *in vivo*, atherosclerosis appears to be a sequel primarily of fluid dynamics applied to the conditions in the circulatory system. The experimental production of atherosclerosis in dogs by altering vascular configurations further corroborates the hemo-dynamic concept of atherosclerosis which considers the laws of fluid mechanics as the primary factor in the etiology and pathogenesis of atherosclerosis.

II. Fluid Dynamics

The motion of fluids may be streamline or turbulent. In streamline or laminar motion the fluid moves in definite layers or paths. In a turbulent flow the fluid moves with an eddying motion and at a given point the velocity varies irregularly from instant to instant. At low velocity the motion of a fluid is usually streamline. As the velocity is increased the laminar motion breaks down and becomes turbulent. When lines of flow converge, as in the arterial tree generally, or in an area of tapering or narrowing due to an atherosclerotic plaque, there is a tendency toward stability or streamline flow. Flow in such tubes with converging boundaries or narrowed lumina is characterized by an in-crease in velocity and a decrease in lateral or static pressure. This de-crease in lateral pressure is predictable in an inviscid fluid on the basis of Bernoulli's Theorem which is:

$$P_1 + \tfrac{1}{2}\rho V_1^2 = P_2 + \tfrac{1}{2}\rho V_2^2 \tag{1}$$

i.e., the sum of the static pressure and the square of the velocity times $\rho/2$ is constant if fluid flows from Point 1 to Point 2 assuming there is no loss of energy between these two points.

Regions of low pressure can readily be discerned in a variety of simple situations:

1. Flow in a Venturi meter (Fig. 1), as in a tube with converging boundaries, causes the lateral pressure to be reduced at the narrow por-tion where the velocity is increased.

2. In curvilinear motion (Fig. 2), the lateral pressure is increased along the outer wall and decreased along the inner wall by virtue of the centrifugal force.

3. Since the velocity of flow at a cross section of a tube (Fig. 3) in-creases from the wall toward the center, division of the more central or axial stream at a site of bifurcation results in a relative increase in velocity and a relative decrease in static pressure at the medial walls of the crotch zone compared with the lateral walls.

4. At areas of external attachment (Fig. 4) the predilection for atherosclerosis is enhanced by the fixation which resists any tendency of the flowing blood to move the wall of the vessel toward the axis of the stream.

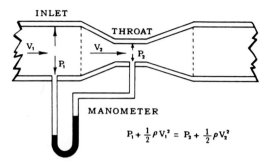

FIG. 1. Venturi meter and Bernoulli's equation.

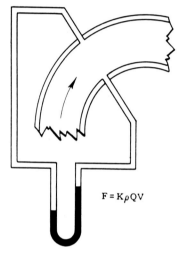

FIG. 2. Elbow flow meter and equation for force developed at a given angle or curvature.

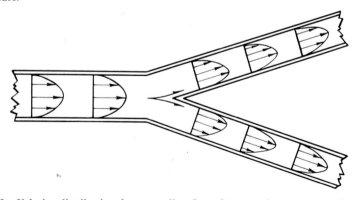

FIG. 3. Velocity distribution for streamline flow along a tube and at a bifurcation.

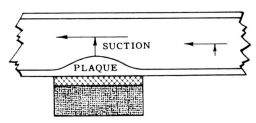

Fɪɢ. 4. Velocity and pressure (suction) changes associated with atherosclerotic plaque at zone of attachment.

5. Sites of branching vary in their anatomical or geometric pattern. Nevertheless, the flow patterns characteristically tend to cause a low pressure region on the inner wall (Points A, Fig. 5), the tendency increasing as the angle of branching or deflection of the stream increases.

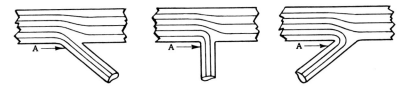

Fɪɢ. 5. Flow patterns at sites of branching.

The flow of rivers and streams, the flight of the airplane, the bird, and the insect, the movement of a ship on the water or a fish in its depths, and the circulation of the blood in our arteries and veins are varied phenomena determined by laws of fluid mechanics. Similarly, physical factors determine the predilection for atherosclerotic lesions to occur at sites of relative decrease in lateral pressure. Such areas in the circulation are characterized by converging boundaries or tapering, curvature, bifurcation, branching, and external attachment. These anatomical patterns can occur in various combinations and variations of geometries. In accordance with the laws of fluid mechanics their common feature is the production of regions of diminished lateral pressure. It is readily apparent that atherosclerosis is not a patchy disease occurring at haphazard or unpredictable areas. The atherosclerotic lesions found at autopsy have been correlated (Texon, 1957) uniformly with their localization as determined by hydraulic principles. The sites of predilection for atherosclerosis are found to be precisely the sites of relative reduction in lateral pressure; they can be predicted by the same principles used by hydraulic engineers.

III. Hydraulic Conditions

The circulation may be considered as a hydraulic system with particular characteristic hydraulic parameters. The relevant hydraulic factors must include the following:

A. Physical Characteristics of the Blood
  1. Viscosity, μ = centipoise
  2. Specific gravity = S, or density = ρ = gm/cc
  3. Homogeneity (particulate size)
  4. Temperature
B. Flow Characteristics
  1. Velocity of flow = V = cm/sec
  2. Lateral pressure = P = dynes/cm^2
  3. Volumetric rate of flow = Q = cm^3/sec
  4. Pulsation of flow
  5. Pulse rate, rhythm, and amplitude
  6. Reynold's number $\mathrm{Re} = \dfrac{VD\rho}{\mu}$
C. Anatomical Pattern (Geometry)
  1. Caliber of lumen = D = cm
  2. Tapering
  3. Bifurcation
  4. Branching characteristics
  5. Curvature
D. Fabric or Local Mural Factors
  1. External attachment
  2. External pressure
  3. Thickness
  4. Elasticity
  5. Porosity
  6. Strength of bond between layers

IV. Sites of Predilection, Localization, and Progressive Changes

The operation of the laws of fluid dynamics under the hydraulic conditions found in the circulatory system gives rise to effects which are prerequisite and conducive to atherosclerosis. The earliest lesions are changes in the intima at certain sites of predilection. These are areas characterized by tapering, curvature, bifurcation, branching, or external attachment. Such locations are subject to a relative decrease in local lateral pressure in accordance with the laws of fluid mechanics (see Section II).

The pressure difference between the outside and the inside of the wall of a blood vessel is the force per unit area which measures the relative tendency to move the wall of the vessel. For a given geometry of curve, taper, bifurcation, branch, or attachment, the maximum pressure difference will be a function of the Reynold's number of the flow and proportional to ρV^2 where ρ is the density and V is the velocity. The localized decrease in lateral pressure at points of predilection produces, in effect, a suction action upon the vessel wall. The intima is here exposed or subject to a lifting or pulling effect upon the endothelial layer and superficial cells. This represents the initial change. The local reaction consists of a reparative process, a thickening due to the proliferation of endothelial cells and fibroblasts from the subjacent layers. See Fig. 9C, p. 184. The thickened intima gradually projects into the lumen, thus creating an increased Venturi effect. The lateral pressure becomes further reduced as the caliber of the lumen diminishes and progressive changes appear. Cellular elements and lipids are added to the intimal fibroblastic proliferation as part of the pathological response *in situ*. The vessel presents an eccentric, or rarely concentric, thickening of the intima corresponding to the composite effects of local hydraulic conditions of flow, curvature, and attachment. This thickened intima gradually assumes the well defined appearance of an atherosclerotic plaque.

The atherosclerotic plaque involves chiefly the intima from its endothelial layer to the basement layer adjacent to the media. The basement areas of the intima present the most active sites of fibroblastic proliferation and the sites of earliest appearance of lipids. The pathological changes may include proliferation of intimal cells, fibroblastic proliferation and deposition of collagen, elastic tissue changes, cellular infiltration, lipid changes, and occasional calcification. Vascularization of the intima may also occur through the growth of capillaries from the adventitia or more rarely from the lumen.

The continued operation of the local hydraulic factors makes further pathological changes inherent and possible. These may be stationary for long periods, slowly progressive, or episodic in nature. A critical stage in the pathology may arrive when a relatively quick or dramatic change takes place. (1) Shearing off or lifting of the superficial layers of an atherosclerotic plaque may occur. A raw or ulcerated surface becomes exposed to the flowing blood elements. These may become deposited to form a thrombus. The thrombus may enlarge to a partially or totally occlusive degree by the accretion of additional blood elements. (2) An intramural or intimal hemorrhage may result from the same hydraulic forces which tend to draw the plaque toward the lumen. The intima is split or torn locally to produce a microscopic hemorrhage in a manner comparable to a gross medial dissecting hematoma of the aorta. Intimal hemorrhages in association with and as part of atherosclerotic plaques are frequent. They vary in size; a small hemorrhage may not be sufficient to affect the caliber of the lumen while a large hemorrhage in the intima may reduce an already narrowed lumen even to the point of total occlusion.

The pathology inherent in atherosclerosis produces occlusive changes of all degrees as the net result of composite local hemodynamic factors. Partial to complete occlusion may result locally from: (1) progressive intimal thickening, (2) acute thrombosis superimposed upon an ulcerated luminal surface of an atherosclerotic plaque, or (3) acute intimal hemorrhage within or in associaton with an atherosclerotic plaque. Although encroachment upon the lumen may be due to any one or any combination of these changes, the most commonly encountered completely occlusive lesion is that in which the lumen is obliterated by progressive thickening of the intima with incorporated old hemorrhage in various stages of transformation (Weinberg and Helpern, 1959).

Partial to complete occlusion distally may result from embolization of the atheromatous content of a plaque by rupture of the overlying intima as it is drawn toward the axial stream.

V. Flow Characteristics in Arteries

The laws of fluid mechanics are most readily applied for steady flow in rigid tubes. In order to determine the flow characteristics in the animal or human circulatory system, the modifications of flow due to the elasticity of the vessels and the pulsatory character of the flow must be considered in addition to modification which may arise from: (1) the anomalous viscous properties of the blood as a suspension of particles in a colloid solution, (2) the complex ejection pattern of blood flow as it enters the aorta, and (3) the flow patterns determined by the intricate anatomical accommodations of structure or geometry which characterize the arterial and venous circulation. A detailed mathematical analysis of flow characteristics throughout the circulatory system is complex but desirable for academic completeness. At the present time such an analysis is not available. Simplification of the analysis of blood flow in arteries is presented here because the major effects pertaining to steady flow in rigid tubes which relate to the development of atherosclerosis also occur in pulsatile flow in the arterial tree.

A. Laminar Flow; Turbulence; Poiseuille's Law; Reynold's Number

Laminar or streamline flow in a circular tube is also called "Poiseuille flow" because Poiseuille (a physician) first studied the steady flow of liquids in cylindrical tubes. Poiseuille's law states that the pressure drop is directly proportional to the length of the tube, to the rate of flow, and to the viscosity, while it is inversely proportional to the fourth power of the radius. If the velocity of flow is increased to a critical point the laminar flow breaks down and becomes turbulent; Poiseuille's law no longer applies. The laws governing pressure-flow relations in turbulent flow are less easily subjected to precise analysis.

The transition from laminar to turbulent flow occurs at critical conditions which depend on the velocity of flow, the density and viscosity of the liquid, and the diameter of the tube. These factors are combined in the Reynold's number defined by:

$$Re = \frac{VD_\rho}{\mu} \tag{2}$$

It is noteworthy that turbulence not only may be due to an increase in velocity of flow but also will occur at a given velocity more readily in larger tubes than in smaller tubes. A Reynold's number of 2000 is usually given as the critical value for transition from laminar to turbulent flow but this value may vary with other conditions of flow such as varying rates of flow and disturbances in flow. The Reynold's number for blood flow in the circulatory system is generally found to be well below the critical level for turbulence.

Because the blood flow is definitely laminar or streamline in all the smaller vessels, their pressure-flow relations can be analyzed with considerable mathematical precision. In the larger arteries, despite the existence of local areas of turbulence during a part of the cardiac cycle, essentially laminar flow can be assumed for calculation of average pressure-flow relations without the introduction of any significant error.

B. Pulsatile Flow; Viscosity; Movement of the Arterial Wall; Pressure-Flow Relations

Arterial flow is characterized by the recurring pulsation imparted by systolic contraction of the heart. Pulsations modify the instantaneous pressure-flow relations found in steady flow (Womersley, 1957; McDonald, 1960). At all frequencies of oscillatory or pulsatile flow a variable lag is produced between the applied pressure and the ensuing movement of the fluid. The laminae nearest the wall have the lowest velocity owing to the effect of viscosity. The flow near the wall has relatively less kinetic energy and reverses easily with each half-cycle. In the more central streamlines the kinetic energy and the velocity are greatest. With reduction in pressure gradient and reversal of flow at the half-cycle the axial streamline may be still flowing forward when reversal of the direction of flow may be occurring in the peripheral laminae. In such conditions the average velocity may approach zero. As the frequency of pulsation increases, the axial stream's velocity is reduced and the parabolic distribution of velocity across the tube flattens.

1. Blood Viscosity

A precise theoretical analysis of the flow of liquids generally assumes the fluid to be homogeneous and of uniform viscosity and that it is a "Newtonian" fluid. Since blood is not a simple fluid the flowing blood presents anomalous viscous properties. In the flowing blood the relatively cell-free zone of plasma which appears close to the wall of a blood vessel causes a local decrease in viscosity. This effect becomes important in the relatively slow rate of capillary blood flow and in vessels of less than 0.5 mm in diameter. Under conditions of relatively high velocity, as in the arteries which develop atherosclerosis, the variable viscosity of the blood does not alter appreciably the pressure-flow calculations. Blood may, in such instances, be considered to behave as a Newtonian fluid. Variation of viscosity, as a physical characteristic of the blood, does not appear to influence significantly the role of hemodynamics in the development of atherosclerosis.

2. Movement of the Arterial Wall

Arteries vary in diameter and length during the cardiac cycle. The transient dilatation following systole is relatively small and its effect on the stability of flow is negligible when compared with effects of the average or peak velocity of flow. Likewise, the longitudinal movement of arteries is usually slight owing to their anatomical attachments. The behavior of the arterial wall as an elastic tube does affect the propagation and damping of the pulse wave but has no appreciable effect on the average pressure-flow relationships which pertain to the development of atherosclerosis. In a larger artery, notably the arch of the aorta, vascular elasticity helps to produce streamline flow by stabilizing the pressure and velocity of flow throughout the cardiac cycle by its action as a surge chamber.

3. PRESSURE-FLOW RELATIONS

In a steady flow the rate of discharge through a tube is directly proportional to the pressure gradient in accordance with Poiseuille's law. The pressure gradient is the difference in pressure between two points in a continuous hydraulic system divided by the distance between the two points. This difference in pressure rather than the absolute values of pressure determines the flow velocity. The chief determinants of the pressure gradient are the force of cardiac ejection (*vis a tergo*) and the peripheral resistance. It is clear that a rise or fall in absolute pressure in a tube will not, *per se*, influence volumetric flow significantly. Similarly, the cyclic change in absolute pressure levels of the arterial tree does not affect appreciably the flow volume. The variable pressure gradient inherent in pulsatile flow produces a variable velocity flow. The peak velocity may be significantly greater than the average velocity with consequently greater effect on the development of atherosclerosis.

An equation relating volumetric flow to a varying pressure gradient may be derived by methods similar to the derivation of Poiseuille's equation. Although steady flow rate is dependent chiefly on the average pressure gradient, pulsatile flow rate is also dependent on the frequency of oscillation of the pulse pressure and its amplitude rather than its absolute value. In brief, Poiseuille's law may be applied to the average arterial oscillatory or pulsatile flow.

The arterial tree branches progressively so that the cross-sectional area of the branches generally increases peripherally. However, the total wall area of the branches, hence the friction or resistance, also increases with the number of branches and causes an increased pressure gradient. The velocity of flow is related to the total cross-sectional area of a vascular bed as well as to the caliber of a single vessel. The velocity of flow may be influenced further by external pressure or arteriolar constriction. Blood flow may then cease or be diverted to alternate channels.

C. Summary

Flow characteristics in a rigid tube, in an elastic tube, and in arteries can be analyzed by applying the same basic equations of fluid dynamics. For practical purposes, the relation between the pressure gradient and flow in arteries can be assumed to be the same as for a rigid tube. The usual variations in rate of flow caused by an oscillating pressure gradient and the cyclic variations in pressure and diameter appear to be significant factors in the development of atherosclerosis. Indeed, given certain hydraulic specifications pulsatile flow may produce conditions even more conducive to the development of atherosclerosis.

VI. Theoretical Calculations; Fluid Mechanics

The forces generated by the flowing blood can be computed. The values calculated will be increasingly reliable as technological instrumentation improves and as the hydraulic specifications are defined.

A. Curvature; Bends

The total force required to deflect a steady stream of fluid through a given angle (Fig. 6) is given by the equation:

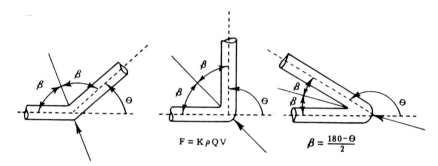

$$F = K\rho QV$$

$$\beta = \frac{180 - \Theta}{2}$$

FIG. 6.   Diagram and equation for hydraulic forces at bends.

$$F = K\rho QV \tag{3}$$

where F = total force in dynes, K = coefficient (see Table I), ρ = density in gm/cm^3, Q = flow rate in cm^3/sec, and V = velocity in cm/sec. The value of the coefficient K depends on the angle θ (Table I). If $\rho = 1$ gm/cm^3, $A = 0.20$ cm^2, $V = 20$ cm/sec, then $Q = AV = 4$ cm^3/sec and from the formula $F = K\rho QV$ at 45°, $F = 61$ dynes; at 90°, $F = 113$ dynes; at 135°, $F = 148$ dynes, and at 180°, $F = 160$ dynes.

TABLE 1

VALUE OF COEFFICIENT K WITH ANGLE θ[a]

θ Degrees	K	θ Degrees	K
0	0	105	1.58
15	0.26	120	1.73
30	0.52	135	1.85
45	0.76	150	1.93
60	1.00	165	1.97
75	1.22	180	2.00
90	1.41	$\beta = \dfrac{180 - \theta}{2}$	

[a] See Fig. 6.

It is clear that at a constant velocity and volumetric flow an increase in the angle θ increases the force required to divert the stream. By halving the diameter and maintaining the volumetric flow the velocity must increase fourfold; thus, the force is increased by increasing the velocity.

The computation of the forces described here, it should be noted, does not describe their distribution. However, it is reasonable to assume that the net effect must be an increased pressure on the outer curvature and a net suction action on the inner curvature. It is this suction effect which causes the atherosclerotic response.

B. Taper

Bernoulli's equation $(P_1 + \frac{1}{2}\rho V_1^2 = P_2 + \frac{1}{2}\rho V_2^2)$ provides the basis for computing the velocity flow and lateral pressure relations in a tapering vessel (Fig. 7). The computations must consider the effect of branch

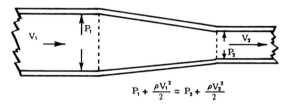

$$P_1 + \frac{\rho V_1^2}{2} = P_2 + \frac{\rho V_2^2}{2}$$

FIG. 7. Tapering tube or vessel.

run-offs if present between the points analyzed. In some instances the effect of gravity must be considered.

C. Attachment

A free elastic tube has no motion of its wall when the pressures on each side of the wall are equal. The flowing blood, whether steady or oscillating, produces a varying imbalance of forces which moves the wall toward the lesser pressure. Motion of a free wall is relatively unrestricted compared to the limitation of motion at zones of attachment. The suction effect of the diminished lateral pressure at sites of attachment (Fig. 4) stimulates intimal proliferation, the initial change in the development of atherosclerosis.

D. Branching

Patterns of blood flow are determined by the anatomical pattern of a branch (Fig. 5) and the peripheral resistance of each branch. The ratios of branch to parent stem's diameter and the angles of branching vary greatly. The flow patterns therefore necessarily vary and change in accordance with the local hydraulic conditions. In each flow pattern of a branch a zone of relatively low pressure is produced. If a sufficient suction effect due to the diminished lateral pressure is produced, an intimal response leading to atherosclerosis will appear. Low pressure areas are identified by the points A in Fig. 5 and correspond precisely to sites of atherosclerotic change.

E. Bifurcation and Trifurcation

The velocity distribution and flow patterns at a bifurcation and a trifurcation are illustrated in Figs. 3 and 8. The sites of relative diminu-

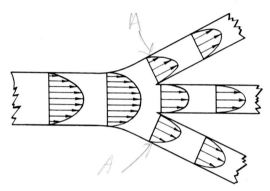

Fig. 8.   Velocity distribution for laminar flow along a tube and at a trifurcation.

tion in pressure or suction are determined in each instance by the relative velocities of flow at the wall of each branch, the angle of branching in relation to the curvature, the anatomical attachments and the ratio of trunk to branch diameter.

In each of the above patterns of flow, in relation to the anatomical design of the arteries, an ideal geometry was described. Minor modifications of flow will be produced by the natural asymmetry or imperfections in the anatomical geometry of blood vessels. Further modifications will be produced progressively as the atherosclerotic process influences the velocity and volumetric flow by encroachment on the lumen.

It should also be emphasized that several hydraulic conditions may be found concurrently. Thus, a tapering vessel may at the same time branch or have an attachment, etc. The composite effect of all the local hydraulic specifications, i.e., curvature, taper, branch, bifurcation, and attachment will influence the velocity and lateral pressure at a given site with respect to its predilection for atherosclerotic change.

VII. Human Atherosclerosis

A. Vascular Embryology and Subsequent Development

The vascular system develops embryologically by means of endothelial sprouts from an early capillary network formed by the growth and co-alescence of blood islands in the mesoderm. The vascular outgrowths are guided in their course by epithelial obstructions which determine the position of the capillary plexuses. Favorable channels enlarge and be-come main arteries and veins sending forth new branches. The hydraulic characteristics change both generally and locally while the anatomical design elaborates in response to the growth needs of the organism as a whole and the needs of individual organs. Hydraulic conditions condu-cive to atherosclerosis appear *in utero* as soon as blood begins to flow in definitive vascular channels. The anatomical design of the vascular sys-tem and the natural laws of fluid mechanics provide hydraulic character-istics which are prerequisite and conducive to atherosclerosis. The earli-est lesions, intimal thickening, are found at certain sites of predilection, namely, regions of relative decrease in lateral pressure such as are pro-duced by curvature, bifurcation, branching, external attachment, or tapering. The continuous operation of local hydraulic forces throughout life makes further pathological changes inherently possible. In fact, atherosclerosis, as a progressive occlusive arterial disease, or its patho-logical complications, is a major cause of human disability and death.

B. Illustrative Examples

The human circulatory system is necessarily characterized by specific hydraulic-biological conditions. The precise correlation of atherosclerotic lesions with their localization at sites of predilection, i.e., regions of diminished lateral pressure, in accordance with the laws of fluid me-chanics is demonstrated by the following specimens.

   (1) The coronary circulation
   (2) The aorta
   (3) Bifurcation of the aorta—common iliac arteries
   (4) Splenic artery
   (5) Pulmonary artery
   (6) Veins

1. THE CORONARY CIRCULATION

The coronary circulation is unique with respect to its hydraulic characteristics. The flow of blood in the coronary arteries is intermittent as a result of systolic contraction. The blood stream is subject to abrupt and rapid changes in velocity, increased velocity and volumetric flow occurring during diastole and reduced velocity and volumetric flow occurring during systole. Retrograde flow or reversal of flow under certain conditions also occurs. The coronary arteries appear to be unique in the body with respect to such wide phasic variations in blood flow. It is noteworthy that the caliber of the extramural coronary arteries tapers rapidly. The anatomical curvatures inherent in the coronary circulation are also notable. The composite effect of these hydraulic factors, namely, the rapid changes in velocity of flow, the nozzle effects of tapering, and the inherent anatomical curvatures seem to be significant factors in the predisposition of the coronary arteries toward atherosclerotic changes. Pathological examination (Texon, 1957, 1960) of coronary arteries reveals

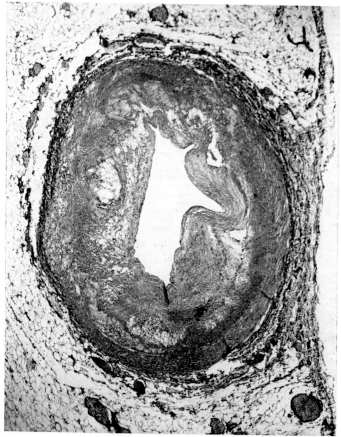

FIG. 9A. Coronary atherosclerosis. Showing concentric occlusive disease, a "converging boundary" or "taper" lesion.

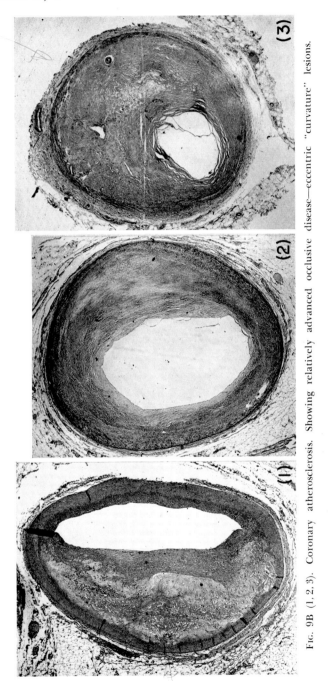

Fig. 9B (1, 2, 3). Coronary atherosclerosis. Showing relatively advanced occlusive disease—eccentric "curvature" lesions.

uniformly that the atherosclerotic process develops at sites of predilection which are determined by the local hydraulic conditions. A free and straight vessel presents correspondingly more concentric atherosclerotic change (Fig. 9A). The forces of blood flow in a zone of curvature determine a greater degree of involvement of the inner wall compared with the outer wall (Figs. 9B 1, 2, and 3 and 9C 1, 2, and 3). The free epicardial arc of a coronary artery may be less affected by atherosclerotic change

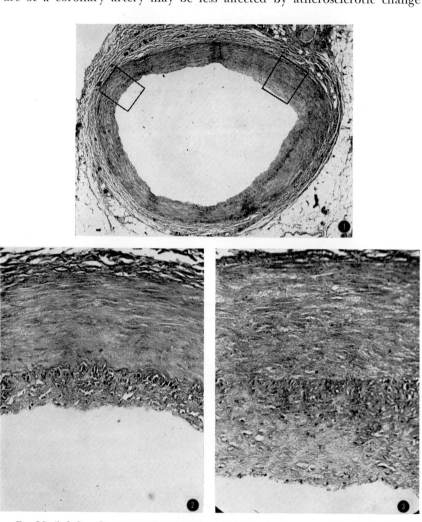

Fig 9C (1, 2, 3). Coronary atherosclerosis. Showing early stage of eccentric intimal proliferation and thickening in a "curvature" lesion. Magnification: (1) 20; (2) 125; (3) 125.

than the tethered or attached myocardial arc. The reduced lumen at the site of atherosclerosis due to curvature or attachment will be, of necessity, eccentrically placed. A frequent finding is a linear atherosclerotic plaque involving the left coronary artery beginning approximately 1 cm from its origin at a point where it curves and continues to form the left anterior descending branch. This is a "curvature" lesion aptly described as a "waterfall lesion."

2. The Aorta

The predilection of the aortic arch for atherosclerotic changes and dissecting hematomata appears to be determined by the increased velocity of blood flow and reduced static pressure or suction effect, characteristic of the hydraulic specifications in this region. A common finding is a large atherosclerotic plaque on the inner curvature of the aortic arch, a "sentinel patch." The sudden release of intra-abdominal pressure in the Valsalva maneuver causes a sudden increase in aortic blood velocity. The accompanying suction effect due to the sudden diminution of lateral pressure may tear the aortic wall by overcoming the bond between the layers and produce a dissecting hematoma. One of the earliest plaques to appear is located at the obliterated exit of the ductus arteriosus, an "attachment" lesion. The thoracic aorta typically and invariably presents atherosclerosis predominantly on the dorsal surface (Fig. 10A and B). The tapering of the aorta results in a relative increase in blood velocity in the abdominal portion of the aorta with consequently more severe atherosclerosis in this area. In advanced instances of atherosclerosis of the aorta, the involvement may be diffuse, affecting both dorsal and ventral walls.

3. Bifurcation of the Aorta and the Common Iliac Arteries

The bifurcation of the aorta divides the more central or axial blood stream. Under such hydraulic conditions a relative increase in velocity and a relative decrease in static pressure are produced at the medial walls of the crotch zone compared with the lateral walls. These forces, as described above, determine the medial walls of the crotch zone as sites of predilection for atherosclerotic changes (Fig. 11A and B). It is notable that the proximal margin of the atherosclerotic changes in the common iliac arteries may be about 1 cm distal to the carina or the margin of bifurcation. It appears that this area, as a stagnation point, is free of atherosclerosis due to the local increase in pressure where impingement of the blood stream occurs. The impingement pressure is less prone to produce atherosclerotic changes than the diminished static pressure at the immediately distal medial walls of the crotch zone.

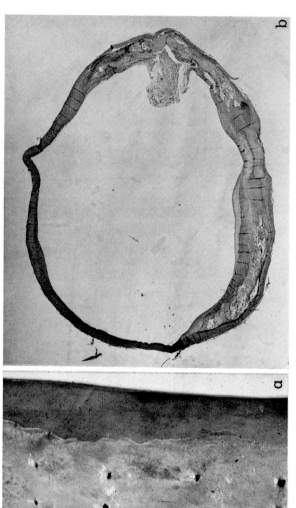

Fig. 10. Atherosclerosis of the thoracic aorta. Showing "attachment" lesion on dorsal surface. a. Gross specimen; b. Microscopic specimen.

The angles of bifurcation of the common iliac arteries vary among different individuals. When the angle of bifurcation is relatively acute the medial wall or "crotch" lesion develops. As the angle of bifurcation increases the lateral walls of the iliac arteries assume their anatomical

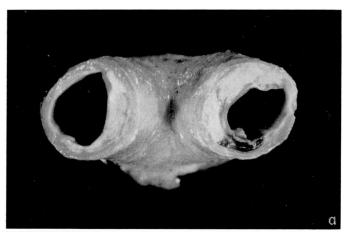

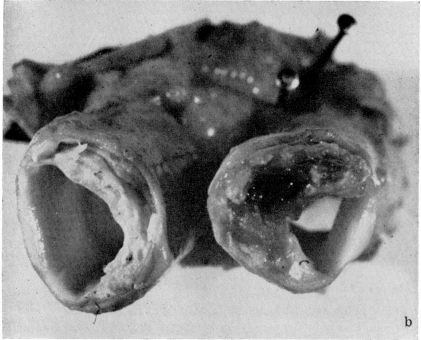

FIG. 11 (a and b). Bifurcation of the aorta. Showing "crotch," "bifurcation," or "Y" lesions of common iliac arteries. (Note intramural hemorrhage.)

importance as inner walls of curvatures in continuity with the aorta. Under such conditions, a "curvature" lesion may appear on the lateral wall of the iliac artery. The geometry or anatomical pattern of the aortic bifurcation will determine the hydraulic characteristics and the sites of predilection for atherosclerosis in each individual.

4. Splenic Artery

The splenic artery is remarkable for its tortuosity and relatively large caliber. The large caliber serves to decrease the velocity of its blood flow. Atherosclerosis is therefore relatively less frequent. Atherosclerosis will be found, nevertheless, as a result of the local hydraulic characteristics

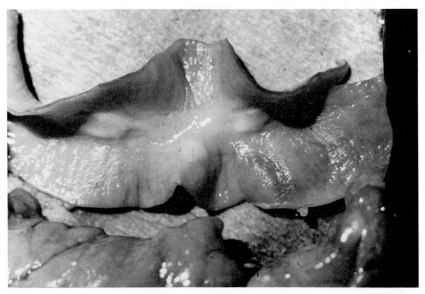

Fig. 12. Splenic artery. Showing "curvature" lesions; atherosclerotic plaque develops on inner wall of curvatures.

in accordance with the laws of fluid mechanics. An atherosclerotic plaque is noted on the inner walls of the curvatures in the specimen illustrated (Fig. 12).

5. Pulmonary Artery

The pulmonary ring and adjacent pulmonary artery have a greater circumference and diameter than the aortic ring and ascending aorta. Since, normally, the same volume of blood per unit time must pass these sections, it is obvious that the velocity of flow is diminished in the pulmonary artery compared with the ascending aorta. Therefore, atherosclerosis due to the suction effect of the blood stream is uncommon or minimized in the pulmonary artery.

6. VEINS

Veins generally present diverging lines of flow and have a larger caliber than arteries. The velocity of blood flow is relatively low and comparatively steady in veins. The suction action upon the walls of veins is therefore minimal, and occlusive sclerotic changes are comparatively rare.

VIII. Experimental Atherosclerosis in Dogs
(Texon *et al.* 1962)

A. Aim of Experiments

An approach to scientific proof that the laws of fluid mechanics are the primary factor in the etiology and pathogenesis of atherosclerosis may be achieved by altering hydraulic characteristics under controlled conditions in order to observe arterial wall changes.

B. Method

Anatomical and hydraulic conditions of the experiment are designed to simulate those operating in human atherosclerosis with respect to curvilinear flow and attachment. S-shaped curvatures are produced surgically by interposing an excised section of the carotid artery as an autograft between the ends of the transected femoral artery. The femoral artery becomes elongated by the autograft and assumes variable S-shaped configurations. Control sections of carotid and femoral arteries are taken at the time of surgery and are compared with sections examined after the dogs have been fed a normal kennel ration for 12 to 36 months.

C. Findings

1. GROSS OBSERVATIONS

The surgically altered femoral arteries, including the carotid artery autografts, are found to be patent, pulsating, and to have assumed varying forms of S-shaped curvatures and attachments to adjacent tissue. The curvatures are identified *in situ* and labeled. The intact specimens are photographed, excised, and examined histologically (Fig. 13).

2. MICROSCOPIC OBSERVATIONS

The control sections of carotid and femoral arteries are normal. At areas of curvature and external attachment of both host and autograft

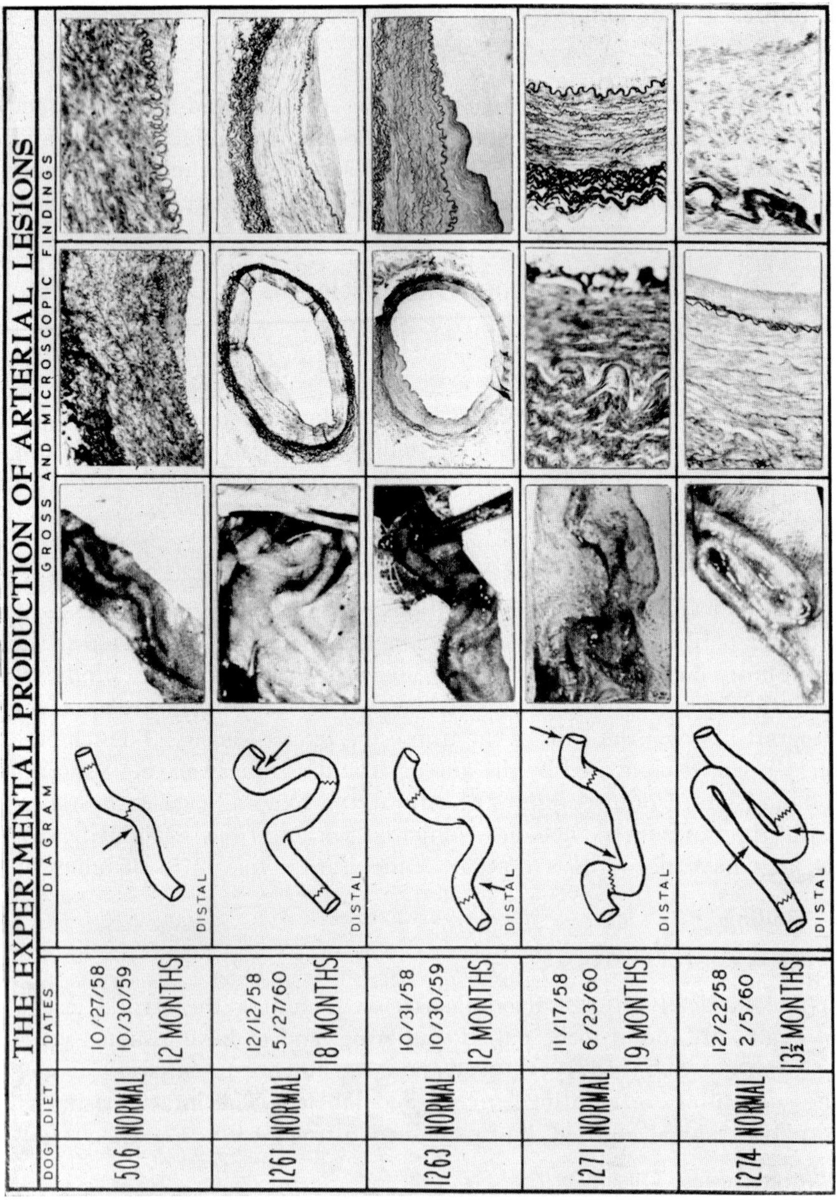

Fig. 13. Hemodynamically produced atherosclerosis in dogs. (Texon *et al.*, 1962.)

vessels, the intima is thickened by plaques of fibroblastic proliferation. The endothelial layer and the internal elastic layer appear intact and unchanged. The thickened intima assumes a crescentic shape with the greatest thickness corresponding to the internal wall of the curvature of the vessel or the zone of external attachment. There is an absence of inflammatory cellular infiltration, vascularization, and lipid formation. The fibroblastic proliferation presents a gradation in the appearance of the nuclei and cytoplasm of the fibroblasts: the nuclei adjacent to the internal elastic layer appear full, rounded, distinct, and surrounded by an area of clear cytoplasm while the nuclei of fibroblasts more removed from the internal elastic layer and approaching the endothelial layer appear shrunken, compressed, and surrounded by relatively dense fibrous tissue. The media is thickened by proliferation of muscular components. The concentric pattern of fibers is altered to an interlacing pattern. The elastic fibers are unevenly separated. The adventitia is also slightly thickened.

The earliest change is an acellular thickening of the intima. Vessels examined after 2 and 3 years reveal more extensive intimal fibroblastic proliferation with progressive diminution of the lumen and lipid formation. The earliest lipid change is noted in the form of minute droplets within fibroblastic cells in the basement zone of the intima. More advanced lesions reveal free lipid droplets which coalesce and extend toward the luminal surface. The predominance of the fibroblastic proliferation is clearly noted.

At the zone of suturing a cellular response is noted in addition to the fibroblastic proliferation. The fibroblastic response not only restores the structural integrity of the interrupted media and adventitia but also produces intimal thickening which encroaches on the vessel's lumen.

D. Discussion

Arterial wall changes are uniformly produced in dogs receiving a normal kennel diet for periods of 12 to 36 months following surgical production of S-shaped vascular configurations. The arterial wall lesions consist of intimal plaques localized at the internal wall of the curvatures and areas of external attachment. The histological change or pathology consists of progressive intimal thickening due to fibroblastic proliferation between the intact endothelial layer and the intact internal elastic layer. The early lesions present no evidence of cellular response, vascularization, or lipid formation. Lipid appears at the basement zone of the intima and becomes more extensive in some plaques as the fibroblastic proliferation increases. Other plaques appear to be free of lipid even when the fibroblastic intimal plaque has produced a marked degree of luminal occlusion.

In these experiments, the intimal plaques, consisting chiefly of intimal fibroblastic proliferation appear to represent the vascular response to the surgically altered hemodynamic characteristics. The plaque appears as a result of the relative decrease in lateral pressure on the inner wall of the curvature region or at a zone of attachment in both host and graft vessels in accordance with the laws of fluid mechanics.

The absence of intimal plaques in control sections and the appearance of naturally occurring plaques at sites of decreased lateral pressure elsewhere in the circulation, in accordance with the local hydraulic characteristics, indicate that the causative common denominator for these lesions—comparable to human atherosclerosis—is primarily the hemodynamic factor. The localization and progressive development of the atherosclerotic lesions does not appear to be dependent on possible differences in local mural lipid or enzymic chemistry. Rather, changes in tissue chemistry must result from the plaque's progressive pathological response to the continuing hydraulic forces.

Time *per se* is not a factor in the production of atherosclerosis, although the composite operation of the laws of fluid mechanics under the hydraulic-biological conditions found in the circulatory system requires time for progressive atherosclerotic changes to appear. Time alone does not produce atherosclerosis unless the prerequisite hydraulic characteristics are present.

Similarly, the roles of contributing atherogenic factors such as sex, race, diet, nutritional status, lipid metabolism, drugs, hormones, associated diseases, hypertension, enzyme systems, and stress must be re-evaluated as secondary factors which may or may not modify significantly the primary hemodynamic mechanism.

E. Conclusion

The experimental production of hemodynamically induced arterial lesions in dogs supports the concept that the laws of fluid dynamics are the primary factor in the localization and pathogenesis of human atherosclerosis.

IX. Summary Discussion

The characteristics of pulsatile flow in arteries can be analyzed by applying the same basic equations of fluid dynamics which apply to flow in rigid tubes. The operation of the laws of fluid mechanics under the hydraulic conditions found in the human circulatory system is prerequi-site and conducive to atherosclerosis.

Atherosclerosis begins as a change in the intima at sites of predilection characterized by tapering, curvature, bifurcation, branching, or external attachment. Such locations are subject to a relative decrease in lateral pressure in accordance with the laws of fluid mechanics. The initial change is the reparative response of the intima to the local suction effect of the flowing blood upon the vessel's wall. The histological reaction is a thickening of the intima due to a proliferation of the endothelial cells and fibroblasts from the subjacent layers. The continued operation of the local hydraulic factors causes further pathological alterations. These may include cellular infiltration, lipid changes, and further fibroblastic proliferation. The plaque thickens and gradually encroaches on the arterial lumen producing varying degrees of occlusion. The hemodynamic mechanism is also described for intimal ulceration, intimal hemorrhage, and dissecting hematoma occurring as complications inherent in the pathogenesis of atherosclerosis.

The variations in the severity of atherosclerosis found in individuals appear to be due principally to individual differences in hydraulic characteristics. The velocity of blood flow, the caliber of the lumen, and the anatomical geometry of design are of importance. A biological factor, namely, the capacity for local reparative response by the intima must also be considered. It is here that genetic differences in tissue or fabric structure may modify the nature and degree of atherosclerotic change.

The possible atherogenic roles of other factors such as age, sex, race, diet, nutritional status, lipid metabolism, drugs, hormones, associated diseases, hypertension, enzyme systems, and stress require re-evaluation as secondary factors which may or may not modify significantly the pri-mary hemodynamic mechanism.

The experimental production of hemodynamically induced arterial lesions in dogs supports the concept that the laws of fluid dynamics are the primary factor in the localization and pathogenesis of atherosclerosis.

X. Conclusion

Based upon the constancy of all the correlated data obtained from human autopsy specimens and the demonstration of the applicable laws of fluid mechanics in models and *in vivo,* atherosclerosis appears to be a sequel primarily of fluid dynamics applied to the natural conditions in the circulatory system. The experimental production of atherosclerosis in dogs by altering the hydraulic characteristics of blood vessels further corroborates the hemodynamic concept of atherosclerosis which considers the laws of fluid mechanics—vascular hemodynamics—as the primary factor in the etiology and pathogenesis of human atherosclerosis.

XI. Significance of Present Findings

The significance of this report rests chiefly upon identifying the primary cause of atherosclerosis and indicating the direction for further research. Hemodynamics is presented as the specific primary factor in the development of atherosclerosis. The correlated data adduced from human autopsy specimens, from the laws of fluid mechanics, from rigid and flexible circulatory models, and from animal experiments in which atherosclerosis was produced by altering vascular configuration compel the conclusion that atherosclerosis is a sequel primarily of fluid dynamics applied to the natural conditions in the vascular system.

Additional or secondary atherogenic factors are described. These may or may not modify the primary hemodynamic mechanism but they cannot, *per se* or in any combination, create atherosclerosis. Secondary factors may influence the atherosclerotic process only by influencing the hydraulic characteristics. If a parallel is drawn to other diseases or pathological conditions one might point out that the response of the host and the size of the stimulus or dose, among other factors, are important. Let us then recognize another parallel—regardless of the response of the host or the size of the dose, the cause of diphtheria or typhoid fever is always the specific organism for that disease. Similarly, regardless of possible modification by altered tissue response, size of stimulus, or other factors, atherosclerosis is invariably the sequel of specific hemodynamic forces in accordance with the laws of fluid mechanics applied to the circulatory system.

The findings presented here identify the research area in which the basic problems of atherosclerosis must be investigated and solved if treatment, cure, or prevention of atherosclerosis is to be achieved. Control of the hydraulic characteristics must be sought in order to control directly the atherosclerotic process.

It may be noted that the hydraulic factors which determine the development of atherosclerosis are not equally amenable to change, manipulation, or control; nor are all the hydraulic factors (see Section III) of equal importance. Thus, the anatomical design or geometry, such as calibers of lumina and angles of curvature and attachments are largely determined by heredity. Similarly, the vascular reaction or biological reparative response of the intima to hydraulic forces is probably determined by heredity as a racial or species characteristic. Each of the hydraulic specifications must be critically analyzed for its relative importance in controlling the atherosclerotic process.

My own interest is directed to the velocity of blood flow. Study of the factors which determine blood velocity may yield data useful in controlling the vascular dynamics and the response of the intima to these hydraulic forces. The blood velocity varies in a given individual under the same or different internal and external environmental conditions and in different areas of the body. The blood velocity also varies from person to person in a highly individualized manner. It is likely that no two individuals have precisely the same hydraulic characteristics. Further study of vascular hemodynamics and its control may be expected to provide the key to the means of solving the problem of atherosclerosis.

ACKNOWLEDGMENTS

The author wishes gratefully to acknowledge the cooperation and encouragement of Dr. Milton Helpern, Chief Medical Examiner of the City of New York, Professor of Forensic Medicine and Chairman of the Department, New York University Post-Graduate Medical School.

Dr. Richard Skalak, Associate Professor of Civil Engineering and Engineering Mechanics at Columbia University reviewed the manuscript and offered helpful suggestions for which the author here records his deep appreciation and thanks.

The author also records his appreciation and gratefully acknowledges the cooperation in the surgical experiments of Dr. Jere W. Lord, Jr., Professor of Clinical Surgery and Dr. Anthony M. Imparato, Assistant Professor of Clinical Surgery, Department of Surgery, New York University Post-Graduate Medical School.

REFERENCES

McDonald, D. A. (1960). "Blood Flow in Arteries." Williams & Wilkins, Baltimore, Maryland.

Texon, M. (1957). *A.M.A. Arch. Internal Med.* **99**, 418.

Texon, M. (1960). *Bull. N. Y. Acad. Med.* **36**, 263.

Texon, M., Imparato, A. M., Lord, J. W., Jr., and Helpern, M. (1962). *Arch. Internal Med.* **110**, 50.

Weinberg, S. B., and Helpern, M. (1959). *In* "Work and the Heart" (F. F. Rosenbaum and E. L. Belknap, eds.), pp. 288-292. Hoeber, New York.

Womersley, J. R. (1957). WADC-TR 56-614.

The Filtration Concept of Atherosclerosis and Serum Lipids in the Diagnosis of Atherosclerosis*

JOHN W. GOFMAN AND WEI YOUNG

I. The General Aspects of the Filtration Concept of Atherogenesis

It is now rare for students of atherosclerosis to regard this process as a necessary concomitant of aging per se. Rather the mounting evidence points strongly to the concept that an overloading type of phenomenon with respect to arterial physiology is operative. It is our purpose here to discuss one view of what the nature of the physiological process may

* The original researches presented in this Chapter were supported by United States Public Health Grant HE-02029-09 and by the United States Atomic Energy Commission.

be, and how such "overloading" comes about. Before considering details of this concept, one issue must be stressed, for this issue has led to much confusion in the field. Atherosclerosis is well known to be, in part, a focal process (Young *et al.*, 1960b), in that the severity of the process shows great variation even in closely contiguous segments of the arterial tree, and in that certain whole regions of the arterial bed are particularly prone to develop severe atherosclerosis in comparison with other major regions of that bed. Such focality has tended to obscure the fact that systemic factors (Gofman, 1959) play a most probable major role in the evolution of the disease. Current concepts in general take cognizance of the strong evidence for the operation of systemic factors, with the view that local arterial or tissue properties, variable from region to region, may grossly intensify or minimize the effect of these systemic factors.

Central in this particular concept of the evolution of atherosclerosis is the thesis that atherogenesis, or at least a most important step in atherogenesis, is represented by the accumulation of "substances" in the subendothelial space of those arteries susceptible to the disease. We shall return to the question of what "substances" and to some of the reasons for conflicting views of pathogenesis that arise from the observations of the chemical or histological structure of atherosclerotic lesions.

Anitschkow (1933), following many years of highly productive investigation of atherosclerosis, held the opinion that the normal artery experiences a constant passage of fluid through its wall in the direction from arterial lumen to adventitia. Further, some of the constituents of such fluid were considered to pass on through along with the fluid vehicle, thus leading to no pathological consequence whatever. Other constituents of the fluid vehicle, for reasons to be considered below, tend to *remain within* the wall of the artery, rather than to pass on through with the fluid in which they were originally suspended or dissolved. Atheroma, it was reasoned, developed, its extent being conditioned by (a) the nature of the substances remaining behind in the arterial wall, and (b) the over-all "responsiveness" of the arterial tissue to these substances.

During the last decade, opportunity for critical evaluation of the Anitschkow concept has greatly increased. Grading of arteriosclerosis in a quantitative fashion has been vastly improved, in contrast to earlier qualitative and semiquantitative measurements. Electron microscopy and related techniques have considerably clarified the structure of arterial wall components, especially such entities as endothelial cells and internal elastic membranes. The concerted attack upon the nature of the lipid-bearing constituents of blood plasma has fabulously advanced our knowledge of these heretofore crudely understood materials—such attack having involved numerous techniques including isotopic labeling, delicate chemical separations, ultracentrifugation, electrophoresis, and electron microscopy. In the ensuing discussion the impact of such advances upon our evaluation of the atherosclerotic process will be outlined. Considerations will center upon three major subjects and their inter-relationship: (a) the general structure of the arterial tree; (b) filtration processes and their relationship to pressure; (c) the critical importance of size of macromolecular entities such as lipoproteins.

A. Filtration Processes in Vascular Beds

The classic work of Landis (1934) established clearly the operation of filtration processes across vascular walls. Since that work the linear relationship between filtration rate and intravascular pressure for the capillaries, at least, has been widely accepted. Pappenheimer (1953) of the same school of investigators, studied the problem of passage of materials from the interior of capillaries to extravascular spaces. His work led him to the conclusion that the data concerning transport across capillaries were most consistent with the existence of a system of pores in the capillary wall. Filtration through such pores, he concluded, did occur but was a relatively slow process of transport of material. Diffusion of water and such small molecules as urea, glucose, and sodium chloride through such pore regions appeared quantitatively much greater as a transfer path than hydrodynamic filtration alone. Some rather special properties of endothelium became apparent in his investigations of a variety of molecules characterized by high lipid:water partition coefficients. For such substances the rate of transfer across capillaries was much greater than would be calculated for molecules of the same size range but of lower lipid:water partition coefficients. The pore concept, thus, did not explain transfer rates for the more hydrophobic molecules, which led Pappenheimer to consider that such molecules were capable of diffusing through regions of the capillary wall which are relatively impermeable to molecules of low lipid solubility. He stated, "It seems reasonable, therefore, to identify the diffusion pathway for lipid-soluble molecules with the plasma membranes of the capillary endothelial cells themselves, as opposed to the system of water-filled pores penetrating through or between these cells, which is capable of accounting for the passage of water and lipid-insoluble molecules."

Kellner (1954) has demonstrated that capillary endothelium is permeable, by some mechanism, to lipid substances, since he was able to demonstrate that lipid was present in the extracellular and tissue fluids obtained by lymphatic cannulation. Further, he showed, by electrophoretic analysis at least, that such lipid in lymph was present in lipoprotein forms similar to those observed for the lipoproteins of plasma. The *concentration* of lipoproteins of lymph was found by Kellner to be lower than that of the lipoproteins of plasma. More recently Courtice and Garlick (1962) in experiments analogous to those of Kellner, perfused capillaries with several species of serum lipoproteins. This work indicated strongly that the size of the lipoprotein molecules represents a crucial factor determining rate of transfer of lipoprotein across the capillary wall. In an almost linear manner, the permeation of lipoprotein was positively related to lipoprotein size.

Inasmuch as the entire vascular system is lined with endothelial cells (which endothelial linings appear permeable to lipoproteins), the major *structural* difference between such vascular entities as arteries, arterioles, capillaries (Fig. 1A), and veins resides in the additional coats of tissue external to this endothelial lining. Coats, such as internal elastic membrane, muscular media, and collagenous adventitia are, in large measure, necessary for the physical strength required to prevent vascular rupture in regions of relatively high intravascular pressure. The general relation of thickness of such coats to intravascular pressure is widely realized.

It appears to us that of all these coats, in addition to the endothelial lining, the internal elastic membrane is of special interest and probable importance for atherosclerosis development. The internal elastic membrane shows the presence of fenestra* (Fig. 1B) an otherwise continuous membrane (Young *et al.,* 1960b). Such fenestra may be anticipated to allow for fluid flow toward the medial and adventitial coats, such fluid having arrived in the subintimal space, along with various solutes, by one or more of the processes of endothelial permeation previously discussed. Presumably, in health, the fenestra provide an adequately competent path for removal of fluid and solutes, including such giant solutes as lipoprotein macromolecules. If, for any reason or set of reasons, the transfer of lipoproteins be impeded through such fenestra *relative* to their influx via the endothelial lining, the stage would be set for an accumulation of lipoproteins within the subintimal space (i.e., between endothelium and internal elastic membrane). The subsequent fate of such entrapped lipoproteins could result in several of what are probably later manifestations of fully developed atherosclerotic lesions. Whether or not fenestra become obstructed by material within the subintimal space, it is clear that the *balance* between influx and endothelium and efflux must be crucial in determination of further accumulation of material. Such

---

* Editors' note: See also Chapter 1 for detailed description and alternate view of importance of fenestra.

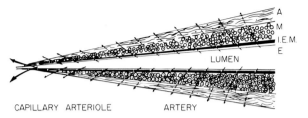

Fig. 1A. Diagram indicating the changing structure of a vascular wall in passing from large artery to capillary. A = adventitia; M = media; I.E.M. = internal elastic membrane; E = endothelium. Points worthy of note are: (a) decreasing thickness of adventitia, media, and internal elastic membrane, (b) incompleteness of internal elastic membrane in arteriole, and (c) absence of internal elastic membrane in capillary.

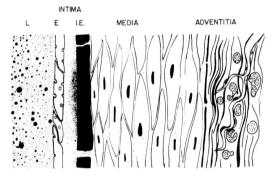

Fig. 1B. Diagram indicating the pertinent structural elements of the arterial wall. L = lumen, E = endothelium, I.E. = internal elastic membrane. Pores and vesicles of endothelium are shown, as are also the fenestra of the internal elastic membrane.

accumulation plus any reactive tissue changes to material already present would be expected to result in a thickening of the subintimal region, with encroachment upon the arterial lumen. In Fig. 2A is shown an arterial section (cerebral artery) with a relatively advanced atherosclerotic lesion present, obviously encroaching markedly upon the vessel lumen. It is of interest to know whether analogous processes may occur *in vitro* in situations where a barrier similar to an unfenestrated elastic membrane exists (in this case providing an absolute barrier to efflux). We have studied a drainage pipe which had been in operation over a 5-year period. Sticky soil has accumulated along the pipe wall, resulting in an ultimate appearance (see Fig. 2B) showing a striking resemblance to the atherosclerotic arterial lesion. The pipe wall, unyielding and without fenestra, presents a barrier to egress via the wall, with a resultant marked narrowing of the drainage pipe lumen.

In the large musculoelastic arteries or the medium muscular arteries,

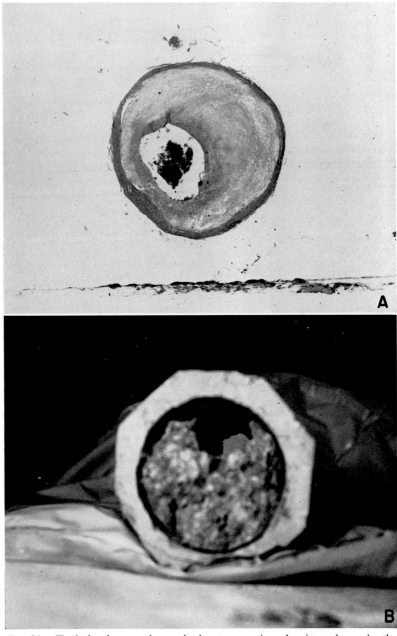

FIG. 2A. Typical atheroma in cerebral artery section showing advanced atherosclerosis.

2B. Accumulated soil debris in rigid drainage pipe, with obliteration of lumen analogous to that in cerebral artery of 2A.

which are both prime candidates for the development of atherosclerosis, a relatively thick internal elastic membrane is always present. This membrane is fenestrated, the area of fenestration representing on the order of 1% of the total membrane area. It would seem unlikely that the unfenestrated region of this membrane would pass substances of the molecular dimensions of lipoproteins. On the other hand, the relatively loose structure of the wall external to this membrane would probably allow such particles as lipoproteins to achieve egress either via lymph channels or vasa vasora.

Numerous authors (see Duff, 1954) have commented upon loss of integrity of the internal elastic membrane as a regular concomitant of the atherosclerotic lesion. The inference is often made that such loss of integrity represents a relatively early stage in the evolution of this disease. Yet the examination of such medium-sized muscular arteries as the coronary and cerebral arteries does not offer any support for this concept. Indeed, in over 5000 sections of coronary and cerebral arteries examined by us thus far, approximately 99% showed the atherosclerotic lesions to be confined to the intimal layer, with intact internal elastic lamellae present. These findings are distinctly in accord with the possible role of a relatively impenetrable internal elastic membrane as a factor in the genesis of the arterial lesion, or at least the early stages of the lesion.

The intriguing question has long existed concerning the predilection of the atherosclerotic lesion for the medium-sized muscular and the larger musculoelastic arteries in contrast with the essential absence of this particular lesion in the arteriole and capillary. Of interest relative to this question are the dimensional features of these several types of arteries.

TABLE I

MEASUREMENT OF DIFFERENT LAYERS OF ARTERIAL WALL
IN RELATIONSHIP TO ARTERIAL SIZE
(All measurements in μ)

Kind of arteries		Intima	Internal elastic membrane	Media	Adventitia	Inner diameter	Outer diameter
Medium-sized artery	(1)	7.36	6.78	104.0	20.9	—	—
	(2)	4.90	6.08	182.0	91.1	1370	2100
	(3)	5.78	3.71	211.5	71.0	1200	2000
	(4)	2.48	4.40	207.0	78.2	1000	2000
Arteriole	(1)	2.71	0.91	18.2	18.2	135	208
	(2)	2.71	Incomplete	5–15	15	—	100
Capillaries		2.7	None	None	None	6–8	15

The data obtained from measurements on sections of such vessels are presented in Table I. The measurements of medium-sized arteries show internal elastic membranes ranging in thickness from 4.4 to 6.8 μ. The arteriole shows a *much* thinner internal elastic membrane (~0.9 μ) and, within the limits of resolution by light microscopy, total absence of this structure in certain parts of the wall. The capillary shows no true elastic membrane, although there does exist the extremely thin basement membrane. Evidence has been presented that this structure of capillaries is permeable to particles of dimensions in the range of 100-200 A (Jennings *et al.*, 1962). The incompleteness of any internal elastic membrane structure in arterioles would be expected to facilitate passage of lipoproteins from the intimal space into the muscularis. Thus the lack of the relatively impenetrable internal elastic membrane could well account for the freedom of arteriole and capillaries from the atherosclerotic process.

B. Blood Pressure, Filtration, and Atherosclerosis

If a filtration process does operate to drive lipoproteins of plasma into the subendothelial space, it would be anticipated, all other factors being equal, that increased hydrostatic pressure intra-arterially would accelerate such filtration, and ultimately, the development of atherosclerosis. This fact would operate to bring into harmony certain features of the process that have appeared paradoxical to some workers. Thus, even though a vast body of evidence indicates that elevation of certain blood lipids (as lipoproteins) is associated with accelerated development of atherosclerosis, it is known that atherosclerosis can develop with relatively moderate blood lipid levels when arterial hypertension is present. If filtration of lipoproteins is involved in the pathogenesis of atherosclerosis, each factor, hypertension or elevated blood lipoprotein levels, would operate independently to accelerate the process. Both factors being in the unfavorable direction would be expected to produce the most marked effect. Since states of lipoproteinemia are essentially unknown in the population at large, the driving force (hypertension) would always have *some* substrate (plasma lipoproteins) upon which it would be operative to produce atherosclerotic disease.

Direct and indirect evidence, both in the human and in experimental animals, support the concept that increased intra-arterial pressure accelerates atherosclerosis development. Primary direct evidence is available through our own studies (Young *et al.*, 1960a) where a significant and reasonably high correlation was proved to exist between ante-mortem blood pressure levels and post-mortem quantitatively assessed atherosclerosis in several arterial beds (see Table II). In early studies (Gofman,

TABLE II

THE RELATIONSHIP OF BLOOD PRESSURE WITH DEGREE OF ATHEROSCLEROSIS
IN THE CORONARY AND CEREBRAL ARTERIES

(A) *Average Degree of Cerebral Atherosclerosis and Blood Pressure*

Age (years)	Cases (no.)	Degree of athero- sclerosis[a]	Blood pressure[b] (mm Hg)	Pearson co- efficient of cor- relation	Signif- icance test (p value)
60–69	19	19.4 ± 13.4	S 156 ± 33	0.71	< 0.001
			D 91 ± 17	0.69	< 0.001
70–79	49	19.5 ± 11.6	S 159 ± 35	0.32	< 0.05
			D 89 ± 15	0.30	∼ 0.05
80–89	27	19.2 ± 10.4	S 151 ± 13	0.40	< 0.05
			D 82 ± 15	0.66	< 0.001
60–89	95	19.4 ± 11.7	S 156 ± 31	0.44	< 0.001
			D 87 ± 15	0.50	< 0.001

(B) *Average Degree of Coronary Atherosclerosis and Blood Pressure*

60–69	19	37.3 ± 9.5	S 156 ± 33	0.56	< 0.01
			D 91 ± 17	0.42	< 0.05
70–79	49	36.9 ± 7.5	S 159 ± 35	0.09	N.S.
			D 89 ± 15	0.11	N.S.
80–89	27	36.3 ± 8.6	S 151 ± 23	0.01	N.S.
			D 82 ± 15	0.33	N.S.
60–89	95	36.8 ± 8.2	S 156 ± 31	0.19	∼ 0.05
			D 87 ± 15	0.27	< 0.01

[a] All values of degree of atherosclerosis are given in units of I/E, where $I =$ area of intimal material and $E =$ total arterial cross-section.

[b] Pressures (S = systolic, D = diastolic) recorded in the arm. All means given ± Standard Deviations.

1959) it was predicted from the blood pressure levels observed in subjects having previously experienced myocardial infarction in contrast to subjects in the population at large, that the risk of myocardial infarction could be calculated as a function of the habitual blood pressure level (see Section II concerning such indirect estimates of atherosclerotic involvement). The only qualification upon such risk estimates was based upon the possibility that the prior occurrence of myocardial infarction may have itself altered the habitual blood pressure level. By direct follow-up studies of a population sample at Framingham, Massachusetts, Dawber *et al.* (1957; Kagan *et al.,* 1962) have directly *measured* risk of coronary disease as a function of habitual blood pressure levels. There is good agreement between the earlier predictions of Gofman and the measured risks of the Framingham study.

Numerous experimental studies, in the dog and rabbit, have provided abundant direct evidence for the positive relationship between elevated blood pressure levels and the acceleration of development of atherosclerosis (Heptinstall and Porter, 1957; Moss *et al.*, 1951). In such studies, hyperlipidemias were present as well as hypertension, but the effect of variation of pressure, at any level of blood lipids, was quite clearly shown.

The effect of pressure in acceleration of filtration processes has been alluded to above and is consistent with this mechanism being considered as a probable basis for the observed associations between hypertension and the development of atherosclerosis, and, in all likelihood, the clinical manifestations of atherosclerosis.

The problem of major concern is one step beyond that of the effect of increased pressure in acceleration of penetration of lipids (as lipoproteins) into the subendothelial region. How long such lipoproteins remain, what changes they undergo there, and specifically how they might provide the basis for all the subsequent steps of atheroma formation are all questions requiring investigation and solution.

Several workers have attempted *in vitro* studies involving relatively acute perfusions of arterial sections (Wilens, 1951; Evans *et al.*, 1952). Goldberg and Morantz (1957) studied lipid infiltration into aortic walls under conditions more physiological than those of earlier studies. In the

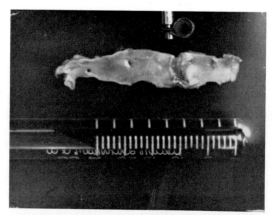

Fig. 3. Rabbit abdominal aorta shown here is the extensive atherosclerosis on the high pressure side of constrictor and the lesser degree of atherosclerosis on the low pressure side. The silver constrictor is shown just above the region of the aorta to which it had been applied during cholesterol feeding. (High pressure side to right of constrictor; low pressure side to left of constrictor.)

main all such *in vitro* studies indicate significant lipid infiltration into arterial walls during short perfusion periods. However, the shortness of the period of perfusion of such studies and the relatively unphysiological conditions employed made it essentially impossible to demonstrate convincingly the development of what might really be termed an atheroma or atherosclerotic lesion. Young (unpublished data) has designed experiments to demonstrate the pressure effect directly utilizing *in vivo* preparations. The abdominal aorta of rabbits was surgically constricted by the use of a silver constrictor (see Fig. 3). The rabbits, postoperatively, were maintained on a diet containing 0.5% cholesterol and 3% Wesson Oil by weight for a period of 6 months. Direct pressure measurements were made just before sacrifice by a cuff-transducer device (not requiring arterial juncture), above and below the constriction. Subsequently, quantitative grading of aortic atherosclerosis was performed in the regions at which the pressure during life had been measured. The results, presented in Table III, indicate clearly a positive association of degree

TABLE III

RELATIONSHIP BETWEEN DIRECT LOCAL PRESSURE MEASUREMENTS AND LOCAL DEGREE OF ATHEROSCLEROSIS (RABBIT AORTA)[a]

	Above constriction	Below constriction
Mean pressure	145 mm Hg	100 mm Hg
Mean degree of atherosclerosis	26.3 I/E units[b]	8.0 I/E units
Mean pulse pressure	33.1 mm Hg	21.3 mm Hg

[a] Pressure differences achieved by Silver Constrictor; 5 Rabbits.

[b] I/E units for degree of atherosclerosis similarly measured as in Table II.

of atherosclerosis with pressure at particular sites of the aorta. Inasmuch as the same blood bathed the regions above and below the constriction, the blood lipid concentration almost certainly must have been identical in the two regions. Our conclusion is that the difference in atherosclerosis is primarily, if not exclusively, related to the difference in pressure. Such data are consistent with observations in human coarctation of the aorta (Boyd, 1943).

In Fig. 4 are presented data relating pressure in the systemic circulation, vessel size, and atherosclerosis development. The degree of atherosclerosis is related to intravascular pressure and to the radius of the artery (Young *et al.,* 1960a).

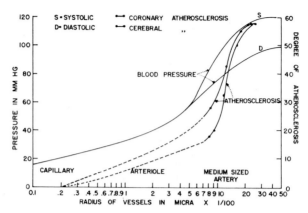

Fig. 4. Schematic diagram of variation of pressure as a function of vessel radius and of mean degree of atherosclerosis (in I/E units) for two critical arterial beds, coronary and cerebral, as a function of vessel radius. (Based upon subjects in the age range 60-100 years).

C. The Relationship of Lipoprotein Size to Atherosclerosis Development

That intravascular lipoprotein lipids do penetrate into the wall structure of arteries seems quite clear, from the evidence discussed above and from supplementary evidence. What mechanism is operative in such transfer? Various pathways have been proposed for the transfer of macromolecules and particles from arterial lumen to the wall structure itself. It has been suggestd that such passage may occur (a) via junction regions between endothelial cells (Chambers and Zweifach, 1947), (b) via some of the "pores" which constitute part of the endothelial lining (Pappenheimer, 1953), or (c) via vesicles of the endothelial cells, revealed by electron microscope studies (Palade, 1956; Bennett, 1956) as an active transport process. No direct estimate is possible concerning the possible influence or lipoprotein size or other properties upon such transfer, since the precise *mechanism* of the transfer is still speculative. However, considerable evidence has accumulated linking size of lipoproteins (and/or other properties that are size-related) with the process of atherosclerosis development. In early studies, Gofman and co-workers (1950) demonstrated that rabbits fed cholesterol develop *de novo* a spectrum of lipoproteins, of various ultracentrifugal flotation rates, such rates being highly related to size of lipoprotein. These observations indicated that certain lipoproteins were much more strongly related to the development of rabbit atherosclerosis than were others. Pierce (1952) confirmed and extended these studies, finding that lipoproteins of the S_f 10-30 class were more strongly associated with atherosclerosis development than were lipoproteins of lower or higher flotation classes (and correspondingly smaller and larger sizes). Furthermore his studies indicated that the mode of induction of hyperlipoproteinemia was not apparently crucial, but rather that the size of the lipoproteins determined the degree of atherosclerosis. These findings help greatly to understand otherwise paradoxical findings with respect to hyperlipoproteinemia and atherosclerosis. Thus, Duff and McMillan had observed (1949) that cholesterol-fed alloxan-diabetic rabbits developed minimal atherosclerosis in spite of hyperlipoproteinemia rarely equaled in other experimental preparations. Pierce determined that the hyperlipoproteinemia induced in this manner was in lipoprotein flotation classes (and size ranges) far higher than those (S_f 10-30 class) which are important for atherosclerosis. No intention exists to consider atherogenicity as *restricted* to a particular size region, or to deny possible importance of other features of the lipoproteins, but rather it is pointed out that atherogenicity seems maximal for S_f 10-30 lipoproteins and falls off markedly for lipoproteins of lower or higher flotation classes. Thus the relatively very small lipoproteins of the high-density classes have never, directly or indirectly, been implicated in atheroma formation. The experimental data in rabbits indicate extremely low atherogenicity for lipoproteins of flotation rates of S_f 100 and higher. If the transition be permissible, such data would argue strongly against a probable role of the extremely large lipoproteins, chylomicrons, which are a common feature of post-prandial lipemia. Certainly no direct evidence has yet been presented for a specific role of chylomicronemia *per se* in atherosclerosis development.

Recent studies of Young, Freeman, and Ng (unpublished data) have extended the observations of rabbit atherosclerosis in relation to lipoprotein level. Feeding to rabbits cholesterol dispersed in a variety of fats resulted in hyperlipoproteinemia. Measurements of degree of atherosclerosis at autopsy compared with lipoprotein level during cholesterol feeding resulted in the data and correlations presented in Table IV. While the banding of ultracentrifugal flotation classes differed somewhat from that of the earlier studies of Pierce, it appears clear that the atherogenicity is more strongly related to lipoproteins in the region of approximately S_f 15-30, falling off on both the low and the high side of this flotation class.

It is unfortunate that direct observations of this type are not yet available in the human. The prerequisites for obtaining such data on human populations make self-evident the reasons for paucity of such data. However, two types of studies in the human are available and both bear upon the question of atherogenicity as a function of lipoprotein type or size.

TABLE IV

CORRELATION OF AORTIC ATHEROSCLEROSIS IN RABBITS VERSUS LIPOPROTEIN CONCENTRATION[a]

Experimental group	Athero-sclerosis versus S_f 0–15 lipo-proteins	Athero-sclerosis versus S_f 15–30 lipo-proteins	Athero-sclerosis versus S_f 30–100 lipo-proteins	Athero-sclerosis versus S_f 100–400 lipo-proteins
19 Rabbits fed cholesterol in olive oil	0.45	0.46	0.61	0.39
18 Rabbits fed cholesterol in hydrogenated olive oil	—0.13	0.12	0.04	—0.15
16 Rabbits fed cholesterol in coconut oil	—0.07	0.58	0.00	—0.11
16 Rabbits fed cholesterol in safflower oil	—0.07	0.43	0.08	0.03

[a] Expressed as Pearson Correlation Coefficient, r.

Hanig and associates (1956) have reported on experimental efforts to isolate lipoproteins from atherosclerotic plaques obtained from freshly isolated human aortas. They found that the isolable lipoproteins were of the ultracentrifugal S_f 12-100 class. The fraction of total lipid present that was in lipoprotein form was small, but this should occasion no surprise since secondary denaturation of lipoprotein within the arterial wall undoubtedly would occur over the time periods required for atheroma formation. Such studies deserve extension and confirmation.

The other type of evidence concerning human atherosclerosis is indirect, but no less pertinent. The Donner Laboratory investigators have previously reported (Gofman *et al.*, 1953, 1954b; Tamplin *et al.*, 1954) the results of *prospective* studies of development of clinically documented coronary heart disease in subjects whose lipoprotein levels had been measured one to several years before the clinical manifestations of coronary disease developed. The series of documented cases of *de novo* coronary disease has now grown to 29 cases. That coronary heart disease and coronary artery atherosclerosis are distinct entities has been amply explained elsewhere (Gofman, 1959). Association of lipoprotein level has been studied in relation to clinical coronary heart disease, with no assumptions whatever concerning the variable *not* directly measurable, namely the quantitative degree of atherosclerosis. The summary of considerations relating atherosclerosis to clinical sequelae is that the probable mechanism whereby lipoprotein level becomes a measure of risk of development of coronary heart disease is via the acceleration of atherosclerosis which results from elevation of such levels. The degree of atherosclerosis, as measured by accumulation of atherosclerotic tissue within the intima, is considered to be a direct function of the integral of lipoprotein levels over time. Expressed otherwise, *rate of accumulation* of atherosclerotic tissue is considered to be *proportional* to the weighted combined level of the lipoproteins involved in the process. *Degree* of atherosclerosis is $= \int_0^t$ rate dt, as a first approximation. This concept in no way denies the importance of any other factors that may be operative. Thus, the local susceptibility of certain arterial beds, or parts of a single bed, well known and well documented, is considered to alter the *constant of proportionality* in the rate equation. Blood pressure level also is considered to operate to determine the constant of proportionality in the rate equation. To be sure it is possible that secondary processes, such as thrombosis, regression, or healing, or intimal hemorrhage might operate to render the rate equation a first approximation (as stated above), rather than a final quantitative estimate.

What is the status of this relationship of lipoprotein level with degree of or rate of development of atherosclerosis? The predictive nature of the association of blood lipoprotein level with a *major consequence of atherosclerosis*—coronary heart disease—is established beyond any reasonable doubt. A vast number of links in the chain of evidence point to a relationship with coronary atherosclerosis as being the intermediary mechanism whereby the clinical disease is predicted by the lipoprotein level. No evidence *inconsistent* with this concept has yet been put forth. No other mechanism that would explain the lipoprotein-coronary heart disease relationship has been proposed. Thus, all factors considered, the *hypothesis* that the mechanism is via lipoprotein level to atherosclerosis is reasonable and useful for further work. As a hypothesis, usefulness is contingent upon the extent to which new phenomena are correctly predicted and to the extent that new phenomena, validly demonstrated, do not conflict with it.

If we accept the license of utilization of this hypothesis, then valuable indirect evidence can be brought to bear upon the question of the role of lipoprotein size (and/or associated properties) in atherogenesis. The lipoproteins of several flotation classes were measured in 4088 healthy subjects that represented the "substrate" out of which developed the above-described 29 cases of documented clinical coronary heart disease. We do not, of course, know the quantitative degree of atherosclerosis in the 29 subjects who developed premature coronary heart disease subsequent to lipoprotein measurement, but our hypothesis would lead to the expectation that the degree of atherosclerosis in the coronary arteries of these 29 subjects is *higher* than in the population substrate out of which they developed. As a first approach to determination of which lipoproteins are most influential in producing the exaggerated degree of atherosclerosis, we can measure the extent to which any particular lipoprotein class is effective in *segregation* of the evolved coronary heart disease sample group from the population at large. It is *not* the difference in concentration of lipoproteins between these groups that determines segregating power, but rather this difference in relationship to the *variability* of lipoprotein level in the substrate population. The ratio

$$\frac{\text{Difference in lipoprotein concentration}}{\text{Standard deviation of distribution}}$$

provides, in standard score units (Guilford, 1956), a valid measure of segregation power. Both sets of data necessary for such calculations are presented for the series of 29 cases of *de novo* coronary disease and for the substrate population in Table V. Inspection of the standard scores of difference in levels (coronary group minus substrate population) shows Standard S_f 12-20 with the largest difference, and the remaining classes in the order Standard S_f 0-12, Standard S_f 20-100, and Standard S_f 100-400. This first approximation undoubtedly places the lipoproteins in the correct order of importance for coronary artery atherosclerosis and provides a reasonable quantitative comparison of importance. A much refined treatment is in order to determine the *independent* quantitative importance of each lipoprotein class. For, it is known from extensive measurement of lipoprotein interrelationships that the levels are correlated (see Table VI), though imperfectly so. The implication of these correlations is that it is possible for the mean level of a particular lipoprotein class to show apparent segregation of coronary atherosclerosis, when truly such apparent segregation results from the correlation of this lipoprotein level with levels of other lipoproteins that *do* show true segregation power. The linear discriminant analysis applied to such problems enables assessment of the independent contribution of each variable to a process such as atherosclerosis. Preliminary application of this method to data for myocardial infarction survivors contrasted with reference populations without overt clinical coronary disease were made using a split at S_f 12, i.e., for the Standard S_f 0-12 class and standard S_f 12-400 class (Gofman, 1954; Gofman *et al.*, 1954a). Those estimates led to a weighting factor of 1.75 for the S_f 12-400 class versus 1.0 for the

TABLE V

SEGREGATION POWER OF LIPOPROTEIN LEVELS FOR DE NOVO CORONARY HEART DISEASE ARISING OUT OF SUBSTRATE POPULATION[a]

Group	Standard S_f 0–12 lipoproteins	Standard S_f 12–20 lipoproteins	Standard S_f 20–100 lipoproteins	Standard S_f 100–400 lipoproteins
De Novo documented male clinical coronary heart disease group (29 cases)	444.1 mg/100 ml	88.5 mg/100 ml	146.9 mg/100 ml	81.0 mg/100 ml
Age-matched healthy male population substrate out of which coronary cases arose (4088 subjects)	386.0 mg/100 ml	57.6 mg/100 ml	110.3 mg/100 ml	68.0 mg/100 ml
Differences in means (de novo coronary cases minus healthy population substrate group)	+58.1 mg/100 ml	+30.9 mg/100 ml	+36.6 mg/100 ml	+13.0 mg/100 ml
p Values	$\ll 0.01$	$\ll 0.001$	< 0.01	~ 0.05
Standard deviation of distribution in healthy population substrate group	84 mg/100 ml	23 mg/100 ml	66 mg/100 ml	91 mg/100 ml
Difference in means expressed in standard score units	0.69	1.34	0.55	0.14

[a] Mean age = 47 years.

TABLE VI

The Correlation of Lipoprotein Levels of Several Classes
in 309 Ostensibly Healthy Men[a]

	S_f^o 0-12[b]	S_f^o 12-20	S_f^o 20-100	S_f^o 100-400	HDL_1	HDL_2	HDL_3
S_f^o 0-12 vs	1.00	+0.54	+0.08	+0.05	—0.01	—0.25	—0.10
S_f^o 12-20 vs	+0.54	1.00	+0.44	+0.22	—0.04	—0.27	—0.04
S_f^o 20-100 vs	+0.08	+0.44	1.00	+0.74	+0.15	—0.26	—0.18
S_f^o 100-400 vs	+0.05	+0.22	+0.74	1.00	+0.41	—0.18	—0.15
HDL_1 vs	—0.01	—0.04	+0.15	+0.41	1.00	—0.05	—0.04
HLD_2 vs	—0.25	—0.27	—0.26	—0.18	—0.05	1.00	+0.41
HDL_3 vs	—0.10	—0.04	—0.18	—0.15	—0.04	+0.41	1.00

[a] (Age group 40-49 years). (Expressed as Pearson Product-Moment Correlation, r).
[b] Standard S_f is abbreviated in the commonly accepted form, S_f^o.

S_f 0-12 class, and to a combined function designated as an "Atherogenic Index" where

$$\text{Atherogenic index (A.I.)} \equiv 0.1 \text{ (Standard } S_f 0\text{–}12) + 0.175 \text{ (Standard } S_f 12\text{–}400)$$

We have previously emphasized the uncertainties in derivation of the independent contributions of the several lipoprotein classes from such data. Foremost among the reservations are: (a) The lack of perfect assurance that the myocardial infarction survivors are truly representative of those who would have grown out of the reference populations studied. (b) The possibility that dietary, pharmacological, or way-of-life alterations may, in the myocardial infarction survivors, have altered the "steady-state" lipoprotein levels of the survivors.

Such reservations do not hold for a group of cases of coronary heart disease arising *prospectively* out of a substrate population. However, other factors militate against accurate assessment of quantitative contributions of the lipoprotein classes. First, the assignment of weighting factors is highly sensitive to the difference in mean levels of each lipoprotein class between the coronary disease group and the reference substrate group. While it is quite clear that the differences in mean levels for the four classes of lipoproteins (coronary minus noncoronary) are all significant, the confidence range on the values for these mean differences is still sufficiently large to make the weighting factors of insufficient reliability. The weighting factors are also sensitive to the magnitude of population variability (as measured by standard deviations) and to lipoprotein level interclass correlations. However, these two data arise out of the very large series of individuals in the substrate population and are much more reliably known than are the critical differences in lipoprotein means between the *de novo* coronary cases and the substrate population.

At this time, it seems preferable to use the relative strength of association of the several lipoprotein classes as measured in standard scores above, and to reserve for later (when the *de novo* series has grown further) an effort at precise assessment of independent contribution and weighting factors.

What emerges, therefore, from these crucial human data is that atherogenicity (at least for the coronary arteries) appears maximal for lipoproteins of the flotation range Standard S_f 12-20 and falls off toward the lipoproteins both higher and lower flotation classes. These evaluations are in close accord with all the data for experiments on rabbits discussed previously.

It was not possible in these particular human studies to make quantitative measurements of the segregation power of lipoproteins of flotation rates above Standard S_f 400, up to and including chylomicra. Of course, it is ultimately desirable to assess the quantitative contribution, if any, of these very large lipoproteins. In the experimental work with rabbits, all the evidence points (see above) to a minimal contribution, if any, of lipoproteins in this range of sizes. The marked fall-off in standard score difference from Standard S_f 12-20 to Standard S_f 20-100 to Standard S_f 100-400 for humans ($1.34 \rightarrow 0.55 \rightarrow 0.14$) suggests that atherogenicity would be anticipated to drop to negligible proportions for the large lipoproteins beyond the Standard S_f 400 class.

Why, both from human evidence and that in the rabbits studied experimentally, should lipoproteins of these intermediary size classes between the very small and very large lipoproteins be of crucial significance with respect to atherogenesis? A considerable body of evidence is by now available from studies of Hayes and Hewitt (1957) and Lindgren *et al.* (1951) dealing with both physical and chemical properties of all the lipoprotein species. Chemical composition studies have shown (Lindgren and Gofman, 1957; Lindgren *et al.,* 1955) that there are large differences extant among the lipoprotein classes in lipid distribution from class to class, as well as in the protein moiety. At present no assessment of the significance of internal chemical composition for atherogenesis is available, if it be pertinent. However, the physical property of size is of great interest. In Fig. 5 are presented data on physical dimensions of lipoproteins in relation to other parameters of interest.

The size ranges for the lipoproteins that show marked atherogenicity is in the range of dimensions of 200 to 800 A. This is comparable with

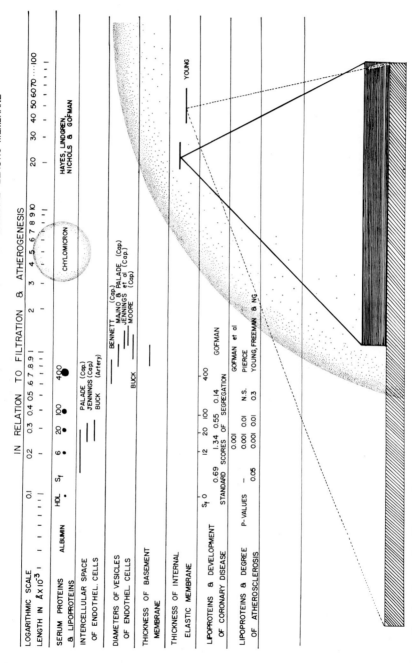

SOME PHYSICAL DIMENSIONS OF LIPOPROTEINS, ENDOTHELIAL CELLS & INTERNAL ELASTIC MEMBRANE
IN RELATION TO FILTRATION & ATHEROGENESIS

Fig. 5. Composite diagram demonstrating several interrelated features pertinent for the filtration concept of atherosclerosis. The dimensional comparison is shown in the hatched area below representing true thicknesses of internal elastic membranes in relation to the dimensions of lipoprotein shown as spheres above.

the general range of dimensions of the intercellular spaces of endo-thelium of capillaries and of similar spaces in arteries (Buck, 1958). Further, as is evident from Fig. 5, these lipoprotein sizes are either smaller or of the order of those of the vesicles of the endothelial cells of arterial walls. If either of these entities (intercellular space or vesicles) represents potential passageway for the lipoproteins into the subendothelial region, it would be clear why *larger* lipoprotein species would be unable even to gain access to the subendothelial region. Of course, this could not explain the lower atherogenicity of the relatively small lipoprotein classes.

Explanation of this latter facet of the problem would have to be sought in the fate of lipoproteins subsequent to entry into the subendo-thelial space. The physical extent to which the fenestrated internal elastic lamella might block passage of lipoproteins *from* subendothelial space as a function of size is at present speculative. It would be anticipated, however, that *if* any obstructive plugging of the fenestrae does occur, the obstruction to passage outward would be greater for S_f 12-30 lipo-proteins than for S_f 0-12, and correspondingly greater for S_f 0-12 than for the much smaller high-density lipoproteins.

On the other hand, passage outward via fenestrae might in general be slow and, in this event, the stability of the various lipoprotein classes against denaturation within the subendothelial space might be quite relevant in determination of which lipoproteins contribute to the ulti-mately accumulated lipid of atherosclerotic lesions.

Clearly, a major effort is still required to understand the fate of lipo-proteins in the region *between* the endothelium and the interal elastic membrane!

II. Serum Lipids in the Diagnosis of Atherosclerosis

A. General Aspects of the Problem of Diagnosis of Atherosclerosis

The simple fact is that atherosclerosis in the living human cannot be directly quantitated. This should serve to make evident the limitations that must surround a question such as the role of serum lipids in the *diagnosis* of atherosclerosis. To be sure, under unusual circumstances, certain surgical procedures might in rare instances provide for a semi-quantitative appraisal of degree of atherosclerosis in certain vascular beds during life, but this can hardly represent any general source of information upon which to base diagnostic studies.

We do not clinically diagnose atherosclerosis, but we are in a posi-tion to assess the quantitative risk of development of at least one of the major clinical consequences of atherosclerosis, namely the risk of future clinical coronary heart disease. In the preceding section of this chapter the basis was presented for believing that the quantity underlying risk of clinical coronary heart disease is very likely the *accumulated degree* of arterial *narrowing* produced by the evolving atherosclerotic process. Such accumulated narrowing is considered by us to represent an integrated value of *rate of accumulation operating over time*. Such rate of accumulation of atherosclerosis appears to be: (a) Proportional to the weighted sum of concentration of those lipoproteins involved in atherosclerosis (Standard S_f 0-12 through Standard S_f 100-400). (b) Proportional to the level of the blood pressure in the arterial region under consideration.

If one refuses to accept this explanation of the mechanism for the clearly established fact that risk of future clinical coronary heart disease is predictable from lipoprotein levels and, separately and independently, from blood pressure levels, then further discussion of serum lipids in the diagnosis of atherosclerosis is irrelevant and purposeless. Even in this event the great implications of lipoprotein levels and blood pressure levels in prediction of risk of clinical manifestations would still remain as valid as ever, since such estimates have been developed with no dependence whatever upon known or suspected relationship between atherosclerosis and clinical arterial disease. We consider the evidence as a whole to support the correctness of the proposed mechanism, namely blood lipoprotein and pressure levels representing *rate* factors in atherogenesis. Since no contradictory evidence is known to us, we shall develop further some of the diagnostic implications of such a mechanism.

Diagnosis is, by its very nature, a practical, clinical problem, although of course its results can be used to further research quests for understanding of disease. In either case, it is perhaps most useful to consider *limitations* upon the use of serum lipoprotein parameters diagnostically and then to consider the positive *contributions* of such use in solving important problems in clinical medicine. Lastly we shall consider possible choices in lipid parameters to be applied in such diagnostic use.

B. Limitations upon Diagnostic Applications of Serum Lipoprotein Measurements

1. THE PATHOLOGY VERSUS THE CLINICAL ENTITY

There are, of course, few individuals in middle or later life who are *free* of atherosclerosis. Thus answers in the form of—atherosclerosis, present or absent—will be essentially nonexistent. At best what might be hoped for would be an assessment, rough or fine, of the rate of atherogenesis and/or the accumulated degree of atherosclerosis. But even here, we are not coming to grips with the true clinical desideratum. A high rate of atherogenesis and/or a high degree of accumulated atherosclerosis may or may not produce a clinical sequel of consequence. There is no question about evaluation of *risk* of clinical consequence for an individual. However, some high-risk individuals will live to an old age, with massive atherosclerosis, only to die of totally unrelated causes. Clearly, in such a case, diagnosis of degree of atherosclerosis or its rate of development, fails to provide what the physician may wish to insist is his need. On the other side, the focal character of the atherosclerotic process, with its dependence upon local features in the arterial anatomy or physiology or both, may result in the death of a relatively young person of coronary heart disease if one critical centimeter of an artery is severely involved, even though over-all atherosclerosis is moderate or minimal. Such cases are definitely *not* the rule, but still they represent diagnostic errors if the serum lipids be expected to diagnose only that atherosclerosis which might lead to clinical sequelae. Indeed, no parameter related to the *general,* or systemic, aspects of atherosclerosis development can possibly overcome the limitation imposed by focality of the disease.

2. VARIABILITY IN BLOOD LIPOPROTEIN LEVEL

Any biological measurement, such as blood lipoprotein level, will show some degree of fluctuation if the measurement is made repeatedly upon the same person. Such fluctuation originates from at least two major sources. The first is what may be regarded as *biological* variation, the result of metabolic alterations within the individual that result in *true* change of the measured variable over a period of time. The second major source of variation is the result of technical error in measurment, and this would be observed even for two identical aliquots of a single specimen of blood. When a measurement is made, we ordinarily perceive directly the combined effect of biological variation and technical error.

If the blood lipoprotein level be considered in the form of the weighted sum of concentrations referred to above as the atherogenic index, and if the blood lipoproteins are to provide diagnostic information, it follows that variation from one sample to another *on the same person* will lead to movement up or down on the scale of predicted rate of devlopment of atherosclerosis, or its consequence, degree of atherosclerosis. The greater such variability in the atherogenic index is, the less valuable will the diagnostic information be, unless a number of repeat observations are made and diagnosis is based upon a mean value for the person. Therefore, it is considerable interest to know quantitatively the character of such variation in human subjects. Studies previously reported (Gofman, 1959) have been made of this variability. Since from other considerations it is known that dietary alterations can grossly influence atherogenic index values, it is desirable to consider this source of variability apart from the other factors described above. These studies were made on a large series of employed males as part of a routine periodic medical examination. Elimination, in some measure, of gross quantitative dietary alterations was achieved by exclusion of all subjects who had gained or lost 5 or more pounds of weight in the 1- to 3-year interval between examinations. There remained 213 men who qualified for study after this exclusion. The best approximation to the "true" atherogenic index value for these cases is the mean of the two measurements made upon each subject. The extent of variation over a 1- to 3-year period (including biological plus technical variation) is present in Table VII. While it is clear that gross misclassification must in

TABLE VII
ATHEROGENIC INDEX VARIATION OVER A 1- TO 3-YEAR PERIOD

Percentage of subjects showing variation	Variation from mean (in A.I. units)
58	Less than 5
25	5-10
13	10-15
4	15 (or more)

general be relatively rare, from the data of Table VII, the variability present is a limitation upon "diagnosis." Of course, one evident approach to minimization of such a source of diagnostic error is the use of multiple determinations to make the diagnostic assessment.

3. RATE OF ATHEROGENESIS VERSUS DEGREE OF ATHEROSCLEROSIS

A diagnostic evaluation from blood lipid measurement would, according to the hypothesis described above, provide information concerning the *rate of accumulation of atherosclerosis*. But, if our diagnostic objective be to know how far the over-all process has advanced in critical arterial regions at a given point in life, it is *degree* of atherosclerosis that is truly the datum needed. If it were known that the relative ranking of a group of individuals upon the variable of *rate* of atherogenesis remained constant, or nearly so, throughout life, it would follow that the relative degrees of atherosclerosis would be correctly predicted from the rates. Insufficient data are at this time available to assess the many possible influences operative over periods of 10 to 40 years of life that might alter the blood lipoproteins, and hence the *rate* measurement. For example, major dietary alterations could materially alter an individual's ranking with respect to rate of atherogenesis at a particular point in life, resulting in an erroneous prediction of degree of atherosclerosis which depends upon rates operative throughout life rather than that measured at a particular time. Other influences upon the rate of atherogenesis may well exist and be unappreciated at the current state of our knowledge.

4. SPECIAL DISEASE CATEGORIES

In certain specific diseases our interest in assessment of degree of atherosclerosis is especially high. Diabetes mellitus and myxedema are good illustrative examples. We are well aware of the profound alterations in lipoprotein levels that occur as a function of control and decontrol if diabetes mellitus (Kolb *et al.*, 1955; Strisower *et al.*, 1958). It is well nigh impossible to determine which degree of control best reflects the "steady state" value for a particular diabetic person. Hence the rate measurement may be too high if measured during relative decontrol, and too low if measured during a period of better than usual control. Parameters such as insulin dosage or dietary pattern may not suffice as indicators since so many factors, known and unknown, appear to influence the level of the metabolic error in the diabetic subject. The considerations in myxedema would follow along analogous lines.

In a sense, this problem is part of the same one of variability in the ostensibly healthy individual. However the difficulties may be magnified in special disease groups such as diabetes or myxedema.

C. Contributions of Serum Lipoprotein Measurement to the Diagnosis of Atherosclerosis

In spite of the limitations described above, there are several situations in which important contributions to the diagnosis of atherosclerosis can be made. Largely such diagnostic contributions are in the realm of false diagnoses based upon other criteria. Some of the prime illustrations are presented in the ensuing discussion.

1. FAMILY HISTORY

The existence of genetically determined *major* disorders in blood lipoprotein levels is known to all workers in this field. One is the Standard S_f 0-20 hyperlipoproteinemia which is frequently accompanied by arcus senilis, xanthelasma, and xanthoma tendinosum. Another is the

S_f 20-400 hyperlipoproteinemia (usually with S_f 0-20 hypolipoproteinemia), frequently accompanied by xanthoma tuberosum (Gofman *et al.,* 1954c). In both these hyperlipoproteinemias the inheritance is such that certain members of a sibship may escape the hypelipoproteinemia. This important fact is often overlooked clinically. The high rate of premature death from the sequelae of atherosclerosis in both types of hyperlipoproteinemia is well documented. As a result numerous persons who belong to families with a history of the disease have been erroneously advised that the unfavorable family history makes their personal outlook poor with respect to premature arterial disease. For those *who have escaped the inheritance* of the hyperlipoproteinemia, such a prognosis is among the most grave of medical errors, since the outlook for these individuals is not that of those with the hyperlipoproteinemia. The proper diagnosis (and prognosis) in such persons is made through the evaluation of serum lipid status, and at present, in no other way. Obviously, if xanthomata are present, the existence of the hyperlipoproteinemia in the particular individual is assured, but otherwise serum lipid analysis can provide the correct information.

In the population at large, exclusive of the extreme derangements of serum lipoprotein levels, it has also been demonstrated that lipoprotein levels represent an important factor related to the familial cardiovascular disease incidence rate (Gofman 1959). Therefore in this circumstance too, an overzealous emphasis upon family history may lead to an erroneous diagnosis of probable excessive atherogenesis. Here, again, certain family members escape the heritable lipoprotein abnormality and may indeed show very favorable serum lipoprotein distributions. For *these* persons, the unfavorable family history is truly irrelevant, at least with regard to that part of the family tendency to excessive atherosclerosis which is the result of the heritable lipoprotein abnormality.

2. DIABETES MELLITUS

Wholly aside from the problem of variability of lipoprotein level as a function of diabetic control and decontrol, there is the larger problem of blood lipoprotein levels in the group of entities known as "diabetes mellitus." In a diffuse way the opinion is widespread that diabetics show premature atherosclerosis and the clinical consequences thereof. The diffuseness is, no doubt, the result of the lack of clear definition of diabetes mellitus as any single entity. In any event, physicians are prone to consider the outlook for atherosclerotic complications unfavorable for the diabetic patient simply because he is diabetic. Indeed, wholly without adequate foundation, it is commonplace for statements to be made that, while insulin has prevented deaths due to keto-acidosis and coma, it has done very little to prevent atherosclerotic complications. Yet, quantitative considerations, within the limits of the available evidence, indicate *that the same factors* are determinative of atherosclerotic complications in the diabetic as are operative in any other patient, namely the level of the critical serum lipoproteins and the level of the blood pressure. No evidence for a *specific diabetes factor* in atherogenesis has yet been presented.

Under such circumstances it is clear that serum lipid measurement can make a positive diagnostic contribution in the case of the diabetic person. If the serum lipids present a favorable picture with respect to atherogenesis rate, then this major aspect of the diabetic's hazard is minimal. There would then remain the problem of blood pressure, but at least a falsely poor prognosis with respect to atherosclerosis could be avoided. Why some patients with diabetes mellitus show extremely unfavorable lipoprotein distributions is an unsolved metabolic problem, but without doubt, a sizable proportion of persons with diabetes mellitus must be developing atherosclerosis at a rate slower than that for many nondiabetic persons in the population at large.

3. HYPERTENSION AND HYPERTENSIVE DISEASE

The hypertensive individual is known to suffer the complications of atherosclerosis with a higher frequency than does the normotensive individual, all other factors being equal. This is, of course, expected since elevated blood pressure ranks along with elevated serum lipoprotein level as a prime, independent factor in determining risk of complications of atherogenesis.

Two important issues deserve emphasis with respect to hypertension:

(a) Atherogenesis rate is proportional both to blood pressure level *and* to lipoprotein level. Thus high levels of both measures imply the poorest prognostic combination with respect to this disease process.

(b) While there is a slight correlation of blood pressure level with serum lipoprotein level, it cannot be overemphasized that the correlation is *very weak*. Thus, essentially, the lipoprotein level is hardly determined at all by the blood pressure level.

Since atherosclerosis is so prominent a hazard for the hypertensive individual, any aid in the diagnosis of atherosclerosis in such subjects is of great clinical importance. Here serum lipids can be very helpful. The hypertensive individual with a very low level of the atherogenically important serum lipoproteins may be regarded as developing atherosclerosis at a slower rate than that half of the population at large ranking above the median atherogenic index value. The hypertensive individual with a high serum lipoprotein level possesses a most unfavorable outlook with respect to atherosclerosis—worse than almost any group save for the cases of genetically determined massive serum lipoprotein distortions. In providing the information upon which a vigorous program of prevention or therapeusis may be based for the hypertensive subject, the serum lipid measurements can prove quite helpful diagnostically.

4. THE "OVERWEIGHT" PROBLEM

No subject has been more controversial with respect to atherosclerosis than that of the role of overweight. Our estimate of the best evidence is that the consequences of atherosclerosis and atherosclerosis itself are more prominent, in a group sense, for overweight persons than those of usual or low relative weight (Dublin, 1930; Dublin and Marks, 1951). However, so imperfect is the association that atherosclerosis can be extreme in underweight individuals and moderate or minimal in overweight persons. The reasonable implication of these findings is that overweight *per se* must be relatively or totally unimportant in acceleration of the process of atherosclerosis. A direct test of the possible independent contribution of overweight has previously been made for a major sequel of atherosclerosis, namely clinical coronary heart disease (Gofman, 1959). This study indicated, first, that overweight is positively, but quite imperfectly, associated with diastolic blood pressure level and with serum lipoprotein level (expressed as atherogenic index value). Indeed, when these two imperfect associations are taken into account, it has been demonstrated that the contribution of overweight to coronary disease is essentially completely explained. No residual *independent* contribution of overweight *per se* to risk of coronary heart disease can be discerned, and for the purposes of this discussion, this would imply that no residual contribution of overweight to *rate* of atherogenesis exists.

The diagnostic implication of these findings is of importance. Countless persons have been left with the impression that their state of overweight is of itself productive of an increased risk of development of premature atherosclerosis. For any individual, however, the imperfection of the overweight-atherogenic index correlation and the overweight-blood pressure correlation is so great, that a truly fat person can have *low* atherogenic index and blood pressure values. No evidence exists that should properly lead to an expectation of excessive atherosclerosis in such a person. Here is an instance where serum lipids can provide valuable diagnostic information: (a) to discern those overweight individuals who have "escaped" the group correlations and who, hence, should not be falsely diagnosed as atherosclerosis-prone and (b) to identify these in whom overweight, via effect upon serum lipoprotein levels, is be-speaking the need for further investigation of atherogenic risk.

5. ATHEROGENESIS IN MEN AND WOMEN

Atherosclerosis is, on the average, more severe in men than in women, especially above the age of 30 years (White *et al.,* 1950; Winter *et al.,* 1958). The consequences of atherosclerosis such as clinical coronary heart disease, are quite clearly more frequent in men than women on an age specific rate basis, even to the eighth decade of life (U.S. Vital Statistics, 1959; Gofman, 1959). So marked is the difference in incidence rate be-tween men and women that clinical impression has exceeded the bounds of the evidence with such statements as, "The consequences of athero-sclerosis are unheard-of in pre-menopausal women," or "post-menopaus-ally, women lose their protection against atherosclerosis and its con-sequences."

The evidence on this question indicates that the major part, and possibly all, of the male-female difference has its origin in the blood lipo-protein and blood pressure differences between the sexes. What the mechanism of the sex difference is upon blood lipoprotein and pressure levels has not been delineated as yet. Some mechanism exists, and it is of the highest importance that future work seek to discover it. For our considerations here, however, the crucial issue is that a diagnostic clean bill of health cannot be given to a pre-menopausal women with respect to atherogenesis, for she may be characterized by a high lipoprotein level, a high blood pressure, or both. Conversely, the post-menopausal woman, as an individual, will frequently be characterized by a low lipoprotein level, a low blood pressure or both. Thus, here again is an area where measurement of serum lipids can make a positive contribution to diag-nosis of status with respect to atherogenesis, where otherwise erroneous generalizations might prevail.

D. The Basis for Possible Choice of Lipid Parameters for Diagnostic Purposes

The literature by this time is overcrowded with studies of serum lipids in the "diagnosis" of atherosclerosis, or more usually in the segregation of subjects with respect to risk of a clinical sequel of atherosclerosis. A high proportion of the reported studies make the claim either that the particular system employed or the parameter measured does a better job of segregation of "atherosclerotics" from "nonatherosclerotics" than do all other tests. And from this the authors go on to state that the particular parameter of their interest must be more closely related to atherogenesis than all others. Specific reference to the host of such studies is hardly worthwhile, inasmuch as the errors, presumptions, and poor quantitative handling of the data invalidate conclusions of any sort.

Instead it may be profitable to consider the general outlines of a rational basis for understanding how a choice might be made if it were desirable to do so. First, we must start with the conclusion that *does* survive the manhandling characteristic of so many studies—namely, that serum lipid levels do provide some information concerning the process of atherosclerosis. The maximal information contained in the serum lipid status is, of course, all one can hope to retrieve no matter what parameter is measured or what system of measurement is used. Further, since measurements are never perfect, it is clear that some information is necessarily lost in the process of measurement. Methodologies differ in extent of information loss, wholly aside from the question of whether the most important parameters are even being measured. A first type of loss is that known as technical error. To the extent that the proper *parameter* is being measured, a method of choice will be one with a minimum technical error, or, alternately, the maximal reproducibility upon repeat measurements of the same sample.

The next type of loss is that which results from biological variation in the parameter measured. Whichever parameter is under consideration, it appears likely that the feature of importance relative to diagnostic information would be the *central* value of the parameter. Whether that central value be the mean over a time period, the median over a time period, the mode, or even some complicated function of the parameter other than these three, it will in any event be true that the information loss in a single measurement will be the larger, the greater is the biological tendency for the parameter to deviate from the central value at one time compared with another. In assessment of such biological variation it is crucial to correct out variation due to technical error.

We may now turn to the entities themselves in which the information resides. The blood lipids exist biologically in the form of a host of lipoproteins, utilizing this term in the broad sense that any entity of blood plasma which contains any lipid substances in some manner bound to protein (or polypeptide) may be regarded as lipoprotein. This would mean that chylomicra as well as albumin-fatty acid complexes can be considered as lipoproteins. An attempt to specify the nature of bonding forces is indeed premature at this time as a criterion for the designation lipoprotein. Atherosclerosis, in so far as it is at all related to serum lipids, must be related to one or more of the following:

(a) Specific lipoprotein entities, as characterized by size, electrical properties, bonding type, or other physical properties.

(b) Ratios of levels of certain lipoproteins.

(c) Specific chemical subconstituents of lipoproteins, such as tri-glycerides, cholesterol, cholesterol esters, phospholipids, fatty acids, etc. Further, each subconstituent represents a melange of further subconstituents (e.g., triglycerides of plasma are subdivided on the basis of the type of fatty acid incorporated into the triglyceride).

(d) Ratios of specific chemical subconstituents.

Many properties included from (a) through (d) are interrelated, although imperfectly so. Hence measurement of one item will, to the extent of such correlation, provide information concerning another item that is imperfectly correlated with it. Should the latter item be the crucial one with respect to atherogenesis, then the measurement of the *former* one, even perfectly executed technically, must necessarily involve a *loss of information* relative to the potential information available.

At the present time there exists no reliable way to estimate what fraction of the total potential information resides in a particular item listed in (a) through (d). A vast sea of knowledge as yet unavailable must be explored before this fraction can be ascertained. The filtration concept of atherogenesis points strongly to the importance of the information content which resides in lipoprotein size. Direct animal experimentation underlies the constructs of the filtration concept. If lipoprotein size be paramount, it would follow that a parameter such as total serum triglyceride, total lipid, or total cholesterol must necessarily provide *less* information than the measurement of the appropriate lipoprotein entities themselves. On the other hand it is entirely possible that chemical constitution of lipoproteins varies even at a particular molecular size, or that chemical bonding internally may vary at a particular size—and that one or both of these features may provide critical information with respect to atherogenesis. Slowly, and laboriously, such points will be evaluated, and the fraction of information retrievable for diagnostic purposes will increase. In the interim, and in the absence of definite final answers, it is both appropriate and useful that various workers will utilize one or more parameters as diagnostics aids. Such use will lead to hypotheses and to experiments designed to test hypotheses. Some hypotheses will be validated, others discarded. Any solid addition to our knowledge of the evolution of the atherosclerotic lesions thereby won will certainly justify the diagnostic utilization of a particular parameter, even though it be imperfectly and indirectly related to atherogenesis.

REFERENCES

Anitschkow, N. (1933). *In* "Arteriosclerosis" (E. V. Cowdry, ed.), p. 271. McMillan, New York.

Bennett, H. S. (1956). *J. Biophys. Biochem. Cytol.* **2** (Suppl.), 99-103.

Boyd, W. (1943). "A Textbook of Pathology," p. 77. Lea & Febiger, Philadelphia, Pennsylvania.

Buck, R. C. (1958). *J. Biophys. Biochem. Cytol.* **4**, 187-190.

Chambers, R., and Zweifach, B. W. (1947). *Physiol. Rev.* **27**, 436-463.

Courtice, F. C., and Garlick, D. G. (1962). *Quart. J. Exptl. Physiol.* **47**, 211-220.

Dawber, T. R., Moore, F. B., and Mann, G. V. (1957). *Am. J. Public Health* **47**, 4-24.

Dublin, L. (1930). *Human Biol.* **2**, 159.

Dublin, L. and Marks, H. (1951). *60th Annual Meeting of the Association of Life Insurance Medical Directors of America* New York, Oct. 11, 12, 1951. **35**, 235-266, 1952.

Duff, G. L. (1954). *In* "Symposium on Atherosclerosis," pp. 33-41. Natl. Acad. Sci., Natl. Res. Council, Washington, D.C.

Duff, G. L., and MacMillan, G. C. (1949). *J. Exptl. Med.* **89**, 611-630.

Evans, S. M., Ihrig, H. K., Means, J. A., Zeit, W., and Haushalter, E. R. (1952). *Am. J. Clin. Pathol.* **22**, 354.

Gofman, J. W. (1954). *Trans. Am. Coll. Cardiol.* **4**, 230-234.

Gofman, J. W. (1959). "Coronary Heart Disease" p. 58. C. C Thomas, Springfield, Illinois.

Gofman, J., Lindgren, F., Elliott, H., Mantz, W., Hewitt, J., Strisower, B., and Herring, V. (1950). *Science* **111**, 166.

Gofman, J., Strisower, B., deLalla, O., Tamplin, A., Jones, H., and Lindgren, F. (1953). *Mod. Med. (Minneapolis)* **21**, 119-140.

Gofman, J. W., deLalla, O., Glazier, F., Freeman, N., Lindgren, F., Nichols, A., Strisower, B., and Tamplin, A. (1954a). *Plasma* **2**, 414-484.

Gofman, J. W., Glazier, F., Tamplin, A., Strisower, B., and deLalla, O. (1954b). *Physiol. Rev.* **34**, 404-411.

Gofman, J., Rubin, L., McGinley, J., and Jones, H. (1954c). *Am. J. Med.* **17**, 514-520.

Goldberg, L., and Morantz, D. J. (1957). *J. Pathol. Bacteriol.* **74**, 1-15.

Guilford, J. P. (1956). "Fundamental Statistics in Psychology and Education," pp. 489-493. McGraw-Hill, New York.

Hanig, M., Shainoff, J. R., and Lowy, A. D. (1956). *Science* **124**, 176.

Hayes, T., and Hewitt, J. (1957). *J. Appl. Physiol.* **11**, 425-428.

Heptinstall, R. H., and Porter, K. A. (1957). *Brit. J. Exptl. Pathol.* **38**, 389.

Jennings, M. A., Marchesi, V. T., and Florey, H. (1962). *Proc. Roy. Soc.* **B156**, 14-19.

Kagan, A., Dawber, T. R., Kannel, W. B., and Revotskie, N. (1962). *Federation Proc.* **21**, 52-57.

Kellner, A. (1954). *In* "Symposium on Atherosclerosis," pp. 42-49. Natl. Acad. Sci., Natl. Res. Council, Washington, D. C.

Kolb, F., deLalla, O., and Gofman, J. W. (1955). *Metab. Clin. Exptl.* **4**, 310-317.

Landis, E. M. (1934). *Physiol. Rev.* **14**, 404-481.

Lindgren, F., and Gofman, J. W. (1957). *Bull. Schweiz. Akad. Med. Wiss.* **13**, 152.

Lindgren, F., Elliott, H., and Gofman, J. W. (1951). *J. Phys. Colloid Chem.* **55**, 80-93.

Lindgren, F., Nichols, A., and Freeman, N. (1955). *J. Phys. Chem.* **59**, 930-938.

Moss, W. G., Kiely, J. P., Neville, J. B., Bourque, J. E., and Wakerlin, G. E. (1951). *Federation Proc.* **10**, 94.

Palade, G. (1956). *J. Biophys. Biochem. Cytol.* **2** (Suppl.), 85-98.

Pappenheimer, J. R. (1953). *Physiol. Rev.* **14**, 404-481.

Pierce, F. T. (1952). *Circulation* **5**, 401.

Strisower, E., Weed, R., Gofman, J. W., Strisower, B., and deLalla, O. (1958). *J. Clin. Endocrinol. Metab.* **18**, 721-735.

Tamplin, A., Strisower, B., deLalla, O., Gofman, J. W., and Glazier, F. (1954). *J. Geront.* **9**, 404-411.

United States Vital Statistics, 1959 Tables. Data on Mortality (1959).

White, N., Edwards, J., and Dry, T. (1950). *Circulation* **1**, 645.

Wilens, S. L. (1951). *Science* **114**, 389.

Winter, M., Sayra, G., Millikan, C., and Barker, N. (1958). *Circulation* **18**, 7.

Young, W., Gofman, J. W., Tandy, R., Malamud, N., and Waters, E. (1960a). *Am. J. Cardiol.* **6**, 294-299.

Young, W., Gofman, J. W., Tandy, R., Malamud, N., and Waters, E. (1960b). *Am. J. Cardiol.* **6**, 300-308.

—7—

The Relationship of Sex and Gonadal Hormones to Atherosclerosis

Jeremiah Stamler

I. The Sex Differential in Atherosclerotic Coronary Disease

In 1912, Herrick made his historic contribution concerning the recognition of nonfatal acute coronary occlusion as a clinical syndrome. In the decades that followed, this disease came to be generally recognized by physicians, and an extensive knowledge was accumulated with respect to its manifestations in patients. Among many observations, a key one related to its sex predilection. A definite impression was recorded that clinical coronary heart disease, particularly myocardial infarction, was far more common among men than women, at least during the middle decades of life (Gertler *et al.*, 1951; Glendy *et al.*, 1953; Katz and Stamler 1953).

Accumulated statistics on large populations have abundantly confirmed this clinical inference. Thus mortality data for the United States reveal that throughout middle-age death rates attributed to arteriosclerotic heart disease are several fold higher in white males than white females (Table I) (Stamler *et al.*, 1960a; Moriyama *et al.*, 1958; Stamler, 1962, 1963). This sex differential gradually decreases, but never disappears completely.

TABLE I

MORTALITY RATES PER 100,000 UNITED STATES POPULATION, 1960, FROM ALL CAUSES,
ARTERIOSCLEROTIC HEART DISEASE, AND OTHER MAJOR CARDIOVASCULAR-RENAL
DISEASES

Sex and color	Age group	All causes	Cardio-vascular renal diseases	Arterio-sclerotic heart disease	Hyper-tensive disease	Cerebro-vascular diseases
All	All	954.7	521.8	275.6	44.1	108.0
White, male	All	1,098.5	604.4	368.0	34.7	102.7
	25–29	152.1	16.3	4.3	0.5	2.6
	30–34	173.2	34.6	15.8	1.5	4.3
	35–39	253.4	81.6	50.1	3.2	8.1
	40–44	417.0	178.3	124.2	6.8	14.7
	45–49	709.3	347.9	254.9	13.4	28.7
	50–54	1,183.3	625.6	462.6	25.7	54.7
	55–59	1,784.6	989.8	719.0	46.4	97.1
	60–64	2,751.4	1,590.5	1,119.1	78.4	189.1
	65–69	4,050.7	2,444.3	1,622.0	136.9	361.0
	70–74	5,909.2	3,734.3	2,291.1	228.3	687.1
	75–79	8,698.7	5,820.0	3,243.2	378.5	1,253.8
	80–84	13,544.3	9,480.0	4,802.5	647.6	2,195.1
	85 & >	21,750.0	15,977.8	7,248.7	1,090.9	3,734.8
White, female	All	800.9	458.1	215.1	43.4	110.1
	25–29	71.6	12.5	1.0	0.4	2.6
	30–34	97.1	17.8	2.7	0.9	4.1
	35–39	147.5	30.3	6.5	1.9	6.7
	40–44	237.9	61.3	19.4	4.7	13.7
	45–49	368.5	109.0	40.8	9.9	25.3
	50–54	560.3	198.0	85.6	18.7	43.3
	55–59	829.7	357.0	183.6	34.4	69.0
	60–64	1,362.2	706.2	384.4	67.8	141.6
	65–69	2,154.9	1,261.5	687.5	123.8	265.1
	70–74	3,583.2	2,330.9	1,211.0	236.8	535.6
	75–79	6,084.2	4,277.1	2,053.9	428.3	1,092.0
	80–84	10,654.3	7,903.0	3,508.1	757.1	2,091.7
	85 & >	19,477.7	14,998.9	6,233.7	1,278.7	3,795.7
Nonwhite, male	All	1,152.0	491.7	190.7	80.5	118.2
	25–29	343.0	44.7	7.4	7.6	7.9
	30–34	428.6	86.1	23.7	16.8	16.2
	35–39	599.2	174.3	62.7	39.1	27.7
	40–44	876.5	331.8	116.1	77.1	63.3
	45–49	1,241.5	546.1	224.8	106.1	119.9
	50–54	1,916.2	923.3	382.1	170.2	200.1

TABLE I *(Continued)*

Sex and color	Age group	All causes	Cardio-vascular renal diseases	Arterio-sclerotic heart disease	Hyper-tensive disease	Cerebro-vascular diseases
	55–59	2,500.5	1,338.3	556.1	233.0	313.3
	60–64	4,053.8	2,293.0	956.0	376.1	547.2
	65–69	5,103.7	2,998.1	1,187.7	496.0	762.9
	70–74	6,493.2	3,996.6	1,565.9	595.7	1,024.2
	75–79	7,628.0	4,813.6	1,849.4	712.5	1,240.6
	80–84	11,017.4	7,295.4	2,716.6	968.2	1,910.2
	85 & >	15,238.7	10,356.8	3,574.5	1,329.7	2,675.3
Nonwhite, female	All	872.6	421.7	131.7	84.2	121.2
	25–29	210.2	46.7	5.4	7.2	11.5
	30–34	307.8	82.9	13.1	17.4	20.6
	35–39	448.1	151.6	31.4	42.5	37.2
	40–44	660.8	275.2	64.2	74.5	73.7
	45–49	919.4	436.1	124.7	106.3	121.2
	50–54	1,419.5	738.3	220.7	176.4	207.9
	55–59	1,951.8	1,138.7	366.2	249.9	330.4
	60–64	3,019.5	1,889.0	636.9	392.0	561.0
	65–69	3,474.4	2,281.3	754.4	455.6	698.1
	70–74	4,742.5	3,281.3	1,110.9	603.2	964.0
	75–79	5,879.2	4,094.7	1,368.1	748.5	1,211.2
	80–84	8,477.5	6,168.3	1,980.1	1,052.7	1,768.8
	85 & >	12,871.2	9,330.6	3,706.3	1,306.0	2,510.2

Recent prospective epidemiological studies in United States living population groups have confirmed that middle-aged women are remarkably insusceptible to heart attacks compared with men. Thus, the National Heart Institute study of over 5000 men and women in Framingham, Massachusetts reported 8-year heart attack rates of 21 and 0 per 1000 men and women respectively age 30-39 at entry. The rates were 48 and 7 respectively at age 40-49; 94 and 20 for men and women respectively at age 50-59 (Kannel *et al.*, 1963).

Analyses of consecutive autopsies have yielded data consistent with the clinical and epidemiological findings concerning the sex differential. Thus, several studies by pathologists demonstrated that fatal coronary atherosclerosis is less common in men than in women of the same age in the United States, and that atherosclerotic lesions are less severe (Clawson and Bell, 1949; White *et al.*, 1950; Ackerman *et al.*, 1950; Roberts *et al.*, 1959).

II. The Theoretical Problem

Modern thinking views atherosclerosis as a disease having multiple causes (Stamler, 1958b, 1959, 1960; Stamler *et al.*, 1963c; Katz *et al.*, 1958). Its etiology involves complex interrelations among many exogenous (environmental) and endogenous (host) factors. What, then, are the factors responsible for the sex differential? More specifically, is it endocrine in origin, attributable to gonadal function? If so, how are the hormonal influences intertwined with other factors implicated in the etiology and pathogenesis of the disease—e.g., diet, cholesterol-lipid-liproprotein metabolism, blood pressure, and smoking? This paper aims to review available evidence bearing upon these significant problems. In addition, it attempts to survey the status of therapeutic efforts based upon research advances concerning the influence of gonadal hormones on the development of atherosclerosis.

III. Animal Experimental Studies

In 1949, animal experiments on these problems were undertaken in chicks (Katz and Stamler, 1953; Stamler, 1958b; Katz *et al.*, 1958; Pick *et al.*, 1952a). They involved an analysis of the effects of estrogens in birds fed atherogenic diets containing significant amounts of cholesterol and fat. It is essential for theoretical clarity to keep firmly in mind the nature of the diets used throughout these studies, i.e., the fact that they were high in cholesterol and fat.

One objective of these investigations was to test the hypothesis that estrogens might have an anti-atherogenic effect. It was recognized that animal-experimental data bearing upon this problem might by inference throw light on the question: Are estrogens responsible for the insusceptibility of women to atherosclerotic disease in middle age?

The initial experiment was of the "prophylactic" type, i.e., estrogens were administered to cockerels simultaneously transferred to an atherogenic diet composed of chick starter mash supplemented with cholesterol plus cottonseed oil. As had been anticipated, the diet induced a hypercholesterolemic hyperlipemia, and the estrogens a marked enhancement of phospholipemia, with consequent maintenance of cholesterol:phospholipid (C:P) ratios at or near normal levels (Pick *et al.*, 1952a). The hormone, given parenterally (1 mg of estradiol benzoate in oil daily), also feminized the cockerels, as indicated by alterations in their combs and other secondary sex characteristics. It should be noted parenthetically that this dosage of estradiol benzoate was arrived at in preliminary studies wherein a trial had been made of varying dosages ranging from 0.1 to 3.0 mg per bird per day. The criterion for desired dosage was the amount of hormone needed to alter the plasma lipid patterns of cockerels to those prevailing in mature, egg-laying, estrogen-secreting hens. Thus an attempt was made to utilize an estrogen dosage that was essentially physiological, based on known endocrine-lipid metabolic interrelations in the female of this avian species.

After several weeks of this experimental regimen the two groups of birds were sacrificed and studied histologically. Gross examination quickly revealed the presence of marked atherogenesis in the aortas of both groups. The estrogen-treated birds had at least as much aorta atherosclerosis as did the controls, similarly fed cholesterol-fat but receiving no hormone. In subsequent detailed histological studies, however, it became apparent that the estrogen-treated birds—in marked contrast to the controls—were practically free of lesions in the coronary arterial tree. Thus, segmental differences in atherogenesis were demonstrated, indicating that both systemic metabolic factors and local factors influence the process of atherogenesis. Incidentally, these findings made it necessary to draw the conclusion that experimentalists cannot rely exclusively upon aorta atherogenesis as an index of the occurrence of lesions throughout the arterial tree. It is noteworthy that to this day, almost 15 years since the original experiments, no adequate explanation has been elucidated for the different effects of estrogens on atherogenesis in the aorta versus the coronary arteries of cholesterol-fat-fed cockerels.

Another significant correlation suggested itself from the findings of this experiment, that is, between C:P ratios and coronary atherogenesis. The data suggested that estrogen-induced inhibition of coronary lesions may be closely interlinked in individual birds with maintenance of C:P ratios below 0.75 to 0.80 (normal: 0.35 to 0.60). Hence this study yielded suggestive (although not definite) experimental support for one of the hypotheses that it was originally designed to test, namely, that C:P ratio elevation (rather than hypercholesterolemia *per se*) is decisive in coronary atherogenesis. This, however, is a problem that is still by no means fully resolved. Thus, it remains a puzzle why—if a systemic lipid metabolic factor is the key—the outcome is different in aorta versus coronary arteries.

Finally, this initial study, by demonstrating that estrogens are capable of preventing experimental cholesterol-induced atherosclerosis in the coronary arterial tree of cockerels, brought forward for the first time experimental evidence supporting the hypothesis that the human sex differential in susceptibility to coronary heart disease may be, at least in part, a resultant of ovarian hormonal secretion.

In subsequent studies it was soon demonstrated that oral administration of mixed conjugated equine estrogens was equally effective in accomplishing the decisive triad of hormone effects: feminization, altered plasma lipid patterns, and prevention of coronary atherogenesis (Katz and Stamler, 1953; Katz *et al.*, 1958; Stamler *et al.*, 1956). In other experiments it was also shown that several synthetic estrogens, given at oral or parental dosage levels adequate to accomplish feminization, also maintained normalization of C:P ratios and prevented coronary atherogenesis in cholesterol-fed cockerels. On the other hand, inability to induce anti-atherogenesis was also recorded with a number of synthetic estrogen analogues of low feminizing potency. Invariably, failure of a compound to feminize in relatively large dosages was associated with an inability to enhance hyperphospholipemia, to normalize C:P ratios, or to prevent coronary lesions in cholesterol-fed birds (Stamler *et al.*, 1956).

These studies reinforced the impression that inhibition of coronary atherogenesis was closely linked to basic biological actions of the estrogens in avian species. Moreover, they pointedly posed the problem of the indissolubility of the triad of estrogen effects. It was subsequently shown, however, that masculinization of secondary sex characteristics (e.g., comb size) could be maintained by combined administration of estrogen plus androgen, while retaining estrogen effects on plasma lipids and inhibition of coronary atherogenesis (Stamler *et al.*, 1953, 1956; Pick *et al.*, 1959a).

As already indicated, the experiments summarized thus far were of the "prophylactic" type. It remained to be seen whether estrogens were effective "therapeutically." Were they able to reverse lesions already induced in the coronary vessels of birds by cholesterol feeding? Studies intended to answer this critical question were designed and carried through, and it was shown that estrogens were fully able to reverse well developed cholesterol-induced plaques in the coronary arteries of chicks. In fact, estrogen "therapeutic" anti-atherogenesis supervened even when the atherogenic diet was continued during the period of institution of hormone administration (Pick *et al.*, 1952b). It should be emphasized that estrogens reversed both the lipid and the fibroblastic components of these atherosclerotic plaques in the coronary vessels.

This is not to say, of course, that estrogens were effective in removing areas of marked hyalinization, advanced fibrosis, calcification, or bone formation. Such advanced lesions were not present in the control birds sacrificed after 5 weeks on the atherogenic diet. Rather, the coronary vessels showed plaques composed only of actively proliferating fibroblastic tissue with moderate collagen deposition, plus lipid and cholesterol, situated extracellularly and in lipophages and fibroblasts. Thus these were relatively "young" plaques that estrogens completely reversed, despite continued feeding of the atherogenic diet during the period of estrogen exhibition. So thoroughgoing was this estrogen "therapeutic" effect that special histological and histochemical studies, using a variety of specific stains on formalin-fixed frozen sections, revealed no deviations whatsoever from normal (other than rare residual lipid infiltration) in the architecture of these coronary vessels. No alterations could be demonstrated in the ground substance (Hojman *et al.,* 1959). This experiment, over and above its significance in demonstrating the "therapeutic" ability of estrogens in chicks, was of further import in that it proved once again—in support of previous observations—that atherosclerotic plaques are, within wide limits, partially and even wholly reversible. Hence the theory of the irreversibility of atherosclerosis was once again refuted. Finally, this experiment—and particularly the special histochemical study accomplished in cooperation with our Argentine colleagues—yielded preliminary evidence suggesting that the mechanism of estrogen antiatherogenesis may perhaps be related, at least in part, to a reticuloendotheliosis induced by the hormone.

Subsequent studies on estrogen-induced reversal of coronary atherosclerosis demonstrated that this effect was partially inhibited by administration of either thiouracil or insulin, i.e., when cholesterol-fat feeding was combined with exhibition of either thiouracil or insulin, the ability of estrogens to influence coronary atherosclerosis was significantly impaired (Stamler *et al.,* 1956, 1960b; Pick *et al.,* 1957b, 1959a).

All the foregoing experiments involved the administration to cockerels of exogenous estrogens, natural or synthetic, oral or parenteral, at a dosage level calculated to yield a plasma lipid pattern typical of the mature, egg-laying hen. In view of the need to determine whether the human sex differential in susceptibility to coronary atherogenesis was significantly a function of estrogen secretion in premenopausal women, it was felt essential to assess male-female differences in coronary atherogenesis in chicks, and to evaluate the effects of the endogenously secreted estrogens of sexually mature hens. Toward this end an experiment was first performed in which 8- to 15-week-old, sexually immature chicks, male and female, were fed an atherogenic diet. Both sexes exhibited significant aorta and coronary atherogenesis; no sex differential in coronary atherogenesis was observed.

A comparison was then made between mature, gonadally active

roosters and hens. It was clearly shown that egg-laying hens, in contrast to roosters of the same age, were remarkably resistant to cholesterol-induced coronary atherogenesis, whereas both sexes were susceptible to aorta atherogenesis (Stamler *et al.,* 1954, 1956; Pick *et al.,* 1959a). This phenomenon in chickens appeared to be a remarkable parallelism to the human preclimacteric sex differential in susceptibility to coronary atherogenesis. Based on this experimental finding, it seemed quite valid to suggest that hens exhibited this "immunity" to cholesterol-induced coronary lesions because of their endogenous estrogen secretion, that they were responding to physiological ovarian hormone secretion like cockerels given exogenous estrogens, and that they were a prototype of the basic physiology of anti-atherogenesis in premenopausal women. These conclusions seemed to be all the more tenable since egg-laying hens had typical estrogenic patterns of plasma lipids, with maintenance of C:P ratios at or near normal levels despite cholesterol feeding.

Before these likely interpretations could be validly projected, however, one or two additional experimental steps were necessary. Thus, in the experiment just described, cholesterol-fed hens had had somewhat lower plasma total cholesterol levels than their rooster counterparts. This fact focused attention on the egg-laying phenomenon and on the possibility that disposal of excess cholesterol-lipid via egg-laying might account, nonspecifically, for freedom from coronary lesions. In order to rule out this possibility, surgical ligation of the oviducts was accomplished in a group of hens in the pre-experimental period, with the result that mature ova were deposited into the abdominal cavity, with subsequent resorption of their lipid content. Such a group of oviduct-ligated, egg-producing, cholesterol-fed hens exhibited plasma cholesterol levels similar to those of an age- and diet-matched group of roosters (Stamler *et al.,* 1954, 1956; Pick *et al.,* 1959a). Nevertheless, these hens—while exhibiting marked aorta atherogenesis—remained almost completely free of coronary lesions. Thus further data were obtained reinforcing the concept that this anti-atherogenesis was a resultant of the endogenous, physiological estrogen secretion of the mature hen.

One further critical experiment remained to be done, that is, removal of the ovary. When such a study was accomplished, mature ovariectomized hens, completely lacking endogenous estrogen secretion, developed grossly elevated C:P ratios and extensive coronary atherosclerotic plaques in response to cholesterol feeding (Stamler *et al.,* 1956; Pick *et al.,* 1957a, 1959a). Ovariectomy had eliminated the "immunity" of hens to cholesterol-induced coronary atherosclerosis. Thus it was definitively demonstrated that the resistance of mature egg-producing hens to cholesterol-induced coronary atherogenesis is a product of ovarian function, particularly estrogen secretion. The possible implications for the human problem are obvious.

Of course, the final assessment of the significance of this series of experiments on estrogens and cholesterol-induced coronary atherosclerosis in chicks can be arrived at only by definitive studies in man (see Sections V and VI). In this connection, one of the important questions arising is: What are the effects of estrogens in cholesterol-fed mammalian—as distinct from avian—species? In this connection, data are available from experiments with rats on an 18-week regimen of estrogens plus an atherogenic diet (a high-cholesterol, high-fat, high-choline, low-protein, low-methionine ration). Rats responded to the administration of estrogens with an enhancement of hyperphospholipemia, so that C:P ratios rose less markedly than in nonhormone-treated animals ingesting a like diet (Moskowitz *et al.*, 1956). This experimental regimen induced a plasma lipid response in rats qualitatively similar to, but quantitatively less marked than, that observed in chicks. In conjunction with this metabolic response, the estrogen-treated rats exhibited significantly less coronary atherogenesis than the controls. The coronary vessels of the estrogen-treated animals showed slight to moderate lipid infiltration, but were practically free of atherosclerotic plaques. Thus in rats, as in chicks, estrogens are apparently capable of enhancing plasma phospholipid levels and inhibiting cholesterol-induced coronary atherogenesis. This evidence from a mammalian species further supports the concept that estrogens may play a significant role in the human female resistance to coronary atherosclerosis, and that this anti-atherogenesis may be related to estrogen-induced alterations in plasma C:P ratios.

Several studies of similar design were also accomplished in another mammalian species, the herbivorous rabbit. In brief, these experiments consistently yielded negative results irrespective of the variations in the level of cholesterol feeding and the route of administering estrogen (Stamler *et al.*, 1956). Estrogen-treated, cholesterol-fed rabbits apparently are as susceptible to coronary atherogenesis as their nonhormone-treated controls ingesting a like atherogenic diet. In association with this inability to inhibit cholesterol-induced coronary atherogenesis in rabbits, estrogens failed to enhance hyperphospholipemia, so that C:P ratios were markedly elevated. Both results were, of course, in significant contrast to findings in chicks and rats as described above. These observations are not inconsistent with data in the earlier literature indicating that cholesterol-fed female rabbits are more susceptible to cholesterol-induced atherosclerosis than males (Katz and Stamler, 1953). They are also confirmed by recent work in ovariectomized, hysterectomized rabbits fed cholesterol and given various dosages of estradiol benzoate (Baczko, 1960). However, partial prevention of aorta atherogenesis was reported in this last study, and in another investigation utilizing intravenous microcrystallized estradiol benzoate and dextran (Malinow, 1960).

Present knowledge is not adequate to determine whether any cause-and-effect relationship exists between failure of estrogens to enhance hyperphospholipemia and their inability to protect the coronary vessels of rabbits against cholesterol-induced atherosclerosis. It is well known that estrogens exert profound biochemical, metabolic, and physiological effects, over and above their influences on plasma lipids-lipoproteins. It is reasonable to hypothesize that these extrahumoral actions may significantly alter the atherogenic process (Katz and Stamler, 1953; Katz *et al.*, 1958; Stamler *et al.*, 1956, 1959, 1961b, 1963b; Werthessen, 1958; Asboe-Hansen, 1958; Malinow, 1960; Malinow *et al.*, 1959; Pincus, 1959). Further work is necessary to clarify the basis for and the significance of the difference in effect of estrogens on coronary atherogenesis in different species.

In addition to these studies on estrogens, the effects of androgens and castration have also been explored in animals. Studies along these lines in cockerels demonstrated that testosterone tended to retard hyper-cholesterolemia in cholesterol-fat-fed cockerels (Pick *et al.*, 1959b). This effect was marked and significant at higher dosage levels, in the order of 10 to 100 mg per bird per day. Despite this influence on cholester-olemia, aorta and coronary atherogenesis were essentially similar in incidence and extent in the control and testosterone-treated groups in several experiments. Gonadectomy was essentially without effect in young male or female chicks. Moderate amounts of testosterone in castrated birds (0.05 to 0.10 mg per bird per day in males, 0.10 to 3.00 in females) were also without apparent effect on hypercholesterolemia and athero-genesis.

Thus, the only positive finding was a partial inhibition of hyper-cholesterolemia induced by testosterone in large dosages. This is in accord with observations in chicks by other workers (Wong *et al.*, 1957). The results were otherwise essentially negative; neither hyperandro-genism nor hypoandrogenism influenced aorta or coronary atherogenesis. However, decreased atherogenesis has been reported in testosterone-treated birds (Wong *et al.*, 1957). In any case, the effects are not the dramatic ones encountered with estrogens. This conclusion seems valid also for the findings on the effects of androgens and of castration in cholesterol-fat-fed rabbits (Katz and Stamler, 1953). Certainly the experimental data do not support the conclusion that androgens are responsible for the susceptibility of men to atherosclerotic coronary heart disease in middle age. It would seem valid to infer that the human sex differential is basically a resultant of estrogen-induced insusceptibility in women, rather than androgen-induced susceptibility in men.

IV. Epidemiological Studies

As indicated at the beginning of the discussion on experimental findings, the influences of gonadal hormones are demonstrable when the animals are fed a high-cholesterol high-fat diet. Epidemiological studies have yielded data consistent with the inference that multiple factors are involved in the sex differential, and—more specifically—that it results from a complex interplay between exogenous and endogenous factors. Several examples are worth citing. First, it is a significant fact that the sex differential in atherosclerotic coronary heart disease, so conspicuous for middle-aged Americans, is apparently absent or manifest only slightly among the peoples of the economically less developed countries. Data to this effect are available, for example, on South African Bantu, Italians, and Japanese. Autopsy studies on Bantu age 50-69 revealed that the percent of all deaths attributable to coronary heart disease was 0.5 and 0.8 for men and women respectively; the corresponding figures for Americans were 10.7% and 5.3% (Stamler 1958a, b, 1959; Katz *et al.*, 1958; Higginson and Pepler, 1954).

In 1950, the coronary heart disease death rate for United States white adults age 45-54 was 330 per 100,000 for males, 67 for females, with a sex differential of about 5 to 1. For Italy, the corresponding data were 130 and 89, with a sex differential of less than 2 to 1. For Japan, the rates were 68 and 57, with a sex differential of only slightly above 1 to 1 (Stamler, 1958a). Correspondingly, autopsy studies revealed a generally lower age specific rate for high grade coronary sclerosis in Japanese, compared with Americans, with the virtual absence of a sex differential (White *et al.*, 1950; Stamler, 1958a; Kimura, 1956). Thus, in the United States over 70% of white males and about 20% of white females had high grade coronary sclerosis at age 55. The corresponding figures for Japanese were below 10% for both males and females.

Therefore, the population of the less developed countries—particularly the men—exhibit less coronary atherosclerosis in middle age, compared to their counterparts in the United States. Consequently the sex differential is small or virtually nonexistent. These data are consistent with the nutritional-metabolic theory of atherogenesis, which holds that a certain nutritional pattern—an habitual diet high in total calories, total fats, saturated fats, and cholesterol—is essential to effect the meta- bolic and humoral prerequisites for atherogenesis in sizable sectors of a population. Without this dietary prerequisite, atherosclerotic disease rarely develops in middle-aged persons of either sex, and the sex differ- ential is absent or slight. This is the situation apparently prevailing in the economically less developed countries, leading to the findings cited from Italy, Japan, and the South African Bantu. When the dietary pre- requisites are present, as in the United States, the susceptibility of the male sex becomes evident. Men are frequently victimized. The female sex, apparently by virtue of the protection afforded through estrogenic secretion, remains resistant in the premenopausal years, and its hormone- induced preferential situation only gradually disappears. Thus, the American female, particularly the white female, exhibits a relatively low coronary disease rate in middle age. However, this rate is apparently higher than that of her counterparts in the economically less developed countries, where the nutritional prerequisites for atherogenesis are vir- tually absent (Stamler, 1958a, 1959).

Data from epidemiological studies in the United States lend support to these concepts. Thus, it has been shown that American women exhibit differentials in risk of middle-aged clinical coronary heart disease, based on the presence or absence of such abnormalities as hypercholesterolemia, hypertension, and diabetes. Given the presence of these risk factors, women experience lower rates than age-matched men with similar find- ings. At the same time, however, such women experience more clinical episodes of coronary disease than women without these abnormalities. Thus, in the Framingham Study men aged 40-59 with serum cholesterol levels less than 210 mg per 100 ml experienced an incidence rate of new coronary disease of 35.2 per 1000 in 6 years, whereas men with levels of 245 mg per 100 ml or greater had a rate of 120.3, i.e., about four times as high (Kannel *et al.*, 1961). The corresponding figures for women of the same age with the same stratification by cholesterol levels were 18.0 and 43.5 per 1000 per 6 years. Qualitatively similar findings were noted in relation to blood pressure. For any given finding with respect to a coronary risk factor, women experienced less events than men, but never- theless demonstrated the role of the abnormality in enhancing coronary proneness. Thus, sex-linked protection remains, but it is not absolute; it is overcome in part by the effect of the coronary risk factors.

The situation with respect to American Negroes, as compared with American whites, is also revealing in this regard. Thus, middle-aged Negro men have death rates for coronary heart disease approximately equal to those of white men in the United States (Table I) (Moriyama *et al.*, 1958; Stamler *et al.*, 1960a, 1961a; Stamler, 1962, 1963). In contrast, rates for Negro women are conspicuously higher than for white women, although they remain somewhat lower than those for Negro or white men. Thus, a sex differential is demonstrable for Negroes, but it is significantly less than for whites. This lower sex ratio, it is worth noting, is not the same qualitatively as that recorded for the economically less developed countries. First, the absolute values in both numerator and denominator are considerably higher for United States Negroes than for Italians or Japanese, for example. Second, the lower sex ratio in United States Negroes is a resultant chiefly of higher rates in the denominator, i.e., higher Negro female rates. In the economically less developed countries the lower ratio results chiefly from lower rates in the numerator, i.e., lower male rates. The end result in both cases is a similar lower ratio, compared with United States whites, but on a different basis.

When these findings on Negroes were related to status with respect to risk factors, it was recognized first that both Negro men and women had considerably higher prevalence rates for hypertension than whites. However, Negro men, particularly those residing in low income communities, had significantly lower prevalence rates of hypercholesterolemia and obesity, singly and in combination, than did middle-aged white men. Prevalence rates for heavy cigarette smoking were also lower. Middle-aged Negro women had higher prevalence rates of hypertension, obesity, and diabetes, and similar prevalence rates of hypercholesterolemia compared with white women (Stamler *et al.*, 1961a). It seemed reasonable to hypothesize that the observed rates of occurrence of coronary disease in Negroes compared with whites could be accounted for by the observed patterns in the four sex-race groups of such risk factors as hypertension, hypercholesterolemia, overweight, diabetes, and heavy smoking, singly and in various combinations. Also it seemed reasonable to theorize that endogenous humoral-metabolic factors operate in Negroes, as in whites —particularly ovarian secretion of estrogens—tending to afford Negro women protection against atherosclerotic coronary heart disease. However, their anti-atherogenic effect is partially overcome in this sex-race group because of the widespread prevalence of abnormalities (hypertension, obesity, diabetes, hypercholesterolemia) tending to accelerate and aggravate atherogenesis. These risk factors operate deleteriously among Negroes just as they do in subgroups of the white female population identified in living population studies.

This interpretation of the data on the sex differential emphasizes the interplay between environmental and host factors (e.g., diet and hormones) in the etiology and pathogenesis of atherosclerotic disease. It is entirely consistent with the previously emphasized observation that estrogenic protection in animals is demonstrable only when a high-cholesterol high-fat diet is fed. That is, it is consistent with the multi-causal nutritional-metabolic theory of atherogenesis. Therefore, the focus of this chapter—on sex and gonadal hormones and their role in athero-sclerosis—should in no sense be viewed as distinct from or in contra-diction to other chapters and other writings, particularly those dealing with nutrition (Stamler, 1958b, 1959, 1960; Stamler *et al.*, 1963c; Katz *et al.*, 1958; also see Chapter 8 by Keys). Extensive knowledge is available demonstrating the role of several factors in the etiology of this disease. It is therefore entirely unnecessary and erroneous to respond with an either-or, yes-no answer to unsoundly formulated questions demanding to know the single cause of atherosclerosis.

V. Clinical Investigations

While the previously described program of research was proceeding on estrogen anti-atherogenesis in cholesterol-fat-fed chickens, significant find-ings were reported concerning the effects of estrogens on man. Thus, it was definitely established that estrogens exert a profound effect on hu-man plasma lipid-lipoprotein levels (Katz and Stamler, 1953; Katz *et al.*, 1958; Pincus, 1959; Stamler *et al.*, 1956, 1963b; Steiner *et al.*, 1955; Barr, 1953, 1955; Eilert, 1949, 1953; Robinson *et al.*, 1956, 1960; Marmorston *et al.*, 1958, 1959; Oliver and Boyd, 1953, 1954, 1955, 1956a, b; Russ *et al.*, 1951). In particular, estrogens increase plasma phospholipids, lower cholesterol (this effect is an inconstant one), reduce cholesterol:phospho-lipid ratios, elevate α-lipoprotein, and increase the ratios α-lipoprotein: β-lipoprotein and α-lipoprotein cholesterol:β-lipoprotein cholesterol. These facts were initially established in women, by comparison between their plasma lipid findings with and without estrogen treatment. They were soon confirmed in men and extended in women by analyses of changes during the menstrual cycle and with menopause (natural or induced).

It was also found that patients with a history of myocardial infarction excreted less urinary estrogens than their controls (Bersohn and Oelofse, 1958; Marmorston *et al.*, 1959). Other studies reported that young ovari-ectomized women, examined several years after surgery, exhibited a sig-nificant loss of the insusceptibility to coronary atherogenesis normally present in women of their age (Oliver and Boyd, 1959; Wuest *et al.*, 1953; Rivin and Dimitroff, 1954; Robinson *et al.*, 1959), a finding not uniformly verified in all investigations (Novak and Williams, 1960; Ritter-band *et al.*, 1962). Further, the occurrence of abnormal electrocardio-grams was found to be lower in estrogen-treated postmenopausal than in untreated women, both naturally postmenopausal and castrated (Davis *et al.*, 1961).

In men, significantly less coronary artery disease was found when the testes were fibrosed, presumably due to high levels of circulating estrogens, than when the testes were normal (Dalldorf, 1961). Correspondingly, eunuchs exhibited female lipid-lipoprotein patterns and less coronary atherosclerosis, compared with normal men (Furman *et al.*, 1956). Further, elderly men, receiving prolonged high-dosage estrogen treatment for prostatic carcinoma, manifested significantly less coronary athero-sclerosis than a matched control group receiving little or no hormone (Rivin and Dimitroff, 1954; Thomas *et al.*, 1961). Estrogenic therapy was also found to induce regression of tuberous xanthomata in some patients with hypercholesterolemic hyperlipemia (Feldman *et al.*, 1959; Russ *et al.*, 1955).

All these findings from clinical investigation strongly indicated that estrogens may be anti-atherogenic in man and may play a key role in accounting for the sex differential in susceptibility to coronary disease.

Several studies with estrogens demonstrated that simultaneous admin-istration of androgens counteracted the effects of the female hormones on plasma lipids-liproproteins (Pincus, 1959; Barr, 1953, 1955; Oliver and Boyd, 1956a; Russ *et al.*, 1955; Furman *et al.*, 1958; Hood and Cramer, 1959). In recent years, clinical studies have also indicated that androgens may have a lowering effect on serum cholesterol-lipids. These findings have stimulated investigations on the possible therapeutic efficacy of androgens, singly or in combination with other drugs (Pincus, 1959; Hellman *et al.*, 1959; Thorp and Waring, 1962; Thorp, 1962). These studies are in their early stages, and a considerable period lies ahead before definitive results may be anticipated.

VI. Studies Evaluating the Long-Term Therapeutic Efficacy of Estrogens in Coronary Disease

On the basis of extensive findings from epidemiological, animal-experimental and clinical research, it was concluded in 1950 that a long-term investigation was essential to determine whether estrogens are ef-fective in the treatment of coronary disease in man. The critical question requiring evaluation was: will estrogens reduce the rate of fatal myo-cardial infarction and increase the survival rate in patients with a history of clinical coronary heart disease? Investigation of this problem was begun late in 1952 and terminated on December 31, 1959 (Katz *et al.*, 1958; Stamler *et al.*, 1956, 1959, 1961b, 1963a, b).

The subjects were 275 men under age 50 with a diagnosis of definite clinical coronary heart disease. Except for 12 patients with chronic coronary disease without a definite clinical infarction, all had had one or more previous myocardial infarctions. Of the 263 men with infarcts, 211 had a history of single infarction, 50 a history of multiple infarction. In 2 patients, 1 in the placebo and 1 in the estrogen group, information was inadequate concerning the number of previous infarctions. All patients with multiple infarction were designated poor risk in relation to long-term prognosis. The men with single infarcts were classified good or poor risk based on the absence or presence during the acute episode of such complications as shock, a pericardial friction rub, a serious arrhythmia, congestive heart failure, a pulmonary infarction, or extension of the myocardial infarction.

The initial design involved three groups, a placebo group, an estrogen group, and an estrogen-androgen group. During the first year of the study, the estrogen-androgen group was abandoned for several reasons (Stamler *et al.*, 1956, 1959) and combined with the estrogen group, which is therefore larger than the placebo group. Otherwise, patients serially entering the study were assigned to the two groups on a double blind basis, using the technique of stratified randomization. Factors considered in the stratified randomization were history of other major diseases (hypertension, diabetes, and hepatic, thyroid, or renal disease), and history of single or multiple infarction. Patients with congestive heart failure persisting after recovery from the acute attack, were excluded from the study; there were no other exclusions. Patient sources were the Michael Reese Hospital, two Chicago Veterans Administration hospitals, and Veterans Administration hospitals throughout the Midwest.

It was most important to assure maximum matching and comparability of the paired groups, since failure to accomplish this objective could conceivably introduce serious biases into the study making impossible any valid conclusions. Accordingly, patients were assigned to treatment or placebo groups on a double blind basis with stratified randomization using the aforementioned criteria.

In addition, extensive auxiliary data, medical and sociological, were collected on each patient and analyzed on a group basis at the end of the study to assess comparability of the groups and possible sources of bias. Information was obtained on race, nationality, religion, occupation, height, weight, and therapeutic regimen, including long-term diet and anticoagulant therapy, both of which were rarely utilized in these patients. Determinations were also made of pretreatment serum cholesterol, phospholipid, and (in some patients) lipoprotein levels. Based on these multiple criteria, analyses of paired groups at the end of the study revealed that the procedure of stratified randomization had generally achieved matching and comparability of paired groups.

From the beginning, a definite minimum therapeutic objective was set, i.e., a mortality rate in the estrogen group no more than one-half that in the control group. Of course, mortality experience—in order to be meaningful in a disease with a natural history such as coronary disease—had to be accrued over a period of several years. In addition, this medically significant result (if it were obtained) had to be evaluated statistically.

In addition to survival and mortality (the critically important end points in evaluation of therapy for coronary heart disease), several other phenomena were followed in the treated and placebo patients—e.g., recurrence of nonfatal myocardial infarction, chest pain and angina pectoris, electrocardiographic patterns, serum cholesterol-lipid-lipoprotein levels, patterns of employment, physical activity, familial relationships, psychological adjustments, etc. For therapeutic evaluation, however, the decisive, critical end point was set as the effect of estrogen on survival rate.

Reported deaths were divided into four categories, based on stated cause, i.e., coronary heart disease, cardiovascular-renal (CVR) disease, uncertain or undetermined cause, and noncardiovascular-renal disease. All deaths were considered as therapeutic failures, except for the few noncardiovascular-renal deaths. In the statistical analysis, these latter cases were treated as losses. Of the 77 deaths total, 68 occurred during the first 5 years after entry into the study. Altogether only 4 deaths were classified as noncardiovascular-renal and counted as losses, 1 in the placebo- and 3 in the estrogen-treated group. The excluded death in the placebo group was a case of fatal Hodgkin's disease in a man age 38 at the time of his single good risk infarction; he entered the study 2 months postinfarction and died 50 months later.

The 3 excluded deaths in the estrogen-treated group were: A man age 38 at the time of his single good risk infarction, entering the study 2 months postinfarction, died of an alcohol-antabuse reaction during the first 2 months in the study, on a dosage of 1.25 mg estrogen. A man age 43 at the time of his first of two infarcts, entering the study 7 months after the second infarct, committed suicide during the first 2 months in the study, on a dosage of 1.25 mg estrogen. A man age 47 at the time of his single good risk infarction, entering the study 25 months postinfarction, died in an automobile accident after 8 months in the study, on a dosage of 10 mg estrogen; at autopsy, no recent myocardial infarction was found; he was not driving the car when the fatal accident occurred. Except for these cases, all other deaths, totaling 73, 64 in the first 5 years of patient follow-up, were known or presumed to be coronary or cardiovascular-renal (CVR) and were counted as fatalities in the statistical analysis. This was the case even for those individuals who dropped out of the study but were found on follow-up to have expired.

An intensive effort was successfully carried out to follow up all dropouts, and to determine their status as of the close-out date (December 31, 1959). Such follow-up was successfully accomplished in 84 of 96 dropouts. In the statistical analyses of over-all survival and mortality, these 84 traced cases were therefore not counted as dropouts. Irrespective of duration off therapy, deaths in the estrogen-treated group among dropout patients were considered as therapeutic failures. In addition to dropout status, adherence was evaluated based on history, breast changes, and α-lipoprotein changes. However, estimate of adherence was in no case used as a basis for excluding any patient from the statistical analyses of survival and mortality.

From the beginning, a definite decision was made to study the effects of a dosage of hormone large enough to produce typical estrogenic effects on serum lipid-lipoprotein patterns and secondary sex characteristics. It was also decided to use natural estrogens, in the form of mixed conjugated equine estrogens (Premarin). At first, a single oral daily tablet of 1.25 mg estrogens was given. The control group, of course, received a daily placebo tablet identical in appearance with the hormone pill. No definitive estrogenic effects were observed with the 1.25 mg dosage nor with 2.5 mg per man per day. They did occur in a high percentage, but not in all, patients given 4.0 per day. To assure a significant effect in all men, the initial and maintenance dosage was raised to 10.0 mg per day in June, 1954. This dosage produced the anticipated side-effects— increase in serum α-lipoprotein and phospholipids, decrease in the cholesterol:phospholipid ratio, gynecomastia, depression of libido and potency —in all estrogen-treated patients. These side-effects undoubtedly account for the higher rate of dropout from the study of estrogen-treated, compared with placebo, patients (40.4% versus 30.3%).

Patients were taken into the study seriatim from September, 1952 to August, 1957. The estrogen-treated patients entering in the earliest phase were started on 1.25 mg per day, and their dosage was increased stepwise to 10.0 mg per day, as successive decisions were made to increase dosage in order to accomplish the aforementioned objectives. New patients randomly assigned to estrogen therapy at later phases were begun on the dosage (e.g., 2.5 mg., 10.0 mg per day) which was at that juncture the established maintenance level. Thus patients entering the study from June, 1954 on were started on 10.0 mg per day when assigned to the treated group. Therefore, estrogen-treated patients entering the study at different times did not have an identical course of drug, in terms of dosage. Originally, this inconsistency in design was deemed to be insignificant. However, it apparently represented a major unanticipated confounding variable, and proved to be a significant shortcoming, compelling detailed attention in the analysis of the data (see below).

In general, patients were considered as suitable for inclusion in the study at a minimum of 2 months following onset of the most recent episode of myocardial infarction. In order to allow a time period for the effects of hormonal therapy to become operative, a decision was incorporated in the original protocol that any episode occurring during the first 2 months of treatment would not be counted as a statistically meaningful event. Since this decision was made for the estrogen-treated group, it obviously had to be applied to the placebo group as well. Four types of events were recorded during this initial 2 months in the study—dropouts, cardiovascular-renal (CVR) and noncardiovascular-renal (non-CVR) deaths, and nonfatal CVR events (i.e., recurrent myocardial infarctions). The rate of such events was considerably greater in the estrogen-treated than in the placebo patients. Unexpectedly, this was true not only for the dropout rate, but also for the rate of fatal and nonfatal CVR events (6.4% and 3.4% fatal events during the first 2 months of the study in the estrogen and placebo groups respectively).

Detailed analysis of this unanticipated finding revealed that most of these CVR events in the estrogen-treated men occurred in patients with a 10.0-mg starting dosage of hormone, instituted within a short time (3 months) of onset of the most recent myocardial infarction. These data strongly indicate that this dosage regimen early postinfarction had a deleterious effect. On the other hand, when this group was excluded from the statistical analysis, the remaining estrogen-treated patients were found to exhibit a rate of nonfatal and fatal CVR events during the first 2 months similar to that of the men receiving placebo. Thus, the group on estrogen therapy, exclusive of men started on 10.0 mg within 3 months of the latest infarction, comprised 96 men, of whom only 4 (4.2%) had a fatal or nonfatal CVR event during the first 2 months; the corresponding data for the placebo group are 4 events in 68 patients (5.9%).

The unanticipated excess of fatal and nonfatal CVR events in estrogen-treated patients during the first 2 months in the study, clustering in
those men started on 10.0 mg shortly after their latest infarction, was
taken into consideration in the statistical analyses in three ways. First,
in accordance with the original design, data on survival and mortality
were analyzed both overall (i.e., including events in the first 2 months),
and excluding such events (conditional survival and mortality). Second,
estrogen-treated patients were evaluated exclusive of the 60 men started
on 10.0 mg within 3 months of the most recent infarction, and were
compared with their corresponding placebo group. Third, insofar as
numbers permitted, a separate analysis was made of patients entering
the study before June, 1954, i.e., before institution of the 10.0-mg starting
dosage. Appropriate comparability tables were made to correspond to
all these analyses.

In addition to this excess of early CVR events with 10.0-mg estrogen
dosage begun within 3 months of latest infarction, and the feminizing
side-effects, the following complications were encountered in hormone-
treated patients: in 1 man, mammary carcinoma, developing in 1962,
after 9 years on estrogens; in 3 men, penile irritation (fibrous cavernitis,
penis plasticus, Peyronie's disease), reversible and nonrecurrent on resumption of treatment with estrogens; in 3 other men, nonspecific ure-
thritis; in 1 other man, a galactocoele; gastrointestinal irritation, lassitude
or malaise were not reported.

The mean duration in the study was 57.2 and 58.8 months for the
placebo and estrogen-treated patients respectively, the minimum being
31 and 30 months and the maximum being 88 and 86 months respectively.
In view of this mean duration, the statistical analyses of survival and
mortality, overall and conditional, focused on the 5-year data (Tables
II-V). In these statistical analyses a comparison was made of all placebo-
treated versus all estrogen-treated patients, poor-risk placebo-treated
versus poor-risk estrogen-treated patients, and single good-risk infarct
placebo-treated versus single good-risk infarct estrogen-treated patients.
The basic method for evaluating the hormone therapeutically was the
life-table method with calculation of survival and mortality with their
standard errors, aided by a program for the IBM 709 computer. The "t"
test was used throughout for evaluation of the statistical significance of
the differences in survival and mortality rates between estrogen-treated
and placebo groups.

Five-year survival and mortality rates were significantly different in
the placebo patients when stratified by risk status (Tables II-V). In the
placebo group with a single good-risk myocardial infarction, the 5-year

survival rate was 79.8 ± 5.3; in the poor-risk placebo group it was 34.0 ± 11.0 (Table II). These are in agreement with results recently reported by other studies on the long-term prognosis of middle-aged men following nonfatal myocardial infarction (Gubner and Ungerleider, 1959; McMichael and Parry, 1960). It may therefore be inferred that the control groups were representative samples of middle-aged postinfarction patients, both good and poor risk.

Overall data on placebo- versus estrogen-treated patients are presented in Table II and Fig. 1. Comparability data, corresponding to the three pairs of groups analyzed in Table II revealed the paired groups to be generally comparable. With the small size of the poor-risk groups, complete comparability was not attained. However, statistical analysis indicated the potential bias to be apparently insignificant. The men started on 10.0 mg estrogen within 3 months of their latest infarction are included in these analyses. As previously indicated, these 60 men had an unexpectedly high incidence of CVR events during the first 2 months on hormone. In association with this phenomenon, the placebo- and estrogen-treated groups—both the good-risk patients and the patients grouped irrespective of risk—exhibited no significant differences in mortality and survival rates. Nevertheless, for these paired groups, the 5-year mortality rates were 15.8% and 30.2% lower, respectively, in the estrogen-treated compared with the placebo-treated patients. Five-year survival and mortality rates were significantly lower in the estrogen-treated poor-risk patients, compared with the placebo-treated poor-risk patients. The mortality rate was 48.2% lower in the estrogen-treated poor-risk patients than in the placebo-treated poor-risk patients.

The data on conditional survival and mortality of placebo and estrogen-treated patients, i.e., survival and mortality excluding events in the first 2 months of the study, are presented in Table III and Fig. 2. Comparability data, corresponding to the three pairs of groups in Table III, revealed the paired groups to be generally comparable. When the men with events in the first 2 months of the study were excluded from the statistical analyses, as provided for in the original protocol, the 5-year survival and mortality rates for the estrogen-treated groups—both poor-risk and irrespective-of-risk—were significantly better than for their matched placebo groups ($P < 0.01$ and < 0.05 respectively). The mortality rates were 59.3% and 46.8% lower respectively in the estrogen-treated groups.

For the good-risk patients, the 5-year survival and mortality rates were also lower in the estrogen-treated than in the placebo-treated groups. The reduction in mortality was 46.7%. However, with the size

TABLE II

FIVE-YEAR SURVIVAL AND MORTALITY RATES, OVER-ALL DATA; PLACEBO- AND ESTROGEN-TREATED GROUPS CLASSIFIED BY RISK STATUS

Group	Number of men	Five-year survival rate (%)	Five-year mortality rate (%)	Standard error	Difference between rates	Standard error of the difference	t	P
1. Placebo—good risk	78	79.8	20.2	5.3	3.2	7.2	0.44	—
2. Estrogen—good risk	88	83.0	17.0	4.8				
3. Placebo—poor risk	34	34.0	66.0	11.0	31.8	13.1	2.43	< 0.02
4. Estrogen—poor risk	50	65.8	34.2	7.2				
5. Placebo—irrespective of risk	119	66.2	33.8	5.2	10.2	6.6	1.55	> 0.10
6. Estrogen—irrespective of risk	156	76.4	23.6	4.0				

TABLE III

FIVE-YEAR CONDITIONAL SURVIVAL AND MORTALITY RATES; PLACEBO- AND ESTROGEN-TREATED GROUPS, CLASSIFIED BY RISK STATUS

Group	Number of men	Five-year survival rate (%)	Five-year mortality rate (%)	Standard error	Difference between rates	Standard error of the difference	t	P
1. Placebo—good risk	72	81.6	18.4	5.3	8.6	6.6	1.30	> 0.10
2. Estrogen—good risk	75	90.2	9.8	4.0				
3. Placebo—poor risk	31	36.2	63.8	11.6	37.8	13.8	2.74	< 0.01
4. Estrogen—poor risk	36	74.0	26.0	7.5				
5. Placebo—irrespective of risk	107	68.8	31.2	5.2	14.6	6.3	2.32	< 0.05
6. Estrogen—irrespective of risk	126	83.4	16.6	3.6				

TABLE IV

FIVE-YEAR SURVIVAL AND MORTALITY RATES: DATA ON ALL PATIENTS EXCEPT MEN ENTERING THE STUDY JUNE 1, 1954 AND THEREAFTER WITHIN 3 MONTHS OF LATEST INFARCTION: PLACEBO- AND ESTROGEN-TREATED GROUPS STRATIFIED BY RISK STATUS

Group	Number of men	Five-year survival rate (%)	Five-year mortality rate (%)	Standard error	Difference between rates	Standard error of the difference	t	P
1. Placebo—good risk	42	82.8	17.2	5.9	10.0	7.2	1.39	> 0.10
2. Estrogen—good risk	54	92.8	7.2	4.1				
3. Placebo—poor risk	20	29.2	70.8	12.3	43.8	16.1	2.08	< 0.02
4. Estrogen—poor risk	24	73.0	27.0	10.4				
5. Placebo—irrespective of risk	68	65.9	34.1	6.2	18.8	7.4	2.54	< 0.02
6. Estrogen—irrespective of risk	96	84.7	15.3	4.1				

TABLE V

FIVE-YEAR SURVIVAL AND MORTALITY RATES: DATA ON PATIENTS ENTERING THE STUDY BEFORE JUNE, 1954: PLACEBO- AND ESTROGEN-TREATED GROUPS CLASSIFIED BY RISK STATUS

Group	Number of men	Five-year survival rate (%)	Five-year mortality rate (%)	Standard error	Difference between rates	Standard error of the difference	t	P
1. Placebo—good risk	25	83.5	16.5	7.6	10.4	8.6	1.21	> 0.10
2. Estrogen—good risk	34	93.9	6.1	4.1				
3. Placebo—irrespective of risk	37	68.8	31.2	7.8	15.0	9.4	1.60	> 0.10
4. Estrogen—irrespective of risk	55	83.8	16.2	5.3				

of these groups and the low number of deaths among the good-risk patients, this substantial difference did not attain statistical significance at the 5% level of probability.

Table IV and Fig. 3 present data on placebo- versus estrogen-treated patients, exclusive of men entering the study June, 1954 and thereafter within 3 months of their latest infarction. Comparability data, corresponding to the three pairs of groups in Table IV, revealed the paired groups to be generally comparable. These analyses were done excluding men started on 10.0 mg estrogen within 3 months of their latest infarc-

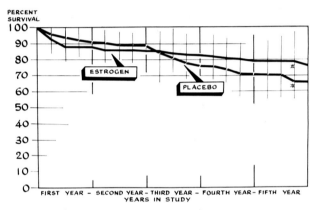

Fig. 1. Survival curves, all patients irrespective of risk; placebo- and estrogen-treated, 119 and 156 men respectively—groups 5 and 6, Table II. * — statistically significant at the 5% level or better.

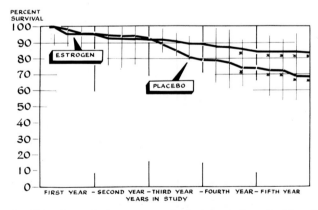

Fig. 2. Conditional survival curves, patients irrespective of risk; placebo- and estrogen-treated, 107 and 126 men respectively—groups 5 and 6, Table III. * — statistically significant at the 5% level or better.

tion, and excluding corresponding placebo patients. Again, the estrogen-treated groups—both poor-risk and irrespective-of-risk—exhibited 5-year survival and mortality rates significantly better than their matched placebo groups (P < 0.02). The mortality rates were 61.9% and 55.2% lower respectively in the estrogen-treated compared with the placebo-treated groups.

For the good-risk patients, the 5-year mortality rate was 58.2% lower in the estrogen-treated than in the placebo-treated group. Again, however, with the small size of the groups and the few deaths in these good

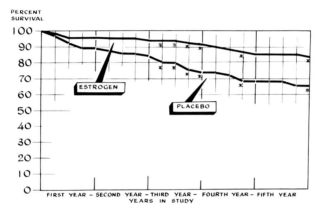

Fig. 3. Survival curves, patients irrespective of risk, except men entering the study June 1, 1954 and thereafter, within 3 months of latest infarction; placebo- and estrogen-treated, 68 and 96 men respectively—groups 5 and 6, Table IV. *—statistically significant at the 5% level or better.

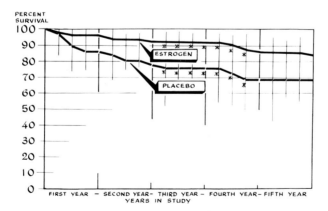

Fig. 4. Survival curves, patients irrespective of risk, entering study before June 1, 1954, placebo- and estrogen-treated, 37 and 55 men respectively—groups 5 and 6, Table V. * — statistically significant at the 5% level or better.

risk patients, this substantial difference was not significant at the 5% probability level.

Table V and Fig. 4 present data on placebo- versus estrogen-treated patients entering the study before June, 1954. Comparability data, corresponding to the two pairs of groups in Table V, revealed the paired groups to be generally comparable. The sizes of the poor-risk groups were too small to warrant statistical analysis. These analyses involved only patients entering the study before June, 1954, i.e., men started on low dosages of estrogen and corresponding placebo patients. The estrogen-treated patients—both good-risk and irrespective-of-risk—exhibited 5-year mortality and survival rates better than those of their matched placebo groups. The mortality rates were 63.1% and 48.2% lower, respectively, in the estrogen-treated than in the placebo-treated groups. However, with the small size of these groups, these substantial differences did not attain statistical significance at the 5% level of probability.

The data of this study on long-term survival and mortality in estrogen-treated patients, as compared with those on placebo, strongly indicate that the hormone exerted a marked beneficial effect. This was true for both poor-risk and apparently also for good-risk patients. The decrease in mortality was generally 50% or greater.

For poor-risk patients, the 5-year survival and mortality rates were highly favorable when compared not only with their paired placebo groups, but also with groups reported in the literature (Gubner and Ungerleider, 1959; McMichael and Parry, 1960).

For the patients with a single good-risk infarct, the recorded 5-year mortality in those treated with estrogen, averaging 6 to 7%, was far below that repeatedly observed in studies on long-term follow-up. Nearly all reports give 5-year mortality rates in the range of 15 to 20%, similar to those observed in the placebo-treated groups of single good-risk infarct patients. The relatively low mortality ratio (observed deaths:expected deaths) of these hormone-treated single good-risk infarct patients, i.e., a 5-year mortality rate about 2.5 times that of the general population of age-race matched men, is virtually without precedent in the literature (Gubner and Ungerleider, 1959; McMichael and Parry, 1960). These results strongly support the general conclusion that the hormone exerted a definitive therapeutic effect.

This conclusion concerning the data of this study is primarily based, it should be emphasized, upon evaluation of the paired groupings established to take into consideration without bias the unexpected deleterious effect of a large (10.0 mg) initial dosage of estrogens begun within 3 months of the most recent infarction. The conclusion that a positive therapeutic effect of estrogens was demonstrated must be tempered by a note of uncertainty and caution relating to this negative phenomenon. No mechanism for this harmful effect of high initial dosage in the early postinfarction period could be ascertained. The excess deaths were attributable largely to recurrent myocardial infarction, not to congestive heart failure. No evidence could be elicited of hypercoagulability and increased tendency to thrombosis as a possible mechanism.

Other remaining areas of uncertainty, incapable of absolute resolution from the data available and therefore qualifying the positive conclusion from this study, include: the higher dropout rates in the estrogen-treated groups and the problem of therapeutic effect in relation to adherence to therapy; the 12 untraced dropouts and the effect of their survival status on the overall statistics; the incomplete comparability of the poor-risk groups, placebo- and estrogen-treated; the failure in the single good-risk infarct groups of the 50% differences in mortality rates to attain statistical significance at the 5% level of probability; and remaining uncertainty as to the mechanism of estrogen action. These difficulties temper the positive evaluation of the results, but do not negate it. They do emphasize the need for one or more repeat studies.

In relation to the findings of the present study, two available clinical reports are particularly relevant. The first is a preliminary paper on a long-term study of low dosage estrogen therapy in men with clinical coronary heart disease (Marmorston *et al.,* 1962). Men recovering from a myocardial infarction were accepted for this investigation irrespective of age. They were assigned by stratified randomization to four groups—control, and for treatment with mixed conjugated equine estrogens, with ethinyl estradiol, or with SC 6924. The two synthetic compounds, although they had estrogenic effects on serum lipids in the low dosages utilized, did not improve survival. However, the interim data from this continuing study indicate that the mixed conjugated equine estrogens increased survival, with the differences between control and treated groups being significant at 12 and 18 months, according to an analysis as of June, 1961. Lesser differences, lacking statistical significance with the number of cases followed, were recorded at 24, 30, and 36 months. The most marked differences were in patients less than 55 years of age. These were statistically significant ($P < 0.05$) at 12, 18, and 24 months; e.g., survivals of 84% and 96% in placebo and estrogen-treated groups, respectively at 24 months. With the dosage of hormone given (in most patients 1.25 or 2.5 mg per day) no alterations in serum lipids were observed, and only minor, tolerable effects on the breasts; i.e., there was an apparent disassociation of lipid, survival, and feminizing effects. The apparent positive influence on survival rate of natural mixed conjugated equine estrogens (at least during the first 2 years of this study), and the absence of such an effect with two synthetic estrogens pose significant questions, particularly since in experimental animals (e.g., chickens) all estrogenically active compounds have proved to be anti-atherogenic.

Two years ago, a final report was published of another long-term study yielding a negative result with ethinyl estradiol in 100 men aged 35 to 64 (50 placebo-treated, 50 estrogen-treated) who had recovered from a single acute myocardial infarction (Oliver and Boyd, 1961). Men with hypertension, angina pectoris preceding the infarct, severe congestive failure after the infarct, obesity, severe hypercholesterolemia, myxedema, and diabetes mellitus were excluded from this study. No detailed mention is made in the report of the risk characteristics of the acute infarction or of the comparability of the two groups in this important aspect, but by personal communication it was established that the patients were all good-risk cases. Ethinyl estradiol, 200-350 µg per day, was utilized in the estrogen-treated group. There were 10 deaths from myocardial infarction in the control group and 13 in the estrogen-treated group.

The reasons for the discrepancy between the results of our study and the foregoing one from Britain are not readily evident. Major apparent differences between the two studies were in drug used, and in number, type, and age of the patients.

In view of the unexplained contradiction in findings of these two studies, and the aforementioned uncertainties, it is evident that no absolute and final conclusion can be drawn concerning the efficacy of estrogens in the long-term treatment of men recovering from myocardial infarction. In any case, it is a fundamental of medical research that positive results of one study must be confirmed by a repeat investigation before final conclusions are drawn. It is our firm conviction that another large-scale, well controlled investigation of the use of mixed conjugated equine estrogens for long-term therapy of myocardial infarction patients should be organized as rapidly as possible. Organizations such as the American Heart Association and the National Heart Institute should make every effort to expedite such an undertaking. This is an urgent matter, since confirmation of the positive results of our study would make it unequivocally clear that estrogens are effective pharmacological agents for increasing survival of patients who have recovered from acute myocardial infarction.

The positive results of our investigation, with the approximately 50% or greater reduction in 5-year mortality rate, lead us to recommend mixed conjugated equine estrogens for use in the long-term management of myocardial infarction. The precautions to be taken, based on our experience, need emphasis. It is probably wise not to start estrogen therapy until 3 months after onset of acute infarction, i.e., after a reasonable recovery and convalescence. In any case, initial dosage should be low (1.25 mg per day) with gradual increase to higher dosage, e.g., stepwise increase at monthly intervals to 2.5, 4.0, and perhaps as much as 5.0 mg per day in men. Higher dosages would appear to be unnecessary.

VII. Conclusion and Perspective

Considerable evidence is available indicating that endogenous ovarian estrogen secretion plays a key role in protecting women against clinical atherosclerotic coronary heart disease. Of all pharmaceutical preparations being evaluated for anti-atherogenic potential, estrogens have been given the most extensive long-term trials, with highly encouraging results. Further work will in the years ahead definitively delineate their place in the therapeutic armamentarium of medicine. In any case, our contemporary epidemic of premature atherosclerotic disease—related as it apparently is to our contemporary mode of life, our habits of eating, smoking, physical inactivity, etc.—cannot be solved by a pharmaceutical "magic bullet," hormonal or otherwise, however useful it may be for the treatment of the seriously afflicted. If proper perspective is to be maintained, this cardinal fact must be kept clearly in mind while further research is proceeding with estrogens and other pharmaceuticals.

ACKNOWLEDGMENTS

The animal-experimental studies with estrogens in chickens, and the long-term clinical evaluation of estrogenic therapy for men with myocardial infarction were carried out in collaboration with Dr. Louis N. Katz, Dr. Ruth Pick, Dr. Alfred Pick, Dr. David M. Berkson, Dr. Benjamin M. Kaplan, and Mrs. Dolores Century of the Cardiovascular Department, Medical Research Institute, Michael Reese Hospital. Much of this work was accomplished during the author's tenure as an Established Investigator of the American Heart Association (1952-1958). Research support was made available by the American Heart Association, the Chicago Heart Association, the Albert D. and Mary Lasker Foundation, the Ayerst Laboratories, the Michael Reese Research Foundation and the National Heart Institute, National Institutes of Health, U. S. Public Health Service (H-626, H-4197, RG-8262).

REFERENCES

Ackerman, R. F., Dry, T. J., and Edwards, J. E. (1950). *Circulation* 1, 1345.
Asboe-Hansen, G. (1958). *Physiol. Rev.* 38, 446.
Baczko, A. (1960). *Polski. Tygod. Lekar.* 15, 3.
Barr, D. P. (1953). *Circulation* 8, 641.
Barr, D. P. (1955). *J. Chronic Diseases* 1, 63.

Bersohn, I., and Oelofse, P. J. (1958). *S. African Med. J.* **32**, 979.

Clawson, B. J., and Bell, E. T. (1949). *A.M.A. Arch. Pathol.* **48**, 105.

Dalldorf, F. G. (1961). *Circulation* **24**, 1367.

Davis, M. E., Jones, R. J., and Jarolim, C. (1961). *Am. J. Obstet. Gynecol.* **82**, 1003.

Eilert, M. L. (1949). *Am. Heart J.* **38**, 472 (Abstr.).

Eilert, M. L. (1953). *Metabolism Clin. Exptl.* **2**, 137.

Feldman, E. B., Wang, C., and Adlersberg, D. (1959). *Circulation* **20**, 234.

Furman, R. H., Howard, R. P., Shetlar, M. R., and Imagawa, R. (1956). *Am. J. Med.* **22**, 965.

Furman, R. H., Howard, R. P., Norcia, L. N., and Kety, E. C. (1958). *Am. J. Med.* **24**, 80.

Gertler, M. M., Garn, S. M., and White, P. D. (1951). *J. Am. Med. Assoc.* **147**, 621.

Glendy, R. E., Levine, S. A., and White, P. D. (1937). *J. Am. Med. Assoc.* **109**, 1775.

Gubner, R. S., and Ungerleider, H. E. (1959). *Am. Heart J.* **58**, 436.

Hellman, L., Bradlow, H. L., Zumoff, B., Fukushima, D. K., and Gallagher, T. F. (1959). *J. Clin. Endocrinol. Metab.* **19**, 936 (Abstr.).

Herrick, J. B. (1912). *J. Am. Med. Assoc.* **59**, 2015.

Higginson, J., and Pepler, W. J. (1954). *J. Clin. Invest.* **33**, 1366.

Hojman, D., Pellegrino-Iraldi, A. A., Malinow, M. R. (Buenos Aires, Argentina), Pick, R., Stamler, J., and Katz, L. N. (Chicago, Illinois) (1959). *A.M.A. Arch. Pathol.* **68**, 533.

Hood, B., and Cramer, K. (1959). *Acta Med. Scand.* **165**, 459.

Kannel, W. B., Dawber, T. R., Kagan, A., Revotskie, N., and Stokes, J., III (1961). *Ann. Internal Med.* **55**, 33.

Kannel, W. B., Barry, P., and Dawber, T. R. (1963). *Proc. 4th World Congr. Cardiol. Mexico City 1962* (in press).

Katz, L. N., and Stamler, J. (1953). "Experimental Atherosclerosis." C. C Thomas, Springfield, Illinois.

Katz, L. N., Stamler, J., and Pick, R. (1958). "Nutrition and Atherosclerosis." Lea & Febiger, Philadelphia, Pennsylvania.

Kimura, N. (1956). "World Trends in Cardiology," Vol. I. Harper (Hoeber), New York.

London, T. W., Rosenberg, S. E., Draper, J. W., and Almy, T. P. (1961). *Ann. Internal Med.* **55**, 63.

McMichael, J., and Parry, E. H. O. (1960). *Lancet* **ii**, 991.

Malinow, M. R. (1960). *Circulation Res.* **8**, 506.

Malinow, M. R., Pellegrino, A. A., and Lange, G. (1959). *Acta Endocrinol.* **31**, 500.

Marmorston, J., Magidson, O., Lewis, J. J., Mehl, J., Moore, F. J., and Bernstein, J. (1958). *New Engl. J. Med.* **258**, 583.

Marmorston, J., Moore, F. J., Magidson, O., Kuzma, O., and Lewis, J. J. (1959). *Ann. Internal Med.* **51**, 972.

Marmorston, J., Moore, F. J., Hopkins, C. E., Kuzma, O. T., and Weiner, J. (1962). *Proc. Soc. Exptl. Biol. Med.* **110**, 400.

Moriyama, I. M., Woolsey, T. D., and Stamler, J. (1958). *J. Chronic Diseases* **7**, 401.

Moskowitz, M. S., Moskowitz, A. A., Bradford, W. L., Jr., and Wissler, R. W. (1956). *A.M.A. Arch. Pathol.* **61**, 245.

Novak, E. R., and Williams, T. J. (1960). *Am. J. Obstet. Gynecol.* **80**, 863.

Oliver, M. F., and Boyd, G. S. (1953). *Clin. Sci.* **12**, 217.

Oliver, M. F., and Boyd, G. S. (1954). *Am. Heart J.* **47**, 348.

Oliver, M. F., and Boyd, G. S. (1955). *Clin. Sci.* **14**, 15.

Oliver, M. F., and Boyd, G. S. (1956a). *Circulation* **13**, 82.

Oliver, M. F., and Boyd, G. S. (1956b). *Lancet* **ii**, 1273.

Oliver, M. F., and Boyd, G. S. (1959). *Lancet* **ii**, 690.

Oliver, M. F., and Boyd, G. S. (1961). *Lancet* **ii**, 499.

Pick, R., Stamler, J., Rodbard, S., and Katz, L. N. (1952a). *Circulation* **6**, 276.

Pick, R., Stamler, J., Rodbard, S., and Katz, L. N. (1952b). *Circulation* **6**, 858.

Pick, R., Stamler, J., and Katz, L. N. (1957a). *Circulation Res.* **5**, 515.

Pick, R., Stamler, J., and Katz, L. N. (1957b). *Circulation Res.* **5**, 510.

Pick, R., Stamler, J., and Katz, L. N. (1959a). *In* "Hormones and Atherosclerosis" (G. Pincus, ed.), p. 229. Academic Press, New York.

Pick, R., Stamler, J., Rodbard, S., and Katz, L. N. (1959b). *Circulation Res.* **7**, 202.

Pincus, G., ed. (1959). "Hormones and Atherosclerosis." Academic Press, New York.

Ritterband, A. B., Jaffe, I. A., Densen, P. M., Magagna, J. F., and Reed, E. (1962). *Circulation* **26**, 668 (abstr.).

Rivin, A. U., and Dimitroff, S. P. (1954). *Circulation* **9**, 533.

Roberts, J. C., Moses, C., and Wilkins, R. H. (1959). *Circulation* **20**, 511.

Robinson, R. W., Higano, N., Cohen, W. D., Sniffen, R. C., and Sherer, J. W., Jr. (1956). *Circulation* **14**, 365.

Robinson, R. W., Higano, N., and Cohen, W. D. (1959). *A.M.A. Arch. Internal Med.* **104**, 908.

Robinson, R. W., Higano, N., and Cohen, W. D. (1960). *New Engl. J. Med.* **263**, 828.

Russ, E. M., Eder, H. A., and Barr, D. P. (1951). *Am. J. Med.* **11**, 468.

Russ, E., Eder, H. A., and Barr, D. P. (1955). *Am. J. Med.* **19**, 4.

Stamler, J. (1958a). *J. Natl. Med. Assoc.* **50**, 161.

Stamler, J. (1958b). *J. Am. Dietet. Assoc.* **34**, 701, 814, 929, 1053, 1060.

Stamler, J. (1959). *Postgrad. Med.* **25**, 610, 685.

Stamler, J. (1960). *Progr. Cardiovascular Diseases* **3**, 56.

Stamler, J. (1962). *Am. J. Cardiol.* **10**, 319.

Stamler, J. (1963). "Epidemiology of Cerebrovascular Diseases" (in press).

Stamler, J., Pick, R., and Katz, L. N. (1953). *Circulation Res.* **1**, 94.

Stamler, J., Pick, R., and Katz, L. N. (1954). *Circulation* **10**, 251.

Stamler, J., Pick, R., and Katz, L. N. (1956). *Ann. N.Y. Acad. Sci.* **64**, 596.

Stamler, J., Pick, R., Katz, L. N., Pick, A., and Kaplan, B. M. (1959). *In* "Hormones and Atherosclerosis" (G. Pincus, ed.), p. 423. Academic Press, New York.

Stamler, J., Kjelsberg, M., Hall, Y., and Scotch, N. (1960a). *J. Chronic Diseases* **12**, 440, 456, 464.

Stamler, J., Pick, R., and Katz, L. N. (1960b). *Circulation Res.* **8**, 572.

Stamler, J., Berkson, D. M., Lindberg, H. A., Miller, W., and Hall, Y. (1961a). *Geriatrics* **16**, 382.

Stamler, J., Katz, L. N., Pick, R., Lewis, L. A., Page, I. H., Pick, A., Kaplan, B. M., Berkson, D. M., and Century, D. (1961b). *In* "Drugs Affecting Lipid Metabolism. Proceedings of the Symposium on Drugs Affecting Lipid Metabolism" (S. Garattini and R. Paoletti, eds.), p. 432. Elsevier, Amsterdam.

Stamler, J., Pick, R., Katz, L. N., Pick, A., Kaplan, B. M., Berkson, D. M., and Century, D. (1963a). *J. Am. Med. Assoc.* **183**, 632.

Stamler, J., Pick, R., Katz, L. N., Pick, A., Kaplan, B. M., Berkson, D. M., and Century, D. (1963b). *In* "Coronary Heart Disease, Proceedings of the Hahnemann Symposium on Coronary Heart Disease" (W. Likoff and J. H. Moyer, eds.), p. 416. Grune and Stratton, New York, N.Y.

Stamler, J., Berkson, D. M., Young, Q. D., Lindberg, H. A., Hall, Y., Mojonnier, L., and Andelman, S. L. (1963c). *Med. Clin. N. Am.* 3.

Steiner, A., Payson, H., and Kendall, F. E. (1955). *Circulation* 11, 784.

Thorp, J. M. (1962). Exhibit, 4th World Congress of Cardiology, Mexico City, 1962.

Thorp, J. M., and Waring, W. S. (1962). *Nature* 194, 948.

Werthessen, N. T. (1958). *Circulation Res.* 6, 759.

White, N. K., Edwards, J. E., and Dry, T. J. (1950). *Circulation* 1, 645.

Wong, H. Y., Johnson, F. B., Wong, A. K., Anderson, J, and Liu, D. (1957). *Circulation* 16, 501.

Wuest, J., Dry, T. J., and Edwards, J. E. (1953). *Circulation* 7, 801.

8

The Role of the Diet in Human Atherosclerosis and Its Complications*

ANCEL KEYS

I. Introduction

No medical question in recent times has provoked more controversy than that of the role of the diet in the development of atherosclerosis

---

* Data from the author's laboratory referred to herein were obtained in research aided by grants from the American Heart Association, New York, and from the U. S. Public Health Service (National Heart Institute, grants number H10 and continuations including HE-04997, and HE-04697).

and its complications, particularly coronary heart disease. Although dietary manipulation has long been the standard method of inducing atherosclerosis experimentally, opinion about the importance of the diet in "natural" atherogenesis in man ranges from the view that it is trivial to the belief that the diet is the primary cause of the epidemic of atherosclerotic disease that now dominates mortality in prosperous populations such as in the United States.

Scientific publications on this subject pour forth endlessly but the data are complex and the evidence is largely indirect. Because commercial stakes are enormous, different segments of the food industry select reports and argument to support their particular interests and bombard us all with propaganda ranging from the most subtle to the crudest claims that governmental regulation may allow. It is no wonder that the medical profession is almost as confused as the general public.

It would be overly optimistic to hope to still the clamor by a critical review of the problem but at least the issues can be clarified and many misapprehensions laid to rest. The literature was reviewed by Rosenthal (1934) and Wilens (1947a, b) and more recently in many monographs and symposia: Groen and van der Heide (1956), Council Symposium (1957), New York Heart Association (1957), Page (1958), Katz *et al.* (1958), Arteriosklerose und Ernährung (1959), Instituto de Cardiologia (1959), Schettler (1961), Jones and Cohen (1961), Fifth International Congress on Nutrition (1961), Myasnikov (1962).

Here we shall discuss findings on man, as contrasted with animal experiments, with emphasis on the most recent data. We shall stress the necessity of evaluating influences rather than causes, and of analyzing statistical probabilities in a situation where both inter-individual and intra-individual variability set traps for the unwary.

II. The Hypothesis of a Major Influence of the Diet

Ten years ago the hypothesis about the effect of the diet was roughly as follows: atherogenesis is promoted by increasing concentration of cholesterol in the blood and the blood cholesterol level is directly influenced by the amount of fat in the diet. Since coronary heart disease is primarily a complication of atherosclerosis, the hypothesis proposed that there are direct, sequential relationships in man between dietary fat and blood cholesterol level, between atherosclerosis and coronary heart disease, and between blood cholesterol level and coronary heart disease (Keys, 1952, 1953).

With the accumulation of new information, the hypothesis should be expanded to accommodate new details: distinction between cholesterol in the α- and β-lipoproteins in the blood, distinction between different kinds of fats, recognition that thrombosis is often involved in the complications of atherosclerosis and may even be related to atherogenesis (cf., e.g., Keys, 1957a, b, 1962a). Moreover, there is increasing evidence that in the same individual the degree of atherosclerosis in different arterial systems is imperfectly correlated and that the influence of the blood cholesterol level on atherosclerosis of the coronary arteries is greater than that in the aorta and cerebral vessels. Currently, the hypothesis may be stated more explicitly:

Atherogenesis in the coronary arteries is promoted by increasing concentration of cholesterol in the β-lipoprotein fraction of the blood plasma and this cholesterol concentration is raised by increasing the proportion of dietary calories supplied by saturated fatty acids, the polyunsaturated fatty acids having a weaker opposing influence. Dietary cholesterol has a slight effect on the blood cholesterol, and some complex carbohydrates in the diet also influence the blood cholesterol level but these effects are small compared with those of the fats. The dietary fats may also affect coagulability and/or fibrinolytic power of the blood so as to influence both coronary atherosclerosis and its complication in the form of coronary heart disease.

The hypothesis does not exclude the influence of other factors, notably heredity, which may operate at any point in the sequence from initial atherogenesis to the clinical catastrophe; it simply postulates a series of important influences that may be expressed as statistical probabilities. Nor does the hypothesis specify or depend upon any postulates as to mechanisms. It is primarily a hypothesis to fit the facts of epidemiology and the natural history of coronary heart disease into a general framework, to stimulate research, and to suggest possibilities for prophylaxis and prevention. The hypothesis is limited to the coronary arteries because, as we shall see, in other arteries the quantitative relationship between pathogenesis and blood composition may be different, although the fundamental mechanisms may be similar. And the hypothesis specifically applies to man, because quantitative relationships may be different in other species.

The hypothesis is consistent with the theory of atherogenesis that emphasizes lipid infiltration into the intima from the blood plasma but it is not dependent on this theory and does not deny the possibility that atherogenesis may begin with the incorporation into the arterial wall of micro-thrombi or fibrin threads from the plasma. It is interesting to recall that the experiments of Duguid (1948, 1949), in support of the latter theory, utilized rabbits with diet-induced hypercholesterolemia.

III. Multifactorial Causation

Much heated debate in the past stemmed from the idea that there is one "cause" to be discovered for atherosclerosis so that espousal of one causal factor would necessarily conflict with a theory implicating another factor. Fortunately, in the modern era of increasing sophistication, single cause theories of the etiology of atherosclerosis have given way to the general concept of a multiplicity of influences that promote the disease. The total atherogenic force is viewed as the sum or resultant of a number of environmental factors operating on the basic genetic endowment. Further, since atherosclerosis is a cumulative, progressive process, it follows that the degree of atherosclerosis attained at a given age must be the summation of these influences continued over time.

This multifactorial concept must be constantly in mind but it does not follow that one factor, e.g., the diet, cannot be important simply because many other factors, some entirely unknown, may also be influential. Nor does agreement that age and heredity are important necessitate a hopeless fatalism. Although atherosclerosis is statistically related to age, the rate of age progression is widely variable among individuals and among populations and there is no evidence that a major part of this variability depends on the genes. Even in the rare families in which the genetic factor is obviously overwhelming (familial hypercholesterolemia), it is reasonable to believe that effective efforts to control the environment—blood composition and circulatory dynamics—should greatly retard atherogenesis. Finally, established atherosclerosis is not necessarily progressive, and some degree of regression seems to be possible, at least in grossly altered metabolism as illustrated in prolonged severe undernutrition (Wilens, 1947a, b; Lober, 1953; Juhl, 1957; Eilersen and Faber, 1960).

Much of what has been said above about atherosclerosis applies also to its complications that are the major concern for both individual and public health—angina pectoris, thrombosis, myocardial infarction, and ventricular fibrillation. The critical factors that precipitate these clinical complications are largely unknown, although they undoubtedly include arterial blood pressure and the circulatory work load on the heart, but there is no reason to believe they are inherently uncontrollable.

In the present discussion on the role of the diet, statistical associations among variables are given prominence. But epidemiological associations do not, of themselves, prove cause and effect; they only provide clues and measures of the consistency of the facts with an hypothesis (Keys, 1957a, 1958). On the other hand, it is indefensible to argue, as did Hilleboe (1957; Yerushalmy and Hilleboe, 1957) that the hypothesis about the importance of dietary fats in the etiology of coronary heart disease is not tenable because it does not perfectly explain all epidemiological data (including inaccurate or inapplicable reports) on the totality of heart disease combined and because mortality from all heart diseases combined is not uniquely associated with the fats in the diet. Although some of the fallacies involved have been exposed (Keys, 1957a, 1958, 1961), they continue to be perpetuated (Yudkin, 1957, 1961; Glatzel, 1960).

The biological significance of the disease and other variables cannot be judged simply by calculating correlation coefficients. Yudkin (1957, 1961) noted significant correlations in international statistics between mortality and "nonsense" variables such as the population use of telephones, radios, and synthetic detergents, from which he inferred that statistical correlations are meaningless and the epidemiological approach is useless. The point to emphasize is that factors to be seriously considered in the etiology of a disease must offer more than "guilt by association"; there must be other evidence and a conceivable mechanism whereby they act as a cause or influence on pathogenesis.

IV. Time Course of Atherogenesis

A major reason for confusion in the past has been failure to take into account the natural history of atherosclerosis and its consequences. Because atherosclerosis in man is generally silently progressive over many years and only its late complications are recognizable in life, it may be unsafe to rely on contemporary observation to identify the characteristics that may have prevailed over the period of atherogenesis.

This difficulty is especially marked in the case of populations that are changing in composition because of migration or that have undergone major dietary changes in the period when severe atherogenesis may tend to develop. A prime example is the analysis of Hilleboe (1957; Yerushalmy and Hilleboe, 1957) who enlarged the original list of countries in the comparison (Keys, 1952, 1953) to twelve by including Israel, Western Germany, and the Netherlands, countries that underwent great dietary changes in the preceding years, Sweden, where the diet also underwent considerable though less extreme change, and Australia, which, like Israel and Western Germany, absorbed a vast number of immigrants with all sorts of dietary backgrounds during the period in question.

Perhaps it is in keeping with the rest of the analysis, that Hilleboe (1957) used 1950-1952 data on mortality ascribed to all heart disease combined and compared these with unofficial estimates of national food balances for the period 1953-1954, i.e., several years *after* the deaths occurred. Moreover, some of the dietary estimates used are at variance with official data as well as being inappropriate for comparison with deaths in 1950-1952. For example, for Canada the diet was stated to be 40% of calories from fats but the actual official figure for the period 1950-1953, inclusive, was 37.5% (Nutrition Division, 1959). For the Netherlands, the figure of 37% fat calories was used but the actual average for 1947-1953, inclusive, was 32.2% (Mulder, 1959). In the Netherlands, of course, severe shortage of dietary fats began in 1941 and starvation conditions prevailed for most of the population in 1944-1945, and a considerable increase of all food, especially fats, had occurred by 1947.

It is well known that, although the mortality on the first "heart attack" is some 25 to 30%, when death from coronary heart disease occurs the disease has already been clinically established for an average of around 5 years (among survivors from the first infarction death occurs some 7 years later on the average). Further, since the basic development of severe atherosclerosis long precedes the first clinical sign, the analysis should emphasize the dietary picture over a period of many years before death.

Somewhat similar considerations apply to comparisons of patients with "controls." In the United States, by middle age most men have severe coronary atherosclerosis (White *et al.*, 1950), so any random group of men who do not happen to exhibit the stigmata of the complications of atherosclerosis will include a majority of men who are actually seriously affected with the disease for which they are supposed to be controls. The fact that many of these "controls" eat high fat diets and have high serum cholesterol values cannot be taken as evidence that the diet and the blood lipids are unimportant.

For both patients and controls the findings at the time of examination may not properly reflect the long time characteristics in respect to other variables besides the diet. Blood pressure is well known to be highly variable so that a measurement on a single occasion has limited significance. The same is true of serum cholesterol. Repeated blood samples over a period of a few weeks show an average intra-individual standard deviation of about 20 to 25 mg per 100 ml, even if all conditions including the diet, are supposed to be unchanged (Keys *et al.*, 1957c). It can be imagined, then, how gross may be the error in estimating the average serum cholesterol level over a lifetime of an individual from a sample of blood drawn in old age, as has been done too often (e.g., Paterson *et al.,* 1956).

V. The Use of Official Statistics

We have already mentioned early efforts to obtain some idea about the possible relationship between the diet and atherosclerosis in populations from official statistics. Besides the obvious necessity of carefully considering the character and history of the population, the validity of the dietary estimates and the general reliability of diagnoses in the country involved, several other matters impose severe limitations.

Death data published in vital statistics are not always comparable in reliability to the diagnostic skill of physicians in the country concerned. In some countries a large proportion of all death certificates are made out by nonmedical functionaries who are guided by ancient custom. This probably explains why in France the vital statistics indicate a very low frequency of coronary heart disease although French physicians insist that the true situation is very different.

The physicians themselves have different attitudes in different countries. In Japan, sudden unexpected death is often labeled cerebral hemorrhage when in the United States the record would read coronary heart disease. In many countries (e.g., Italy, Japan), death associated with the diagnostic picture of chronic valvular heart disease ends up with the label chronic endocarditis, natural heart disease, etc. (not specified as rheumatic), and in the statistics they bear the international list number 421. But in the United States and some other countries the physician usually adds the word "rheumatic" in such a case, even though no direct evidence is available as to the origin of the lesion, and the case is classified in the number 410-416 series of the international list. In the United States, deaths in category number 421 are generally lumped with those in numbers 420 and 422 to make a broad category of coronary heart disease. Application of this custom to vital statistics of other countries can lead to serious errors, for example, the implication that young women in Japan are very prone to die from coronary heart disease.

In regard to the diet the problems are more numerous. Apart from the question of estimating an average *per caput* food intake from the national food balance estimated from many sources of information on food production, import and export, and diversion of foods to use by industry and animals, there are other problems. First, there is the obvious question of waste, which differs among food items and among countries. Perhaps even more serious is the fact that there is no information about the distribution of the food consumption within the population by age and sex, by socio-economic class, by occupation, and usually little or no information about the food disappearance in different regions of the country.

In a few countries, notably Japan, the attempt is made to correct some of these deficiencies by annual national dietary surveys (cf. Ministry of Health and Welfare, 1962) but so far such additional information has not been applied to studies, using official statistics, on the epidemiology of atherosclerosis as related to diet. In my own research in several countries it has been possible to measure all foods consumed in a series of households and, separately, that part consumed by the heads of the households; this often turns out to be significantly different in composition from the average for the household. On the island of Crete, for example, the percentage of calories supplied by fats in the diet of the husbands averaged 32 while that for the whole households was nearly 37.

In view of the fact that the effect of dietary fat depends on its fatty acid composition, the absence of information on the fatty acids in official statistics on national food data produces serious questions when different populations are compared. Laborious computations for each food item, using recently available tables of food composition that specify fatty acids, can help a great deal, but work of this kind is only beginning and has not been applied in any detail to the estimation of national diets from data in official statistics.

In spite of all these seemingly insuperable difficulties in the use of official statistics in the study of the relationship of the diet to atherosclerosis, some crude pictures emerge, and these are improving in clarity since the first attempts (Keys, 1952, 1953). Jolliffe and Archer (1959) classified into rough categories of saturation the total fats consumed in different countries and found a remarkably good correlation between percentage of calories from saturated fats and the mortality rate ascribed to coronary heart disease. They also observed some significant correlations involving other classes of nutrients, but by more detailed statistical analysis it appeared that the percentage of saturated types of fats was a central variable, with animal protein an important intercorrelated variable. Their analysis is easily improved by making allowance for some obvious differences among "saturated type" and "unsaturated type" of fats and more sophisticated analyses may be expected in the future.

VI. Limitations of Animal Experiments

The present discussion is limited to human atherosclerosis and its complications. Although spontaneous atherosclerosis occurs in many species, the picture is anything but clear (Vastesaeger and Delcourt, 1961). Experiments on animals have been extremely important in advancing knowledge about atherogenesis but they have serious limitations in application to the situation in man. Besides the question as to whether experimental atherosclerosis in animals is really comparable to the "natural" disease in man (Detweiler, 1962), extreme caution is necessary in extrapolating to man the findings on the effect of the diet in experiments on animals. Although some of the lesions produced may be considered similar to those observed in the human disease, their character, their distribution, and their frequent association with other lesions (e.g., renal infarcts besides myocardial infarcts), produces argument (cf. Prior *et al.*, 1961; Naimi *et al.*, 1962). And species differences in quantitative metabolism raise equally grave questions. Among many possible illustrations of metabolic differences, two should suffice.

Cholesterol in the diet, the agent first used to produce experimental atherosclerosis, has so little effect in man compared with the rabbit or the chick, that in many studies on man no significant effect could be proved (Keys *et al.*, 1950, 1956), although a slight average effect can be demonstrated when large cholesterol dose differences are maintained (Beveridge *et al.*, 1959, 1960; Connor *et al.*, 1961; Anderson *et al.*, 1962).

Species differences in the effect of dietary fatty acids on blood cholesterol are equally significant. Although oleic acid in the diet has little or no effect in man (Keys *et al.*, 1958a), in the rat it appears to be at least as productive of hypercholesterolemia as the saturated fatty acids (Hegsted *et al.*, 1959). Linoleic acid in the diet, which lowers the serum cholesterol level in man, may raise the level in the rat when added to a low fat diet (Grande *et al.*, 1957).

But one rule in animal experiments is so universal that there is no reason to doubt its relevance to man. So far, experimental atherosclerosis closely resembling that in man has been associated, almost without exception, with marked, in most cases extreme, hypercholesterolemia (Stamler, 1960). Further, the severity of the atherosclerosis in experimental animals is correlated with the concentration of cholesterol in the serum (e.g., Tennent *et al.*, 1957). This relationship may not be so clear when comparison is made only among animals all of whom have fantastically high degrees of hypercholesterolemia, but such comparisons are improper.

VII. Atherosclerosis and Myocardial Infarction

A major stimulus to work on atherosclerosis is its relationship to coronary heart disease and myocardial infarction. In the present discussion it is not possible to offer many data directly relating the diet to atherosclerosis itself. Unfortunately, it is not now possible to evaluate directly, let alone to measure, atherosclerosis in life, so recourse is therefore made to the reverse identification. Patients with coronary heart disease are often considered to represent severe coronary atherosclerosis. Certainly myocardial infarction seldom occurs unless there is far advanced disease in the coronary arteries. And in comparisons of populations that differ in the frequency of myocardial infarction, parallel differences appear in the frequency of severe coronary atherosclerosis (Kimura, 1956; Gore *et al.*, 1960; Scott *et al.*, 1961; Hirst *et al.*, 1962).

However, it is not safe to infer the absence of coronary atherosclerosis from the absence of coronary heart disease or other clinical complications nor to estimate the degree of atherosclerosis in one set of arteries from observations in another. Within individuals there is a far from perfect correlation between the degree of atherosclerosis in the coronary arteries and in the aorta (Bjurulf, 1960; Crawford, 1961). In general, populations differ much more in the frequency of severe coronary atherosclerosis than in regard to the lesion in the aorta (Laurie and Woods, 1958; Schroeder, 1958; Gore *et al.*, 1960; Hirst *et al.*, 1962).

Accordingly, the limitations of the present discussion must be recognized. To a large extent the available data on man in respect to dietary effects relate to coronary atherosclerosis which is inferred from clinical coronary heart disease. While the diet may well influence atherogenesis in other parts of the body, the evidence from man is scanty. Further, it is possible that the frequency of myocardial infarction in a population may not always be a good indication of the frequency of severe coronary atherosclerosis in that population. Morris (1951), on what seems to be quite inadequate evidence, concluded that in London the frequency of death from coronary heart disease increased greatly over a period of 40 years but the incidence of severe coronary atherosclerosis did not. More relevant may be modern data indicating an increase in infarctions disproportionate to the change in frequency of severe atherosclerosis (Bansi *et al.*, 1955; Schettler, 1954).

VIII. Evidence from World War II and After

During the latter part of World War I in Germany, Aschoff (1933) observed a substantial decline in the finding of severe atherosclerosis at autopsy which he subsequently attributed to the low fat content of the diet, but more impressive evidence came from the period of World War II and after. The first, and still in some respects the best, evidence came from Scandinavia. Biörck (1956) summarized some of the data.

In Finland, changes in the mortality pattern were observed during the two wars with Russia beginning in the winter of 1939-1940 (Vartiainen, 1946) but more important data emerged from a detailed analysis of causes of death and from autopsy findings in Helsinki (Vartiainen and Kanerva, 1947). Deaths ascribed to arteriosclerosis began to decline in 1942 and fell to about one-third the prewar level in the years 1943-1946. At autopsy the frequency of fatty streaking was unchanged but moderate degrees of atherosclerosis decreased somewhat while the frequency of finding severe and complicated lesions decreased markedly, especially at ages 30-60. The Finnish investigators concluded that the food shortage, especially of fats, was perhaps involved and the data suggested that arteriosclerosis "possibly could be treated or prevented by dietary methods."

Vital statistics and hospital records from the war period in Norway showed substantial and progressive reductions in deaths from arteriosclerotic heart disease, especially in Oslo where the dietary privation, especially of fats, was most severe (Strøm, 1948, 1954; Strøm and Jensen, 1950, 1951). From a careful analysis of the diet in Oslo, where the best data in Norway were available, Pihl (1952) concluded that "at the present time it seems justified to recommend to people suffering from cardiovascular disease or threatened by it, a lean diet low in calories but otherwise adequate. Such a diet will, incidentally, be moderate in cholesterol as well." Malmros (1950) pointed out that arteriosclerotic disease mortality declined during World War II in Sweden too, but not in Denmark, and that the changes noted in Scandinavia were associated with the fat and cholesterol content of the diets and not with the strain of being at war and other nondietary factors associated with the war.

In Rotterdam, from 6527 autopsies including 230 cases of myocardial infarction, Schornagel (1953) found that there was a slow and gradual decline in mortality from coronary heart disease during World War II, with a rapid increase thereafter, and this was associated with marked changes in the fat content of the diet. Since both men and women showed similar changes, Schornagel concluded that tobacco smoking could not be involved; women in the Netherlands rarely smoked at any time.

In Germany, too, the incidence of coronary heart disease was affected by World War II but the changes—decline and subsequent sharp increase—were delayed in comparison with those in the Netherlands and Scandinavia (Bansi et al., 1955; Pezold, 1959; Jahnke and Breitbach, 1959); this corresponds to the later period of fat deprivation in the diet and subsequent refeeding in Germany. However, Bansi et al. (1955) emphasized that the difference in the autopsy findings was much more in the frequency of myocardial infarction than in the incidence of atherosclerosis, a point also noted by Schettler (1954) in 5000 autopsies at Marburg. But Bansi *et al.* noted that in only 4 out of 329 infarctions was there relative freedom from coronary atherosclerosis.

Data from the war period in other countries (e.g., Greece, Italy, France, Japan) are in general agreement with the thesis that a sharp reduction in the diet, especially in fats, produces decreased mortality attributed to arteriosclerotic disease but that where only slight dietary changes were involved, the war period was not associated with important changes in this disease (e.g., United States, Great Britain, Denmark). The case of Denmark has been misinterpreted (e.g., by Yudkin, 1961). As Biörck (1956) pointed out, although the total fat disappearance in the Danish retail market fell somewhat during World War II, there was a large substitution of butter, locally produced, for margarine, which depended on oil imports, so the concentration of saturated fatty acids in the dietary fat rose during the war while that of *trans* acids fell. Egg consumption also apparently rose and undoubtedly the Danes, like the Dutch in the same period, managed to consume more fat than the statistics, intended for the German occupation, showed.

The evidence from World War II and after has been criticized on various grounds—because of the obvious fact that variables other than the fat in the diet were also altered at the same time, because of the rapidity of the changes in mortality, and for less acceptable reasons based on faulty data and specious reasoning (Glatzel, 1960; Yudkin, 1961; Barnes, 1961). It is true that the diet was not the only variable and the fat in the diet was not the only dietary variable in the picture, but no other factor comes close to fitting all the situations so well in all populations on whom there are acceptable data. It can certainly be insisted that in every population undergoing a drastic decrease in dietary fat there was, in time, a major decline in coronary heart disease with a subsequent increase following the resumption of a high fat diet.

Various critics have been unhappy about the data from World War II and after because the reductions in mortality were more rapid than might be expected simply from a decline or even cessation in the progress of atherogenesis. Major changes in mortality were evident after less than 2 years of dietary reduction in some populations. It seems probable, indeed, that besides an effect on atherogenesis, other important changes, e.g., vascular ulceration and thrombogenesis, were associated with continued subsistence on a diet reduced in calories and sharply restricted in fats. A possible influence of the fall in blood pressure produced by dietary restriction and a sharp rise on refeeding, as reported from the siege of Leningrad, must also be considered (Brozek *et al.*, 1946).

IX. Migrating Populations: Israel

Populations migrating from one region or country to another frequently change their diets, particularly when they move from food restriction to abundance, retaining some customs of flavoring and cookery, perhaps, but eventually adopting the ways of their new homeland. The most studied of such populations in the present connection are the Yemenites and other groups moving into Israel, but Japanese and Italians moving to the United States also provide instructive data.

Among Jews migrating to the new Jewish State, those from Yemen were strikingly different from the "western" Jews in several ways, particularly in their diet, and this difference was associated with a remarkably low incidence of myocardial infarction (Asher, 1948; Dreyfuss, 1953; Dreyfuss *et al.*, 1957). "Oriental" Jews in general were found to be much less susceptible to arteriosclerotic heart disease than the Western Jews, although they were somewhat more prone to cerebrovascular disorders (Kallner, 1958). But these peculiarities diminished with continued stay in Israel and the gradual adoption of Western ways. Among recently migrated Yemenites the "atherosclerotic mortality rate" for men of equal age was only about one-fourth that of earlier Yemenite settlers and far lower than among European Jews in Israel (Toor *et al.*, 1960). The differences in the incidence of myocardial infarction were much more striking. Relative rates for men of the same age were 0.1 for recent Yemenites, 1.6 for early Yemenites, 5.2 for all immigrants of Eastern origin, and 17.7 for immigrants of Western origin (Toor *et al.*, 1960).

Major differences among Jews from various origins were observed in the concentration of cholesterol and other lipids in the serum and these differences were shown to be associated with differences in the incidence of severe atherosclerosis and its complications (Toor *et al.*, 1957; Brunner and Loebl, 1958). One of the most important features of these data was the finding that the longer the Yemenites and other "Oriental" Jews remained in Israel, the more they came to resemble the Western Jews in serum cholesterol level, and in the character of the diet as well as in the frequency of arteriosclerotic heart disease. In a study of 2200 persons in Israel, among men aged 45-54 the serum cholesterol averages (in mg per 100 ml) were: recent Yemenites, 158; semi-recent Yemenites, 180; early Yemenites, 197; European manual workers, 190; European middle class, 248 (Toor *et al.*, 1960).

The diet in Israel has fluctuated with war and economic conditions but in general the Israelis of Western origin maintain a European-American type of nutrient distribution, that is to say a diet in which fats contribute up to 40% of calories and rarely fall below 30%. In contrast, the diet of the recently arrived Yemenites averaged only 16% fat calories but with longer stay in Israel the average rose to around 23% while total calories also increased (Toor *et al.*, 1960).

X. Migrating Populations: The Japanese

A very low frequency of arteriosclerotic heart disease in Japan is indicated by both vital statistics and the reports of medical travelers, but extensive autopsy studies were needed to prove that the frequency of severe coronary atherosclerosis in Japan is, indeed, very low (Kimura, 1956; Gore *et al.*, 1960), a finding fully in accord with detailed sampling surveys of morbidity (Kusukawa, 1956). This is not a racial peculiarity because Japanese who migrated to Hawaii are much more often affected, while Japanese Nisei (second generation) in California tend to resemble other Americans in their susceptibility to atherosclerosis and its complications (Larsen, 1957; Keys *et al.*, 1958b; Larsen and Bortz, 1959, 1960).

In regard to vascular disease mortality, "Japanese in Hawaii tend to occupy an intermediate position between the Japanese of the United States and Japan" (Gordon, 1957), as they do also in regard to dietary habit and serum cholesterol level (Keys *et al.*, 1958b). A similar gradient may tend to exist in regard to physical exercise but sedentary Japanese in Japan also have lower serum cholesterol levels and fewer myocardial infarctions than their relatives in Hawaii and California. Dietary experiments in Japan, incidentally, indicate that Japanese respond in serum cholesterol to dietary fats just as do men in Minnesota (Keys *et al.*, 1957b).

XI. Migrating Populations: Italians and Others

In Italy, especially in the south, coronary heart disease is relatively uncommon as compared with the situation in the United States and this peculiarity is associated with low serum cholesterol values and subsistence on a diet low in saturated fats (Keys *et al.*, 1955; Keys, 1956, 1957b; White, 1956). These characteristics are not observed among Italo-Americans, even among those whose ancestral home was in the south of Italy (Miller *et al.*, 1958; Jankelson *et al.*, 1962).

Data on incidence of atherosclerosis and its complications are inadequate for exact comparisons but certainly Italo-Americans are not remarkably different from other Americans in this respect and Italo-Americans tend to eat a diet much higher in saturated fats, and to have much higher serum cholesterol values, than do their relatives in Italy.

It seems probable, although proper data are lacking, that these statements would also apply to Greek-Americans, Yugoslav-Americans, and other groups whose relatives in their homelands eat diets low in saturated fats, have relatively low serum cholesterol values, and are less prone to the clinical complications of atherosclerosis.

XII. Tales from Medical Travelers

Snapper (1941) is a fine example of the astute medical traveler who returns from a short period of careful observation in a foreign land with a host of impressions, many of them close to the truth, about the frequency and character of diseases in the population he has seen. In recent years, the ease of travel has encouraged some single-handed "epidemiological surveys" covering half the world, at jet speed, with innocence of the customs and languages of the countries "covered" at a rate of one or more per week. Of necessity, the only information gleaned comes from brief discussions with the few English-speaking local physicians to whom they have access.

This can make an amusing holiday but it is unfortunate that in some instances the result is a publication in which selected impressions are readily mistaken for evidence by the unwary or are cited as verity to serve an argument. Two examples may be mentioned.

Schroeder (1958) talked with pathologists who showed him autopsy summaries from which he derived conclusions about the frequency and severity of atherosclerosis and the character of the diets in many millions of people from Japan to the Mediterranean. The burden of his thesis is that atherosclerosis is ubiquitous and is not obviously related to dietary fats. Such data as he actually quoted—and almost none is statistically acceptable—indicate that among old people aortic atherosclerosis is common everywhere. It is interesting that in all populations whose diets are low in fats the complications of coronary atherosclerosis were reported to be far fewer, in comparison with the complications of aortic or cerebral atherosclerosis, than is the experience in the United States or other high-fat diet areas.

Pollak's (1959) account of a trip to the Far East has the virtue of being short and unburdened with statistics (good or bad), but the concentration per page of broad generalizations and of highly questionable "information" is not lower than in Schroeder's report. Both reports, of course, will long be cited by anyone who is interested in confusing the issue.

XIII. Coronary Heart Disease and Serum Cholesterol

Patients exhibiting clinical complications of atherosclerosis tend to be characterized by relatively high concentrations of cholesterol in the blood serum. The significance of this fact for causal interpretations remained debatable until it could be shown that the lipid peculiarity actually preceded the appearance of the disease. The first clear evidence of this sequence was obtained by following 3462 men for 2 years after measuring cholesterol in the blood serum (Technical Group, 1956). During the follow-up, 57 of these men developed "definite" coronary heart disease, of whom 41 had cholesterol values above the median for all men at the outset, a distribution that would occur by chance with $p = 0.01$. Among other things, this study disposed of claims for the prognostic superiority of ultracentrifugal analysis.

Long before the "Technical Group" began the study mentioned above, other prospective studies were started and findings from these and other similar studies now permit more detailed analysis (Keys *et al.*, 1963a). Fifteen years of follow-up on Minnesota business and professional men initially aged 45-55 gave essentially the same result as obtained in an 8-year follow-up of a sample of the general population of men aged 30-59 initially in Framingham, Massachusetts (Dawber *et al.*, 1957; Dawber, 1962), and a 6-year follow-up of male civil service employees of the state of New York, initially aged 40-55, in Albany, New York (Doyle *et al.*, 1957; Doyle, 1962). In all, there are data on 4069 men among whom 251 developed definite coronary heart disease.

Within each area and age group, the incidence of new coronary heart disease rose steadily with the pre-disease serum cholesterol level and for the entire material the risk of future disease proved to be a direct function of the third power of the cholesterol value (Keys *et al.*, 1963a). There is no particular critical level for increasing risk but, in general, men with cholesterol values over 260 have 3 or 4 times the risk of men with pre-disease cholesterol values of the order of 220 or less.

All evidence is in agreement so it appears that in the United States, at least, very high significance must be given to the serum cholesterol level in regard to the incidence of clinical disease, although there are still no data directly relating to atherosclerosis itself. It should be observed, further, that these follow-up findings are, in general, based on analysis of single blood samples so that misclassifications of some of the men in respect to cholesterol level must be considered. Spontaneous intra-individual variability in serum cholesterol concentration is far from trivial; for American men leading a supposedly constant life, including the diet, the intra-individual standard deviation is of the order of 20-25 mg of cholesterol per 100 ml of serum (Keys *et al.*, 1957a). This value is for repeated blood samplings in a period of a few weeks; larger variability must prevail over the years. The inference, of course, is that these follow-up studies underestimate the degree of relationship between long-time, average pre-disease cholesterol level and subsequent incidence of the disease.

XIV. Fats in the Diet and the Serum Cholesterol Level

We have already referred to many epidemiological studies—and scores more could be cited—which indicate a marked relationship between the serum cholesterol level and the fats in the diet. Much more definite and detailed data are available from numerous controlled dietary experiments on man. In summary, they show that saturated fatty acids in the diet elevate the serum cholesterol level, while polyunsaturated fatty acids have the opposite effect, about 2 gm of linoleic acid being required to counter the effect of 1 gm of the ordinary saturated fatty acids in human diets (Keys *et al.*, 1957c, 1959). Oleic acid, and perhaps other natural mono-enes, is neutral in this respect and may be isocalorically exchanged for starch in the diet without affecting the cholesterol in the blood (Keys *et al.*, 1958a).

There has been some confusion, in respect to effect on serum cholesterol, between the iodine number and the fatty acids of fat in the diet. Ahrens proposed that the effect of dietary fat in man may be simply determined by the iodine number (cf. Page, 1958, p. 222). The iodine number of a fat is simply a measure of the average number of double bonds in it. Accordingly, a mixture of equal parts of linoleic acid (two double bonds per molecule) and stearic acid (saturated) has the same iodine number as pure oleic acid (one double bond). As noted above, oleic acid is neutral in respect to effect on serum cholesterol in man, while saturated and polyunsaturated fatty acids have opposite effects. But the cholesterol effect of the common saturated fatty acids (12 to 18 carbon atoms per molecule) is about twice as great, per gram, as that of ordinary poly-enes, such as linoleic acid (Keys *et al.*, 1957a, 1959). Further, the effect of the fatty acids with four or more double bonds, such as in fish oils, is hypocholesterolemic but not notably more so than linoleic acid.

Hence, although iodine numbers of mixtures of ordinary fats is often a good rough guide, it cannot substitute for a more detailed breakdown of composition. Moreover, it is always necessary to consider the total amount of fat, as percentage of total calories, in the diet. In general, the average effect of changing the fat in the diet of man is indicated by the equation:

$$\text{Chol.}_2 - \text{Chol.}_1 = 2.7\ (S_2 - S_1) - 1.3\ (P_2 - P_1)$$

where chol. is milligrams of total cholesterol per 100 ml on the second and first diets, and S and P refer to percentage of total diet calories provided by glycerides of saturated and of polyunsaturated fatty acids, respectively, in the two diets.

Confirmation in the data from experiments elsewhere of predictions on the above basis indicates the generality of the relationships (cf. Keys *et al.*, 1959; Malmros and Wigand, 1957; Turpeinen *et al.*, 1960; Hashim *et al.*, 1960). But it should be observed that these are *average* effects in groups of men. Individual predictions require many analyses to eliminate spontaneous variations and, further, allowance may be necessary for innate differences among individuals as indicated by the fact that one man may tend to have much higher cholesterol values than another man on the same diet. In general, the higher the inherent cholesterol level of the individual, the greater is his response to a dietary change (Keys *et. al.*, 1959).

Most of the controlled experiments from which these relationships emerged were limited to a few weeks or months but more prolonged experiments show no diminution of the diet fat effect (cf. Antonis and Bersohn, 1961, 1962). Studies on populations habitually subsisting on different diets suggest, if anything, an enhanced effect over the years, but the basic relationships seem to be of the same character (Keys, 1962a, Keys *et al.*, 1963b).

When the diet contains substantial amounts of hydrogenated fats, the effect of the *trans* isomers they contain must be considered. The *trans* acids tend to elevate the serum cholesterol level as compared with equal amounts of the natural *cis* isomers in the diet, and a still greater effect on the serum triglycerides is observed (Anderson *et al.*, 1961).

The chain length of the saturated fatty acids also has an effect but this has little importance in natural diets (Grande *et al.*, 1961). Saturated fatty acids with 10 or fewer carbons in the chain have little or no effect while the most powerful cholesterol-raising effect is observed with the 12-carbon lauric acid.

The effect of dietary cholesterol was mentioned earlier in this chapter. In man, in contrast with the rabbit and the chick, the effect of change of cholesterol in the diet is small. Changing from a natural human diet with a high cholesterol content, say 800 mg per day, to a diet otherwise identical but low in cholesterol, say only 300 mg per day, may produce a fall of the order of 15 mg of cholesterol per 100 ml of serum (cf. Connor *et al.*, 1961; Anderson *et al.*, 1962).

XV. Nonfat Nutrients and the Lipids in the Blood

Many other nutrients have been investigated as to effect on the serum cholesterol. Various claims for vitamin effects have been made but, with exception of the pharmacological action of huge (nondietary) doses of nicotinic acid, these have not been confirmed. Claims emanating from Russia about vitamins have been discussed elsewhere (Simonson and Keys, 1961).

Magnesium in the diet caused a short-lived flurry of interest but there is no longer reason to think it is of interest (Garcia de los Rios, 1961). A more interesting but unresolved set of questions is raised by the report of a statistical association between the mortality rate ascribed to coronary heart disease and the "hardness" of the water in the local supply system (Schroeder, 1960a, b; Morris *et al.*, 1961).

Both in the United States and in England and Wales, there is a general tendency for the cardiovascular mortality rate to be inversely related to the hardness of the local water. Although there is no evidence from theory or experiment to indicate what is involved, the statistical correlation is "significant"—of the order of $r = 0.4$ to 0.5 for males—in each of the two national areas. The correlation is less with coronary heart disease than with all other cardiovascular disease and, in England and Wales, the correlation with chronic bronchitis is also significant and that with cerebrovascular disease is higher than with coronary heart disease (Morris *et al.*, 1961). In England and Wales the correlation between hardness of water and industrial air pollution was also significant ($r = -0.22$, $p < 0.05$ with 83 pairs of observations). Some experiments on animals are reported to be in general support of the thesis that soft water is "bad" but they add little to useful knowledge (Neal and Neal, 1962).

One difficulty in attempting to evaluate these purely paper-work observations is the fact that water "hardness" is a composite description of the combined effect of many variables in the chemical composition. Strain (1961) has pointed out the fact that in many natural waters in the United States "hard" waters tend to be high in vanadium and that if there is any causative relationship between hard water and relatively low incidence of atherosclerosis and its consequences, this element may be involved. But perhaps enough has been said to indicate the complexity of the problem.

Dietary proteins have attracted interest. Controlled experiments on man show that within a wide range of natural human diets, variations in animal protein in the diet have no effect on serum cholesterol (Keys and Anderson, 1957). When diets of populations are compared, the intake of (animal) protein is often found to be highly correlated with the intake of saturated fats so, as would be expected, the average serum cholesterol level in these populations is found to be correlated with animal protein as well as with fat in the diet. This fact has been widely misrepresented as indicating an independent effect of protein on atherogenesis (e.g., Yerushalmy and Hilleboe, 1957; Yudkin, 1957, 1961; Glatzel, 1960; Barnes, 1961).

Finally, some complex carbohydrates, including pectin and the carbohydrates in legumes, in the diet have a moderate cholesterol-lowering effect which may help to explain the low cholesterol levels in some populations (Keys *et al.*, 1960, 1961; Luyken *et al.*, 1962). Fiber, however, is unimportant in this respect (Keys *et al.*, 1960, 1961).

XVI. "Nibbling" versus Meal Eating

In addition to the amount and composition of the diet, there appears to be a small effect on the serum cholesterol according to the pattern of eating, whether the day's food is mainly eaten in one or two meals or distributed in a number of small meals (nibbled). In several animal species nibbling produces a different body composition than the same diet fed in meal eating (Cohn and Joseph, 1959; Feigenbaum *et al.*, 1962), and lower degree of atherosclerosis is reported when the diet is nibbled (Cohn *et al.*, 1961). In a controlled study on women, "nibbling" 7 meals a day resulted in a fall in the serum cholesterol level from the value on the same diet eaten mainly in two meals a day (Lowry *et al.*, 1963).

XVII. Diet, Cholesterol Level, and Risk of Individuals

The data discussed above seem to explain most or all of the diversity of serum cholesterol levels when averages of populations or dietetically discrete groups are compared. The link with atherosclerosis is less clear but an important relationship between the fat content of the habitual diet and the risk of clinical coronary heart disease is difficult to deny. However, every dietary experiment shows a wide range of cholesterol levels of individuals who are all on the same diet. Although a given dietary change provokes the same kind of response in almost all persons, the individuality of the setting of the "cholesterolstat" is obvious.

Elucidation of the reasons for such innate differences among individuals remains as one of the most important problems to be answered but in the meantime we can ask: How much of the inter-individual variation in cholesterol level in a population can be ascribed to individual differences in dietary habit? The answer, of course, depends upon, among other things, the validity of the dietary and cholesterol data and the intra- and inter-individual variability in respect to both variables. Until now, these questions have not received adequate attention in the few studies that have been reported in the literature.

Where the dietary variation among the individuals is small, little or no correlation with serum cholesterol is to be expected. Among elderly women in an institution no correlation was found between the individual serum cholesterol and the individual total fat intake (Walker *et al.*, 1956). There were no data on the dietary fatty acids in this study, incidentally.

In general, attempts to examine this question with dietary data obtained by interviews have failed to show significant correlations between serum cholesterol and estimates of total fat in the diet in restricted population groups—London busmen (Morris, 1962b), employees of a corporation in Chicago (Paul *et al.*, 1963). Dawber *et al.* (1962) concluded that dietary data from careful interviews can be useful in epidemiological studies and this is probably the case when it is only desired to distinguish groups that offer a substantial contrast. But it is unlikely that the interview or recall method will ever suffice for analyses involving small differences among individuals. In any case, in view of the intra-individual variability in serum cholesterol, it is essential that blood sampling, preferably repeated on several occasions, be strictly contemporary with the period covered by the dietary information.

Some relationships can be discerned even when this last requirement is not met, as was the case in a study of 54 middle-aged men in a small town in the Netherlands. Data on actual food intake were obtained by weighing all items eaten for 7 days, with subsequent chemical analysis of composites for each man's diet (Dalderup *et al.*, 1963). In that study the serum cholesterol level failed to show significant correlation with the dietary fats as estimated from tables of food composition applied to interview data but there was a significant correlation ($r = 0.4$) when the data from chemical analysis were used. When allowance was made for analytical error and intra-individual variability it appeared that the true correlation coefficient should be of the order of $r = 0.6$. This is for a population with a relatively high degree of dietetic homogeneity; with greater dietary variations among individuals the correlation should be higher still, of course.

XVIII. Serum Triglycerides, Diet, and Atherosclerosis

Patients who have had myocardial infarctions tend to differ from "controls" in respect to serum triglyceride level in much the same way that they differ in respect to cholesterol (Albrink *et al.,* 1961; Albrink and Man, 1959; Carlson, 1960; Horlick, 1961). Although no pre-disease data (prospective studies) are available, it is proposed that triglycerides, like serum cholesterol, are involved in the etiology of atherosclerosis and its complications. If this is so, it is important to ask what may be the effect of the diet on the serum triglyceride level.

Change from the usual high-fat American diet to a diet very low in fats promptly produces an increase in serum triglycerides (Ahrens *et al.,* 1959; Dole *et al.,* 1959), a result prematurely proclaimed to indicate a hazard in eating low-fat diets. The first obvious fact, without any information about serum triglycerides, is that populations habitually on low-fat diets have a *low,* not a high, incidence of severe atherosclerosis and its consequences. The second fact is that in populations on low-fat diets the serum triglyceride level is not unduly high and may be definitely low (Antonis and Bersohn, 1960; Fidanza *et al.,* 1963).

Prolonged dietary experiments explain the apparent discrepancy in the reports on the effect of dietary fat on serum triglycerides. If the diet is abruptly changed from very high to very low in fat, the serum triglyceride does, indeed, tend to rise promptly. But as the low-fat diet is continued this effect is seen to be temporary, the serum triglycerides tend to fall after a few weeks and in a few months the level is generally as low or is lower than on a high-fat diet (Antonis and Bersohn, 1961).

XIX. Obesity and Atherosclerosis

Obesity, whether produced by under-expenditure of energy or plain overeating, is always a reflection of a relative excess of dietary intake. It is widely believed, on the basis of life insurance data, that obesity is a prime promotor of atherosclerosis and its consequences but the evidence is not so clear when it is examined critically (Keys, 1954, 1955). The insurance data refer to overweight, which is not equivalent to obesity (fatness), and until recently to "heart disease," which is far from synonymous with atherosclerosis. Lately the actuaries have reported that the mortality rate ascribed to coronary heart disease is elevated among men who are unusually heavy for their height (Society of Actuaries, 1959) but there are still no data on obesity (body fatness) from insurance experience.

In an analysis of 1250 cases at post-mortem, Wilens (1947a, b) reported a significant correlation between relative body fatness ("lean," "normal," "obese" bodies) and the degree of atherosclerosis, particularly coronary atherosclerosis. Faber and Lund (1949) failed to confirm this in an autopsy analysis in which the ratio of body weight to height was the measure of "obesity" and the bodies were matched in respect to the presence or absence of hypertension before death. More severe atherosclerosis was reported for obese than for lean persons by Sjövall and Wihman (1934) and by Henschen (1959).

Bjurulf (1959) measured body fatness by the thickness of the subcutaneous fat and by the size of the fat cells and evaluated atherosclerosis in aorta and coronary arteries by an objective scheme. The severity of coronary atherosclerosis was slighty but significantly correlated with both measures of fatness ($r = +0.31$ to $+0.32$) but aortic atherosclerosis was not ($r = +0.17$ to $+0.18$). Bjurulf's material contained only 19 cases of myocardial infarction so the question of a relationship between this condition and obesity could not be decided.

It appears then, that in some populations there is some direct relationship between body fatness (and therefore relative excess of dietary calories) and atherosclerosis, but the correlation is of a low order and is only proved in regard to the coronary arteries. Further, none of these investigators attempted to examine the relationship, if any, between atherosclerosis and the prevailing degree of fatness over most of the life before mortal illness.

Autopsy findings are almost always severely limited by the character of the sample and the possibility of changes associated with the course of illness. The latter is most significant in some cases. Many investigators agree that it is usual to find reduced degrees of atherosclerosis in patients dying after a prolonged period of cachexia (Sjövall and Wihman, 1934; Wanscher *et al.*, 1951; Lober, 1953; Juhl, 1955, 1957; Henschen, 1959). It appears that ordinary variations in obesity, and the diet it depends on, have no great effect on atherosclerosis but that prolonged, severe undernutrition does have an effect. Extreme cachexia seems to promote regression as well as stop progression of atherosclerosis.

Epidemiological evidence on the relationship between obesity and atherosclerosis and its complications must be examined carefully because in some populations the degree of obesity is correlated with several other variables that in themselves are suspected of playing a role in etiology. For example, in Naples patients with coronary heart disease tend to be fatter than their fellows; they are also characterized by higher serum cholesterol concentrations, a better socio-economic status, and tend to be a richer (i.e., fatter) as well as having a higher calorie diet than the general population (Keys and Fidanza, 1960). In the Framingham study, coronary heart disease developed with undue frequency among the most overweight men but most of this relationship disappeared when men with hypertension were excluded (Dawber and Kannel, 1961). In the Minnesota study no relationship was observed between risk of coronary heart disease and either relative body weight or body fatness (Keys *et al.*, 1963a).

XX. Eskimos, Navajos, Trappists, and Others

The literature—scientific, pseudo-scientific, and popular—on the relationship of the diet to atherosclerosis is replete with misinformation and plain nonsense about special population groups that are supposed to refute the hypothesis under review in this chapter. The idea that there are exotic, simple populations who are mysteriously spared from common ills because of or in spite of their diets has an appeal that keeps alive tall tales about the "happy Hunza" and the like.

The Eskimo, popularly pictured as maintaining robust health on a diet of nothing but fat meat and blubber, is frequently cited as evidence that dietary fat does not necessarily have anything to do with the etiology of atherosclerosis and its complications (Stefansson, 1956, 1958; Myasnikov, 1962). On the contrary, Ehrström (1951), who actually tried to make estimates, concluded that arteriosclerosis is exceedingly *common* among primitive Eskimos, but his evidence is not impressive. The fact is that even if a proper study on atherosclerosis among Eskimos were carried out—and so far none has been attempted—it is improbable that the results would contribute significantly to the debate on the diet-atherosclerosis hypothesis (Keys, 1957b).

The Eskimos have always been a tiny population among whom at no time have there been more than a few hundred surviving to the age when they would be candidates for the complications of severe atherosclerosis. There are simply not enough primitive Eskimos beyond the years of youth to meet statistical requirements for comparative epidemiology. Moreover, their ancient primitive diet, although often very high in fat (Krogh and Krogh, 1914-1915), comprised quite different fats than those we are concerned about in the modern Western World—no beef, pork, eggs, or butterfat in any form but fats dominated by polyunsaturated fatty acids—and their diet in the last 40 years is apt to be considerably lower in fat than that of the average contemporary American (Bertelsen, 1935, 1937, 1940; Sinclair, 1953; Rodahl, 1956; Mann *et al.*, 1962c).

It was once stated that "Navajos usually eat a typically American diet . . . (but) coronary heart disease among them is rare" (Gilbert, 1954; Page *et al.*, 1956), and this statement is often quoted (*e.g.*, Myasnikov, 1962). It is true that on the Navajo Indian Reservation, severe atherosclerosis and myocardial infarction is less common than elsewhere in the United States, although "rare" may be an exaggeration, and this is what would be expected from the predominance of low serum cholesterol values in the population (Keys, 1957b; Streeper *et al.*, 1960). But it is also abundantly clear that the diet of the Navajo Indian is grossly different from the usual American diet (Darby *et al.*, 1956; Keys, 1957b; Kositchek *et al.*, 1960); this is consistent with the blood lipid picture. Whereas the Eskimo tells us nothing either way, the Navajo seems to provide positive evidence that is consistent with the hypothesis.

Trappist monks have attracted attention in this connection because of their Spartan lacto-vegetarian diet. Both in the Netherlands (Groen and van der Heide, 1956; Groen *et al.*, 1961) and in the United States (McCullagh and Lewis, 1960; Barrow *et al.*, 1960), it is agreed that Trappist monks have lower serum cholesterol values than men of the same age in the general population or in the Benedictine order (which does not have such dietary rules). The average difference—of the order of 30 mg of cholesterol per 100 ml of serum—is about what would be predicted from the fat composition of the diets concerned (Keys, 1962b). But the claim has been made that their diet (and the cholesterol level it produces) does not "offset the advance of cardiovascular degeneration and arterial hypertension" (McCullagh and Lewis, 1960), and the data from the Netherlands have been cited to mean "there was no significant difference as regards changes that may be attributed to atherosclerosis" (van Buchem, 1962).

Analysis of the actual data provides no basis whatever for these conclusions (Keys, 1962b). In the Netherlands prevalence was judged from medical examination of far too few monks to afford any significant comparisons. In the study of McCullagh and Lewis the data concerned blood pressure and minor eyeground changes from which it appeared that Trappists, too, can have high blood pressure, although there is no reason why this should be relevant to the question of dietary fat and atherosclerosis. The limited mortality data, however, show that, compared with other white Americans of the same age, the death rate from coronary heart disease among Trappists is remarkably low. Detailed analysis shows that if this is not the case, then we must conclude that Trappists are extraordinarily prone to die from cancer! (Keys, 1962b). The far more extensive study of Barrow *et al.* (1960) is indicating that Trappists are relatively protected against coronary heart disease. Among 1253 Benedictines and 684 Trappists, age-matched, 23 Benedictines and only 3 Trappists show evidence of complications of atherosclerosis (Barrow, 1961).

In East Africa some nomadic tribes subsist on a diet dominated by milk consumed in large amounts in the periods of abundance that alternate with times of "frank inadequacy" (Shaper *et al.*, 1961). These nomads are reputed to have a high level of energy expenditure and their average general level of dietary adequacy is indicated by the fact that they are extremely thin. Even though the caloric intake may be high, the nutritional plane is that of bare subsistence.

Serum cholesterol values reported from these tribes show striking contrasts. Samples from the cattle-herding Samburu people of northern Kenya show relatively low values (average = 190 mg per 100 ml), while the nearby camel-herding Rendille show cholesterol values (average = 233 mg per 100 ml) fully as high as United States averages (Shaper *et al.*, 1961; Shaper and Jones, 1962). It has been estimated that at the time of blood sampling the percentage of calories from fats may have been 20-25% for the Samburu and 35-40% for the Rendille (Gordon, 1959). Such diets, consumed at a bare subsistence level, would be consistent with the serum cholesterol values observed.

There are no acceptable data from which it is possible to conclude anything about metabolic peculiarities, let alone atherosclerosis or its complications, among these primitive nomads. However, there will be no lack of irresponsible assertions that these people show that a high intake of saturated fatty acids does not lead to high serum cholesterol levels and the promotion of atherosclerosis.

XXI. The Diet, Thrombosis, and Fibrinolysis

One theory attributes the initiation of atherogenesis to micro-thrombi or fibrin threads and it is certain that many of the clinical complications of atherosclerosis arise from thrombosis on an atheromatous base. Moreover, there is increasing agreement that "atherosclerotic patients" (i.e., with clinical complications) tend to have blood that, in comparison with that of "controls," is hyper-coagulable *in vitro* (McDonald, 1957; Mustard, 1958; Spittel *et al.*, 1960; Murphy and Mustard, 1962). Accordingly, the question arises as to the influence of the diet on thrombogenesis and fibrinolysis.

This has long been a controversial field of inquiry; there is little agreement about methods and even the results of apparently comparable experiments often disagree (cf. Hashim and Clancy, 1958). In man, after a fatty test meal the coagulation time of plasma recalcified in the presence of Russell's viper venom ("Stypven time") is consistently shortened (Fullerton *et al.,* 1953; Maclagen and Billimoria, 1956; Poole and Robinson, 1956; Sohar *et al.,* 1957; Merskey and Nossel, 1957; Mandel *et al.,* 1958; Nitzberg *et al.,* 1959); but the effect on other clotting tests has been disputed. However, although Merskey and Nossel (1957) and Nitzberg *et al.* (1959) disagree, most of the more recent reports agree that a fatty meal accelerates whole blood clotting in a siliconized system, or the prothrombin time, or both (Buzina and Keys, 1956; Mustard, 1957; Pilkington, 1957; Keys *et al.,* 1957c; Kingsbury and Morgan, 1957; McDonald and Fullerton, 1958). Under the same conditions inhibition of fibrinolysis has been reported (Thomas and Scott, 1957; Greig, 1957) but again universal agreement is lacking.

The experiments mentioned above refer only to the lipemic phase after a fatty meal; the effect of different diets on the blood of man drawn in the fasting state is also uncertain although it has been less studied. McDonald and Edgill (1958) observed no effect on coagulation in patients from subsistence on a low-fat diet for 4 to 5 weeks but they did observe a decrease in platelet "stickiness." This is interesting in view of reports that patients with coronary heart disease tend to have blood with a high degree of platelet stickiness (Harders, 1957; Goldrick, 1962). Mayer and Ford (1958) observed lengthened clotting time in patients in whose diets corn oil was substituted for animal fat. Similar exchange of soybean oil for animal fat in the diet of 23 patients in a home for the aged in Copenhagen produced *increased* coagulability (Ollendorf *et al.,* 1961).

In the largest scale test so far, apparently important results were obtained in mental hospitals in Helsinki (Buzina *et al.,* 1961). After 6 months there was no change in the whole blood clotting time of 57 patients who continued on the unchanged hospital diet but there was a highly significant prolongation in 53 patients whose dietary fat was changed to have a ratio of saturated to polyunsaturated fatty acids of 2.0:1 from the control level of 6.6:1.

The purpose of the long-range programs in Copenhagen and Helsinki is to see whether a change from saturated to polyunsaturated fatty acids in the diet will reduce the incidence of thrombo-embolic and other vascular disorders. The Helsinki group have not yet reported the clinical experience but it can be said that it is "encouraging" (Karvonen *et al.,* 1962). At Copenhagen, among 133 patients on the unchanged diet there have been 5 myocardial infarctions and 9 other patients have suffered major thrombo-embolic events, while among an equal number of age-matched patients in whose diets soybean oil replaced most of the animal fat, only 2 patients suffered thrombo-embolic events.

Comparisons of population samples in regard to blood coagulability and fibrinolysis are fraught with hazard unless the groups are compared in the same laboratory at the same time. With this kind of control, Buzina and Fidanza (1958) observed shorter whole blood clotting and prothrombin times among Neapolitan businessmen on a relatively high-fat diet than among Neapolitan laborers on a low-fat diet. A similar difference was observed in comparisons of sedentary and physically active men in Minneapolis, although no important difference in the diet was apparent (Buzina *et al.*, 1957).

The Bantu, famed for relative immunity to coronary atherosclerosis and thrombosis, exhibits a puzzling mixture of differences in blood coagulation factors as compared with Europeans in South Africa which do "little to explain the Bantu's freedom from coronary artery disease" (Merskey, 1957). More extensive studies have been made on Papuans, who seem to resemble the Bantu in relative freedom from coronary pathology as well as in subsistence on a low-fat diet, and on healthy and "atherosclerotic" Australians (Goldrick, 1962). Besides the expected marked differences in serum cholesterol level, there were highly significant differences in coagulation and fibrinolysis. The Papuans averaged some 30% *faster* in whole blood clotting time but they were even more remarkable in having blood that was some 70% more fibrinolytic than the Australians.

These observations call to mind the fact that apparently susceptibility to coronary atherosclerosis and to thrombo-embolic phenomena in general go hand in hand, both being low in populations on low-fat diets (van Unnik and Straub, 1953; Wang, 1956; Keating, 1956; Keys, 1957b).

In regard to the effect of the diet on thrombosis and fibrinolysis, as in the question of the dietary effect on atherogenesis, reports from experiments on animals often seem to contribute more confusion than light to the problem in man. At least quantitative comparability is usually lacking. It is claimed that by suitable adjustment of the fats in the diet fed to rats, atherosclerosis or thrombosis, or both, can be induced (Gresham and Howard, 1960, 1961). The general idea is that large amounts of saturated fat in the diet produce thrombosis and myocardial infarction (such as reported by Thomas *et al.*, 1960a), while a diet containing large amounts of linoleic acid and a small amount of saturated fatty acid produces atherosclerosis. But all the diets in these experiments contained 5% cholesterol, 2% cholic acid, 0.3% thiouracil, and 40% fat and it is questionable whether the results have any relevance to "natural" atherogenesis *or* thrombosis in man.

Grossly artificial diets fed to animals *can* produce atherosclerosis, thrombosis, changes in coagulability and fibrinolytic power of the blood, and infarcts, especially when the diet is so extreme as to produce generalized lipidosis. But as pointed out by Naimi *et al.* (1962), it is difficult to perceive a clear cause-and-effect relationship between the changes in the blood lipids, the changes in coagulation and fibrinolysis, and the cardiovascular-renal lesions, including atheromatous lesions in the arteries and myocardial and renal infarcts.

XXII. Summary

The area of controversy about the role of the diet in atherosclerosis and its complications has lately been substantially reduced by new data and better understanding of the questions at issue. Although new problems, providing fresh ground for argument, arise, many older problems are no longer seriously disputed.

Confusion is reduced by appreciating reasons for past debate. Now it is agreed that instead of a single cause for atherogenesis it is necessary to consider the contributions of a number of influences, including the diet. Moreover, since much of the evidence on man concerns clinical complications from which atherosclerosis is often inferred, factors that promote clinical complications, notably coronary heart disease, need attention; these factors are not necessarily identical to those involved in atherogenesis.

It is now realized that, because atherogenesis commonly has a long silent course before coronary heart disease is evident, observations limited to the diet contemporary with the clinical event may not accurately portray the situation during atherogenesis. Further, it is now realized that, in both man and animals, the degree of atherosclerosis in one artery is often poorly correlated with that in other arteries. In man, there is increasing evidence that the diet tends to be much more closely related to atherosclerosis in the coronary arteries than to that in the aorta.

So far no animal experimental model closely mimics the details of pathology in the body, its distribution, and the time course of the "natural" disease in man. Further, major differences among species in lipid metabolism and in the influence of the diet on it make it unsafe, and often misleading, to extrapolate from diet experiments on animals to the natural situation in man.

The fats in the diet clearly have a large effect on the blood lipids, especially cholesterol, of man. On the average, the effect of a change in diet fat on the serum cholesterol level is predictable from information on the amount and kind of fatty acids in the diet. Such information explains most of the average differences in blood cholesterol observed when populations are compared. But within a population that is dietetically relatively homogeneous, differences among individuals in blood lipids are often reflections of unknown, nondietary factors, including heredity.

In the United States the risk of future coronary heart disease is strongly related to the pre-disease serum cholesterol level. And when populations are compared, the frequency of coronary heart disease proves to be related to the average serum cholesterol level in the populations. The evidence for the same relationship between serum cholesterol and the frequency of severe atherosclerosis is less extensive.

The frequency of coronary heart disease in populations has often been observed to respond to major dietary change in a few years but such dietary changes are generally associated with other changes in the mode of life as well. In man, dietary changes induced in hope of a prophylactic effect regularly lower the blood cholesterol level but as yet there is no convincing evidence of reduced frequency of future complications of atherosclerosis and no data at all on atherogenesis.

In the lipemic phase after fatty meals some changes in coagulation and fibrinolysis are observed *in vitro*. There are reports that seem to link these factors to atherosclerotic disease, particularly to thrombotic complications, but interpretations are controversial.

All of the evidence so far is consistent with the hypothesis that, in man, the fats in the habitual diet, operating largely through their effect on the blood cholesterol and related lipids, play a major role in the development of coronary artery and coronary heart disease. Application of this hypothesis to preventive programs involves no hazard but the benefit that may be gained is uncertain, especially when the disease is already clinically manifest. Since there is little prospect that this uncertainty can be soon resolved by rigorously controlled experiments on man, practical decisions must be made on the basis of weighing the probabilities suggested by less direct evidence.

REFERENCES

Ahrens, E. H., Jr., Miller, T., and Thomasson, H. J. (1959). *Lancet* i, 115.
Albrink, M. J., and Man, E. B. (1959). *A.M.A. Arch. Internal Med.* **103**, 4.
Albrink, M. J., Meigs, J. W., and Man, E. B. (1961). *Am. J. Med.* **31**, 4.
Anderson, J. T., Grande, F., and Keys, A. (1961). *J. Nutr.* **75**, 388.
Anderson, J. T., Grande, F., Chlouverakis, C., Proja, M., and Keys, A. (1962). *Federation Proc.* **21**, 100.
Antonis, A., and Bersohn, I. (1960). *Lancet* i, 998.

Antonis, A., and Bersohn, I. (1961). *Lancet* **i**, 3.

Antonis, A., and Bersohn, I. (1962). *Am. J. Clin. Nutr.* **10**, 484.

Arteriosklerose und Ernährung (1959). *Wiss. Veroeffentl. Deut. Ges. Ernaehrung* **3**, 246 pp.

Aschoff, L. (1933). *In* "Arteriosclerosis" (E. V. Cowdry, ed.). Macmillan, New York.

Asher, G. (1948). *Dapim Refjuim (Israel)* **7**, 199.

Bansi, H. W., Neth, R., and Schwarting, G. (1955). *Verhandl. Deut. Ges. Kreislauf-forsch.* 21 *Tagung*, 139.

Barnes, B. O. (1961). *Scientific Exhibit, American Medical Association Meeting*, Denver, Colorado.

Barrow, J. G. (1961). Personal communication.

Barrow, J. G., Quinlan, C. P., Cooper, G. R., Whitner, V. S., and Goodloe, M. H. R. (1960). *Ann. Internal Med.* **52**, 386.

Bertelsen, A. (1935). *Medd. Groenland* **117**, 83 pp.

Bertelsen, A. (1937). *Medd. Groenland* **117**, 248 pp.

Bertelsen, A. (1940). *Medd. Groenland* **117**, 234 pp.

Beveridge, J. M. R., Connell, W. F., Haust, H. L., and Mayer, G. A. (1959). *Can. J. Biochem. Physiol.* **37**, 575.

Beveridge, J. M. R., Connell, W. F., Mayer, G. A., and Haust, H. L. (1960). *J. Nutr.* **71**, 61.

Biörck, G. (1956). *In* "Cardiovascular Epidemiology" (A. Keys and P. D. White, eds.), p. 8. Harper (Hoeber), New York.

Bjurulf, P. (1959). *Acta Med. Scand. Suppl.* **349**.

Brozek, J., Wells, S., and Keys, A. (1946). *Am. Rev. Soviet Med.* **4**, 69.

Brunner, D., and Loebl, K. (1958). *Ann. Internal Med.* **49**, 732.

Buzina, R., and Fidanza, F. (1958). Personal communication.

Buzina, R., and Keys, A. (1956). *Circulation* **14**, 854.

Buzina, R., Taylor, H. L., and Keys, A. (1957). To be published.

Buzina, R., Karvonen, M. J., Roine, P., and Turpeinen, O. (1961). *Lancet* **ii**, 287.

Carlson, L. A. (1960). *Acta Med. Scand.* **167**, 399.

Cohn, C., Pick, R., and Katz, L. N. (1961). *Circulation Res.* **9**, 139.

Cohn, D., and Joseph, D. (1959). *Am. J. Physiol.* **196**, 965.

Connor, W. E., Hodges, R. E., and Bleiler, R. E. (1961). *J. Lab. Clin. Med.* **57**, 331.

Council Symposium (1957). "Fats in Human Nutrition," 131 pp. Am. Med. Assoc., Chicago, Illinois; *J. Am. Med. Assoc.* **164**.

Crawford, T. (1961). *J. Atherosclerosis Res.* **1**, 3.

Dalderup, L., van Buchem, F. S. P., and Pol, G. (1963). To be published.

Darby, W. J., Salsbury, C. G., McGanity, W. J., Johnson, H. F., Bridgforth, E. B., Sandstead, H. R., Adams, C. M., Pollard, M., Dalton, E., McKinley, P., Smith, H. H., Timeche, L., Stockell, A. K., Sandstead, J. A. E., Houk, N., and Tracy, L., (1956). *J. Nutr.* **60** (Suppl. 2), 1.

Dawber, T. R. (1962). Personal communication.

Dawber, T. R., and Kannel, W. B. (1961). *Mod. Concepts Cardiovascular Disease* **30**, 671.

Dawber, T. R., Moore, F. E., and Mann, G. V. (1957). *Am. J. Public Health* **47**, 4.

Dawber, T. R., Pearson, C., Anderson, P., Mann, G. V., Kannel, W. B., Shurtleff, D., and McNamara, P. (1962). *Am. J. Clin. Nutr.* **11**, 226.

Detweiler, D. K. (1962). *J. Chronic Diseases* **15**, 867.

Dole, V. P., James, A. T., Webb, J. P. W., Rizack, M. A., and Sturman, M. F. (1959). *J. Clin. Invest.* **38**, 1544.

Doyle, J. T. (1962). Personal communication.

Doyle, J. T., Heslin, A. S., Hilleboe, H. E., Formel, P. F., and Korns, R. F. (1957). *Am. J. Public Health* **47**, 25.

Dreyfuss, F. (1953). *Am. Heart J.* **45**, 749.

Dreyfuss, F., Toor, M., Agmon, J., and Zlotnick, A. (1957). *Cardiologia* **30**, 387.

Duguid, J. B. (1948). *J. Pathol. Bacteriol.* **60**, 57.

Duguid, J. B. (1949). *Lancet* **ii**, 925.

Ehrström, M. C. (1951). *Acta Med. Scand.* **140**, 416.

Eilersen, P., and Faber, M. (1960). *Arch. Pathol.* **70**, 103.

Faber, M., and Lund, F. (1949). *A.M.A. Arch. Pathol.* **48**, 351.

Feigenbaum, A. S., Fisher, H., and Weiss, H. S. (1962). *Am. J. Clin. Nutr.* **11**, 312.

Fidanza, F., Keys, A., and others (1963). To be published.

Fifth International Congress on Nutrition (1961). *Federation Proc.* **20**, 115, 121, 127, 135, 146, 152, 161.

Fullerton, M. W., Davie, W. J. A., and Anastasopoulos, G. (1953). *Brit. Med. J.* **II**, 250.

Garcia de los Rios, M. (1961). *Am. J. Clin. Nutr.* **9**, 315.

Gilbert, J. (1954). *Calif. Heart Assoc., San Francisco,* 7 pp.

Glatzel, H. (1960). *Deut. Med. Wochschr.* **85**, 1296.

Goldrick, R. B. (1962). Doctoral Thesis, Univ. Sydney, Sydney, Australia.

Gordon, H. (1959). *Post Grad. Med. J.* **35**, 186.

Gordon, T. (1957). *U. S. Dept. Health Educ. Welfare Public Health Rept.* **72**, 543.

Gore, I., Robertson, W. B., Hirst, A. E., Hadley, G. G., and Koseki, Y. (1960). *Am. J. Pathol.* **36**, 559.

Grande, F., Anderson, J. T., Glick, D., Grunbaum, B., and Geary, J. R., Jr. (1957). *Proc. Soc. Exptl. Biol. Med.* **94**, 613.

Grande, F., Anderson, J. T., and Keys, A. (1961). *J. Nutr.* **74**, 240.

Greig, H. B. W. (1957). *Brit. Med. J.* **II**, 708.

Gresham, G. A., and Howard, A. N. (1960). *J. Exptl. Pathol.* **41**, 395.

Gresham, G. A., and Howard, A. N. (1961). *J. Exptl. Pathol.* **42**, 166.

Groen, J., and van der Heide, R. M. (1956). "Atherosclerose en Coronairthrombose." Gezondheids organisatie T.N.O., Uitgevers, Rotterdam.

Groen, J., Tjiong, B. K., Koster, M., Verdouk, G., Perlot, R., and Willebrands, A. F. (1961). *Ned. Tijdschr. Geneesk.* **105**, 222.

Harders, H. (1957). *Thromb. Diath. Haemorrhag.* **1**, 482.

Hashim, S. A., and Clancy, R. E. (1958). *New Engl. J. Med.* **259**, 1115.

Hashim, S. A., Arteaga, A., and van Itallie, T. B. (1960). *Lancet* **i**, 1105.

Hegsted, D. M., Gotsis, A., Stare, F. J., and Worcester, J. (1959). *Am. J. Clin. Nutr.* **7**, 5.

Henschen, F. (1959). *Svenska Läkartidn.* **56**, 1674.

Hilleboe, H. E. (1957). *J. Chronic Diseases* **6**, 210.

Hirst, A. E., Jr., Piyaratn, P., and Gore, I. (1962). *Am. J. Clin. Pathol.* **38**, 162.

Horlick, L. (1961). *Am. J. Cardiol.* **8**, 459.

Instituto de Cardiologia do Estado de Sao Paulo (1959). "O Metabolismo Lipidico e o Enfarte do Miocardio" Secr. Saude e Assist. Soc., Sao Paulo, Brazil.

Jahnke, K., and Breitbach, A. (1959). *In* "Symposium der Deutschen Gessellschaft für Ernährung in Bad Neuenahr," p. 170. Steinkopf, Darmstadt.

Jankelson, O. M., Stefanik, P. A., and Stare, F. J. (1962). *Am. J. Clin. Nutr.* 11, 134.

Jolliffe, N., and Archer, M. (1959). *J. Chronic Diseases* 9, 636.

Jones, R. J., and Cohen, L. (1961). "Chemistry and Therapy of Chronic Cardiovascular Disease," 200 pp. C. C Thomas, Springfield, Illinois.

Juhl, S. (1955). *Acta Pathol. Microbiol. Scand.* 37, 167.

Juhl, S. (1957). *Acta Pathol. Microbiol. Scand.* 41, 99.

Kallner, G. (1958). *Lancet* i, 1155.

Karvonen, M. J., Turpeinen, O., Roine, P., and others (1962). Personal communication.

Katz, L. N., Stamler, J., and Pick, R. (1958). "Nutrition and Atherosclerosis," 146 pp. Lea & Febiger, Philadelphia, Pennsylvania.

Keating, V. (1956). *Brit. Med. J.* II, 851.

Keys, A. (1952). *Voeding* 13, 539.

Keys, A. (1953). *J. Mt. Sinai Hosp.* 20, 118.

Keys, A. (1954). *Am. J. Public Health* 44, 864.

Keys, A. (1955). *In* "Weight Control," pp. 18, 108. Iowa State Coll. Press, Ames, Iowa.

Keys, A. (1956). *In* "Cardiovascular Epidemiology" (A. Keys, and P. D. White, eds.), p. 50. Harper (Hoeber), New York.

Keys, A. (1957a). *J. Chronic Diseases* 6, 552.

Keys, A. (1957b). *J. Am. Med. Assoc.* 164, 1912.

Keys, A. (1958). *Proc. 3rd World Congr. Cardiol., Brussels 1958*, p. 397.

Keys, A. (1961). *Deut. Med. Wochschr.* 86, 2490.

Keys, A. (1962a). *Cardiol. Prat.* 8, 225.

Keys, A. (1962b). *Malattie Cardiovascolare* 3, 33.

Keys, A., and Anderson, J. T. (1957). *Am. J. Clin. Nutr.* 5, 29.

Keys, A., and Fidanza, F. (1960). *Circulation* 22, 1091.

Keys, A., Mickelsen, O., Miller, E. v. O., and Chapman, C. B. (1950). *Science* 112, 79.

Keys, A., Fidanza, F., and Keys, M. H. (1955). *Voeding* 16, 492.

Keys, A., Anderson, J. T., Mickelsen, O., Adelson, S., and Fidanza, F. (1956). *J. Nutr.* 59, 124.

Keys, A., Anderson, J. T., and Grande, F. (1957a). *Lancet* ii, 959.

Keys, A., Kimura, N., Kusukawa, A., and Yoshitomi, M. (1957b). *Am. J. Clin. Nutr.* 5, 245.

Keys, A., Buzina, R., Grande, F., and Anderson, J. T. (1957c). *Circulation* 15, 274.

Keys, A. Anderson, J. T., and Grande, F. (1958a). *Proc. Soc. Exptl. Biol. Med.* 98, 387.

Keys, A., Kimura, N., Kusukawa, A., Bronte-Stewart, B., Larsen, N. P., and Keys, M. H. (1958b). *Ann. Internal Med.* 48, 83.

Keys, A., Anderson, J. T., and Grande, F. (1959). *Circulation* 19, 201.

Keys, A., Anderson, J. T., and Grande, F. (1960). *J. Nutr.* 70, 257.

Keys, A., Grande, F., and Anderson, J. T. (1961). *Proc. Soc. Exptl. Biol. Med.* 106, 555.

Keys, A., Taylor, H. L., Blackburn, H., Brozek, J., Anderson, J. T., and Simonson, E. (1963a). *Circulation,* In press.

Keys, A., Fidanza, F., Buzina, R., van Buchem, F. S. P., Roine, P., and others. (1963b). International collaborative studies on the diet and blood cholesterol in populations. To be published.

Kimura, N. (1956). *In* "Cardiovascular Epidemiology" (A. Keys and P. D. White, eds.), p. 22. Harper (Hoeber), New York.

Kingsbury, K. J., and Morgan, D. M. (1957). *Lancet* **ii**, 212.

Kositchek, R. J., Wurm, M., and Straus, R. (1960). *Circulation* **23**, 219.

Krogh, A., and Krogh, M. (1914-1915). *Medd. Groenland* **51**, 1.

Kusukawa, A. (1956). *In* "Cardiovascular Epidemiology" (A. Keys and P. D. White, eds.), p. 159. Harper (Hoeber), New York.

Larsen, N. P. (1957). *A.M.A. Arch. Internal Med.* **100**, 436.

Larsen, N. P., and Bortz, W. (1959). *Hawaii Med. J.* **19**, 159.

Larsen, N. P., and Bortz, W. (1960). *J. Am. Geriat. Soc.* **8**, 867.

Laurie, W., and Woods, J. D. (1958). *Lancet* **i**, 231.

Lober, P. H. (1953). *A.M.A. Arch. Pathol.* **55**, 357.

Lowry, J., Anderson, J. T., and Keys, A. (1963). To be published.

Luyken, R., Pikaar, N. A., Polman, H., and Schippers, F. A. (1962). *Voeding, Jaargang 1962*, p. 447.

Maclagan, N. F., and Billimoria, J. D. (1956). *Lancet* **ii**, 235.

McCullagh, E. P., and Lewis, L. A. (1960). *New Engl. J. Med.* **263**, 569.

McDonald, L. (1957). *Lancet* **ii**, 457.

McDonald, L., and Edgill, M. (1958). *Lancet* **ii**, 996.

McDonald, C. A., and Fullerton, H. W. (1958). *Lancet* **ii**, 598.

Malmros, H. (1950). *Acta Med. Scand. Suppl.* **246**, 137.

Malmros, H., and Wigand, G. (1957). *Lancet* **ii**, 1.

Mandel, E., Mermall, H. L., Preston, F. W., and Silverman, M. (1958). *Am. J. Clin. Pathol.* **30**, 11.

Mann, G. V., Scott, E. M., Hursh, L. M., Heller, C. A., Youmans, J. B., Consolazio, C. F., Bridgforth, E. B., Russell, A. L., and Silverman, M. (1962c). *Am. J. Clin. Nutr.* **11**, 31.

Mayer, G. A., and Ford, W. (1958). *Circulation* **18**, 496.

Merskey, C. (1957). *Leech* **28**, 45.

Merskey, C., and Nossel, H. L. (1957). *Lancet* **i**, 806.

Miller, D. C., Trulson, M. F., McCann, M. B., White, P. D., and Stare, F. J. (1958). *Ann. Internal Med.* **49**, 1178.

Ministry of Health and Welfare (1962 and previous years). "Nutrition in Japan." Tokyo.

Morris, J. N. (1951). *Lancet* **i**, 69.

Morris, J. N. (1962a). *Proc. Roy. Soc. Med.* **55**, 693-695.

Morris, J. N. (1962b). *Cardiol. Prat.* **8**, 85.

Morris, J. N., Crawford, M. D., and Heady, H. A. (1961). *Lancet* **i**, 860.

Mulder, T. (1959). *Voeding* **20**, 105.

Murphy, E. A., and Mustard, J. F. (1962). *Circulation* **25**, 114.

Mustard, J. F. (1957). *Can. Med. Assoc. J.* **77**, 308.

Mustard, J. F. (1958). *Can. Med. Assoc. J.* **79**, 554.

Myasnikov, A. L. (1962). "Atherosclerosis: Occurrence, Clinical Forms, Therapy" (Translation from the Russian). 634 pp. Natl. Heart Inst., Natl. Inst. Health, Bethesda, Maryland.

Naimi, S., Goldstein, R., Nothman, M. M., Wilgram, G. F., and Proger, S. (1962). *J. Clin. Invest.* **41**, 1708.

Neal, J. B., and Neal, M. (1962). *Arch. Pathol.* **73**, 400.

New York Heart Association (1957). "Conference on Atherosclerosis and Coronary Heart Disease," 133 pp. N. Y. Heart Assoc., New York; *J. Chronic Diseases* **4** (4).

Nitzberg, S. I. (1959). *Circulation* **19**, 676.

Nitzberg, S. I., Peyman, M. A., Goldstein, R., and Proger, S. (1959). *Circulation* **19**, 676.

Nutrition Division (1959). Canadian Food and Nutrition Statistics, 1953 to 1956. Queen's Printer, Ottawa, Canada. Cat. No. H58-2959.

Ollendorff, P., Geill, T., Astrup, T., and Lund, F. (1961). *Acta Med. Scand.* **170**, 351.

Page, I. H., ed. (1958). "Chemistry of Lipids as Related to Atherosclerosis," 342 pp. C. C Thomas, Springfield, Illinois.

Page, I. H., Lewis, L. A., Gilbert, J. (1956). *Circulation* **13**, 675.

Paterson, J. C., Cornish, B. R., and Armstrong, E. C. (1956). *Circulation* **13**, 224.

Paul, O., Lepper, M. H., Phelan, W. H., Dupertuis, C. W., MacMillan, A., McKean, H., and Park, H. (1963). *Circulation*, **28**, 20.

Pezold, F. A. (1959). "Arteriosklerose und Ernährung," p. 162. Steinkopf, Darmstadt.

Pihl, A. (1952). *Scand. J. Lab. Clin. Invest.* **4**, 122.

Pilkington, T. R. E. (1957). *Clin. Sci.* **16**, 261.

Pollak, O. J. (1959). *Am. J. Clin. Nutr.* **7**, 502.

Poole, J. C. F., and Robinson, D. S. (1956). *Quart. J. Exptl. Physiol.* **41**, 31.

Prior, J. T., Kurtz, D. M., and Ziegler, D. D. (1961). *Arch. Pathol.* **71**, 672.

Rodahl, K. (1956). *Hawaii Med. J.* **16**, 131.

Rosenthal, S. R. (1934). *A.M.A. Arch. Pathol.* **18**, 473, 660, 827.

Schettler, C. (1954). *Verhandl. Deut. Ges. Inn. Med.* **60**, 883.

Schettler, C., ed. (1961). "Arteriosklerose." Thieme, Leipzig.

Schornagel, H. E. (1953). *Doc. Med. Geograph. Trop.* **5**, 173.

Schroeder, H. A. (1958). *J. Chronic Diseases* **8**, 287.

Schroeder, H. A. (1960a). *J. Chronic Diseases* **12**, 586.

Schroeder, H. A. (1960b). *J. Am. Med. Assoc.* **172**, 1902.

Scott, R. F., Daoud, A. S., Florentin, R. A., Davies, J. N. P., and Coles, R. M. (1961). *Am. J. Cardiol.* **8**, 165.

Shaper, A. G., and Jones, K. W. (1962). *Lancet* ii, 1305.

Shaper, A. G., Jones, M., and Kyobe, J. (1961). *Lancet* ii, 1322.

Simonson, E., and Keys, A. (1961). *Circulation* **24**, 1239.

Sinclair, H. M. (1953). *Proc. Nutr. Soc. (Engl. Scot.)* **12**, 69.

Sjövall, H., and Wihman, G. (1934). *Acta Pathol. Microbiol. Scand. Suppl.* **20**.

Snapper, I. (1941). "Chinese Lessons to Western Medicine." Interscience, New York.

Society of Actuaries (1959). "Build and Blood Pressure Study," 2 Vols. Chicago, Illinois.

Sohar, E., Rosenthal, M. C., and Adlersberg, D. (1957). *Am. J. Clin. Pathol.* **27**, 503.

Spittel, J. A., Jr., Pascuzzi, C. A., Thompson, J. H., Jr., and Owens, C. A., Jr. (1960). *Proc. Staff Meetings Mayo Clinic* **35**, 37.

Stamler, J. (1960). *Cardiovascular Disease* **3**, 56.

Stefansson, V. (1956). "The Fat of the Land," 339 pp. Macmillan, New York.

Stefansson, V. (1958). *Science* **127**, 16.

Strain, W. H. (1961). *In* "Symposium on Geochemical Evolution—the First Five Billion Years," Amer. Assoc. Adv. Sci., Denver, Colorado.

Streeper, R. B., Massey, R. U., Lin, G., Dillingham, C. H., and Cushing, A. (1960). *Diseases Chest* **38**, 305.

Strøm, A. (1948). *Acta Med. Scand. Suppl.* **214**.

Strøm, A. (1954). *Akad. Trykningssentral*, Oslo, 41 pp.

Strøm, A., and Jensen, R. A. (1950). *Nord. Hyg. Tidskr.* **31**, 5, 125.

Strøm, A., and Jensen, R. A. (1951). *Lancet* i, 126.

Technical Group of Committee on Lipoproteins and Atherosclerosis and Committee on Lipoproteins and Atherosclerosis of National Advisory Heart Council. (1956). *Circulation* **14**, 691.

Tennent, D. M., Siegel, H., Gunther, W. K., Ott, W. H., and Mushett, C. W. (1957). *Proc. Soc. Exptl. Biol. Med.* **96**, 679.

Thomas, W. A., and Scott, R. F. (1957). *Proc. Soc. Exptl. Biol. Med.* **96**, 24.

Thomas, W. A., Davies, J. N. P., O'Neal, R. M., and Dimakulangan, A. A. (1960a). *Am. J. Cardiol.* **5**, 41.

Thomas, W. A., Hartroft, W. S., and Neal, R. M. (1960b). *J. Nutr.* **69**, 325.

Toor, M., Katchalsky, A., Agmon, J., and Allalouf, D. (1957). *Lancet* **i**, 270.

Toor, M., Katchalsky, A., Agmon, J., and Allalouf, D. (1960). *Circulation* **22**, 265.

Turpeinen, O., Roine, P., Pekkarinen, M., Karvonen, M., Rautanen, Y., Runeberg, J., and Alivirta, P. (1960). *Lancet* **i**, 196.

van Buchem, F. S. P. (1962). *Nutr. Dieta* **4**, 122.

van Unnik, J., and Straub, M. (1953). *Doc. Med. Geograph. Trop.* **5**, 261.

Vartiainen, I. (1946). *Ann. Med. Internae Fenniae* **35**, 234.

Vartiainen, I., and Kanerva, K. (1947). *Ann. Med. Internae Fenniae* **36**, 748.

Vastesaeger, M. M., and Delcourt, R. (1961). *Nutr. Dieta* **3**, 174.

Walker, G. R., Morse, E. H., and Potgieter, M. (1956). *J. Nutr.* **60**, 517.

Wang, C. (1956). *Bull. Assoc. Harvard Med. Alumni.*

Wanscher, O., Clemmesen, J., and Nielsen, A. (1951). *Brit. J. Cancer* **5**, 172.

White, N. K., Edwards, J. E., and Dry, T. J. (1950). *Circulation* **1**, 645.

White, P. D. (1956). *In* "Cardiovascular Epidemiology" (A. Keys and P. D. White, eds.), p. 62. Harper (Hoeber), New York.

Wilens, S. L. (1947a). *Am. J. Pathol.* **23**, 793.

Wilens, S. L. (1947b). *A.M.A. Arch. Internal Med.* **79**, 129.

Yerushalmy, J., and Hilleboe, H. E. (1957). *N.Y. State J. Med.* **57**, 2343.

Yudkin, J. (1957). *Lancet* **ii**, 155.

Yudkin, J. (1961). *Practitioner* **187**, 150.

ADDITIONAL REFERENCES

Adelson, S. F., and Keys, A. (1962). *U. S. Dept. Agr.* ARS **62-11**, 280 pp.

Ahrens, E. H., Jr., Insull, W., Blomstrand, R., Hirsch, J., Tsaltas, T-T., and Peterson, M. L. (1957). *Lancet* **i**, 943.

Albrink, M. J., Meigs, J. W., and Granoff, M. A. (1962). *New Engl. J. Med.* **266**, 484.

Beaumont, V., Beaumont, J.-L., and Lenegre, J. (1958). *Rev. Franc. Etudes Clin. Biol.* **3**, 746.

Beveridge, J. M. R., Connell, W. F., and Mayer, G. A. (1956). *Can. J. Biochem. Physiol.* **34**, 441.

Biörck, G., Blomqvist, G., and Sievers, J. (1960). *Acta Tertii European Cardiovascular Sci. Conv. (Roma) A* p. 63.

Brunner, D., Loebl, K., Fischer, M., and Schick, G. (1955). *Harlefuah* **48**, 1.

Cohn, C., Pick, R., and Katz, L. N. (1959). *Circulation* **20**, 969.

Danaraj, T. J., Acker, M. S., Danaraj, W., Ong, W. H., and Yam, T. B. (1959). *Am. Heart J.* **58**, 516.

Dodds, C., and Mills, G. L. (1959). *Lancet* **i**, 1160.

Fischer, F. W. (1957). *Klin. Wochschr.* **35**, 373.

From Hansen, P., Geill, T., and Lund, E. (1962). *Lancet* **ii**, 1193.

Gopalan, C., Srikantia, S. G., Jagannathan, S. N., and Ramanathan, K. S. (1962). *Am. J. Clin. Nutr.* **10**, 332.

Grant, F. W., and Groom, D. (1959). *J. Am. Dietet. Assoc.* **35**, 910.

Groom, D. (1961). *Ann. Internal Med.* **55**, 51.

Groom, D., McKee, E. E., Webb, C., Grant, F. W., Pean, V., Hudicourt, E., and Dallemand, J. (1959). *Ann. Internal Med.* **51**, 270.

Katz, L. N., and Stamler, J. (1953). "Experimental Atherosclerosis," 375 pp. C. C Thomas, Springfield, Illinois.

Keys, A., and White, P. D., eds. (1956). "World Trends in Cardiology: I. Cardiovascular Epidemiology," 193 pp. Hoeber & Harper, New York.

Kinsell, L. W., Partridge, J., Boling, L., Margen, S., and Michaels, G. (1952). *J. Clin. Endocrinol. Metab.* **12**, 909.

Kinsell, L. W., Michaels, G. D., and Dailey, J. P. (1957). *Circulation* **16**, 479.

Lew, E. A. (1957). *J. Chronic Diseases* **6**, 192.

Luyken, R., and Jansen, A. A. J. (1960). *Doc. Med. Geograph. Trop.* **12**, 145.

Mann, G. V., Munoz, J. A., and Scrimshaw, N. S. (1955). *Am. J. Med.* **19**, 25.

Mendez, J., Tejada, C., and Flores, M. (1962). *Am. J. Clin. Nutr.* **10**, 403.

Morris, J. N. (1961-1962). *Yale J. Biol. Med.* **34**, 359-369.

Muir, C. S. (1960). *Brit. Heart J.* **22**, 45.

Orvis, H. H., Thomas, R. E., Fawal, I. A., and Evans, J. M. (1961). *Am. J. Med. Sci.* **241**, 167.

Paterson, J. C., Dyer, L., and Armstrong, E. C. (1960). *Can. Med. Assoc. J.* **82**, 6.

Pezold, F. A., ed. (1961). "Lipide und Lipoproteide im Blutplasma," 399 pp. Springer, Berlin.

Scrimshaw, N. S., Trulson, M., Tejada, C., Hegsted, D. M., and Stare, F. J. (1957). *Circulation* **15**, 805.

Sinclair, H. M. (1956). *Lancet* i, 521.

Tamayo, R. P., Brandt, H., and Ontiveros, E. (1961). *Arch. Pathol.* **71**, 113.

Tejada, C., Gore, I., Strong, J. P., and McGill, H. C. (1958). *Circulation* **18**, 92.

Toor, M., Agmon, J., and Allalouf, D. (1954). *Bull. Res. Council Israel* E4, 202.

Wainwright, J. (1961). *Lancet* i, 366.

— 9 —

Interrelationships of Lipids in Blood and Tissues

Leon Swell and C. R. Treadwell

I. Introduction

Considerable data of diverse types have accumulated in recent years which indicate that the lipids may be of prime importance in the etiology of arterial disease. The evidence for the participation of lipids, in particular, cholesterol, in arterial disease is based on the following general observations: (a) a common factor in all experimental procedures for producing atherosclerosis in animals is the feeding of cholesterol; (b) populations with high serum lipid levels have a higher incidence of heart disease than groups without elevated levels; (c) there is a greater incidence of atherosclerosis in individuals with abnormal lipid metabolism, such as diabetes, xanthomatosis, and nephrosis; (d) analysis of atheromatous lesions indicates the presence of large amounts of lipids. The basic question which cannot be answered at present is whether the disease process is primarily the result of abnormal lipid metabolism in the aorta, blood, or other tissues or whether the accumulation of lipids is a secondary phenomenon following some primary damage to the vessel wall.

Many of the metabolic pathways in lipid metabolism have been elucidated, others are being intensively studied, while still others are being re-examined in the light of newer information. The question of the origin, regulation, and transport of lipids has also received considerable attention, but much remains to be elucidated. Several developments have provided new experimental approaches for the study of these areas of lipid metabolism. One observation was that the ingestion of polyunsaturated fatty acids lowers the blood cholesterol level in man; this provided an impetus for studies on the role of the essential fatty acids in atherogenesis and cholesterol metabolism. Another was the development of a reliable technique (gas-liquid chromatography) for the identification and determination of the fatty acids.

The present discussion will be concerned with the interrelationships of the blood and tissue lipids and will primarily consider data on the origin of the lipids in blood, liver, and aorta and their fatty acid compositions. Particular emphasis has been placed on the more recent data in these areas of lipid metabolism and their significance to the atherosclerosis problem.

II. Fatty Acid Composition of the Lipids in Blood

A. Cholesterol Esters

This and the succeeding sections on lipid fatty acid composition refer to data on the individual lipid fractions, and references to results obtained on the fatty acid composition of total lipids are omitted.

Kelsey and Longenecker (1941) carried out the first detailed study on the fatty acid composition of the plasma cholesterol esters which formed the basis for the general belief that the blood cholesterol esters contain a high proportion of polyunsaturated fatty acids. These workers reported that the cholesterol ester fatty acid (CEFA) composition of cow plasma was as follows: linoleic 62%, saturated 15%, oleic 8%, linolenic 9%, and arachidonic 2%. Mukherjee et al. (1957) determined the CEFA composition of normal rat blood by the alkali isomerization technique; they found 56% saturated, 25% dienoic, 10% tetraenoic, and no oleic. These findings on rat blood cholesterol esters were not confirmed by later workers (Howton and Hashimoto, 1960; Swell et al., 1960c; Klein and Dahl, 1961; Albers and Gordon, 1962; Carroll, 1962; Apostolakis et al., 1962) who found that arachidonic acid constituted 50-68% of the CEFA. Lough and Garton (1957) and Duncan and Garton (1962) examined the CEFA of ox plasma and found a high percentage of linolenic acid. The occurrence of this acid in large amounts is of interest since in the serum cholesterol esters of other species only small amounts occur. As pointed out by the authors, this may be the result of a high content of linolenic acid in their feed lipids. Since the advent of newer techniques human plasma CEFA composition has been extensively investigated in normal and diseased subjects. The data agree in that plasma cholesterol esters of normal subjects are high in polyunsaturated fatty acids and that linoleic acid is the major acid (Dole et al., 1959; Bjorntorp and Hood, 1960; Hallgren et al., 1960; Hanahan et al., 1960a; Riley and Nunn, 1960; Swell et al., 1960a, d, 1962c; Böttcher and Woodford, 1961; Lawrie et al., 1961a; Schrade et al., 1961). The blood CEFA composition of several species is shown in Table I. The polyunsaturated fatty acids comprise a major portion of the total fatty acids; in most species linoleic acid is the major fatty acid. The most notable exceptions are the rat, in which arachidonic acid is the major acid, and the goose and chicken where the percentage of oleic acid tends to predominate slightly over linoleic acid. As can be seen, the over-all fatty acid spectrum varies from species to species. The factors determining this species variation are unknown, although one might speculate that diet and essential fatty acid metabolism are

TABLE I

THE SERUM OR PLASMA CHOLESTEROL ESTER FATTY ACID COMPOSITION OF VARIOUS SPECIES

(Data given in terms of % of total fatty acids)

Major fatty acids[b]	Species[a]										
	Man (1)[c]	Rat (2)[c]	Dog (2)[c]	Guinea pig (2)[c]	Pig (2)[c]	Goose (2)[c]	Chicken (2)[c]	Rabbit (3)[c]	Mouse (4)[c]	Ox (5)[c]	Gerbil (6)[c]
Palmitic	15.6	12.4	12.2	18.6	12.8	17.2	15.1	21.7	5.0	5.5	5.4
Palmitoleic	3.7	2.4	2.9	2.4	2.9	1.7	6.9	3.9	1.5	2.8	6.8
Stearic	2.4	2.6	3.2	0.5	4.2	2.4	6.1	3.9	1.2	1.5	—
Oleic	21.8	9.8	18.1	14.8	30.8	40.0	35.8	27.2	6.0	5.6	22.8
Linoleic	47.5	19.5	44.9	57.9	45.4	31.3	29.3	36.4	50.1	52.4	65.1
Linolenic	0.5	0.3	—	0.2	0.4	0.3	0.3	0.6	—	22.9	—
Arachidonic	5.9	50.0	17.0	1.1	1.8	5.8	5.2	1.8	29.9	4.6	—

[a] Represents values obtained on normal animals.

[b] Determined by gas-liquid chromatography.

[c] Reference code: (1) Swell et al. (1962c), (2) Swell et al. (1960b), (3) Swell et al. (1962b), (4) Rehnborg et al. (1961), (5) Duncan and Garton (1962), (6) Albers and Gordon (1962).

intimately involved. Another interesting aspect concerning the plasma cholesterol esters, particularly of man, is that in a given individual or group there is very little fluctuation in the fatty acid composition over periods for as long as 1 year (Swell *et al.,* 1962c, d). This is in contrast to the wide fluctuation in the level of the serum cholesterol which may occur even from day to day.

The early work which demonstrated that the serum cholesterol esters contain a high proportion of polyunsaturated fatty acids led to speculation that one important function of cholesterol is to transport those fatty acids to the tissues. It is now known that cholesterol and essential fatty acid metabolism are closely interrelated. Alfin-Slater *et al.* (1954) and Achaya *et al.* (1954) found an accumulation of cholesterol esters in the livers of essential fatty acid-deficient rats containing primarily saturated and oleic acids. These findings suggested that the alternate possibility also exists; namely, that the essential fatty acids are of importance in the transport of cholesterol. Similar findings were also noted in chicks maintained on a fat-free diet (Dam *et al.,* 1955). Other studies have shown that the feeding of a fat-free diet with cholesterol hastens the development of essential fatty acid deficiency in rats (Holman and Peifer, 1960; Gambal and Quackenbush, 1960). This depletion of the reserve of essential fatty acids by cholesterol further supports the contention that the essential fatty acids are required for the transport of cholesterol.

The possible importance of essential fatty acids in cholesterol metabolism provided an impetus for a number of studies of their effect on the blood cholesterol level. It is now well documented that ingestion of diets high in polyunsaturated fatty acids will produce a decrease in the serum cholesterol of man and animals under a variety of conditions. Such diets also lead to an increased proportion of polyunsaturated fatty acids (mostly linoleic acid) in the serum lipid fractions (Holman *et al.,* 1957; Kinsell *et al.,* 1958; Ahrens *et al.,* 1959; Patil and Magar, 1960; Swell *et al.,* 1962c). In Table II are shown some results obtained in a recent study (Swell *et al.,* 1962d) on the effect of a high linoleic acid diet on the serum cholesterol level, CEFA, and triglyceride fatty acid composition of normal subjects. There was a highly significant increase in the proportion of linoleic acid in the serum cholesterol esters with proportional drops in saturated and oleic acids. These results suggest that there is an inverse relationship between the serum cholesterol level and the percentage of linoleic acid in the cholesterol ester fraction.

The effect of polyunsaturated fatty acids on the serum cholesterol

TABLE II

INFLUENCE OF A HIGH LINOLEIC ACID DIET ON SERUM LIPID FATTY ACID COMPOSITION

Major fatty acids[a]	Cholesterol esters (% of total fatty acids)		Triglycerides (% of total fatty acids)	
	Before dietary change	On diet 52 weeks	Before dietary change	On diet 52 weeks
Palmitic	16.7	12.0	33.5	27.5
Palmitoleic	3.8	2.6	3.4	4.3
Stearic	3.4	0.9	5.8	3.7
Oleic	24.5	16.2	40.2	35.0
Linoleic	42.9	58.1	11.6	23.6
Arachidonic	4.4	6.5	0.7	0.9
Serum cholesterol (mg/100 gm)	293	230	—	—

[a] Represents the average of 16 subjects; taken from Swell *et al.* (1962d). Determined by gas-liquid chromatography.

level and the suggested role of those acids in cholesterol transport led Sinclair (1956) to propose that atherosclerosis might result from a chronic deficiency of the essential fatty acids, and in particular, arachidonic acid. According to this view, if insufficient essential fatty acids were available, cholesterol would become esterified with more saturated and unnatural fatty acids, and those esters tend to be deposited in the aorta and other tissues. A number of studies have been carried out in man and animals to test this hypothesis. These reports have been concerned with the changes in the fatty acid composition of the lipid fractions in blood and aorta associated with the development of atherosclerosis; changes in the fatty acid composition of the blood lipid fractions will be considered first.

James *et al.* (1957) noted that the serum acetone-soluble lipids (cholesterol esters plus triglycerides) of subjects with coronary artery disease had a slightly higher percentage of monounsaturated acids than those of normal subjects. These findings might have been more significant had the cholesterol esters been separated from the triglycerides. Lewis (1958) found that the serum cholesterol esters of patients with coronary artery disease had significantly less linoleic acid and more saturated fatty acids than normal subjects. A comparable relationship between the serum cholesterol esters of normal and atherosclerotic subjects was also reported by Wright *et al.* (1959) and Bjorntorp and Hood (1960). Schrade and co-workers (1961) and Böttcher and Woodford (1961), employing gas-liquid chromatography, also reported that the serum cholesterol esters of subjects with atherosclerosis contain a lower percentage of linoleic acid than healthy subjects. On the other hand, Lawrie *et al.* (1961a, b) did not observe any differences in the serum CEFA composition between healthy subjects and patients with ischemic heart disease.

Aging has also been shown to affect the proportions of fatty acids of the serum cholesterol esters. Swell *et al.* (1960d) found that the serum cholesterol esters of children (6-10 years old) had a higher percentage of linoleic acid and less oleic acid than that serum fraction of older subjects (aged 67-72 years). Schrade and co-workers (1961) have carried out some excellent detailed studies in which the serum lipid fatty acid distribution of healthy subjects of different ages was compared with subjects with atherosclerosis and hyperlipemia. In older subjects (46-71 years) the proportion of linoleic and arachidonic acids was lower and the monounsaturated fatty acids higher in the serum cholesterol esters than in younger subjects (19-42 years).

The results of the above studies (although there is by no means complete agreement) have provided evidence that subjects with heart disease and atherosclerosis tend to have a lower percentage of linoleic acid and a higher proportion of monounsaturated acids (mostly oleic) in their serum cholesterol esters than normal individuals, and second, that older subjects show changes in the same direction when compared with young subjects. Here, as in other aspects of metabolism, the available data do not allow a clear-cut distinction between the processes of aging and atherosclerosis.

Recent data are also available on the serum CEFA composition or normal and cholesterol-fed rabbits. Some of these data are shown in Table III. The results obtained by Zilversmit *et al.* (1961b), Swell *et al.* (1961b, 1962b), and Evrard *et al.* (1962) are in general agreement that the plasma cholesterol esters of the cholesterol-fed rabbit with atherosclerosis contain a higher percentage of oleic acid and a lower percentage of linoleic acid than animals receiving diets without cholesterol.

Another interesting aspect of the role of essential fatty acids in atherosclerosis was reported in a study (Swell *et al.*, 1960b) in which the percentages of arachidonic acid in the serum cholesterol esters of several different species were compared. It was noted (Table I) that those species (rat and dog) which are resistant to the development of atherosclerosis have a high percentage of arachidonic acid in their serum cholesterol esters, while those species (rabbit, dog, goose, chicken, and guinea pig) which are susceptible to atherosclerosis and develop the disease spontaneously have small proportions of that acid in their serum cholesterol esters. The gerbil appears to be an exception to this rule since it has a low level of arachidonic acid and does not develop atheroscle-

TABLE III

THE SERUM OR PLASMA AND AORTA CHOLESTEROL ESTER FATTY ACID COMPOSITION OF CHOLESTEROL-FED RABBITS

(Data given in terms of % of total fatty acids)

Major fatty acids[a]	Normal rabbits		Cholesterol-fed rabbits					
	Serum (1)[b]	Plasma (2)[b]	Aortic intima (3)[b]	Aortic intima (2)[b]	Aorta (1)[b]	Serum (1)[b]	Plasma (2)[b]	Plasma (3)[b]
Palmitic	21.3	18.2	13.5	14.4	31.0	20.5	15.8	17.8
Palmitoleic	4.7	2.5	4.5	2.5	4.1	5.4	3.1	5.1
Stearic	3.9	3.4	2.9	4.0	6.7	4.3	4.6	4.3
Oleic	23.2	33.6	54.9	57.4	39.4	40.6	50.2	44.2
Linoleic	39.6	39.2	16.1	18.5	11.8	22.3	24.2	24.3
Arachidonic	1.5	—	—	—	0.3	0.8	—	—

[a] Determined by gas-liquid chromatography.

[b] Reference code: (1) Swell *et al.* (1961b), (2) Evrard *et al.* (1962), (3) Zilversmit *et al.* (1961b).

rosis (Albers and Gordon, 1962). This relationship suggests that arachidonic acid may play a significant role in the prevention of cholesterol deposition in tissues. Clearly, further studies are needed to ascertain the role of the essential fatty acids in cholesterol metabolism and atherosclerosis.

The data of the studies on man or the rabbit indicate that the fatty acid composition of the serum cholesterol esters changes under varying dietary conditions and atherosclerosis. These changes are confined chiefly to the percentages of oleic and linoleic acids. These findings suggest that a derangement of cholesterol oleate metabolism may be of prime significance in atherosclerosis. This possibility will be discussed further in connection with the aorta (Section IV, E).

B. Triglycerides

Practically all of the absorbed dietary fat appears in the lymph as chylomicron triglyceride and then passes into the blood via the thoracic duct. Since more triglyceride is contained in the chyle following the ingestion of the usual meal than is present in the blood at any given time, it might be expected that the blood triglyceride would soon acquire the fatty acid composition of the chyle and dietary fat. Several studies have been carried out to examine this point. Fernandes *et al.* (1955) studied a child with chylothorax and found that the pattern of chyle fatty acids was influenced by the type of dietary fat, but there was always a significant difference in fatty acid composition between the lymph and dietary fat. Blomstrand and Dahlback (1960) fed several different diets to subjects with a thoracic lymph fistula. Examination of the lymph triglycerides indicated that they rapidly acquired the pattern of the dietary fat. Dole *et al.* (1959) found that neither the chylomicron fraction of serum nor any other fraction acquired the pattern of the dietary fat during alimentary lipemia. Contrary to these findings, Bragdon and Karmen (1960, 1961) observed that the fatty acid composition of chylomicrons of rat lymph, rat serum, and human serum mirrored the fatty acid composition of the dietary fat (corn oil or coconut oil). These discrepancies between the two groups might have been caused by differences in the technique for preparing chylomicrons. In connection with these studies, it is important to distinguish between endogenous plasma glycerides present principally in the lipoprotein fractions of fasting serum and the exogenous fraction present as chylomicrons. The latter fraction has been shown to be rapidly removed from the circulation.

The fasting serum or plasma triglyceride fatty acid composition of several species is shown in Table IV. In general, the fatty acid composition is characteristic of the individual species. However, three fatty acids (palmitic, oleic, and linoleic acids) account for 80-90% of the total fatty acids of the blood triglyceride fraction of man, rabbit, and rat; the plasma triglycerides of the ox are unusual in that they contain 30% stearic acid. The ratio of oleic to linoleic acid is also of interest. This ratio is approximately 4 for man and 1 for the rabbit and the rat. The comparable values for the normal diets of the species are approximately 3 for man, 2 for the rabbit, and 1 for the rat. Thus, the fatty acid composition of the blood triglycerides does bear a relationship to the percentage of oleic and linoleic acids present in the dietary fat. In addition to variations in the proportions of individual fatty acids in serum triglycerides, there is the problem of localization of fatty acids on specific positions of the triglyceride molecules. Beef, horse, sheep, and human fat resemble vegetable fat in that positions 1 and 3 contain predominantly saturated fatty acids. Linoleic acid appears to have a strong affinity in most species for the 2-position. The significance of this specificity in determining the fatty acid composition of the triglycerides remains to be explored. Likewise, the possibility of abnormal triglycerides that might be present in the tissues of certain disease states requires investigation.

Schrade *et al.* (1961) reported no significant differences in serum triglyceride fatty acid composition between normal and atherosclerotic subjects.

The effect of cholesterol feeding in rabbits on the blood triglyceride fatty acid composition has also recently been reported. Zilversmit and co-workers (1961b) and Swell *et al.* (1961b, 1962b) did not find any major differences in the fatty acid composition of the plasma triglycerides between rabbits fed diets with and those fed diets without cholesterol. While the feeding of a diet containing cholesterol has no influence on the blood triglyceride fatty acid composition, the type of fat present in the diet with cholesterol does have an effect. Swell *et al.* (1962b) showed that addition of 8% corn oil to a high-cholesterol diet significantly increased the percentage of linoleic and reduced the proportion of saturated fatty acids in the serum triglycerides when compared with animals consuming their regular chow diet; also, the addition of 8% olive oil to such a diet greatly increased the percentage of oleic and decreased the percentage of linoleic acid.

TABLE IV

THE SERUM OR PLASMA TRIGLYCERIDE AND PHOSPHOLIPID FATTY ACID COMPOSITION OF SEVERAL SPECIES

(Data given in terms of % of total fatty acids)

Major fatty acids[a]	Triglyceride				Phospholipid			
	Man (1)[b]	Rabbit (2)[b]	Rat (3)[b]	Ox (4)[b]	Man (5)[b]	Rabbit (2)[b]	Rat (6)[b]	Ox (4)[b]
Palmitic	24.9	38.0	30.1	24.0	31.0	32.9	22.0	16.2
Palmitoleic	6.2	2.6	3.5	4.8	3.5	1.2	1.8	1.1
Stearic	4.0	5.6	9.6	30.0	12.5	15.1	20.1	26.8
Oleic	41.4	23.4	22.5	24.3	15.0	25.3	11.8	16.3
Linoleic	10.9	25.2	26.5	4.6	21.2	15.6	19.4	14.1
Arachidonic	0.8	0.5	4.3	—	8.1	2.4	24.0	9.7

[a] Determined by gas-liquid chromatography.

[b] Reference code: (1) Hallgren et al. (1960). (2) Swell et al. (1961b). (3) Swell et al. (1961a). (4) Duncan and Garton (1962). (5) Schrade et al. (1961), (6) Carroll (1962).

C. Phospholipids

A summary of some data on the fatty acid composition of plasma or serum phospholipids is shown in Table IV. The saturated acids comprise close to 50% of the total acids with palmitic generally the major saturated acid. The unsaturated fatty acids are oleic, linoleic, and arachidonic acids. Oleic and linoleic acids vary somewhat from species to species; in man, linoleic predominates. Lis and Okey (1961) and Carroll (1962) reported that arachidonic acid was a major component (about 25%) of rat plasma phospholipids while Swell *et al.* (1961a) reported a lower value (6%) for that acid. The phospholipid fraction contains small amounts (3-8%) of the long chain fatty acids (C_{22} and longer). Perhaps of more significance is the availability of data on the individual human and bovine plasma phospholipids (Hanahan *et al.*, 1960a). Lysolecithin contains almost all saturated fatty acids while lecithin contains about equal proportions of saturated and unsaturated fatty acids. Sphingomyelin contains predominantly saturated fatty acids with a significant proportion of the long chain (22:0 and 24:0) fatty acids. The unsaturated fatty acids have been shown to occur principally in the β-position of lecithin (Hanahan *et al.*, 1960b).

The fatty acid composition of human serum phospholipids is not significantly altered by advancing age, atherosclerosis, alimentary lipemia, or diet (Schrade *et al.*, 1961; Swell *et al.*, 1962c). However, in rabbits fed high cholesterol diets, the percentage of linoleic increases at the expense of oleic acid in the serum phospholipid fraction (Swell *et al.*, 1961b).

D. Nonesterified Fatty Acids

Reliable data on the fatty acid analysis of the nonesterified fatty acids (NEFA) of human plasma were first reported by Dole *et al.* (1959). The major fatty acids were palmitic, stearic, oleic, linoleic, and arachidonic acids. The results of three recent studies are shown in Table V. Of particular interest is the high percentage (30-40%) of saturated acids in this plasma lipid fraction. The differences in NEFA composition between the several reports may be in part attributed to the different techniques for isolating the plasma NEFA. The plasma NEFA compositions of the sheep, cow, pig, horse, and chicken have also been determined and found to have a fairly consistent pattern; this is interesting in view of the different diets eaten by these species (Dole *et al.*, 1959).

Schrade *et al.* (1961) did not find any significant changes in NEFA composition with advancing age. However, in subjects with atheroscle-

TABLE V

THE FATTY ACID COMPOSITION OF THE NONESTERIFIED FATTY ACIDS OF HUMAN PLASMA

Major fatty acids[a]	Nonesterified fatty acids (% of total)		
	(1)[b]	(2)[b]	(3)[b]
Palmitic	23.2	27.5	22.9
Palmitoleic	2.4	7.3	4.8
Stearic	12.9	15.3	10.6
Oleic	28.9	25.4	37.2
Linoleic	14.5	13.4	8.6
Arachidonic	4.7	2.4	0.5[c]

[a] Fatty acids determined by gas-liquid chromatography.

[b] Reference code: (1) Dole *et al.* (1959), (2) Schrade *et al.* (1961), (3) Hallgren and Svanborg (1962).

[c] Includes small amounts of $C_{20:3}$ and $C_{20:5}$.

rosis the percentage of saturated fatty acids in that plasma fraction was higher and linoleic and arachidonic acids lower when compared to normal healthy subjects.

E. Interrelationships of Lipids in Blood

The transport of the lipids in blood presents the organism with a special problem due to their insolubility in aqueous media. It is now definitely established that the lipids of the blood are transported as lipoprotein complexes. There are four main lipoprotein types for the transport of plasma lipids. These are (1) low-density β-lipoproteins, (2) high-density α-lipoproteins, (3) chylomicrons, and (4) fatty acids bound to albumin. The over-all composition in terms of lipid types and fatty acid composition is determined by both the structure of the individual lipoproteins and the amounts of each of these fractions present.

A comparison of the fatty acid composition of the several lipid fractions in normal animals indicates that (a) the cholesterol ester fraction contains the highest percentage of polyunsaturated fatty acids, (b) the glyceride fraction simulates the fatty acid composition of the dietary fat to a large degree, (c) the phospholipid fraction contains equal amounts of saturated and unsaturated fatty acids. Thus, all three major lipid fractions have a different and specific fatty acid composition. The reasons for these differences in fatty acid composition are largely unknown. This is an area in need of intensive study.

III. Fatty Acid Composition of the Liver Lipids

A. Cholesterol Esters

The CEFA composition of whole liver of several species is shown in Table VI. Palmitic and stearic acids are the principal saturated fatty acids and account for 32-53% of the total fatty acids. The proportion of oleic acid in the liver cholesterol esters is variable; it is highest in man (37.3%) and lowest in the rat (20.3%). The percentage of polyunsaturated fatty acids in the liver cholesterol esters varies from 16 to 22%. In general, the liver cholesterol esters in the species studied are characterized by a high level of saturated and monounsaturated and a low level of polyunsaturated fatty acids. The cholesterol esters of individual cellular fractions of rat liver have also been studied (Getz *et al.*, 1962). The mitochondrial and microsomal cholesterol esters are similar in fatty acid composition. There also do not appear to be any marked differences in CEFA composition between these fractions and whole rat liver.

The fatty acid composition of the liver cholesterol esters has been shown to be influenced by dietary fat and cholesterol feeding. Klein (1958) showed that the percentage of polyunsaturated fatty acids in the liver cholesterol esters is directly related to the level of dietary polyunsaturated fatty acids. Klein (1959) also showed that the addition of 0.5% cholesterol to a diet fed to rats produced a marked decrease in the level of polyunsaturated fatty acids in the liver ester fraction compared with animals receiving comparable diets without cholesterol. Evans *et al.* (1959) fed cholesterol with tallow or corn oil to rabbits and noted that the monounsaturated fatty acids became the principal fatty acids of the liver cholesterol esters. This was particularly true in animals receiving the cholesterol-tallow diet. Swell *et al.* (1962b) reported similar observations in rabbits fed cholesterol diets with corn oil or olive oil. In the animals receiving the olive oil diet, oleic acid comprised 69% of the liver CEFA. The above studies suggest that the composition of the liver cholesterol esters is intimately related to the nature of the dietary fatty acids and the availability of essential fatty acids for the transport of cholesterol.

It is important to distinguish between the essential fatty acids, linoleic and arachidonic acids. The former has its origin in the diet while the latter is synthesized in the body from linoleic acid; very little arachidonic acid is ingested in the diet. Virtually nothing is known about the metabolism of arachidonic acid. The greatest amounts of arachidonic acid are found in the liver phospholipids, adrenal lipids, and testes. In view of the observations that cholesterol esters accumulate in

TABLE VI

The Liver Lipid Fatty Acid Composition of Several Species

(Data given in terms of % of total fatty acids)

Major fatty acids[a]	Per cent in cholesterol ester			Per cent in triglyceride			Per cent in phospholipid		
	Man (1)[b]	Rat (2)[b]	Rabbit (3)[b]	Man (5)[b]	Rat (4)[b]	Rabbit (3)[b]	Man (5)[b]	Rat (4)[b]	Rabbit (3)[b]
Palmitic	24.1	32.5	28.3	29.2	31.4	37.6	34.2	30.1	23.5
Palmitoleic	5.5	3.0	2.9	6.4	3.5	2.0	3.0	1.3	1.0
Stearic	8.4	21.9	18.0	9.1	4.5	4.4	23.6	27.4	25.7
Oleic	37.3	20.1	29.4	35.9	23.8	20.5	16.3	9.8	9.6
Linoleic	16.3	12.2	15.2	15.9	28.8	30.2	16.9	15.7	26.6
Arachidonic	3.0	8.8	0.8	2.1	6.0	0.3	8.3	9.5	4.5

[a] Determined by gas-liquid chromatography.

[b] Reference code: (1) Swell *et al.* (1960a). (2) Swell *et al.* (1960c). (3) Swell *et al.* (1961b). (4) Swell *et al.* (1961a). (5) Takahashi and Tanaka (1961).

the livers of animals fed high-cholesterol or essential fatty acid-deficient diets, it is suggested that arachidonic acid utilization and metabolism is intimately involved in these processes. Perhaps in the case of the cholesterol fatty liver, insufficient arachidonic acid is available to metabolize and utilize the excess cholesterol entering the liver; cholesterol then becomes esterified with saturated and oleic acids. This condition may be similar to the one in which cholesterol esters accumulate in the liver of essential fatty acid-deficient animals. Of particular significance is the observation made by Klein (1959) that the feeding of cholesterol to rats leads to a virtual disappearance of cholesterol arachidonate from the serum.

B. Triglycerides

The liver triglyceride fatty acid composition of several animals is shown in Table VI. Three fatty acids (palmitic, oleic, and linoleic) account for 85-90% of the total fatty acids of the liver triglyceride fraction. Palmitic acid is the major saturated acid and comprises approximately one-third of the total fatty acids. The most variable aspect of the fatty acid composition of the liver triglycerides is the ratio of oleic to linoleic acid. The level of linoleic acid in the liver triglycerides bears a direct relationship to the proportion of linoleic acid present in the diet. For example, the total fat in the diet of man generally contains about 9-11% linoleic acid while the diets of the rat and rabbit contain a greater proportion (29-49%) of that acid (Swell et al., 1960b, 1962b). The studies of Getz et al. (1962) have shown that the triglycerides of rat liver mitochondria and microsomes have essentially the same fatty acid composition.

Short-term feedings (4-18 hours) of corn oil or olive oil to rats have essentially no effect on the liver triglyceride fatty acid composition (Dittmer and Hanahan, 1959). However, the feeding of diets high in a particular fatty acid does alter the fatty acid composition of the liver triglyceride fraction, i.e., the liver triglycerides of rabbits fed an 8% olive oil diet contain a high percentage (47%) of oleic acid (Swell et al., 1962b).

C. Phospholipids

Early studies established that the liver phospholipids of different species contain a high percentage of saturated fatty acids (palmitic and stearic acids); the principal polyunsaturated fatty acids identified in this fraction were linoleic, arachidonic, docosopentaenoic, and docosohexaenoic acids. Recently, Okey and Harris (1958) provided some quantitative data on rat liver phospholipids which indicated that this fraction contained as much as 27% arachidonic acid. Evans *et al.* (1959) and Swell *et al.* (1961b) have reported a level of 5-10% of arachidonic acid in the liver phospholipids of rabbits; Swell *et al.* (1961a) reported a level of about 10% arachidonic acid in the liver phospholipids of rats. Table VI shows the fatty acid composition of the liver phospholipid fraction of man, rat, and the rabbit. The major fatty acids are palmitic, stearic, oleic, and linoleic acids. Fatty acid analyses have also been carried out on the individual liver phospholipids and each has a characteristic fatty acid spectrum (Dittmer and Hanahan, 1959).

Getz *et al.* (1962) have presented data on the fatty acid analyses of the individual phospholipids of the subcellular fraction of rat liver. These data confirm the findings of Dittmer and Hanahan (1959) in that they show that the cephalins contain a higher proportion of arachidonic and docosohexaenoic acids than the other lipids.

Okey *et al.* (1961) reported that the feeding of diets containing corn oil or coconut oil, with or without cholesterol, has very little effect on the liver phospholipid fatty acid composition. Evans *et al.* (1959) and Swell *et al.* (1961b) have also noted very little change in the liver phospholipid fatty acid composition of rabbits fed diets containing different fats with cholesterol. Unfortunately, no data are available on the effect of such diets on the fatty acid composition of the individual liver phospholipids. The measurement of the fatty acid composition of the total phospholipid fraction would mask any changes occurring in the individual phospholipid fractions.

D. Interrelationships of Liver Lipids

As with the serum, each lipid class of the liver has a characteristic fatty acid spectrum. Of particular interest is the fact that the percentage of saturated fatty acids is high in all of the liver lipid fractions. The liver triglyceride fatty acid composition simulates the fatty acid composition of the dietary fat while the polyunsaturated fatty acids are highest in the phospholipid fraction. In terms of total amounts of individual fatty acids present in the liver lipid fractions, the largest amounts of all fatty acids, and in particular, of the polyunsaturated fatty acids, are found in the phospholipid fraction since the latter comprises about 75% of the total liver lipids. Nothing is known about the mechanisms involved in determining and regulating fatty acid composition of the liver lipid fractions. The differences in fatty acid composition may be related to any number of factors such as the relative specificity of the enzyme systems involved in the formation of the liver lipids and/or the pool sizes of the individual fatty acids from which the fatty acid components of the liver lipid fractions are synthesized. There is some evidence with respect to the triglyceride fraction that a common mechanism is involved since the triglycerides of the liver, serum, and adipose tissue have essentially the same fatty acid composition.

IV. Fatty Acid Composition of Human Aortic Lipids

A. Introduction

Before describing the recent data on the fatty acid composition of human aorta, several remarks are in order regarding the problems associated with the analysis of aortic lipids. In normal aorta, the intima accounts for a relatively small portion of the aortic tissue; the media accounts for the greatest portion of the aorta. In order to delineate clearly the changes associated with atherosclerosis, the various layers of the aorta should be separated before analysis, though one must admit that it is difficult to obtain discrete layers or portions of the aorta. There are differences in the lipids of the intima and media, from the standpoint of both lipid and fatty acid composition. Changes in the lipid fractions associated with the development of atherosclerosis may be obscured by not analyzing the intima and media separately; this is particularly true in so-called normal aortic tissue where the media will contribute a greater proportion of lipids than the intima. In diseased aorta, the inclusion of the media with the diseased intima will dilute out or mask any inherent differences in lipid composition attributable to the atherosclerotic process. The discrepancies in the literature, particularly on the fatty acid analysis of the aorta, could in large part be caused by failure to carry out separate analyses of the layers of the aorta. Another factor complicating the role of lipids in atherosclerosis is the process of aging. Some workers have looked upon the aging and atherosclerotic processes as distinctively different, the aging process being associated chiefly with the media and the atherosclerotic process with the intima. If such differences do exist, it can readily be seen why separate analyses of the aorta are essential for distinguishing between the two processes.

B. Cholesterol Esters

Mounting evidence that implicates cholesterol, dietary fats, and essential fatty acids in cardiovascular disease has provided an impetus for studies on the qualitative and quantitative aspects of the lipid constituents of aorta and in particular, the cholesterol esters. A number of studies have been carried out in which the fatty acid composition of the cholesterol esters has been determined in aortas with varying degrees of atherosclerosis. The results obtained by a number of these workers are summarized in Table VII. The data are by no means in general agreement and this is undoubtedly caused by several factors such as differences in methodology and the lack of uniformity in the region of the aorta analyzed. In evaluating the data on aorta, the term atheromatous or normal aorta refers to aorta preparations consisting of intima (normal or diseased) plus media, while plaques, plaque lipids, and intima refer to those regions of the aorta that are essentially free of media. Examination of the data on the CEFA of atheromatous aorta indicates that the studies of Wright *et al.* (1959), Böttcher *et al.* (1960a), Mead and Gouze (1961) are in general agreement from a quantitative standpoint. The major CEFA are palmitic, oleic, and linoleic acids; monounsaturated and linoleic acids occur in approximately equal proportions (30-35%). The results of Luddy *et al.* (1958) do not fall in line with the above data and show the presence of a large proportion of monoenoic acids (61.5%), and a very small proportion of saturated acids. The studies of Böttcher *et al.* (1960a) and Mead and Gouze (1961) on the CEFA composition of normal aortic tissue are not in agreement. A possible explanation for these differences has recently been offered by Böttcher and Woodford (1962). The normal aortic tissue analyzed by Böttcher *et al.* (1960a) were from younger individuals than those obtained by Mead and Gouze (1961). Changes in CEFA composition caused by aging may occur in the same direction as atherosclerosis (Böttcher and Woodford, 1962); older individuals have a certain degree of atherosclerosis while only very young individuals are essentially free of the disease.

Böttcher *et al.* (1960a) observed that the aortic cholesterol esters became progressively more unsaturated with advancing atherosclerosis; the principal changes were an increase in the percentage of linoleic and a decrease in saturated acids. Contrary to the findings of those authors, Mead and Gouze (1961) found that the CEFA of the aorta were similar at early and late stages of atherosclerosis. Lewis (1958) and Böttcher *et al.* (1960b) examined the CEFA composition of atheromatous coronary arteries. Lewis (1958) found a high proportion of saturated and monounsaturated fatty acids in the cholesterol esters of atheromatous coronary arteries. On the other hand, Böttcher *et al.* (1960b) found that the cholesterol esters of diseased coronary and cerebral arteries had a higher proportion of polyunsaturated fatty acids than the cholesterol esters of normal vessels.

TABLE VII

THE CHOLESTEROL ESTER FATTY ACID COMPOSITION OF HUMAN AORTA

(Data given in terms of % of total fatty acids)

Major fatty acids	Normal aorta[a]		Atheromatous aorta[a]				Plaques (early)[a]	Plaques (advanced)[a]				Media[a]		Serum[a]
	(1)[b]	(2)[b]	(1)[b]	(2)[b]	(3)[c]	(4)[c]	(5)[b]	(4)[c]	(5)[b]	(6)[b]	(7)[b]	(5)[b]	(7)[b]	(8)[b]
Saturated[d]	31.2	12.4	17.0	13.1	4.2	26.1	22.5	26.2	22.0	9.7	27.5	20.0	23.7	20.0
Monoenoic[e]	39.9	33.9	36.7	33.0	61.5	35.1	43.1	34.3	44.4	41.3	44.9	33.5	31.2	25.5
Linoleic	24.5	41.2	36.0	42.1	23.6	29.5	28.8	30.0	28.1	38.3	25.1	37.9	39.4	47.5
Arachidonic	2.2	6.5	4.7	7.3	7.0	4.7	3.9	5.0	3.7	9.7	1.8	7.2	5.1	5.9

[a] Reference code: (1) Böttcher et al. (1960a), (2) Mead and Gouze (1961), (3) Luddy et al. (1958), (4) Wright et al. (1959), (5) Swell et al. (1960e), (6) Tuna et al. (1958), (7) Swell et al. (1960a), (8) Swell et al. (1962c).

[b] Determined by gas-liquid chromatography.

[c] Determined by alkali isomerization.

[d] Saturated acids include principally palmitic and stearic.

[e] Monoenoic acids include palmitoleic and oleic.

Another approach used by several workers has been to examine the CEFA from different areas of the same aorta; namely, normal and diseased intima and media. The CEFA of advanced plaques have been shown by Tuna *et al.* (1958), Wright *et al.* (1959), and Swell *et al.* (1960a, e) to contain a high percentage (34-45%) of monounsaturated fatty acids (principally oleic). The saturated and linoleic acids occur in about equal proportions (22-30%); the results of Tuna *et al.* (1958) are not in agreement with those of the other studies and indicate a much lower percentage (10%) of saturated fatty acids. The percentage of arachidonic varies from 1.8 to 9.7%. Early and advanced plaques were shown by Swell *et al.* (1960e) to have essentially the same CEFA composition.

A comparison of the CEFA composition of plaques with normal aorta has been made by Wright *et al.* (1959) using the alkali isomerization technique. They found no differences between the CEFA of the two regions of the aorta. On the other hand, Nelson *et al.* (1961) found that the CEFA of the intima with fatty streaking in young subjects had a higher percentage of oleic acid in the area of the lesion than in the adjacent normal tissue.

Swell *et al.* (1960a, e) compared the CEFA composition of media alone versus plaques. They found marked differences in CEFA of those two regions of the aorta. The cholesterol esters of the media were found to contain significantly more linoleic and less saturated fatty acids than plaques; the major fatty acid of plaques was oleic acid (44%) and of the media, linoleic acid (39%). These findings on the differences in CEFA composition of plaques and media may account for the lack of agreement in the several studies in which intima and media were not analyzed separately.

C. Triglycerides

The major fatty acids of the triglycerides (Table VIII) from normal and atheromatous aorta are palmitic, oleic, and linoleic acids; the first two acids occur to the extent of about 40% while the latter accounts for only about 10% of the total acids. The studies of Böttcher *et al.* (1960a) have shown that there is an increase in the percentage of polyunsaturated and a decrease in saturated fatty acids of the aorta triglycerides with advancing atherosclerosis. The changes in the triglyceride fraction were much less significant than the changes in the aorta cholesterol esters. On the other hand, Swell *et al.* (1960e) did not find any significant differences in the triglyceride fatty acid composition of media, early plaques, and advanced plaques. The data in general seem to indi-

TABLE VIII

THE TRIGLYCERIDE FATTY ACID COMPOSITION OF HUMAN AORTA

(Data given in terms of % of total fatty acids)

Major fatty acids	Normal aorta[a] (1)[b]	Atheromatous aorta[a] (1)[b]	Atheromatous aorta[a] (2)[c]	Plaques (early)[a] (3)[b]	Plaques (advanced)[a] (3)[b]	Media[a] (3)[b]	Adipose tissue[a] (4)[b]	Serum[a] (3)[b]
Saturated[d]	44.9	35.3	22.2	42.3	43.8	46.2	37.3	39.1
Monoenoic[e]	40.4	43.3	67.4	46.1	44.3	44.0	54.3	47.8
Linoleic	9.6	12.6	7.0	9.8	10.4	8.2	7.0	11.6
Arachidonic	2.7	3.9	2.3	0.8	0.7	0.8	1.0	0.8

[a] Reference code: (1) Böttcher et al. (1960a), (2) Luddy et al. (1958), (3) Swell et al. (1960e), (4) Kingsbury et al. (1961).

[b] Determined by gas-liquid chromatography.

[c] Determined by alkali isomerization.

[d] Saturated acids include principally palmitic and stearic.

[e] Monoenoic acids include palmitoleic and oleic.

cate that atherosclerosis has very little effect on the composition of the aorta triglycerides.

D. Phospholipids

A summary of data on the fatty acid composition of the phospholipid fraction of human aorta is shown in Table IX. Phospholipid fatty acids of the aorta are characterized by a high percentage of saturated fatty acids. Böttcher *et al.* (1960a) have reported that the atheromatous aorta has a smaller percentage of polyunsaturated fatty acids than the normal aorta. Swell *et al.* (1960e) noted that early and advanced plaques have the same phospholipid fatty acid composition. A comparison of plaque with medial phospholipids revealed that the latter had significantly more arachidonic acid than the former. Here, as with the cholesterol ester fraction, inclusion of the media with the intima could mask any differences in phospholipid fatty acid composition attributable to the disease process. Another important feature of the aortic phospholipid fraction is that it consists of three major classes (lecithins, cephalins, and sphingomyelins). Böttcher and van Gent (1961) determined the relation of the fatty acid patterns of the individual aorta phospholipids to the degree of atherosclerosis. In normal aorta, lecithins contain 37% saturated, 19% monounsaturated, and 44% polyunsaturated (mostly arachidonic) fatty acids; sphingomyelins contain 60% saturated (with 24% C_{22} and C_{24}), 24% monounsaturated, and 16% polyunsaturated fatty acids. The other fractions (lysolecithins, plasmalogens, and cephalins) were also analyzed and found to have characteristic fatty acid spectra. Comparison of the phospholipid fractions of normal and atheromatous aortas indicated that with advancing atherosclerosis there was an increase in the amount of sphingomyelin; there was also a decrease in the percentage of polyunsaturated fatty acids (particularly arachidonic acid) in the lecithins and sphingomyelins with a concomitant increase in the percentage of the saturated acids.

These data provide suggestive evidence that changes in the phospholipid distribution and fatty acid patterns do occur with advancing atherosclerosis; it is clear that further studies are needed to more clearly define these changes in the lesion. It would be of interest to determine the fatty acid composition of the individual phospholipids in the media, and in the normal and diseased intima.

E. Interrelationships of Lipids in Blood and Aorta of Man

Several basic questions may be posed concerning the changes in the fatty acid composition of aortic lipids during the development of athero-

TABLE IX

THE PHOSPHOLIPID FATTY ACID COMPOSITION OF HUMAN AORTA

(Data given in terms of % of total fatty acids)

Major fatty acids	Normal aorta[a]	Atheromatous aorta[a]		Plaques (early)[a]	Plaques (advanced)[a]	Media[a]	Serum[a]
	(1)[b]	(1)[b]	(2)[c]	(3)[b]	(3)[b]	(3)[b]	(4)[b]
Saturated[d]	55.2	62.0	32.2	55.8	50.4	59.0	44.2
Monoenoic[e]	19.4	16.6	55.7	25.4	27.8	21.8	18.5
Linoleic	5.0	4.2	7.2	7.4	8.7	5.6	21.2
Arachidonic	9.9	7.4	2.6	2.6	1.8	10.2	8.1

[a] Reference code: (1) Böttcher et al. (1960a), (2) Luddy et al. (1958), (3) Swell et al. (1960e), (4) Schrade et al. (1961).

[b] Determined by gas-liquid chromatography.

[c] Determined by alkali isomerization.

[d] Saturated acids include principally palmitic and stearic.

[e] Monoenoic acids include palmitoleic and oleic.

sclerosis. Do changes in the proportions of the essential fatty acids in the aorta lipid fractions occur as a result of atherosclerosis? What relationship do the aortic lipids bear to the lipids of the blood? If the lipids of aorta and blood were to have the same fatty acid composition, this might supply supportive evidence for the indiscriminate deposition (filtration theory) of lipids from the blood into the intima. The data available at the present time have not provided a definite answer to these questions, but some general trends can be considered. A comparison of the CEFA of normal and diseased areas of the aorta with that fraction of serum is made in Table VII. The data of Böttcher *et al.* (1960a) show that normal aortic CEFA have a much lower percentage of linoleic and a higher percentage of oleic and saturated acids than serum CEFA. On the other hand, Mead and Gouze (1961) showed that the cholesterol esters of both normal aorta and serum were similar in fatty acid composition. A comparison of the results obtained by Luddy *et al.* (1958), Lewis (1958), Wright *et al.* (1959), Böttcher *et al.* (1960a), and Mead and Gouze (1961) on the CEFA of atheromatous aorta with serum do not provide clear-cut differences. The data suggest that the percentage of linoleic acid is lower and oleic acid higher in the cholesterol esters of atheromatous aorta than in those of the serum fraction.

The data on the cholesterol esters of the separate regions of the aorta (intima, plaques, media), when compared with the serum cholesterol esters, have shown more definitive differences in fatty acid composition. The results of the studies of Tuna *et al.* (1958), Wright *et al.* (1959), and Swell *et al.* (1960a, 1962d) are in general agreement that plaque cholesterol esters contain a higher percentage of monounsaturated fatty acids (principally oleic) and a lower percentage of linoleic acid than the serum cholesterol ester fraction. Also, except for the study of Tuna *et al.* (1958), the several reports agree that there is a higher percentage of saturated and a lower percentage of arachidonic acid in the plaque cholesterol esters than in the serum cholesterol esters. A comparison of media with serum CEFA has been made by Swell *et al.* (1960a, e); both have approximately the same CEFA composition. This latter finding is of particular significance and may partially explain the lack of agreement between the studies of the several workers who analyzed the cholesterol esters of intima plus media.

The dissimilarity in the CEFA composition of the plaques and serum suggests that indiscriminate deposition of serum cholesterol esters in the aorta does not occur or that the aorta selectively retains certain cholesterol esters. The process appears to be selective since there is a preferential deposition (or retention) of saturated and monounsaturated cholesterol esters in the intima at the expense of linoleic and arachidonic esters. However, all of the usual cholesterol esters occur in the vessel wall. The one cholesterol ester which stands out above all others as generally increased in both blood and plaques is cholesterol oleate. A derangement in the metabolism of this ester may be of paramount importance in the atherosclerotic process and could arise from a relative deficiency of lino-leic and arachidonic acids (as suggested by Sinclair, 1956) or by some other defect in cholesterol ester metabolism. Clearly, further studies are needed on the metabolism of cholesterol esters in serum, aorta, and other tissues. In the past, not enough attention has been given to the fatty acid moiety of the cholesterol ester fraction. It will undoubtedly be necessary to study the metabolic aspects of each individual cholesterol ester.

The data on the triglyceride fatty acid composition of normal and diseased aorta, plaques, and media, as reported by Luddy *et al.* (1958), Böttcher *et al.* (1960a), and Swell *et al.* (1960e), when compared with the triglycerides of serum, are in general agreement and reveal that all of those regions of the aorta have essentially the same tri-glyceride fatty acid composition. It does not appear that a specific tri-glyceride is deposited in the aorta from the blood or as shown in rabbit aorta (Section VIII, B), the triglycerides may be synthesized *in situ*.

The several reports (Böttcher *et al.*, 1960a; Swell *et al.*, 1960e; Böttcher and van Gent, 1961) on aortic phospholipids indicate that normal and diseased aortic phospholipids contain a higher percentage of saturated and a lower percentage of polyunsaturated fatty acids than the serum phospholipid fraction. The differences between aortic and serum phospholipid may be due to preferential deposition of a specific phospholipid such as sphingomyelin or alternatively may indicate that the phospholipids are synthesized by the aorta. Further studies are needed on the fatty acid composition of the individual phospholipids of normal intima, plaques, and media to make a judgment on the former possibility. The latter possibility will be discussed below (Section VIII, C).

V. Fatty Acid Composition of Animal Aortic Lipids

A. Cholesterol Esters

Studies have also been carried out on the changes in aortic and blood lipid fatty acid composition associated with the production of experi-mental atherosclerosis in rabbits and chickens. The data of the several studies on rabbits are summarized in Table III. The reports of Swell *et al.* (1961b), Zilversmit *et al.* (1961b), and Evrard *et al.* (1962) are in general agreement that the aortic and intimal cholesterol esters of cholesterol-fed rabbits have a high percentage (39-57%) of oleic and a low percentage (12-19%) of linoleic acid. The diets fed in those studies contained cholesterol with essentially no added fat (Swell *et al.,* 1961b), small amounts of peanut oil (3%) (Evrard *et al.,* 1962), or hydrogenated fat (2.6%) (Zilversmit *et al.,* 1961b). The type of fat added to the diets at these low levels had no appreciable effect on the CEFA of aorta. However, Swell *et al.* (1961b) reported that the aortic CEFA is influenced by the nature of the dietary fat when fed to rabbits at the 8% level in a high cholesterol diet. The aortic cholesterol esters of rabbits fed 8% olive oil had a lower percentage of linoleic acid than rabbits receiving a similar diet with 8% corn oil. However, in both groups oleic acid still remained the major acid of the cholesterol ester fraction. Blomstrand and Christensen (1961) reported that the aortic cholesterol esters of chickens fed a high-cholesterol diet had a higher percentage of oleic and a lower percentage of saturated acids than normal animals. Addition of peanut oil to the diet produced a further increase in the percentage of oleic acid in the aortic cholesterol esters. The findings of the latter two studies suggest that the cholesterol esters deposited in the aorta are not of constant composition, but are dependent to a certain extent on the level and type of fat fed with cholesterol.

The results obtained by Swell *et al.* (1961b, 1962b) and Evrard *et al.* (1962) indicate that the aortic cholesterol esters of cholesterol-fed rabbits contain a much higher percentage of oleic and a lower percentage of linoleic acid than the plasma cholesterol esters of normal animals. Similar, but smaller differences exist when the findings made by Zilversmit *et al.* (1961b), Swell *et al.* (1961b, 1962b), and Evrard *et al.* (1962) on the fatty acid composition of plasma and aortic cholesterol esters of cholesterol-fed rabbits are compared.

The studies summarized above in the rabbit and the chicken point up one common factor associated with the cholesterol ester fraction during the development of atherosclerosis, namely, the increased percentage of oleic acid in the plasma and aortic cholesterol esters. In both man and the rabbit the data thus far indicate that the changes in plasma and aortic cholesterol esters are principally at the expense of linoleic acid. The high concentrations of cholesterol oleate and low concentration of linoleate in the plasma and aorta cannot be explained on the basis that the diet is deficient in linoleic acid since it has been shown that such differences exist in rabbits fed diets containing cholesterol with 8% corn oil (Swell *et al.,* 1962b). If these views are correct, then the deposition of cholesterol esters from the serum into the aorta may not be random, but may result from a local disturbance in the aorta of cholesterol ester metabolism or some as yet unknown process which favors the deposition of plasma cholesterol oleate or both.

B. Triglycerides

Zilversmit *et al.* (1961b) and Swell *et al.* (1961b, 1962b) have shown that the aortic and serum triglycerides of normal and cholesterol-fed rabbits are similar in fatty acid composition when fed high-cholesterol diets containing no added fat or 2.6% hydrogenated cottonseed oil. Swell *et al.* (1962b) fed high-cholesterol diets containing 8% corn oil or 8% olive oil. The aortic and serum triglyceride fatty acid composition mirrored the fatty acid composition of the dietary fat. The available information on the serum and aortic triglyceride fatty acid composition in rabbits agrees with the findings in man and suggests that the plasma and tissue triglycerides are derived from similar fatty acid pools; no alteration in the specificity of triglyceride synthesis which might result in the formation of a particular triglyceride is apparent.

C. Phospholipids

Swell *et al.* (1961b) and Blomstrand and Christensen (1961) noted that the feeding of cholesterol diets to rabbits and chickens had very little effect on the fatty acid composition of the aortic phospholipids. However, a comparison of the serum and aortic phospholipids of cholesterol-fed rabbits did show differences in fatty acid composition (Swell *et al.*, 1961b). The aortic phospholipids had a lower percentage of polyunsaturated fatty acids than the plasma fraction; these changes were at the expense of saturated and oleic acids. Zilversmit *et al.* (1961b) determined the fatty acid composition of the individual phospholipid fractions of rabbit aorta and plasma. These workers found pronounced differences in the fatty acid composition of intimal and plasma lecithins, sphingomyelins, and lysolecithins in the normal and cholesterol-fed rabbit. A pertinent observation was that the phospholipid fractions of the plasma had a higher percentage of polyunsaturated fatty acids than those fractions of the intima.

The limited data available indicate that differences exist in the fatty acid composition of plasma and arterial phospholipids of normal and cholesterol-fed rabbits. As with aortic cholesterol esters, it appears that the aortic phospholipids are not merely random deposits of the plasma phospholipids, but are selectively deposited from the plasma or are synthesized *in situ*.

VI. The Origin of the Plasma Lipids

A. Introduction

The plasma lipids are derived from two sources, namely, endogenous synthesis and the diet. The levels of the various lipids present in the plasma and the proportions of those lipids derived from exogenous and endogenous sources are governed by a number of factors such as the intake and nature of the dietary fat and the rate of tissue lipid synthesis and catabolism. The level of dietary fat markedly influences the proportion of lipids synthesized by the tissues and released into the blood.

The origin of the plasma lipids is a complex problem owing to the contribution of the various tissues to the lipid pool of plasma. Furthermore, the lipids entering the blood via the lymph serve as an important source of the plasma lipids. It is important that the plasma lipids be viewed as a unit since they occur in definite proportions, have fixed fatty acid compositions, and are always in combination with protein.

B. Total Cholesterol

The plasma cholesterol is derived from several sources, notably, the liver, extrahepatic tissues, and the diet via the lymph. It is important to first point out the experimental approaches that have been used to study the origin of the plasma cholesterol. These have been: (a) *in vitro* studies to ascertain the ability of tissues to synthesize cholesterol from precursors such as acetate and mevalonate, (b) the effect of removal of organs such as the liver and the gastrointestinal tract on the plasma cholesterol, (c) equilibration and turnover rates of plasma and tissue cholesterol following the administration of labeled cholesterol or labeled acetate. The origin of the plasma cholesterol will be considered in the light of these approaches.

Virtually all tissues examined to date have been shown to possess the capacity to synthesize cholesterol from acetate. The most active tissues have been shown to be the liver, intestine, skin, and adrenal. The rate of liver cholesterol synthesis is under homeostatic control and is governed by the intake of cholesterol in the diet. It has been amply demonstrated that surviving liver slices prepared from rats, dogs, and monkeys previously fed a high-cholesterol diet show a depression in the incorporation of acetate-1-C^{14} into cholesterol. Conversely, if cholesterol is withdrawn from the body via a lymph or bile fistula, the rate of liver cholesterol synthesis is markedly increased.

The early *in vitro* work led to the view that the liver might be the chief source of the plasma cholesterol. In order to assess the role of this tissue in regulating the plasma cholesterol level, *in vivo* experiments have been carried out in hepatectomized animals. A comment is in order on the use of hepatectomized animals in experiments on the origin of plasma lipids. The removal of the liver from an animal produces an interrupted metabolism in other tissues; e.g., the animal can no longer produce bile, which is known to be essential for cholesterol absorption, and transformations in the chylomicrons and lipoproteins coming via the lymph can no longer take place. Also, the liver is the chief source of the protein portion of the plasma lipoproteins; lipids from other sources would not be available to the blood owing to a defective lipid transport system in the hepatectomized animal. Friedman *et al.* (1951) concluded that the liver was the chief source of plasma cholesterol when they observed that the plasma cholesterol level of plasmapheresed rats did not rise to normal levels in hepatectomized rats. Byers *et al.* (1951) found that the rise in blood cholesterol which occurs after ligation of the bile duct was partially or completely blocked after hepatectomy. Harper *et al.* (1953) and Eckles *et al.* (1955) injected C^{14}-acetate into normal and hepatectomized dogs and noted that no significant amount of tagged cholesterol appeared in the plasma of hepatectomized animals. Tennent *et al.* (1957) carried out studies on the ability of the liver to contribute cholesterol to the blood in an isolated system. Labeled acetate was introduced into the blood of dog heart, lung, and liver preparations. In was shown that the specific activity of the cholesterol isolated from the blood was less than that from the liver, but greater than that from the heart or lung, indicating that the blood C^{14}-cholesterol was derived from the liver.

Experiments to assess *in vivo* the contribution of dietary and endogenously synthesized cholesterol to the serum cholesterol pool have been carried out in the rat and man. The premise for these experiments is based on the previously mentioned observations that the intake of dietary cholesterol regulates the rate of endogenous synthesis. Morris *et al.* (1957) fed rats (for varying periods up to 6 weeks) diets containing either 0.05% or 2% C^{14}-cholesterol. It was estimated from the ratio of the specific activity of the serum cholesterol to that of the dietary cholesterol that in rats fed the low-cholesterol diet endogenous synthesis contributed from 67 to 80% to the serum cholesterol. In animals fed the 2% C^{14}-cholesterol diet, from 10 to 26% of the serum cholesterol was derived from endogenous synthesis. In another study, Morris and Chaikoff (1959) fed similar diets to rats and studied the origin of cholesterol in the liver. In rats fed a 0.5% C^{14}-cholesterol diet, endogenous sources contributed 70-80% of the cholesterol in the liver, while in the animals receiving a 2% C^{14}-cholesterol diet, the cholesterol derived from endogenous synthesis ranged from 10 to 30%. This approach to the role of the diet as a source of serum cholesterol has also been used in man (Taylor *et al.*, 1960). Human subjects ingested cholesterol-rich diets labeled with C^{14}-cholesterol. The ratio of the specific activity of the serum cholesterol to the dietary cholesterol indicated that 24-31% of the serum cholesterol was derived from the diet. Presumably, at least 75% of the serum cholesterol in those human subjects was derived from cholesterol synthesis in extrahepatic tissues.

The available data suggest that the liver plays an important role as a contributor and prime regulator of the plasma total cholesterol. The question of how much of the plasma cholesterol is derived from the liver is still open to question. Particularly in the case of man, it appears that a large proportion of the plasma cholesterol may be derived from sources other than the liver.

C. Free Cholesterol

In considering the plasma cholesterol, it is important to differentiate between the free and esterified cholesterol fractions. There is ample evidence to indicate that the free and esterified cholesterol fractions of the blood and tissues are derived in part from different sources and have different functions.

The approaches to the problem of the origin of the plasma free cholesterol fraction are basically the same that have been used in studying the origin of the plasma total cholesterol. Harper *et al.* (1953) and Eckles *et al.* (1955) injected C^{14}-acetate into normal and hepatectomized dogs and observed that no significant amount of labeled free cholesterol appeared in the plasma. However, labeled free cholesterol was isolated from a number of tissues. These studies suggest that while extrahepatic tissues can synthesize cholesterol, only the liver can furnish free cholesterol to the plasma. Eckles *et al.* (1955) obtained serial liver biopsies in dogs following the injection of C^{14}-acetate and compared the specific activities of the liver and plasma free cholesterol fractions. The liver free fraction reached a peak in about 40 minutes and the plasma free fraction reached its peak in about an hour. The rates of equilibration between the free fractions in the liver and plasma, expressed as half-times, were estimated to be about 20 minutes. LeRoy *et al.* (1957) carried out similar experiments in human subjects in which tissue biopsy samples were obtained shortly after the administration of C^{14}-acetate. The C^{14}-specific activities of the liver and plasma free fractions were found to be approximately the same at 1½ hours after the administration of C^{14}-acetate. These findings indicate that in man and in dog, the liver and plasma free cholesterol fractions come into very rapid equilibrium and for practical purposes may be looked upon as a single compartment. Since the plasma and liver free cholesterol come into such rapid equilibrium, Gould and co-workers (1955) have used this as a measure of hepatic synthesis of cholesterol in man. They have estimated a rate of interchange between free cholesterol of liver and plasma of 0.87 gm per hour in each direction. Field *et al.* (1960) have confirmed and extended these observations in man. Cholesterol-4-C^{14} was administered orally to a number of human subjects with limited life expectancies and a number of tissues were obtained at autopsy. The plasma and liver free cholesterol fractions were in equilibrium at the earliest time (2½ days) and thereafter the liver and plasma free cholesterol fractions had the same specific activity. On the other hand, the free cholesterol fraction of a number of other tissues examined came into equilibrium with the plasma free fraction at much later dates. These data strongly suggest that a major portion of the plasma free cholesterol is derived from the liver. The exchange of free cholesterol between the plasma and extrahepatic tissues occurs at a very slow rate and at least a portion of the free cholesterol in those tissues may be derived from the plasma.

The free cholesterol fraction of the plasma is also derived, in part, from the intestine since a portion of the lymph cholesterol (usually 10-30%) is in the free form. This arises partly from the reabsorption of endogenous cholesterol secreted in the bile and also from synthesis by the intestine. Thus, the intestine contributes some free cholesterol to the plasma. This is both direct and indirect since the chylomicron, which would contain most of the free cholesterol from the intestine, is removed from the circulation by the liver which, in turn, may then release the free cholesterol fraction into the plasma.

D. Cholesterol Esters

The problem of the esterified cholesterol fraction is complicated since it is composed of a number of individual cholesterol esters which may have independent origins and different metabolic functions. Free cholesterol is the precursor of the esterified cholesterol fraction in the plasma and tissues. However, the sites of esterification and, in particular, whether the cholesterol esters synthesized in a given tissue contribute to the plasma ester pool have not been entirely clarified. The plasma cholesterol esters may have their origin from one or more sources; namely, the liver, intestine, blood, and other extrahepatic tissues.

One line of approach to the study of the origin of the plasma cholesterol esters has been to investigate cholesterol esterification *in vitro.* The investigations of Nedswedski (1935), Yamamoto *et al.* (1949), Swell and Treadwell (1950a), Hernandez and Chaikoff (1957), and Korzenovsky *et al.* (1960) have provided evidence that the pancreas contains an enzyme which is very active in the esterification of cholesterol. It has been shown that this enzyme has the requisite specificity for the synthesis of the physiological cholesterol esters and in the proportions in which they occur in blood and other tissues (Swell *et al.,* 1955). Attempts to demonstrate an esterifying cholesterol esterase in other tissues, using natural or artificial substrate mixtures of cholesterol and fatty acid, have also been made. In general, with the exception of dog serum and rat intestinal mucosa, the data suggest a very low order of enzymic activity in other tissues. Cholesterol esterase, therefore, appears to play its major role in the absorption of cholesterol from the intestine. The cholesterol esterase of serum has been the subject of sporadic studies since Sperry (1935) first demonstrated that the incubation of human serum leads to a decrease in free and an increase in the esterified cholesterol fractions. Swell and Treadwell (1950b) have questioned the significance of the serum enzyme since the enzymic activity was found to be of a very low order; also, the system in human serum is unusual in that it was not influenced by the concentration of added substrate or end-product and the esterification reaction did not occur when serum was diluted more than 1:5. Several mechanisms have been proposed for the esterification reaction in serum. Le Breton and Pantaleon (1944) suggested that the fatty acid of the newly formed cholesterol ester arose from lecithin by a coupled reaction of lecithinase and cholesterol esterase on their respective substrates. Recently, Glomset *et al.* (1962) have also reported that a fatty acid donor in the cholesterol esterase reaction of rat and human plasma is lecithin. The reaction appears to involve a direct transfer of the fatty acid from lecithin to cholesterol and is carried out by a transferase. At the present time, the role of the serum esterifying enzyme in the formation of cholesterol esters *in vivo* is not clear, but if it has one it is probably of minor importance.

With the clarification of the pathways for the synthesis of the triglycerides and phospholipids, it became apparent that related processes might be involved in the synthesis of cholesterol esters; most notably, a reaction between cholesterol and a fatty acid CoA derivative. Mukherjee *et al.* (1958) observed that whole liver homogenates formed cholesterol palmitate from cholesterol and either ATP plus CoA or palmityl CoA; the reaction proceeded at a greater rate in the presence of palmityl CoA.

Swell *et al.* (1962a; unpublished observations; Swell and Treadwell, 1962) have confirmed and extended these observations. It was shown that whole rat liver homogenates can form C^{14}-cholesterol esters from C^{14}-acetate and C^{14}-mevalonate as well as esterify cholesterol-4-C^{14}. Studies on subcellular fractions of rat liver have provided evidence that microsomal, mitochondrial, and soluble fractions can all esterify added cholesterol-4-C^{14}. The microsomal system has thus far been most thoroughly studied and requires ATP and CoA. However, different CoA esters could not entirely replace ATP and CoA. Deykin and Goodman (1962) have also recently demonstrated that rat liver mitochondria or microsomes can esterify cholesterol in the presence of ATP and CoA. However, those authors observed that fatty acid CoA esters could entirely replace ATP and CoA in the microsomal system. Of particular importance has been the recent identification (Swell *et al.*, unpublished observations) of the C^{14}-cholesterol esters formed in the liver microsomal system. The C^{14}-cholesterol esters synthesized have approximately the following fatty acid composition: saturated 25-30%, monounsaturated (principally oleic) 45-50%, linoleic 10-15%, arachidonic 3-7%. This fatty acid composition bears a closer relationship to the fatty acid composition of the cholesterol esters present in the liver than in the serum. Dailey *et al.* (1962) have recently observed that dog adrenal homogenates synthesize cholesterol esters by a mechanism similar to the system identified in liver microsomes. Thus, the available data indicate that the liver and other tissues contain one or more enzymic systems capable of forming cholesterol esters. However, additional studies are needed to further clarify the mechanisms involved in these reactions. The formation of plasma cholesterol esters will next be considered from an *in vivo* standpoint.

Harper *et al.* (1953) and Eckles *et al.* (1955) reported that no C^{14}-cholesterol esters appeared in the plasma or tissues of hepatectomized dogs following the administration of C^{14}-acetate. Friedman and Byers (1955) showed that the rate of replacement of an experimentally reduced plasma cholesterol ester was very low in drastically hepatectomized rats; on the other hand, the rate of replacement of plasma ester in animals without their gastrointestinal tract and kidneys was not appreciably affected. Also, the disappearance of injected esterified cholesterol occurred only in the presence of functioning liver tissue. From these findings, the above authors concluded that the liver serves as the chief source of plasma cholesterol ester. However, the alternate possibility exists that a portion of the liver cholesterol esters might be derived from other sources and undergo alteration by the liver before being released back into the plasma.

A more direct approach to the site of formation of the plasma cholesterol esters has been to examine the specific activity relationships of the plasma and liver esterified cholesterol following the administration of labeled cholesterol or acetate. In short-term studies, Eckles *et al.* (1955), LeRoy *et al.* (1957), and Swell *et al.* (1958) observed that in man, the dog, and the rat, following the administration of C^{14}-acetate, the liver free cholesterol had a higher specific activity than the esterified fraction in the liver or plasma. These findings support the contention that the free cholesterol is the precursor of the esterified cholesterol fraction in liver and serum. A further study of a more detailed nature was carried out by Field *et al.* (1960) in which the specific activity relationships of the plasma and liver cholesterol were compared at varying times in the livers of subjects who had received cholesterol-4-C^{14}. Whereas the free cholesterol of the liver and plasma came into very rapid equilibrium, the esterified fraction of the plasma and liver did not acquire the same specific activity until 18-27 days had elapsed. Calculation of the turnover times and turnover rates from the data showed that the turnover time of the esterified cholesterol fraction of the liver was twice as long as that fraction in the plasma. If all of the cholesterol esters of the plasma were derived from the liver, the turnover rate of the esterified cholesterol fraction of the liver should have been at least 10 times as great as was found.

The data described above on the esterified cholesterol fractions of plasma and liver have considered the esterified cholesterol fraction as a unit. However, cholesterol is esterified with a number of different fatty acids and there is evidence that those esters are metabolized at different rates and perhaps have different functions. Klein and Martin (1959a) studied the heterogeneity and turnover rates of rat liver cholesterol esters. Following the administration of C^{14}-acetate to rats, it was shown that the liver cholesterol esters at early times (30 minutes) had different specific activities; in order of decreasing activity were esters of oleic, linoleic, saturated, and arachidonic acids. In another study (Klein and Martin, 1959b), these workers fed tritiated cholesterol to rats for varying periods of time up to 7 days and noted that the individual liver cholesterol esters had different specific activities; the cholesterol oleate pool was found to expand in comparison to the other ester pools. These findings are of particular importance since they point up the heterogeneous character of the plasma and liver cholesterol esters. To further complicate the picture, Klein and Dahl (1961) have reported that the turnover of the individual cholesterol esters is altered by stress. Additional evidence for the nonhomogeneity of the plasma and liver cholesterol esters is apparent from their fatty acid compositions. The plasma cholesterol esters of man, the rat, and the rabbit contain a high proportion of polyunsaturated fatty acids (50-70%), whereas the liver cholesterol ester fraction contains principally saturated and monounsaturated fatty acids with a much lower proportion of polyunsaturated fatty acids (20-25%). These differences are most striking in the case of the rat, in which the major cholesterol ester of the plasma is cholesterol arachidonate, while rat liver cholesterol esters have a small percentage of cholesterol arachidonate, the major esters of the liver being cholesterol oleate, stearate, and palmitate. In order to account for the liver as the major source of serum cholesterol arachidonate in the rat, the turnover of that liver ester would have to be rather high. In fact, the presently available *in vitro* and *in vivo* data on the synthesis of liver cholesterol esters indicate that the monounsaturated cholesterol esters have the highest turnover rate while cholesterol arachidonate appears to have the slowest turnover. This raises the question of where a large part of the plasma cholesterol arachidonate is synthesized in the rat.

Another important source of the cholesterol esters in the blood and tissues is the intestine, as a result of absorption and synthesis. Most of the cholesterol in the lymph is in the esterified form (70-90%) as an integral part of the chylomicron. In the rat, 10-20 mg of cholesterol ester per day enter the circulation via the lymph. This amount of cholesterol ester exceeds that present in the blood and liver pool. Furthermore, if the cholesterol esters derived from the lymph are withdrawn from the body via a fistula, there results a greatly increased synthesis of cholesterol esters in the tissues and, in particular, the liver. In lymph fistula animals, there is a marked decline in the percentage of polyunsaturated fatty acids in the serum cholesterol esters and an increase in the percentage of saturated fatty acids in the liver ester fraction. Of particular significance are the recent observations by Swell *et al.* (1960c) and Apostolakis *et al.* (1962) that in the rat the cholesterol esters of the lymph, plasma, and liver have different fatty acid compositions. All of these factors, taken together, indicate that the liver, plasma, and lymph cholesterol ester pools are not homogeneous. Much remains to be clarified regarding the role of the intestine as a source of cholesterol esters. However, it is apparent that the intestine does, in some manner, influence plasma cholesterol ester metabolism.

While the studies to date indicate that the liver and the intestine play an important role in the regulation of the plasma cholesterol ester fraction, there are other discrepancies which remain to be explored. The liver undoubtedly occupies a central position in cholesterol ester metabolism in that it may alter cholesterol esters entering from other tissues via the blood and lymph, selectively excrete certain esters into the blood, and retain other esters in the liver ester pool. A considerable amount of work is needed on the fate and turnover of the individual cholesterol esters from the standpoint of both the cholesterol and fatty acid moieties.

E. Triglycerides

The plasma triglyceride fraction is derived from exogenous and endogenous sources. Dietary fat is absorbed from the intestine and enters the lymph as part of the chylomicron structure; approximately 88% of the chylomicron is triglyceride. Following the entrance of chylomicron triglycerides into the blood, they are rapidly removed by the liver where they may follow several pathways; triglycerides may undergo partial or complete hydrolysis or re-enter the plasma as part of the lipoproteins. The studies of Byers and Friedman (1960), Stein and Shapiro (1960), and Havel and Goldfien (1961) have indicated that the liver plays an important role in the regulation of the plasma triglyceride. Hepatectomized dogs given labeled free fatty acids have virtually no labeled triglyceride in their plasma and hepatectomized rats do not show any accumulation of plasma triglyceride after triton injection as compared to a large increase in normal animals. Adipose tissue also serves as an important indirect reservoir of plasma triglycerides. Current evidence indicates that adipose tissue releases free fatty acid bound to albumin into the plasma which is transported principally to the liver. A portion of the free fatty acids is then incorporated into liver triglyceride and released back into the plasma. Thus, the plasma triglyceride is derived from at least several sources, namely, diet, adipose tissue, and liver; the liver plays a central role in plasma triglyceride regulation.

F. Phospholipids

Fishler *et al.* (1943) and Entenman *et al.* (1946) demonstrated, with the aid of P^{32} that phospholipid synthesis occurred in kidney and small intestine of hepatectomized and normal dogs, but only very small amounts of labeled phospholipids appeared in plasma of liverless dogs. Goldman *et al.* (1950) confirmed these observations with palmitic acid-1-C^{14}. It appears that although other tissues can synthesize phospholipids, only the liver can serve as the principal source of the plasma phospholipids. The liver is also concerned with the removal of the plasma phospholipids. Hepatectomized dogs (Entenman *et al.*, 1946) injected with labeled phospholipids showed a greatly reduced rate of removal of the labeled plasma phospholipids.

Another source of the plasma phospholipid is the intestine. While it has now been established that the phospholipids are not intermediates in the absorpion of fat, there is evidence to indicate that there is an increase in lymph phospholipids during triglyceride and cholesterol absorption. This increased phospholipid synthesis in the intestine is undoubtedly related to the formation of chylomicrons, of which phospholipids are an integral component. In this connection, McCandless and Zilversmit (1957) observed that during alimentary lipemia in dogs, there is an increase in plasma phospholipids. Furthermore, the increase (15-30%) in plasma phospholipid can be accounted for in terms of the phospholipid entering the plasma via the lymph. From these data and the earlier studies, it would be expected that the plasma of fasting dogs would contain very little phospholipid of intestinal origin.

While the present information suggests that the plasma total phospholipids have their primary origin in the liver, not enough data are available on the origin of the individual phospholipids. Also, the experiments with P^{32} are open to criticism since they do not indicate the origin and fate of the individual fatty acids.

VII. The Origin of Human Aortic Lipids

A. Introduction

Before considering the relative proportions of the aortic lipids derived from the plasma and synthesis *in situ,* some general statements are in order. All extrahepatic tissues have the capacity to synthesize lipids to a limited extent. Considerable significance has been attached to the fact that the aorta of a number of species can synthesize cholesterol from acetate and other percursors. The important question which remains to be answered is how much of the cholesterol and other lipids associated with the atherosclerotic lesion are synthesized by the aorta. In this connection, several theories have been advanced to account for the accumulation of lipids in the aorta. One was proposed many years ago and is known as the filtration theory. It briefly states that at some point the plasma cholesterol becomes elevated and this increased level of cholesterol in the blood leads to a precipitation or accumulation of cholesterol and its esters in the aortic intima; triglycerides and phospholipids are deposited to a lesser extent from the blood. Perhaps the most significant support for this theory stems from the work of Hirsch and Weinhouse (1943) who, in an elegant study, compared the lipid composition of several regions of the aorta and plasma lipids; a marked similarity in the lipid composition of plaque and plasma lipids was observed. This theory accounts for deposition of plasma lipids in the aortic intima on an indiscriminate basis and does not take into account the possibility that specific cholesterol esters, triglycerides, and phospholipids may be deposited in the aorta. Another theory recently advanced regarding the origin of the atheroma lipids has been the local formation theory which briefly states that the lipids are synthesized *in situ* in the aorta. In this respect, atherosclerosis may be looked upon as the result of a derangement in lipid metabolism of the aorta. Studies on the dynamic aspects of lipid metabolism in the aorta of man and animals have provided important information on the relative contribution of the plasma lipids versus aortic lipid synthesis to the lipids of the atherosclerotic lesion.

B. Free and Esterified Cholesterol

The few studies that have been carried out in man on the origin of the aortic cholesterol have been concerned with the appearance of administered labeled cholesterol in the aorta. The interpretation of the results in such studies is based on the following considerations: that the administered labeled cholesterol is indistinguishable chemically from endogenous cholesterol present in the plasma, that the aortic and plasma cholesterol interchange freely, and that the aorta does not contribute appreciable amounts of cholesterol to the plasma.

Biggs *et al.* (1952) reported that H^3-cholesterol was present in the aorta of a subject with atherosclerosis 43 days after feeding H^3-cholesterol. Kurland *et al.* (1961) also found C^{14} activity in the aorta in one of three subjects given intravenous infusions of C^{14}-cholesterol who died 15 days later; the specific activity of the aortic cholesterol was much less than that fraction of the plasma, liver, adrenal, testes, and muscle. Rabinowitz *et al.* (1960) examined several regions of the aorta of 5 subjects who expired 2-10 days after receiving C^{14}-cholesterol intravenously. Intima had a higher cholesterol specific activity than media; plaque areas had a much lower cholesterol specific activity than intima with less atherosclerotic involvement. Field *et al.* (1960) have carried out the most extensive studies to date on the dynamic aspects of cholesterol metabolism in different areas of the aorta and other tissues in man. Estimations of free and esterified cholesterol turnover and interchange of those fractions between plasma and the aorta indicated that: (a) The turnover of cholesterol (free and ester) is much slower in early plaques than in normal appearing intima; the cholesterol of advanced plaques is relatively inert and has essentially no turnover. (b) The esterified cholesterol fraction of the different layers of the aorta turns over at a slower rate than the free fraction. (c) The cholesterol (free and ester) of normal appearing intima is derived in large part (60-65%) from the plasma cholesterol; the remainder is derived from synthesis *in situ*. (d) Of the tissues studied (liver, adrenal, ventricular muscle, kidney, skeletal muscle), the aorta has the slowest cholesterol turnover.

The presently available data on the origin of the aortic cholesterol in man suggests that a large portion of the cholesterol of the aorta is derived from the serum. Whether human aorta can esterify free cholesterol to form at least a portion of its own cholesterol esters is presently unknown. The one outstanding feature of the aortic cholesterol turnover data is the inertness of advanced plaques. This logically raises the question of whether far advanced plaques can be reabsorbed or has the atherosclerotic process at this stage gone past the point of reversibility. On the other hand, since thickened intima does appear to have a cholesterol turnover, this early stage of atherosclerosis may be reversible. The alternate possibilities exist that thickened intima has a greater uptake of plasma cholesterol than far advanced plaques and that the cholesterol of diseased areas of the aorta may not be freely interchangeable with the plasma cholesterol.

C. Triglycerides

The proportions of human aortic triglyceride derived from the plasma and synthesis *in situ* are unknown. Rabinowitz *et al.* (1962) reported that aortic intima obtained from one subject synthesized C^{14}-fatty acids from C^{14}-acetate. The significance of this observation in relation to atherogenesis must await further studies.

D. Phospholipids

The only pertinent study in man on the origin of the aortic phospholipids was carried out by Zilversmit *et al.* (1961a). Following the injection of P^{32}-phosphate into patients with vascular disease, considerable quantities of labeled phospholipids were recovered in the intima and adventitia of the abdominal aorta as well as peripheral vessels with atherosclerotic lesions. A comparison of arterial plaque and plasma phospholipids indicated that in several instances (particularly at the early times) the plaque phospholipid specific activity exceeded that in the plasma. According to those workers, these findings suggest that the phospholipids of the plaque are derived from synthesis by the arterial wall. Further studies are needed in this area, particularly in regard to the origin of the individual phospholipid fractions in human aorta, utilizing C^{14}-acetate as well as P^{32}-phosphate.

VIII. The Origin of Animal Aortic Lipids

A. Free and Esterified Cholesterol

To ascertain the contributions of exogenous and endogenous cholesterol to the atherosclerotic lesion of cholesterol-fed rabbits, Biggs and Kritchevsky (1951) compared aortic cholesterol in animals fed H^3-cholesterol or H^3-enriched water. They observed that rabbit atherosclerotic aorta derives the bulk of its plaque cholesterol from the plasma rather than endogenous synthesis. Dury and Swell (1960) and Schwenk and Stevens (1960) also noted the entrance of endogenous cholesterol-4-C^{14} into the aortas of cholesterol-fed rabbits. In addition, Schwenk and Stevens (1960) estimated that only a very small amount (0.03 mg) of the fed cholesterol (900 mg) was laid down in the aorta per day; there was also a continuous exchange of cholesterol between the tissues and blood. Newman *et al.* (1961) have studied the origin of the cholesterol fractions in rabbit aorta. Cholesterol-fed rabbits were injected with C^{14}-acetate and the specific activity of the cholesterol fractions in the plasma and intima determined. The results indicated that in rabbit aorta there was a very small incorporation of C^{14}-acetate into digitonin-precipitable material. Also, the rate of incorporation was lower for the esterified cholesterol than for the free fraction. The specific activity relationships of the free and esterified cholesterol fractions in terminal plasma and intima indicated that the intimal cholesterol was derived predominantly from the plasma. In a later report, Newman *et al.* (1962) studied the movement of cholesterol and cholesterol ester in and out of the aorta of cholesterol-fed rabbits. These studies revealed, as in the previous report, that the plasma was the primary source of the cholesterol in the atheromatous aorta. The accumulation of cholesterol in the atherosclerotic lesion was found not to be a static process, but subject to continuous turnover; larger quantities of cholesterol in the lesion were associated with higher influxes of cholesterol. Also, relative to their concentration in the plasma, the rate of free cholesterol entering the intima was found to be greater than that of the cholesterol ester fraction. The authors state that a simple filtration of blood constituents entering the blood of the aorta cannot account for the above findings. Dayton (1959) studied the turnover of cholesterol in the arterial walls of chickens. In the normal animal it was observed that plasma cholesterol is the major source of the cholesterol in the arterial wall, but local synthesis may contribute a significant fraction.

The studies in rabbits tend to confirm the observations in man, namely, that most of the aortic cholesterol is derived from the plasma. There appear to be differences in the rate of movement of free and esterified cholesterol fractions into the aorta. At the present time, no data are available on the movement of the individual cholesterol esters into and out of the aorta.

B. Triglycerides

The study of Newman *et al.* (1961) suggests that the triglyceride fatty acids of cholesterol-fed rabbits may be synthesized *in situ* by the aorta. The specific activity of intimal triglycerides was found to be higher than the plasma triglycerides following the injection of C^{14}-acetate to cholesterol-fed eviscerated rabbits.

C. Phospholipids

The experiments of Zilversmit *et al.* (1954), Shore *et al.* (1955), McCandless and Zilversmit (1956) and Newman *et al.* (1961) have provided convincing evidence that in the cholesterol-fed rabbit the aorta accumulates lipids containing appreciable amounts of phospholipids. Furthermore, by injecting P^{32}-phosphate and C^{14}-acetate into cholesterol-fed eviscerated and noneviscerated rabbits and following the specific activity relationships of the plasma and aortic phospholipids, it was shown that most of the excess phospholipids are derived by synthesis in the aorta; only about 10% of the excess aortic phospholipids are derived from the plasma. Comparison of the specific activities of individual plasma and intimal phospholipids showed that all intimal phospholipids had higher specific activities than corresponding terminal plasma phospholipids (Newman *et al.,* 1961). Of particular interest is the observation (Zilversmit, 1959) that when cholesterol is removed from the diet and hyperlipemia disappears, the lesions persist and phospholipid synthesis in the aorta remains as high as that observed in hypercholesterolemic rabbits. These findings suggest (Zilversmit, 1959) that the defective lipid metabolism of the aorta initiated by cholesterol feeding is not readily reversed by decreasing the serum lipid levels.

IX. Conclusions

The last few years have added significantly to our knowledge of the interrelationships of the lipids in blood and tissues. This has come about primarily from the newer data on the fatty acid composition of lipids and also from information obtained with the aid of isotopes on the dynamic aspects of lipid metabolism. However, many basic problems still remain to be solved and many inconsistencies in the experimental data have yet to be adequately clarified. Moreover, the available data on interrelationships of lipids is still largely of a descriptive type. As pointed out in this review, there is a mass of data on the levels and fatty acid composition of the tissue lipid fractions, but little is known about the processes of metabolism and transport which underlie these data. For example, the cholesterol esters of the plasma are always high in polyunsaturated fatty acids. How and where these esters are formed and what happens to the fatty acid moieties of this fraction are presently unknown. It is apparent that future studies on cholesterol ester metabolism will have to be concerned with the individual esters. Likewise, the metabolism of the specific triglycerides and phospholipids must also be studied.

The enigma of the role of the essential fatty acids in tissue metabolism and why they are primarily esterified to cholesterol must also be clarified. It is possible that the highly unsaturated cholesterol esters are involved in the transfer of the essential fatty acids across the cell membrane; the polyunsaturated cholesterol esters, upon entering the tissue, may be hydrolyzed, releasing the essential fatty acids for other biological processes and the free cholesterol being returned to the blood. Of paramount importance in regard to the essential fatty acids is their role in the atherosclerotic process.

When more is known about the function and transport of lipids, the significance of the interrelationships among the tissue lipids and the relationship of lipids to the development of atherosclerosis will be more clearly understood. The evidence at hand strongly suggests that there is either a primary or a secondary defect in cholesterol ester metabolism in atherosclerosis.

REFERENCES

Achaya, K. T., Alfin-Slater, R. B., and Deuel, H. J., Jr. (1954). Unpublished results. Cited *In* "The Lipids," H. J. Deuel, Jr. (1957). Vol. III, p. 825. Interscience, New York.

Ahrens, E. H., Jr., Insull, W., Jr., Hirsch, J., Stoffel, W., Peterson, M. L., Farquhar, J. W., Miller, T., and Thomasson, H. J. (1959). *Lancet* i, 115-119.

Albers, H. J., and Gordon, S. (1962). *Proc. Soc. Exptl. Biol. Med.* **109**, 860-863.

Alfin-Slater, R. B., Aftergood, L., Wells, A. F., and Deuel, H. J., Jr. (1954). *Arch. Biochem. Biophys.* **52**, 180-185.

Apostolakis, M., Grimmer, G., Glaser, A., and Voigt, K. D. (1962). *Biochem. Z.* **336**, 1-9.

Biggs, M. W., and Kritchevsky, D. (1951). *Circulation* **4**, 34-42.
Biggs, M. W., Kritchevsky, D., Colman, D., Gofman, J. W., Jones, H. B., Lindgren, F. T., Hyde, G., and Lyon, T. P. (1952). *Circulation* **6**, 359-366.
Bjorntorp, P., and Hood, B. (1960). *Circulation Res.* **8**, 319-323.
Blomstrand, R., and Christensen, S. (1961). *Nature* **189**, 376-378.
Blomstrand, R., and Dahlback, O. (1960). *J. Clin. Invest.* **39**, 1185-1191.
Böttcher, C. J. F., and van Gent, C. M. (1961). *J. Atherosclerosis Res.* **1**, 36-46.
Böttcher, C. J. F., and Woodford, F. P. (1961). *J. Atherosclerosis Res.* **1**, 434-443.
Böttcher, C. J. F., and Woodford, F. P. (1962). *Federation Proc.* **21**, 15-19.
Böttcher, C. J. F., Woodford, F. P., ter Haar Romeny-Wachter, C. C., van Houte, E. B., and van Gent, C. M. (1960a). *Lancet* **i**, 1378-1383.
Böttcher, C. J. F., van Houte, E. B., ter Haar Romeny-Wachter, C. C., Woodford, F. P., and van Gent, C. M. (1960b). *Lancet* **ii**, 1162-1166.
Bragdon, J. H., and Karmen, A. (1960). *J. Lipid Res.* **1**, 167-170.
Bragdon, J. H., and Karmen, A. (1961). *J. Lipid Res.* **2**, 400-402.
Byers, S. O., and Friedman, M. (1960). *Am. J. Physiol.* **198**, 629-631.
Byers, S. O., Friedman, M., and Michaelis, F. (1951). *J. Biol. Chem.* **188**, 637-641.
Carroll, K. K. (1962). *Can. J. Biochem. Physiol.* **40**, 1115-1122.
Dailey, R. E., Swell, L., and Treadwell, C. R. (1962). *Arch. Biochem. Biophys.* **99**, 334-337.
Dam, H., Prange, I., and Sondergaard, E. (1955). *Acta Physiol. Scand.* **34**, 141-146.
Dayton, S. (1959). *Circulation Res.* **7**, 468-475.
Deykin, D., and Goodman, D. S. (1962). *Biochem. Biophys. Res. Commun.* **8**, 411-415.
Dittmer, J. C., and Hanahan, D. J. (1959). *J. Biol. Chem.* **234**, 1976-1982.
Dole, V. P., James, A. T., Webb, J. P. W., Rizack, M. A., and Sturman, M. F. (1959). *J. Clin. Invest.* **38**, 1544-1554.
Duncan, W. R. H., and Garton, G. A. (1962). *J. Lipid Res.* **3**, 53-55.
Dury, A., and Swell, L. (1960). *Am. J. Physiol.* **198**, 363-365.
Eckles, N. E., Taylor, C. B., Campbell, D. J., and Gould, R. G. (1955). *J. Lab. Clin. Med.* **46**, 359-371.
Entenman, C., Chaikoff, I. L., and Zilversmit, D. B. (1946). *J. Biol. Chem.* **166**, 15-23.
Evans, J. D., Oleksyshyn, N., Luddy, F. E., Barford, R. A., and Riemenschneider, R. W. (1959). *Arch. Biochem. Biophys.* **85**, 317-322.
Evrard, E., van den Bosch, J., De Somer, P., and Joossens, J. V. (1962). *J. Nutr.* **76**, 219-222.
Fernandes, J., Kramer, J. H. van de, and Weijers, H. A. (1955). *J. Clin. Invest.* **34**, 1026-1036.
Field, H., Jr., Swell, L., Schools, P. E., Jr., and Treadwell, C. R. (1960). *Circulation* **22**, 547-558.
Fishler, M. C., Entenman, C., Montgomery, M. L., and Chaikoff, I. L. (1943). *J. Biol. Chem.* **150**, 47-55.
Friedman, M., and Byers, S. O. (1955). *J. Clin. Invest.* **34**, 1369-1374.
Friedman, M., Byers, S. O., and Michaelis, F. (1951). *Am. J. Physiol.* **164**, 789-791.
Gambal, D., and Quackenbush, F. W. (1960). *J. Nutr.* **70**, 497-501.
Getz, G. S., Bartley, W., Stirpe, F., Notton, B. M., and Renshaw, A. (1962). *Biochem. J.* **83**, 181-191.
Glomset, J. A., Parker, F., Tjaden, M., and Williams, R. H. (1962). *Biochim. Biophys. Acta* **58**, 398-406.
Goldman, D. S., Chaikoff, I. L., Reinhardt, W. O., Entenman, C., and Dauben, W. G. (1950). *J. Biol. Chem.* **184**, 727-733.

Gould, R. G., LeRoy, G. V., Okita, G. T., Kabara, J. J., Keegan, P., and Bergenstal, D. M. (1955). *J. Lab. Clin. Med.* **46**, 372-384.

Hallgren, B., and Svanborg, A. (1962). *Scand. J. Clin. Lab. Invest.* **14**, 179-184.

Hallgren, B., Stenhagen, S., Svanborg, A., and Svennerholm, L. (1960). *J. Clin. Invest.* **39**, 1424-1434.

Hanahan, D. J., Watts, R. M., and Pappajohn, D. (1960a). *J. Lipid Res.* **1**, 421-432.

Hanahan, D. J., Brockerhoff, H., and Barron, E. J. (1960b). *J. Biol. Chem.* **235**, 1917-1923.

Harper, P. V., Jr., Neal, W. B., Jr., and Hlavacek, G. R. (1953). *Metab. Clin. Exptl.* **2**, 69-80.

Havel, R. J., and Goldfien, A. (1961). *J. Lipid Res.* **2**, 389-395.

Hernandez, H. H., and Chaikoff, I. L. (1957). *J. Biol. Chem.* **228**, 447-457.

Hirsch, E. F., and Weinhouse, S. (1943). *Physiol. Rev.* **23**, 185-202.

Holman, R. T., and Peifer, J. J. (1960). *J. Nutr.* **70**. 411-417.

Holman, R. T., Hayes, H., Malmros, H., and Wigand, G. (1957). *Proc. Soc. Exptl. Biol. Med.* **96**, 705-709.

Howton, D. R., and Hashimoto, S. (1960). *Am. J. Clin. Nutr.* **8**, 50-52.

James, A. T., Lovelock, J. E., Webb, J., and Trotter, W. R. (1957). *Lancet* i, 705-708.

Kelsey, F. E., and Longenecker, H. E. (1941). *J. Biol. Chem.* **139**, 727-740.

Kingsbury, K. J., Paul, S., Crossley, A., and Morgan, D. M. (1961). *Biochem. J.* **78**, 541-550.

Kinsell, L. W., Michaels, G. D., and Fukayama, G. (1958). *Proc. Soc. Exptl. Biol. Med.* **98**, 829-833.

Klein, P. D. (1958). *Arch. Biochem. Biophys.* **76**, 56-64.

Klein, P. D. (1959). *Arch. Biochem. Biophys.* **81**, 382-389.

Klein, P. D., and Dahl, R. M. (1961). *J. Biol. Chem.* **236**, 1658-1660.

Klein, P. D., and Martin, R. A. (1959a). *J. Biol. Chem.* **234**, 1685-1687.

Klein, P. D., and Martin, R. A. (1959b). *J. Biol. Chem.* **234**, 3129-3132.

Korzenovsky, M., Diller, E. R., Marshall, A. C., and Auda, B. M. (1960). *Biochem. J.* **76**, 238-245.

Kurland, G. S., Lucas, J. L., and Freedberg, A. S. (1961). *J. Lab. Clin. Med.* **57**, 574-585.

Lawrie, T. D. V., McAlpine, S. G., Pirrie, R., and Rifkind, B. M. (1961a). *Clin. Sci.* **20**, 255-261.

Lawrie, T. D. V., McAlpine, S. G., Rifkind, B. M., and Robinson, J. F. (1961b). *Lancet* i, 421-424.

Le Breton, E., and Pantaleon, J. (1944). *Compt. Rend. Soc. Biol.* **138**, 38-39.

LeRoy, G. V., Gould, R. G., Bergenstal, D. M., Werbin, H., and Kabara, J. J. (1957). *J. Lab. Clin. Med.* **49**, 858-868.

Lewis, B. (1958). *Lancet* ii, 71-73.

Lis, E. W., and Okey, R. (1961). *J. Nutr.* **73**, 117-125.

Lough, A. K., and Garton, G. A. (1957). *Biochem. J.* **67**, 345-351.

Luddy, F. E., Barford, R. A., Riemenschneider, R. W., and Evans, J. D. (1958). *J. Biol. Chem.* **232**, 843-851.

McCandless, E. L., and Zilversmit, D. B. (1956). *Arch. Biochem. Biophys.* **62**, 402-410.

McCandless, E. L., and Zilversmit, D. B. (1957). *Am. J. Physiol.* **191**, 174-178.

Mead, J. F., and Gouze, M. L. (1961). *Proc. Soc. Exptl. Biol. Med.* **106**, 4-7.

Morris, M. D., and Chaikoff, I. L. (1959). *J. Biol. Chem.* **234**, 1095-1097.

Morris, M. D., Chaikoff, I. L., Felts, J. M., Abraham, S., and Fansah, N. O. (1957). *J. Biol. Chem.* **224**, 1039-1045.

Mukherjee, S., Achaya, K. T., Deuel, H. J., Jr., and Alfin-Slater, R. B. (1957). *J. Biol. Chem.* **226**, 845-849.

Mukherjee, S., Kunitake, G., and Alfin-Slater, R. B. (1958). *J. Biol. Chem.* **230**, 91-96.

Nedswedski, S. W. (1935). *Z. Physiol. Chem.* **236**, 69-72.

Nelson, W. R., Werthessen, N. T., Holman, R. L., Hadaway, H., and James, A. T. (1961). *Lancet* **i**, 86-88.

Newman, H. A. I., and Zilversmit, D. B. (1962). *J. Biol. Chem.* **237**, 2078-2084.

Newman, H. A. I., McCandless, E. L., and Zilversmit, D. B. (1961). *J. Biol. Chem.* **236**, 1264-1268.

Okey, R., and Harris, A. G. (1958). *Arch. Biochem. Biophys.* **75**, 536-537.

Okey, R., Shannon, A., Tinoco, J., Ostwald, R., and Miljanich, P. (1961). *J. Nutr.* **75**, 51-60.

Patil, V. S., and Magar, N. G. (1960). *Biochem. J.* **74**, 441-444.

Rabinowitz, J. L., Myerson, R. M., and Wohl, G. T. (1960). *Proc. Soc. Exptl. Biol. Med.* **105**, 241-243.

Rabinowitz, J. L., Skerrett, P. V., and Riemenschneider, R. W. (1962). *J. Am. Med. Assoc.* **179**, 153-155.

Rehnborg, C. S., Nichols, A. V., and Ashikawa, J. K. (1961). *Proc. Soc. Exptl. Biol. Med.* **106**, 547-549.

Riley, C., and Nunn, R. F. (1960). *Biochem. J.* **74**, 56-61.

Schrade, W., Biegler, R., and Bohle, E. (1961). *J. Atherosclerosis Res.* **1**, 47-61.

Schwenk, E., and Stevens, D. F. (1960). *Proc. Soc. Exptl. Biol. Med.* **103**, 614-617.

Shore, M. L., Zilversmit, D. B., and Ackerman, R. F. (1955). *Am. J. Physiol.* **181**, 527-531.

Sinclair, H. M. (1956). *Lancet* **i**, 381-383.

Sperry, W. M. (1935). *J. Biol. Chem.* **111**, 467-478.

Stein, Y., and Shapiro, B. (1960). *J. Lipid. Res.* **1**, 326-331.

Swell, L., and Treadwell, C. R. (1950a). *J. Biol. Chem.* **182**, 479-487.

Swell, L., and Treadwell, C. R. (1950b). *J. Biol. Chem.* **185**, 349-355.

Swell, L., and Treadwell, C. R. (1962). *Proc. Soc. Exptl. Med.* **110**, 55-57.

Swell, L., Boiter, T. A., Field, H., Jr., and Treadwell, C. R. (1955). *Am. J. Physiol.* **181**, 193-195.

Swell, L., Trout, E. C., Jr., Field, H., Jr., and Treadwell, C. R. (1958). *J. Biol. Chem.* **230**, 631-641.

Swell, L., Field, H., Jr., Schools, P. E., Jr., and Treadwell, C. R. (1960a). *Proc. Soc. Exptl. Biol. Med.* **103**, 651-655.

Swell, L., Field, H., Jr., and Treadwell, C. R. (1960b). *Proc. Soc. Exptl. Biol. Med.* **104**, 325-328.

Swell, L., Law, M. D., Field, H., Jr., and Treadwell, C. R. (1960c). *J. Biol. Chem.* **235**, 1960-1962.

Swell, L., Field, H., Jr., and Treadwell, C. R. (1960d). *Proc. Soc. Exptl. Biol. Med.* **105**, 129-131.

Swell, L., Field, H., Jr., Schools, P. E., Jr., and Treadwell, C. R. (1960e). *Proc. Soc. Exptl. Biol. Med.* **105**, 662-665.

Swell, L., Law, M. D., Schools, P. E., Jr., and Treadwell, C. R. (1961a). *J. Nutr.* **74**, 148-156.

Swell, L., Law, M. D., Schools, P. E., Jr., and Treadwell, C. R. (1961b). *J. Nutr.* **75**, 181-191.

Swell, L., Law, M. D., and Treadwell, C. R. (1962a). *Proc. Soc. Exptl. Biol. Med.* **109**, 176-179.

Swell, L., Law, M. D., and Treadwell, C. R. (1962b). *J. Nutr.* **76**, 429-434.

Swell, L., Schools, P. E., Jr., and Treadwell, C. R. (1962c). *Proc. Soc. Exptl. Biol. Med.* **109**, 682-685.

Swell, L., Schools, P. E., Jr., and Treadwell, C. R. (1962d). *Proc. Soc. Exptl. Biol. Med.* **111**, 48-50.

Takahashi, Y., and Tanaka, K. (1961). *J. Biochem.* **49**, 713-720.

Taylor, C. B., Patton, D., Yogi, N., and Cox, G. E. (1960). *Proc. Soc. Exptl. Biol. Med.* **103**, 768-772.

Tennent, D. M., Zanetti, M. E., Atkinson, D. I., Kuron, G. W., and Opdyke, D. F. (1957). *J. Biol. Chem.* **228**, 241-245.

Tuna, N., Reckers, L., and Frantz, I. D., Jr. (1958). *J. Clin. Invest.* **37**, 1153-1165.

Wright, A. S., Pitt, G. A. J., and Morton, R. A. (1959). *Lancet* ii, 594-597.

Yamamoto, R. S., Goldstein, N. P., and Treadwell, C. R. (1949). *J. Biol. Chem.* **180**, 615-621.

Zilversmit, D. B. (1959). *In* "Hormones and Atherosclerosis" (G. Pincus, ed.), pp. 145-155. Academic Press, New York.

Zilversmit, D. B., Shore, M. L., and Ackerman, R. F. (1954). *Circulation* **9**, 581-585.

Zilversmit, D. B., McCandless, E. L., Jordan, P. H., Jr., Henly, W. S., and Ackerman, R. F. (1961a). *Circulation* **23**, 370-375.

Zilversmit, D. B., Sweeley, C. C., and Newman, H. A. I. (1961b). *Circulation Res.* **9**, 235-241.

—10—

Naturally Occurring Arteriosclerosis in Animals: A Comparison with Experimentally Induced Lesions

S. Lindsay and I. L. Chaikoff

I. Introduction

Arteriosclerosis in humans and animals is an extremely complex disease. Undoubtedly numerous interrelated processes in the vascular wall are involved, only some of which concern lipids. Nonetheless, since Anitschkow's (1913) early demonstration that the feeding of massive amounts of cholesterol induces atherosclerosis in rabbits, unusually great emphasis has been placed on the lipid aspects of the disease in man. Despite claims to the contrary, the experimental lesion produced by cholesterol feeding does not closely resemble the naturally occurring lesion in any animal species, including man. Thus, the modern tendency to regard arteriosclerosis merely as a disease of lipid origin has led to an oversimplification in recent concepts dealing with its nature, etiology, and treatment. The lipid phase observed in the human lesion is almost unique in the animal kingdom. The primary degenerative aspects of the arterial disease—those that occur before excess lipids appear—cannot be disregarded, nor should it be assumed that they are of little or no consequence in the etiology of arteriosclerosis.

Studies of the cardiovascular apparatus of many species of mammals and birds in this and other laboratories have clearly demonstrated that, as these animals age, basic alterations take place in the walls of their arteries—changes that may lead to advanced arteriosclerosis. The basic vascular changes in all species seem to be similar, but variations in the sequences of development of the arteriosclerotic lesions in different species may lead to different end results.

A survey of naturally occurring arteriosclerosis in animals—its histogenesis and development—is presented here. An attempt has been made to relate the naturally occurring disease to experimentally induced arteriosclerosis. It will be shown that certain lesions described as having been produced experimentally are, in fact, naturally occurring lesions that were modified in some fashion by the experimental process.

II. Description of Arteriosclerotic Lesions in the Class Aves

A. Domestic Chicken *(Gallus)*

In 1944 Dauber reported that the structure and location of naturally occurring arteriosclerotic lesions differed in male and female chickens. In the hen, lipid was found within intimal cells of both thoracic and abdominal portions of the aorta before fibrosis or other alterations appeared. In the rooster, on the other hand, fibrosis was the earliest change detected in the abdominal aortic intima, accompanied only occasionally by lipid. Dauber (1944) suggested a dual origin for spontaneous arteriosclerosis in chicks: in the rooster, initiated by fibrosis with secondary accumulation of lipid; in hens, beginning as an accumulation of lipid in the intima and followed by fibrosis. Dauber compared this latter development of arterial disease with that produced by cholesterol feeding, and stressed the similarities in the foam cell characteristics of these naturally occurring and experimentally induced lesions (Dauber and Katz, 1942, 1943).

Chaikoff *et al.* (1948) compared naturally occurring arteriosclerosis in male chickens with that artificially induced by prolonged feeding of cholesterol and with that induced by injections of diethylstilbestrol.* In young male birds, the naturally occurring lesions in the thoracic aorta were characterized by lipid droplets within the intima and adjacent media. Although Dauber (1944) had indicated that this primary lipid lesion was to be found only in the female chicken, Lindsay and Chaikoff (unpublished) also found it in roosters and capons (Figs. 1 and 2) over 5 years of age, and were able to accentuate its development in young male birds by either cholesterol feeding or diethylstilbestrol injections, experimental procedures that induce a hyperlipidemia (Chaikoff *et al.,* 1948). The naturally occurring plaques in the abdominal aorta contained small amounts of lipid material some of which was probably cholesterol. These plaques were modified by extensive deposition of lipids and cholesterol in the birds that were fed cholesterol or injected with diethylstilbestrol. We have repeatedly stressed that the cholesterol-induced lesion should be considered as part of a widespread cholesterol storage process and therefore as an artificial arterial disease.

Additional studies of the naturally occurring disease in male chickens were carried out by Lindsay *et al.* (1955) who demonstrated that the thoracic aortic lesion resulted from an accumulation of lipids that first

---

* Lipid metabolism in the bird is unique in that it is under ovarian control. Injections of estrogens have been shown to raise the concentrations of certain lipid constituents in the blood stream of the chicken to extraordinary heights (Lorenz, 1954).

appeared in the intima and later in the media. Proliferation of intimal foam cells then led to intimal thickening and development of plaques. In the abdominal aorta the initial change was fragmentation of the internal elastic membrane, followed by deposition of acid mucopolysaccharide. Proliferation of intimal fibroblasts and further deposition of

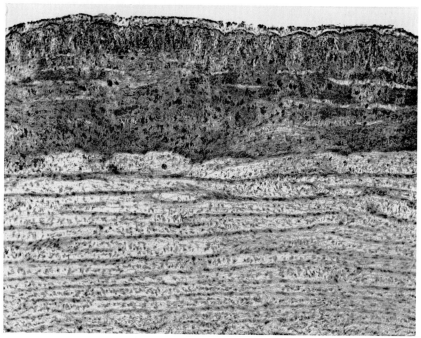

FIG. 1. Thoracic aorta (female chicken, age 5). Magnification: 125. Sudan IV-hematoxylin stain. Considerable lipid infiltration is noted in the inner third of the media Accumulations of lipid-containing foam cells have resulted in slight intimal thickening. Polarized light showed moderate numbers of cholesterol crystals in the intima and media.

mucoid substances resulted in formation of intimal plaques. Deposition of lipids did occur later in the deep portions of these plaques, but they apparently played no part in the pathogenesis of the earliest lesions.

It has also been shown that feeding of dihydrocholesterol or Δ^4-cholestenone to young cockerels resulted in the development of severe aortic arteriosclerosis that was identical with that resulting from feeding of cholesterol. These sterols appeared as crystalline deposits in the arterial wall, but did not give positive Schultz reactions for cholesterol (Nichols et al., 1955, 1960).

Weiss and Fisher (1959) evaluated sex and segmental differences in naturally occurring arteriosclerosis in chickens. Aortic cholesterol was highly correlated with plasma cholesterol, and aortic hydroxyproline with blood pressure levels. Weiss (1959) studied the development of spontaneous aortic arteriosclerosis in white Leghorn chickens up to 5 years of age. On the basis of severity of aortic disease and cholesterol content

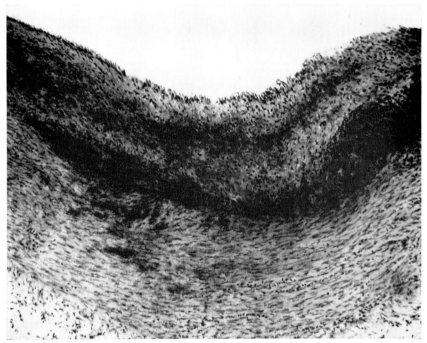

Fig. 2.   Abdominal aorta (capon, age 5). Magnification: 125. Sudan IV-hematoxylin stain. Moderate intimal fibrous thickening with plaque formation is present. Abundant lipid deposits are noted in the thickened intima, especially in the deeper portions, and smaller amounts of lipid are also present in the adjacent media. Few foam cells are noted. Polarized light revealed many anisotropic, spindle-shaped crystals, characteristic of cholesterol in this intimal layer.

and weight of the aorta, arteriosclerosis became progressively severe with age in both male and female birds maintained on a nonatherogenic diet. The abdominal aorta was more affected than the thoracic, as much as a fourfold difference being observed in the oldest birds. The abdominal aorta in the male was only slightly more affected than that in the female. Cholesterol concentration increased progressively in the atherosclerotic segments, but at a slower rate, in the male, than did fibrotic proliferation. Weiss concluded that the distribution of naturally occurring lesions and of cholesterol content along the aorta was the reverse of that occurring with cholesterol feeding or estrogen injections in male chickens. The elevated levels of cholesterol caused spontaneous abdominal lesions resembling those typically characteristic of atheroma, whereas little gross fibrotic proliferation occurred in the thoracic aorta despite high or increasing levels of cholesterol.

A high incidence of spontaneous arteriosclerosis in coronary arteries of male chickens was reported by Paterson et al. (1948). According to these investigators, lesions occurred more frequently in the coronary vessels than in the aorta, and consisted of foci of hydropic degeneration in the media. They suggested that the lesions might be of infectious origin. Cholesterol feeding resulted in secondary lesions in which lipid and cholesterol were believed to have been deposited at sites of the naturally occurring disease, thus accelerating the arteriosclerotic process and resulting in formation of stenosing plaques of the atherosclerotic type. In a later report Paterson et al. (1949) found that the severity of this naturally occurring disease in the coronary arteries was not in- fluenced by protecting the birds from infection. It was suggested that the primary medial lesion in the coronary arteries was not due to hyper- sensitivity nor to dietary agents. Intravenous injections of staphylococci or of staphylococcal toxin failed to produce these medial lesions or to accelerate those of the spontaneous variety.

In their study on coronary arteries of white Leghorn cockerels, Lind- say and Chaikoff (1950) concluded that the hydropic degeneration of the media described by Paterson et al. (1948) was an artifact and did not represent pathological lesions of arteriosclerosis. No evidence was found to support the view that a medial degeneration precedes the appearance of intimal disease in normal birds or, for that matter, in birds fed cho- lesterol or injected with diethylstilbestrol.

Regression of arteriosclerosis produced by cholesterol feeding has been observed by Horlick and Katz (1949). Cessation of cholesterol feed- ing after 10 weeks resulted in a gradual decrease in the severity of the lesions during the next 14 weeks. The early lesions were completely resorbed. The more advanced lesions in both thoracic and abdominal aortas underwent regressive and reparative changes consisting of fibrosis, disappearance of or diminution in foam cells and lipid, and calcification of the atheromas. Lindsay et al. (1955) also studied regression of aortic arteriosclerosis that had been induced in male chickens by cholesterol feeding and stilbestrol injections. Regression of the thoracic lesions was characterized by a decrease in size and number of intimal plaques, and by decreased amounts of lipids and increased amounts of intercellular fibrillary substance in the lesions. These workers found little evidence of regression of the experimentally induced lesions in the abdominal aortas. The late lesion in the abdominal aorta was recognized as a naturally occurring plaque, modified by pronounced accumulation of lipids, including cholesterol, that closely resembled the late arteriosclerotic lesions observed in human muscular arteries. This finding raises the question whether dietary or other procedures for lowering plasma lipids in man would bring about regression of a well established, severe arteriosclerotic lesion.

Orma (1957) studied the effect of physical activity on atherogenesis in cockerels. The incidence and severity of atherosclerosis were more pronounced in an inactive, cholesterol-fed group than in an active, cholesterol-fed group, and were believed to be related to lower thyroid activity in the inactive, cholesterol-fed chickens.

Gey and Pletscher (1961) investigated the influence of dietary corn oil on spontaneous arteriosclerosis of old hens, and reported that visible lesions as well as the total lipid and cholesterol contents of the aorta were not influenced by the corn oil treatments. Fisher *et al.* (1959) also studied the effects of different fats as well as of varying levels of protein and carbohydrates in chickens. In growing roosters, the feeding of a low-protein diet containing 0.3% cholesterol and 10% corn oil resulted in a less severe arteriosclerosis than that induced by the feeding of a high-protein diet containing 2% cholesterol and 10% corn oil. In hens, the feeding of saturated fat (tallow) hastened the development of aortic lesions. These investigators did not comment upon the differences in pathogenesis of thoracic and abdominal lesions, nor on the possible differences in naturally occurring disease of the two sexes. It was shown, however, that fatty acid composition of the thoracic aortic lesions resembled that of dietary fat, whereas fatty acids of the abdominal aorta remained constant, irrespective of dietary fat.

Chaikoff *et al.* (1961) examined the role of protein intake on naturally occurring aortic arteriosclerosis that develops in chickens fed low-cholesterol diets (similar to those ingested by man). No differences were noted in the gross size of arteriosclerotic plaques nor of microscopic lipid deposition in the thoracic and abdominal portions of the aortas of birds fed two levels of protein, 7.3% and 14.5%. However, more pronounced intimal thickening was observed in the abdominal aortas of birds fed the lower level of protein. It was suggested that a disturbance of protein metabolism caused by suboptimal protein intake may have interfered with regeneration of elastic tissue in the abdominal aorta, thereby promoting the arteriosclerotic intimal thickening.

B. Domestic Pigeon (Columba)

Naturally occurring arteriosclerosis in various breeds of pigeons has been studied by Clarkson et al. (1959). Intimal plaques covering approximately 10% of the surface of the thoracic aorta were found in Autosexing Kings, Silver Kings, and White Carneau pigeons, but the thoracic aortas of Racing Homers and Show Racers were almost devoid of such lesions. Most of the plaques were yellow and elevated, and were found at the distal end of the thoracic aorta; central hemorrhage and ulceration were present in some of the plaques. These workers regarded the microscopic features of these lesions as nearly identical with those observed in human beings. Fibrous connective tissue plaques contained deep accumulations of intracellular and extracellular neutral fat, cholesterol crystals, and calcium salts. The amounts of acid mucopolysaccharides were increased in the plaques, and the internal elastic membrane beneath them was disrupted. Coronary arteriosclerosis was found in a single instance. No relation to sex, diet, or exercise was observed.

In 1962 Prichard et al. described the effects of fat and cholesterol feeding in young male and female pigeons of susceptible and resistant breeds. After 6 or 7 months, all of the susceptible White Carneau pigeons had aortic atherosclerosis, whereas only 18% of the Carneau controls were atherosclerotic. Only 10% of Racing Homers, a nonsusceptible breed that was fed cholesterol, developed a few plaques; the control birds did not show aortic arteriosclerosis. Quantitative histological differences among the breeds were observed in coronary atherosclerotic plaques: the lesions in Carneau pigeons consisted of fibrocytic proliferation; those in Show Racers were almost entirely fatty in nature with little fibrocytic proliferation. Although the histological descriptions of lesions in the pigeon are not extensive, it seems likely that both naturally occurring and experimentally induced lesions are similar to those described in chickens (Chaikoff et al., 1948).

Lofland and Clarkson (1959) dealt with some biochemical aspects of spontaneous arteriosclerosis in the two susceptible breeds, White Carneau and Silver Kings, and in the two nonsusceptible breeds, Racing Homers and Show Racers. The incidence and severity of aortic atherosclerosis seemed unrelated to blood levels of total, free, and ester cholesterol, and total phospholipids, and to the ratio of cholesterol to phospholipids. Aortic weight and aortic cholesterol content did, however, parallel the severity of the disease. No relation of the severity of the disease to age, sex, diet, and physical activity was observed.

Lofland et al. (1961) also studied the effects of dietary fat, protein, and cholesterol on the atherosclerosis of susceptible breeds of pigeons.

Cholesterol feeding elevated serum cholesterol and increased the cholesterol content of the aorta and the severity of arteriosclerosis. In cholesterol-fed birds, corn oil feedings lowered blood cholesterol. Suggestive evidence was obtained that the severity of arteriosclerosis was influenced by the type of dietary fat, by the level of protein in the diet, and by the presence or absence of cholesterol in the diet.

C. Wild Birds in Captivity

1. STRUTHIONIFORMES (OSTRICHES); RHEIFORMES (RHEAS); CASUARIIFORMES (EMUS, CASSOWARIES)

Fox (1933) examined 13 ostriches, 14 rheas, and 22 cassowaries. In a number of these birds he found lesions consisting of flat atheromatous plaques that appeared to arise near the aortic valves and extended to the renal arteries. In two other South African ostriches he found advanced aortic calcification. Vestesaeger (1959a) observed intimal fibrous

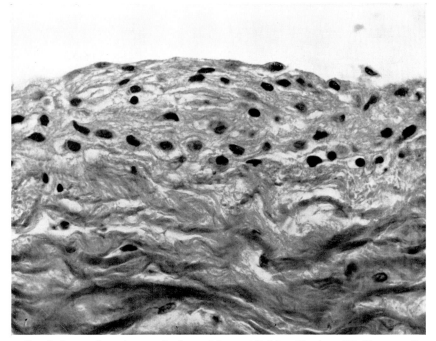

FIG. 3. Lower thoracic aorta (male ostrich, age 10). Magnification: 500. Hematoxylin-eosin stain. Early intimal plaque composed of vacuolated fibroblasts and collagen fibers. Coarse and fine intracellular lipid deposits were present in this lesion (Sudan IV stain).

thickening in the right coronary artery of an emu; foamy cells were found in the depths of the intima in the vicinity of the media. Lindsay and Chaikoff (unpublished) observed aortic arteriosclerosis in 7 male and female ostriches ranging in age from 1 to 17 years (Figs. 3-6). Similar disease was found in an old female rhea (Fig. 7), but none was present

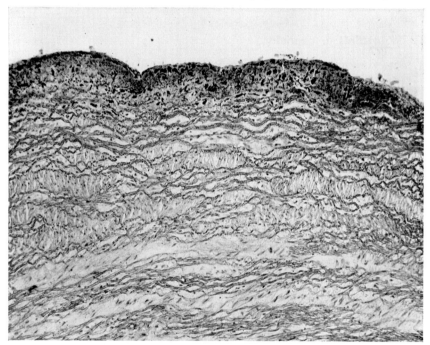

Fig. 4. Lower thoracic aorta (male ostrich, age 10). Magnification: 125. Sudan IV-hematoxylin stain. The intima and superficial layer of the media contain coarse lipid droplets. A few cholesterol crystals were demonstrable with polarized light.

in a 2-year-old, female rhea. Most lesions were characterized by elevated, coalescing yellow or yellow-gray plaques involving much of the aorta, and appearing most prominently in the lower thoracic and abdominal aortas. Microscopically the lesions were found to consist of foamy macrophages, but showed considerable intimal fibrosis. The lesions were regarded as comparable with those observed in domestic chickens.

2. PELECANIFORMES (PELICANS, CORMORANTS)

Fox (1933) found nodular and confluent lesions in the aortas of old birds of this group. Mural atherosclerosis involving the media, fraying and rupture of the elastica, and calcification deep in the media were observed.

3. CICONIIFORMES (HERONS, EGRETS, STORKS, IBISES)

Arterial disease ranging from mild atheromatous patches in the sinus of Valsalva to stiff, firm arteries without definite intimal lesions was observed in these birds (Fox, 1933). In one bird, fibrillar thickening

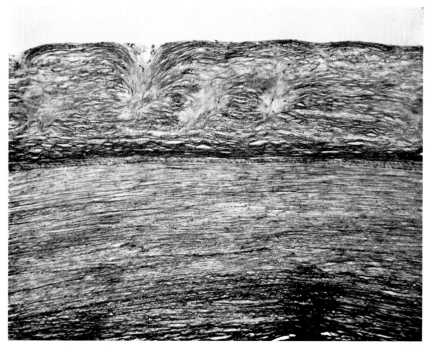

FIG. 5. Lower thoracic aorta (male ostrich, age 10). Magnification: 125. Weigert-van Gieson stain. The intima is widened and many coarse elastic fibers are present.

of the intima and calcific deposits in the media were found, and in a second bird, intimal atheroma of moderate grade and medial calcification.

4. PHOENICOPTERIFORMES (FLAMINGOS)

Coronary arteriosclerosis in a Chilean flamingo (Lindsay and Chaikoff, unpublished) is shown in Figs. 8 and 9.

5. ANSERIFORMES (DUCKS, GEESE, SWANS, SCREAMERS)

In ducks, geese, and swans, arteriosclerosis, according to Fox (1933), was found most prominently in the sinus of Valsalva, and at the origins of the brachiocephalic and renal arteries. The lesions ranged from a simple fibrillar increase in the intima, with splitting of the elastica, to complete atheromas containing hyaline and fatty substances, calcium, cartilage, bone, and even bone marrow. Eventually the internal elastic membrane disintegrated and the media became progressively thinner.

Vastesaeger *et al.* (1959a) found arteriosclerosis of the anterior de-

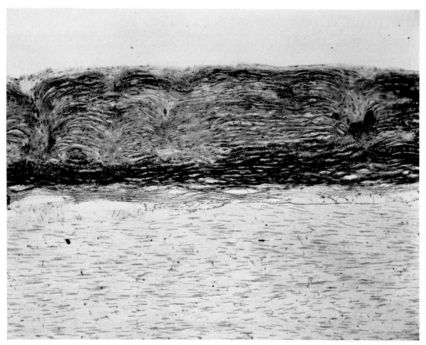

FIG. 6. Lower thoracic aorta (male ostrich, age 10). Magnification: 125. Sudan IV-hematoxylin stain. The thickened intima contains abundant, extracellular, lipid appearing as fine droplets distributed along elastic fibers. No foam cells are present. Cholesterol is absent (polarized light).

scending coronary artery in a Javanese swan. Considerable intimal fibrous thickening was observed, and much of the internal elastic membrane either was stretched and no longer undulating or was absent. The lumen of the posterior descending artery was narrowed by pronounced intimal fibrous thickening, and the internal elastic membrane of that vessel had disappeared. Similar fibrous thickening was observed in the anterior descending coronary artery of a snow goose.

Wolffe *et al.* (1949) found that naturally occurring atheromatosis appeared much less frequently in wild ducks than in domesticated ducks and geese. Both atheromatosis and atherohepatosis were produced in force-fed geese. The arterial lesions were believed similar to those of the human being.

Fox (1933) found a yellow, aortic plaque near the renal arteries in 1 of 7 screamers that he examined.

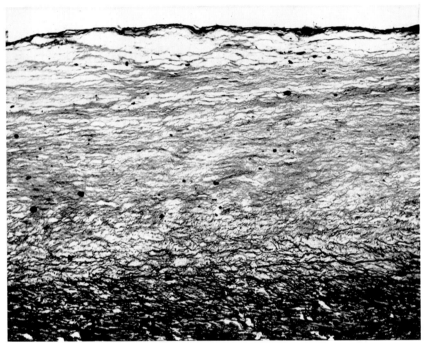

FIG. 7. Abdominal aorta (female rhea, age 6). Magnification: 125. Weigert-van Gieson stain. Pronounced intimal thickening and plaque formation are noted. Elastic fibers are more numerous in the deeper portion of the plaque, whereas the superficial portion is mucoid. Considerable extracellular lipid is present, distributed mainly along elastic fibers (Sudan IV stain). No cholesterol was demonstrable with polarized light.

6. FALCONIFORMES (EAGLES, HAWKS, BLACK AND TURKEY VULTURES)

Fox (1933) asserts that the incidence of arteriosclerosis is low in eagles and Old World vultures. He found atheromatous plaques principally in the sinus of Valsalva and in the brachiocephalic arteries of black and turkey vultures. The thoracic aorta and celiac and mesenteric arteries were less involved. The atheromatous lesions contained calcific granules. Extension of the atheroma through the media caused fraying of elastic fibers and thinning of the media, which in two cases resulted in aneurysmal bulging.

Aronson (1962) has described acute myocardial infarction with endocardial mural thrombosis in a bald eagle (*Haliacetus leucocephalus*). The intramural coronary arteries were diffusely involved by an obliterating intimal proliferation. The lesions were practically devoid of lipids.

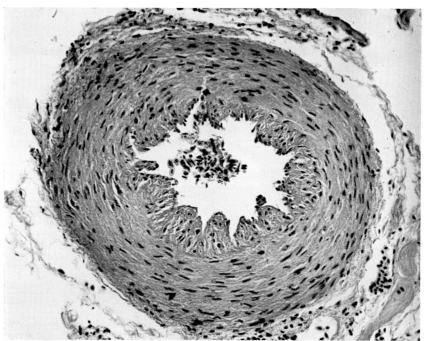

Fig. 8. Coronary artery (Chilean flamingo, age 8). Magnification: 250. Hematoxylin-eosin stain. Concentric fibrous thickening of the intima is noted. No lipid (Sudan IV stain) is present.

7. Galliformes (Grouse, Pheasants, Turkeys, etc.)

Fox (1933) found arterial disease in wild birds of this order. The process was an atherosclerosis, but the medial changes were more prominent than those in the intima. Gresham et al. (1962) briefly described arteriosclerosis in the abdominal aorta of a male turkey. The thickened, collagenous intima contained extracellular metachromatic material and abundant lipid.

The common occurrence of aortic rupture in 12- to 20-week-old male turkeys, associated with atherosclerotic plaques at the site of rupture, has been reported by Howard et al. (1962). It was suggested that atherosclerosis led to aortic weakening and rupture and that hypertension in some breeds of turkeys might be a contributing factor. These investigators also studied the effects of various fat supplements in the diets in

1-day-old turkeys. No significant differences were observed in severity of atherosclerosis in birds fed either a commercial turkey starter, a commercial turkey starter plus 20% beef tallow, a commercial turkey starter

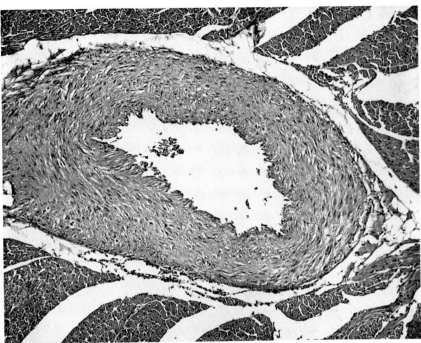

FIG. 9. Coronary artery (Chilean flamingo, age 8). Magnification: 125. Hematoxylin-eosin stain. Mild intimal fibrous thickening is present mainly on the left side. No lipid (Sudan IV stain) is noted in the vascular walls.

plus 20% arachis oil, or a synthetic diet containing 20% beef tallow. Atherosclerotic lesions in all groups bore close histological and histochemical similarities to those of man.

8. GRUIFORMES (CRANES, TRUMPETERS)

Fox (1933) described yellow aortic streaks and slightly elevated, thin yellow plaques in birds of this order. The intimal process was characterized by a fibrillar increase, vacuolated cells, and calcific deposits. The media was not damaged by the process. Vastesaeger *et al.* (1959a) observed intimal fibrous thickening in the coronary arteries of a Senegalese crane. The internal elastic membranes had lost their undulating characteristics, and some segments were absent.

9. Columbiformes (Doves, Pigeons)

Only two birds in this group were found by Fox (1933) to display small, yellow intimal plaques in the thoracic and upper abdominal portions of the aorta.

10. Psittaciformes (Parrots)

Fox (1933) found significantly higher prevalence of lesions in males of this order than in females. Elevated yellow plaques were observed in the thoracic and abdominal aortas, the brachiocephalic arteries, and at times in the iliac and celiac arteries. Coronary arteries, particularly those on the left side, were often affected. Atheromatous deposits containing lipids caused intimal thickening. The intimal internal elastic membrane was penetrated, and the lesion extended into the media. Fox did not observe ulceration or thrombosis in these arteriosclerotic lesions in the larger vessels of parrots, but did note several instances in which even the smallest arteries contained grossly visible, stiff intimal plaques.

Finlayson and Hirchinson (1961) fed cholesterol to female budgerigars. Slight intimal sudanophilic stippling led to development of multiple, creamy white or yellow, lipid-containing nodules and plaques that involved both the intima and inner media. Intimal thickening resulted from accumulations of foam cells which extended into the media of the aorta. Small coronary arteries were occluded by these intimal foam cells.

11. Strigiformes (Owls)

According to Fox (1933), the incidence of arteriosclerosis in this order is low. The lipid-containing, yellow, thickened intima resulted in slight stiffening of the thoracic and abdominal segments of the aorta.

12. Coracciformes (Motmots and Hornbills) and Piciformes (Toucans)

Fox (1933) stated that atheromas were most prominent at the apex of the aortic arch in these birds, but that they also extended into the brachiocephalic and sometimes into the renal and iliac arteries. The atheromas contained crystals, vacuoles, and calcific deposits; rupture of the elastic laminas and encroachment of the plaques on the media were observed. Arborization of delicate elastic fibers had extended from the media through the thickened intima.

13. Passeriformes (Perching, Song Birds)

Fox (1933) described stiff or firm thickening of the great vessels in song birds. Yellow, firm plaques were found in the brachiocephalic vessels and along the posterior wall of the thoracic aorta. The iliac and coronary arteries were rarely involved. One bird with massive atheromas showed extension of fat into the inner media, cartilaginous metaplasia, and frayed elastic laminas.

14. MISCELLANEOUS OBSERVATIONS

Rigg *et al.* (1960) reported arteriosclerosis in 16 of 35 birds examined at the London Zoo. Lesions resembling those of human atherosclerosis were found in four parrots, a parakeet, slender-billed cockatoo, peahen and peafowl, crested screamer, touraco, scarlet macaw, red-billed hornbill, Bahama duck, American widgeon, and an African cattle egret. The lesions consisted of atheromas of the thoracic aorta and brachiocephalic arteries, formed by loosely arranged, fibrous tissue with a considerable lipid content. An excess of mucopolysaccharide was often demonstrated. Lipid was found both extracellularly and intracellularly, mainly in the superficial layer of the intima just below the endothelium, but some was also present in the deeper intimal layers. Crystalline lipid material which yielded a positive Schultz reaction for cholesterol was found mainly in the deeper intimal layers. Some lipid-containing lesions were almost free of fibrosis, whereas some fibrous lesions contained only a little lipid. Elastic fragmentation, lipid deposition, and calcification were seen in the media of some birds. Coronary arterial lesions were not found.

Ratcliffe *et al.* (1960) found striking atheromas in the thoracic aorta and brachiocephalic arteries of birds, especially in parrots and their relatives. Convulsive seizures experienced by parrots were attributed to brachiocephalic arterial occlusion by these lesions. Relatively large atheromas had also developed in the thoracic aortas and brachiocephalic arteries of ducks and geese, pheasants, carnivorous birds, and the bird of paradise. The microscopic appearances of the atheromas were characterized by loosely arranged fibrous tissue with a considerable lipid content. The bases of these lesions usually extended into the medial coats, often as far as the inner half. Ratcliffe *et al.* (1960) stated that, within a year after improved diets had been fed at the Philadelphia Zoo, large atheromas of the thoracic aorta and brachiocephalic arteries became rare in birds of all groups. The lesions observed after the improvement of diets were smaller and more compact atheromata, usually located in the abdominal aorta and its branches. Secondary involvement of the media was rarely observed. It was concluded that dietary improvement had resulted in changes in the character and location of arterial lesions in birds.

III. Arteriosclerotic Lesions in the Class Reptilia

Rigg *et al.* (1960) found no macroscopic lesions in the hearts and aortas of 9 reptiles (tortoises, snakes, crocodiles, and an iguana) that they examined. Microscopic sections of the aorta appeared normal.

IV. Arteriosclerotic Lesions in the Class Mammalia

A. Monotremata (Platypus, Echidnas or Spiny Anteaters)

Arteriosclerosis has not been studied in this order. Because monotremes lay large, heavily yolked eggs, a study of their vascular lesions would be of extreme interest.

B. Marsupialia (Kangaroos, Wallabies, Bandicoots, Dasyures, etc.)

The marsupial family with the highest incidence of arteriosclerotic lesions was found by Fox (1933) to be the kangaroo, but other animals of this order also exhibited arterial disease of a similar character. In the arch, along the thoracic aorta and, less often, in carotid and abdominal arteries, Fox observed granular lesions or diffuse opacities consisting of medial degeneration with calcification. The overlying intima displayed fibrous thickening, but elastic fibers were not prominent. Fox concluded that the media rather than the intima appeared to be the primary site of arteriosclerosis in marsupials.

Rigg *et al.* (1960) found small, grayish intimal plaques and nodules in the aortas of 3 wallabies. The lesions consisted of focal fragmentation and calcium encrustation of the elastic fibers at the junction of the intima and the media. Comparable, though less pronounced, lesions were found in a coronary artery of one of the animals. These workers concluded that these lesions bore no resemblance to the human atheroma. Ratcliffe *et al.* (1960) described the occurrence of arteriosclerosis in the aortas and coronary arteries of 10 herbivorous marsupials that included kangaroos, wallabies, and wallaroos.

C. Insectivora (Moles, Hedgehogs, Shrews); Dermoptera (Colugos, etc.); Chiroptera (bats)

Arteriosclerotic lesions have not been described in these orders of mammals.

D. Primates

1. LEMURIDAE (LEMURS)

No arteriosclerosis was observed by Fox (1933) in members of this order. Vastesaeger *et al.* (1959a) found no arteriosclerosis in the coronary network in a black lemur.

2. NEW WORLD MONKEYS

a. *Hapalidae (Marmosets).* Arteriosclerosis was not found in the 63 marmosets that Fox (1933) examined.

b. *Cebidae (Squirrel, Capuchin, Spider, Woolly, and Other Monkeys).* Fox (1933) found a single case of arteriosclerosis among 204 Cebidae that he studied. Vastesaeger *et al.* (1959a) failed to observe coronary artery disease in a woolly monkey, but Ratcliffe *et al.* (1960) have described both coronary and aortic arteriosclerosis in New World monkeys that they examined.

Arteriosclerosis has been induced by Mann *et al.* (1953) in the *Cebus fatuella* by cholesterol feeding; the entire aorta and proximal portions of the carotid and femoral arteries were involved, but the lesions in the coronary vessels were minimal. These cholesterol-induced lesions in cebus monkeys were characterized by lipid-filled macrophages, which brought about intimal thickening and fibrosis that extended into the media layer. These lesions were clearly of lipid origin and were associated with fatty livers and accumulation of lipids in spleens and tubular epithelium of the kidneys.

Wissler *et al.* (1962) compared the effects of feeding butterfat, coconut oil, and corn oil to young adult cebus monkeys for 45 weeks. Gross or microscopic fatty intimal lesions of the aorta were found in 3 of 4 monkeys consuming butterfat, in all monkeys that received coconut oil, and in none fed corn oil.

3. CERCOPITHECIDAE (OLD WORLD MONKEYS, MACAQUES, BABOONS)

Fox (1933) did not include the *Rhesus macaque* in his study of Old World monkeys, but in other members of this order he found superficial atheromatous plaques in the arch and thoracic portions of the aorta; the abdominal aorta was only rarely involved. The early lesions showed subendothelial, fibrillar thickening with fine lipid droplets. The more advanced form of the disease exhibited intimal widening, hyalinization, a minimal amount of calcification, and splitting and fraying of the internal elastic membrane. Fox regarded these lesions as atheromas.

Lindsay and Chaikoff (unpublished) observed well developed aortic arteriosclerosis in 6 rhesus monkeys that were over 20 years old (Figs. 10-12), but found no gross evidence of arterial disease in 46 young members of this group. Lindsay and Chaikoff (unpublished) have also noted aortic arteriosclerosis in pig-tailed and moor macaques (Figs. 13-15). Ratcliffe *et al.* (1960) did not state whether rhesus monkeys were included in the Old World monkeys that they examined.

Rinehart and Greenberg (1949, 1951) described widespread arteriosclerosis of the aorta and many smaller arteries of rhesus monkeys that had been subjected to prolonged pyridoxine deficiency. The lesions consisted of split and reduplicated internal elastic membranes and coarse intimal collagenous sclerosis that led to intimal thickening. Accumulation of mucinous material in the intima was followed by cellular proliferation and formation of collagenous and elastic fibers. In a few in-

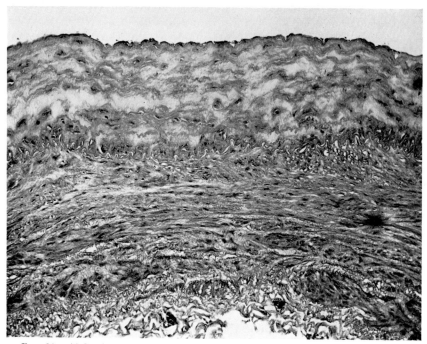

Fig. 10. Abdominal aorta (female rhesus monkey, age 15). Magnification: 125. Hematoxylin-eosin stain. This intimal plaque consists of mucoid connective tissue. The internal elastic membrane is fragmented and reduplicated. Only a few fine lipid droplets lie along the deep elastic fibers (Sudan IV stain).

stances, fat droplets and calcification were observed in the deeper portions of the intimal plaques. These lesions closely resembled naturally occurring disease observed in rhesus monkeys 20 to 25 years of age (Chaikoff and Lindsay, unpublished; Figs. 10-12).

McGill et al. (1961) induced aortic arteriosclerosis in rhesus monkeys by feeding them lard and making them hypertensive by the Goldblatt procedure. Two types of lesions were observed: (1) simple fatty streaks, usually more numerous in the descending portion of the thoracic aorta; and (2) glistening, circumscribed, pearly plaques that did not stain for fat. In the fatty streaks the intima was thickened by elongated spindle cells separated by unstained or faintly eosinophilic and metachromatic ground substance. Few macrophages containing fat were found. The pearly plaques had a similar structure but contained more numerous intercellular substances; not all of these lesions contained fat, but when present, it was found in the deeper portions. All of the experimental

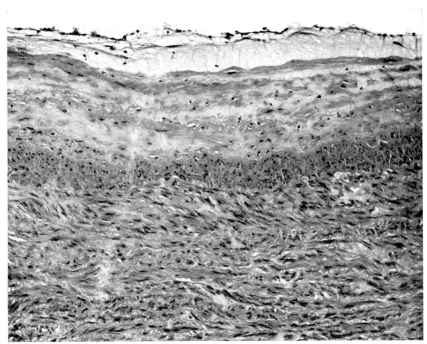

FIG. 11. Abdominal aorta (female rhesus monkey, age 22). Magnification: 125. Hematoxylin-eosin stain. Two distinct layers are present in this intimal plaque. The deeper layer is fibrous and condensed; the superficial layer is distinctly mucoid. Lipid deposition is limited to fine droplets clustered along the internal elastic membrane (Sudan IV stain).

animals developed lipid-containing lesions, but more were found in those animals made hypertensive. All animals with fibrous plaques were hypertensive, suggesting that hypertension was associated with or was responsible for increased lipid deposition with final conversion into pearly, fibrous plaques. These authors concluded that this experimental lesion bore little resemblance to human lesions but did resemble the arteriosclerosis in rhesus monkeys described by Rinehart and Greenberg (1949, 1951).

Taylor *et al.* (1962) observed hypercholesterolemia and fatty deposits in aortas of rhesus monkeys that had been fed a high-fat, high-cholesterol diet for 3 to 65 months. The lesions consisted of lipid droplets diffusely distributed in the interstitial areas throughout the intima. Later, these lipid droplets were phagocytosed by macrophages, and intimal fibrosis developed; the internal elastic membrane and media were progressively

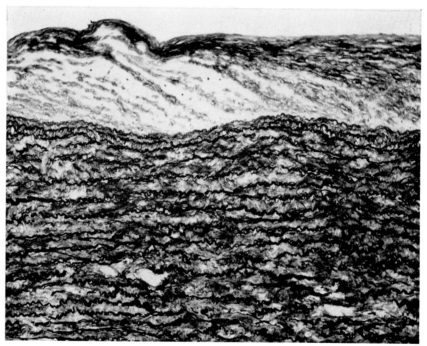

FIG. 12. Thoracic aorta (female rhesus monkey over 20 years of age). Magnification: 125. Weigert-van Gieson stain. Elastic tissue appears first in the intima adjacent to fibroblasts. Coarse elastic fibers are present on the right. The thickened intima contains moderate numbers of fine extracellular, lipid droplets; fewer are found throughout the media (Sudan IV stain). Cholesterol is absent (polarized light).

destroyed and replaced by lipid-containing macrophages. In control animals only a minimal amount of lipid infiltration of the intima was infrequently encountered, and arteriosclerosis was not observed. These investigators did not comment on the conditions of other tissues. Earlier studies of cholesterol feeding in rhesus monkeys failed to reveal arteriosclerosis (Kawamura, 1927; Sperry et al., 1944; Heuper, 1946).

Arteriosclerosis in baboons has been extensively studied. A single baboon examined by Fox (1933) had an atheromatous protrusion partially obstructing the orifice of the right anterior coronary artery. Lindsay and

Chaikoff (1957) studied the aortas and iliac and coronary arteries of 2 male 20-year-old baboons (*Papio anubis*). Diffuse, gray, fibrous intimal thickening or discrete, white, fibrous plaques were observed in the thoracic and abdominal portions of the aorta, and linear yellow streaks were present in the thoracic portions. Both fibrous and fatty plaques

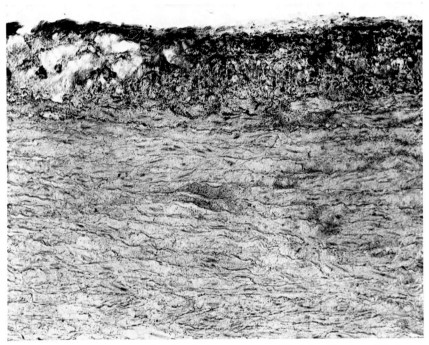

Fig. 13. Thoracic aorta (male pig-tailed macaque, age 27). Magnification: 125. Sudan IV-hematoxylin stain. Large lipid deposits are noted in the thickened intima and less is seen in the media. The lipid deposits are mainly extracellular. No foam cells are present. Cholesterol is absent (polarized light).

were found in an iliac artery of 1 animal. The vascular lesions seemed to be initiated by degeneration of the internal elastic membrane or inner medial elastic layer, accompanied by fragmentation, splitting, and reduplication. This degenerative phase was followed first by deposition of increased amounts of polysaccharide substance, and then by proliferation of fibroblasts that produced reticulum, collagen, and elastic fibers. This proliferative reaction often led to development of distinct intimal plaques. Lipid infiltration appeared mainly on or near intimal elastic tissue and seemed to be preceded by degeneration of this tissue. Affinity of the lipid for intimal mucopolysaccharide material was observed. Lipid within the cytoplasm of fibroblasts and lipid-containing macrophages eventually appeared. Cholesterol was identified in the lesions.

Gillman and Gilbert (1957) studied the aortas of 59 female and 26 male baboons, aged 3 to 26 years, that had been fed a low-cholesterol

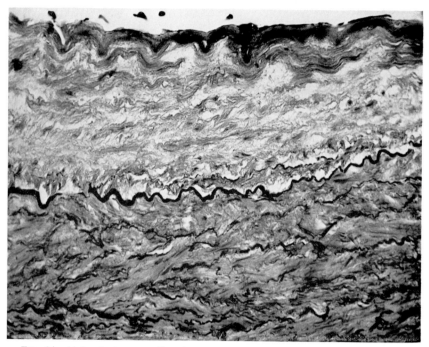

Fig. 14. Abdominal aorta (female moor macaque, age 20). Magnification: 250. Weigert-van Gieson stain. Segment of intimal plaque. Elastic fibers are condensed in the superficial portion. Coarse and fine lipid droplets (Sudan IV stain) are demonstrable in this lesion, especially adherent to elastic fibers. Foam cells are absent.

diet. They concluded that atherosis was related to and preceded by modification of the structure of intimal fibers and cells, which included elastosis and fibrosis, without an increase in cellularity of the intima. According to these investigators, elastic degeneration and injury promoted increased combining capacity for lipid and calcium. The first detectable change was the appearance of lipid globules on elastic fibers. In some cases the lesions progressed and spread to the media. In others they underwent repair during which lipid disappeared and the destroyed elastic tissue was replaced by collagenous connective tissue.

In a later report, Gilbert and Gillman (1960) described the coronary arterial system of 133 domesticated baboons of both sexes, ranging in age from birth to 18 years. Coronary disease was not found in animals under 1 year of age, but did appear in those between 1 and 4 years of age. There was no evidence to indicate that the severity of coronary arteriosclerosis in the baboon is related to age or to the extent of the disease

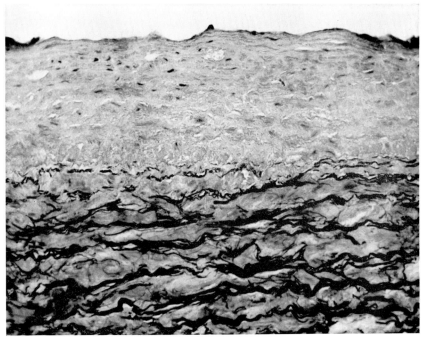

Fig. 15. Thoracic aorta (male moor macaque, age 20). Magnification: 250. Weigert-van Gieson stain. Relatively acellular, fibrous, intimal plaque. Note absence of elastic fibers. Abundant large and small lipid droplets are present in the intima (Sudan IV stain) and many fine droplets in the media.

in the aorta. These investigators found that coronary arterial lesions in the baboon were almost identical with those described in Portuguese East Africans (Gillman *et al.,* 1960). The stages of the disease were: lysis and reduplication of the elastic lamina; cellular infiltration in the intima from the underlying media; collagenization and progressive broadening of the intima; and finally, lysis or necrosis of collagenous fibers with deposition of cholesterol and calcium.

After McGill *et al.* (1960) found naturally occurring arteriosclerosis in a 16-year-old baboon that had been kept in a zoo, they studied arteriosclerosis in 163 wild baboons (*Papio doguera*) of all ages that had been trapped in Kenya, Africa. Some degree of aortic intimal lipid deposition was noted in 75% of adult baboons, as judged by gross staining with Sudan IV, but extensive fatty streaks were found in only a few of the baboons. In most animals, 1-10% of the intimal surface showed lipid infiltration. Small, elevated, translucent, glistening pearly plaques were

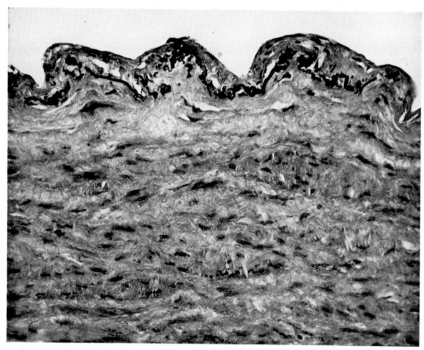

FIG. 16. Abdominal aorta (female chimpanzee, age 20). Magnification: 250. Hematoxylin-eosin stain. Early arteriosclerotic lesion characterized by severe degeneration and fragmentation of internal elastic membrane. Granular calcific deposits are present in some segments of the membrane. Minimal intimal fibrous thickening is also noted. Lipid is not present at this stage (Sudan IV stain).

also present. Large and small lipid droplets were found in the intima and at times in the media, both intracellularly and in the interstitial spaces. Lipid was also found in macrophages and in the cytoplasm of the smooth muscle cells of the intima. Fine lipid droplets were encrusted on the elastic laminas. No gross lesions were observed in the coronary arteries, but a few small musculofibrous intimal plaques were found in these vessels. McGill *et al.* concluded that arteriosclerosis in the baboon increases with age but is not related either to sex or to pregnancy. Their illustrations reveal fragmentation and reduplication of the internal elastic membranes identical with those reported by Lindsay and Chaikoff (1957) and Gillman and Gilbert (1957).

4. PONGIDAE (GIBBONS, ORANGUTANS, CHIMPANZEES, GORILLAS)

Fox (1933) did not observe arteriosclerosis in members of this group that he examined. Manning (1942) described coronary arteriosclerosis

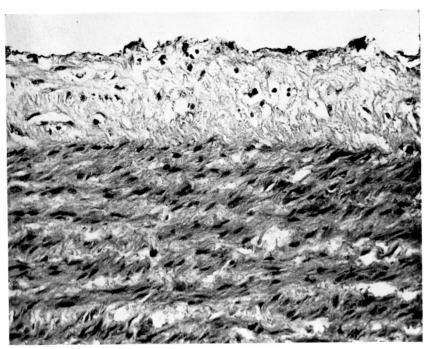

FIG. 17. Thoracic aorta (female chimpanzee, age 20). Magnification: 250. Hematoxylin-eosin stain. The thickened intima consists of mucoid connective tissue. Delicate fibrils and a few fibroblasts are noted. This lesion contains coarse lipid droplets in the vacuolated fibroblasts (Sudan IV stain). A few cholesterol cystals were demonstrable with polarized light.

and myocardial infarction and fibrosis that resulted in death of an 8-year-old female ape, presumably a chimpanzee. Subendothelial intimal thickening was prominent in the medium and smaller coronary arteries, but atheromatous lesions and thrombosis were not observed. Ratcliffe *et al.* (1960) observed coronary arteriosclerosis in all 7 members of Pongidae that they examined, but aortic disease was found in only 1 of them. Intimal fibrous thickening of intramural branches of the coronary arteries was illustrated in a male orangutan, 18 years of age. Perivascular fibrosis and occlusion of a lateral branch of an artery were also noted. Although Vastesaeger *et al.* (1959a) failed to detect arteriosclerosis in a gibbon, an orangutan, and in 2 dwarf chimpanzees, atheromatous lesions similar to those of man were observed in 2 pale-faced chimpanzees (*Pan schweinfurtii*). The right coronary artery of a 4-year-old female

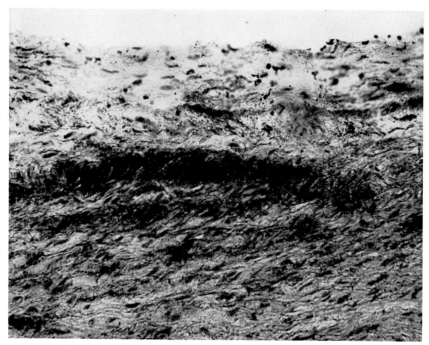

FIG. 18. Thoracic aorta (female chimpanzee, age 20). Magnification: 250. Sudan IV-hematoxylin stain. Most of the lipid is extracellular and in the media concentrated along the medial elastic fibers. Few droplets are noted in the very slightly thickened intima. No cholesterol is present (polarized light).

showed intimal fibrous thickening associated with fragmentation of the internal elastic membrane. The lumen had become practically obliterated by eccentric intimal thickening. Occlusion was completed by an adherent thrombus near a segment of intima that contained numerous cholesterol crystals. In an older, pale-faced chimpanzee, these workers observed narrowing of the right coronary lumen by an eccentric intimal fibrous thickening that contained cholesterol crystals. The anterior descending artery of this same animal showed moderate intimal fibrous thickening associated with an intact internal elastic membrane. Our studies of primate arteriosclerosis (Lindsay and Chaikoff, unpublished) have revealed well developed arteriosclerotic lesions in the aortas of several old chimpanzees (Figs. 16-19).

Vastesaeger *et al.* (1959a) did not find coronary arteriosclerosis in a mountain gorilla and in a coastal gorilla that they examined. Steiner *et al.* (1955) examined a giant lowland gorilla (*Gorilla gorilla*). Approxi-

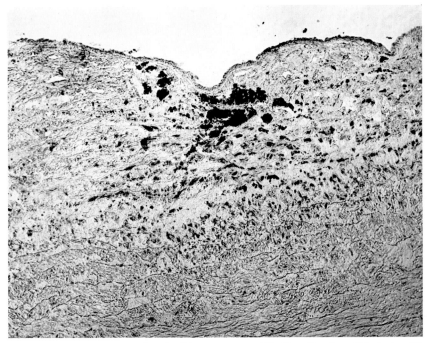

FIG. 19. Thoracic aorta (female chimpanzee, age 20). Magnification: 125. Sudan IV-hematoxylin stain. The large lipid deposits in the intima are mainly intracellular. Few foam cells are present. Minimal lipid is present in the adjacent media.

mately 10% of small coronary arteries in the myocardium showed hyaline fibrosis that involved chiefly the media but sometimes all layers. In the more severe lesions the internal elastic membrane had degenerated. Microscopic examination of other vessels revealed sclerotic changes only in those of the nervous system. Although the aorta appeared normal grossly, microscopic examination showed areas of intimal fibrous thickening. A similar plaque was observed in the celiac artery. Steiner *et al.* (1955) concluded that the arteriosclerotic lesions in this animal were likely due to a dietary deficiency, on the basis of the changes in other tissues, especially the nervous system.

E. Edentata (Sloths, Armadillos, True Anteaters)

Arteriosclerosis has not been studied in this order of mammals.

F. Pholidota (Pangolins, Scaly Anteaters)

Vastesaeger et al. (1959a) described early arteriosclerosis in the posterior descending coronary artery of a giant pangolin. Successive layers of elastic tissue had proliferated between the endothelium and internal elastic membrane, producing cushion-like lesions that projected into the lumen. Distinct fragmentation of the internal elastic membrane was illustrated. The other layers of the artery appeared normal.

G. Lagomorpha (Rabbits, Hares)

Fox (1933) has summarized the principal reports that appeared before 1930, dealing with naturally occurring arteriosclerosis in rabbits. An incidence as high as 34% was reported in a variety of strains. The lesions were most prominent in the thoracic aorta, where they appeared as elevated intimal granulations or large, flat plaques. The intimal thickening, which resulted from proliferation of elastic fibers, contained small amounts of lipids and calcific deposits. Some authors regarded naturally occurring arteriosclerosis in the rabbit as very much like that of the human being.

Bragdon (1952a) extended the work of Solowjew (1932) who first observed focal deposits of subanophilic material in the aortic intima of suckling rabbits. After weaning, lipids in the endothelial cells and in the intercellular intimal matrix gradually disappeared, first from the former and later from the intima. New, spontaneous lesions, identical in distribution and histological structure, appeared in older rabbits of both sexes. Bragdon regarded these lesions as identical with those that develop in rabbits in the early periods of cholesterol feeding. It should be noted, however, that these lesions were not sclerotic, and possibly resulted from transient periods of mild hypercholesterolemia.

That changes with aging may be responsible for intimal lipid deposition in older rabbits has been suggested by Waugh et al. (1956) who examined aortas of female rabbits of two age groups (3 months and 46 months) corresponding to human childhood and middle age. In the older rabbits the water, sodium, calcium, nonlipid phosphorus, and possibly cholesterol contents of the aorta were increased. These authors concluded that the lower levels of total lipid and cholesterol in the rabbit aortas, as compared with those of man, probably account, at least in part, for the relative freedom of the rabbit from naturally occurring arteriosclerosis.

Duff *et al.* (1957) have described three types of naturally occurring focal lesions in the aortas of rabbits. One consisted of a focal accumulation of polymorphonuclear leucocytes in the intima and media. A second type involved medial degeneration, a process related to aging, which in advanced cases had converted the aorta to a wide, calcific tube with irregular fusiform dilatations. The intima was thickened by fibroblastic proliferation, and the elastic laminas and muscularis of the media were destroyed or disorganized by varying numbers of mononuclear cells that rarely contained Sudan IV-staining droplets. The third was an uncommon naturally occurring lesion consisting of clumps of mononuclear cells immediately under the endothelium. No fat stainable with Sudan IV was present in these lesions. Duff *et al.* (1957) were unable to find naturally occurring, lipid-containing lesions similar to those reported by Bragdon (1952a).

Arteriosclerosis experimentally induced by cholesterol feeding has been extensively studied in the rabbit. Duff *et al.* (1957) studied early cholesterol-induced lesions by the surface-examination technique, and found the smallest, and presumably the earliest, lesions to consist of a few intimal cells containing fat droplets. Fat was also deposited in otherwise normal appearing fibroblasts and histiocytes and rarely in subendothelial monocytoid cells. As the lesions grew larger, histiocytes and monocytoid cells accumulated in the intima, and the amounts of demonstrable fat increased. Not only were more fat-containing cells present, but the individual cells had also ingested greater quantities of lipid. The lesions spread peripherally as more fibrocytes and histiocytes came to contain fat droplets. The fat was mostly intracellular, but no abnormality was found in the endothelium. Duff *et al.* (1957) concluded that the monocytoid cells in the lesions entered the intima from the blood, and that some macrophages originated from this cell type, although it was believed that the number of histiocytes increased mainly by mitosis. There was no evidence to support Leary's theory (1949) that lipid was carried to the intima by phagocytes, nor Duguid's theory (1952) of intimal incorporation of thrombi.

Prior *et al.* (1961) compared the late effects of prolonged cholesterol feeding in rabbits with the naturally occurring disease in control animals. They also failed to find the lipid-containing lesion in normal rabbits described by Bragdon (1952a), but they did note naturally occurring aortic and iliac medial calcification which apparently represented degeneration of the elastic medial fibers with secondary calcification. The control animals (noncholesterol fed) also displayed intimal thickening in the pulmonary arteries, associated with an increased number of elastic fibers. The medial layers were considerably thickened and the internal elastic membrane was frequently frayed and split. After prolonged feeding of cholesterol, extensive deposition of this substance was found not only in the arterial system but also in many organs and tissues. Foam cell plaques that had become fibrotic, and extension of the lipid process into the medial layer were observed. Xanthomatous lesions in other organs and tissues suggested the resemblance of this process to other forms of storage disease described by Heuper (1942). This study emphasized the fact that, although the vascular lesions found in the cholesterol-fed animals somewhat resembled certain stages of human disease, the experimentally produced lesions were irregularly distributed, and differed in their histogenesis and complications from the disease found in man. It was emphasized that the widespread storage disease in hypercholesteremic rabbits is not analogous to that observed in man except for that seen in essential hypercholesterolemia.

In a study of the ultrastructure of coronary arteries of rabbits, Parker (1958) found that the endothelial cells sent filiform processes toward the media through fenestrae in the internal elastic membrane. The endothelial cells contained small surface invaginations that formed caveolae, with transitions to oval, thin-walled vesicles believed analogous to pinocytosis, suggesting a role in nutritive transport. The fenestrated internal elastic membrane appeared as a sheet of moderately thick material consisting of two components, the first a homogeneous, tenacious matrix and the second, embedded within the matrix, consisting of numerous fibrils without periodicity. Elastic strands branching from the internal elastic membrane extended into the media between smooth muscle cells. The smooth muscle of the media did not appear syncytial, and the cells had well defined basement membranes. Collagenous and elastic fibers were interposed between smooth muscle cells. Loosely packed collagen with typical periodicity and elastic fibers made up the bulk of the adventitial layer. This author pointed out that the exact nature of the elastic tissue matrix of the internal elastic membrane was not clear, but suggested that it consisted of a tangle of long, macromolecular protein chains similar to the elastic chains of rubber.

Buck (1962), by means of the electron microscope, studied the structure of rabbit atherosclerotic lesions produced by feeding cholesterol. The endothelium formed a continuous, single layer separated from the tunica media by a thick layer of modified smooth muscle cells and extracellular material. The endothelial cells differed from normal cells by prominence of their cytoplasmic organelles, particularly the Golgi apparatus, suggesting that these cells were more active metabolically than were normal endothelial cells. The presence of material of moderate density in the dilated cisternae of the endoplasmic reticulum was not thought to be a stage in the imbibition of lipoprotein from the serum. After these rabbits had been fed a normal diet for 2 years, the amount of collagenous and elastic fibers was much greater, and typical foam cells and macrophages were rarely observed. The predominant cell in the intima was a modified smooth muscle cell. Its role in the pathogenesis of rabbit arterial disease was considered significant, but was not understood. It was believed that a large proportion of the extracellular material in the intima consisted of mucopolysaccharide. Cholesterol could not be visualized.

Higginbotham and Higginbotham (1958) studied regression of rabbit aortic atheromatosis in intraocular transplants. When atheromatous aortic tissues were transplanted into untreated, healthy hosts, the number of foam cells and the amounts of subanophilic material in the atheromatous transplants were reduced and these cells were replaced by fibrous connective tissue. Cholesterol esters appeared to have been converted to cholesterol crystals. Similar regressive changes were reported by Horlick and Katz (1949) and by Lindsay *et al.* (1955) for plaques in intact chickens after normal diets had been substituted for atherogenic diets.

Arterial disease has been induced in rabbits by means other than the feeding of cholesterol. Oester *et al.* (1955) compared the arteriopathy produced by injections of epinephrine and thyroxine, by intravenous administration of cholesterol suspensions, and by a combination of these injections. Of 84 untreated rabbits, only 1 showed arteriopathy. Of 48 animals that received injections of epinephrine and thyroxine, 43 showed nonatheromatous, mainly medial disease which, in some cases, was severe and characterized by almost complete disappearence of the media. These lesions resembled human medial arteriosclerosis or arterionecrosis. Infrequently, the lesions also showed a proliferating intima. Of 32 animals that received cholesterol injections, 23 showed macroscopic aortic lesions. These were found in the intima, were atheromatous, and were less extensive than those induced by epinephrine and thyroxine. Rabbits that had been injected with a combination of epinephrine, thyroxine, and cholesterol had severe sclerosis which appeared to be a combined form of disease. When intimal proliferation appeared in these latter animals, it was usually more extensive than in those fed cholesterol alone.

Hass *et al.* (1960) induced arteriosclerosis in rabbits by feeding them excessive amounts of irradiated ergosterol. A generalized disorder characterized by bone resorption and by abnormal deposition of calcium salts in many extraosseous tissues was observed. Calcium appeared first in the inner media of the aortic arch. With time, the calcific deposits spread in depth and in the direction of blood flow along the aorta and its major branches. The histological alterations consisted of inflammatory, degenerative, and calcific sequences with subsequent repair reactions. The principal changes appeared in the internal elastic membrane and the media, while the fibroblastic intimal proliferative reactions and vascularized stromal resorption of the media were the principal manifestations of repair. These investigators concluded that the lesion was similar to that of Mönckeberg's sclerosis in the human being.

Arteriosclerosis has been induced in rabbits by the intravenous injection of papain (Tsaltas, 1962). Animals so treated developed raised, white, circumscribed plaques in the arch and descending portions of the aorta and in its major branches. The lesions usually involved the subintimal portions of the media, but some extended through the entire wall. The elastica was fragmented, and the lesions contained an abundance of periodic acid-Schiff positive material and calcium. Connective tissue proliferation and cartilagenous and osseous metaplasia were also observed.

H. Rodentia (Rats, Mice, Squirrels, Guinea Pigs, etc.)

Fox (1933) did not observe arterial disease in wild rodents, and he was unable to find reports of naturally occurring disease in the common guinea pig.

Bragdon (1954) studied hyperlipemia and atheromatosis in a species of hibernating squirrel, *Citellus columbianus*. These animals exhibited extremely high fat levels in the blood, with triglycerides predominating. Cholesterol and phospholipid levels were said to be among the highest recorded in any mammals. Cholesterol feeding did not produce hypercholesterolemia. In approximately one-third of the animals fed a high-fat diet and of those with severe lipemia, there were focal deposits of sudanophilic material in the intima. These deposits appeared as fine droplets along the inner surface of the internal elastic membrane, and in only two instances were there foam cell accumulations. Usually no tissue reaction was present. Altschul and Fedoroff (1960) studied hypercholesterolemia in the prairie gopher (ground squirrel, *Citellus richardsonii* Sabine). Although hypercholesterolemia resulted from cholesterol feeding, only 2 of 22 animals had discrete vascular lesions of the aorta and coronary arteries consisting of accumulations of foam cells in and beneath the endothelium. These investigators suggested that the vulnerability of the vascular system to hypercholesterolemia in this species was either very slight or missing, thus supporting the view that, in other genera, including man, hypercholesterolemia is secondary and is not the primary factor in atherogenesis.

Naturally occurring arteriosclerosis has not been described in the mouse; nevertheless, aging in this species has been shown to be associated with certain degenerative lesions in the aorta. According to Smith *et al.* (1951), aging in the mouse is accompanied by an increase in amounts of ground substance in the aorta and in the number and density of elastic and reticular interlamellar fibers. These authors inferred that the structure of the aging mouse aorta meets decreasing efficiency of its elastic membranes by increasing the amount of elastin, by forming fine interlamellar fibrils, by developing circular reticular or collagenous fibers, and by maintaining resiliency with an increased amount of ground substance. Karrer (1961) studied the ultrastructure of the tunica media in aging mice and found gradually increasing amounts of collagen, rarefactions and interruptions of the elastic membranes, disconnections between smooth muscle cells and elastic layers, and a peculiar fraying or fragmentation of the innermost elastic membrane. A subendothelial proliferative lesion consisting of elongated cells and newly formed collagen and elastin was interpreted as possibly being similar to the initial lesion of arteriosclerosis. Aging subendothelial elastic fibers became denser, and new elastic fibers formed between the inner elastic membrane and endothelium. Numerous collagen fibers appeared to arise from proliferative connective tissue cells rather than from the endothelium. This was regarded as comparable with the process observed in early arteriosclerosis.

Arteriosclerosis, both naturally occurring and experimentally induced, has been more extensively investigated in rats than in other rodents. Although the rat appears to be less susceptible than do other animals to development of naturally occurring or experimentally induced arterial disease, two forms of arteriosclerosis have been described.

Wilens and Sproul (1938a) found coronary arterial lesions in 60% of 487 albino rats that had resulted in loss of smooth muscle and medial replacement by fibrous tissue. Medial calcification was infrequent and no lipid deposits were observed. The internal elastic membrane was straightened but intact. The incidence of this coronary disease in the rat was twice as high in males as in females, and paralleled the incidence of myocardial fibrosis. Disease in the aorta and other arteries was also investigated by Wilens and Sproul (1938b). Calcific deposits in the inner third of the aortic media protruded into the lumen through disrupted elastic lamellae. Similar medial calcification was observed in many arteries, sometimes impregnating elastic fibers. These arterial lesions were found in animals of both sexes and over 700 days of age.

Malinow *et al.* (1956) studied the aortas, hearts, and kidneys of male, white, William strain rats between 15 and 24 months of age. Arterial lesions were found in 17 of 30 rats, but in only 50 of the more than 10,000 arterial sections examined. These lesions consisted of endothelial and/or subendothelial infiltration of sudanophilic, Liebermann-Burchard positive material that sometimes extended into the media. Proliferation of endothelial and/or subendothelial cells formed tiny plaques protruding into the vascular lumens. This study indicated that endothelial cells of the rat can react to give rise to an atheromatous lesion just as they do in the rabbit and bird.

Wexler and Miller (1958) described severe arterial disease of the aorta and coronary and other arteries in discarded, female breeder, Sprague-Dawley rats that had been injected with corticotropin (ACTH). The larger arteries showed senile ectasia with pronounced thickening, and the aorta was severely stiffened. Similar changes were observed in the cerebral vessels, peripheral arteries, and coronary arteries. Although the disease was restricted mainly to the medial layer, intimal swelling and proliferation were also observed. The media was hypertrophied and there were extensive calcific deposition and/or necrosis of the medial elastic tissue. Cartilaginous metaplasia was observed in some lesions. Swelling and fragmentation of elastic fibers resulted in herniation of arterial walls. The intimal plaques contained minute droplets of intracellular and extracellular fat. The coronary arteries contained recanalized thrombi, and multiple ventricular infarcts were observed in some animals. The control animals in this study consisted of young rats, and no lesions were found in them. Identical lesions were observed by Lindsay and Gherman (unpublished) in untreated, 1- to 2-year-old Long-Evans female breeder rats, and administration of ACTH and/or cholesterol to groups of these rats did not alter the basic arterial disease.

Wilgram and Ingle (1959) also studied aortic arteriosclerosis in old female Sprague-Dawley rats that had been injected with ACTH or subjected to neuromuscular stress. They failed to find significant differences in pathological lesions in the experimental and control groups, and called attention to the lack of control animals in the studies of Wexler and Miller (1958). The aortic lesion observed by Wilgram and Ingle (1959) consisted of medial sclerosis with calcification and splitting of the elastic membranes; disintegration of muscular layers with replacement by necrotic and calcifying debris suggested a pattern of Mönckeberg's sclerosis. Wexler and Miller (1959) studied coronary arteriosclerosis in discarded female breeder rats subjected to unilateral nephrectomy and injected with ACTH; 75% of these rats showed some degree of arteriosclerosis of the coronary arteries; the intima was thickened by intimal hyperplasia. Deposition of basophilic ground substance, possibly acid mucopolysaccharide, in the intimal and medial layers had occurred. Some coronary arteries were virtually occluded and some contained foamy giant cells. In a third report, Wexler *et al.* (1960) dealt with arteriosclerosis induced in both male and female, Sprague-Dawley rats, 2 months of age, by repeated breedings, ACTH injections, and unilateral nephrectomy. Early arteriosclerotic lesions in the aortas of repeatedly bred rats of both sexes were observed, consisting of subintimal accumulations of acid mucopolysaccharide and proliferating fibroblasts. Later, fibrosis, endothelial hyperplasia, and lipid and calcific deposition occurred. Lipids and calcium were found in the more advanced lesions, and showed an affinity for areas rich in mucopolysaccharide. Elastic tissue changes were believed to be independent and to occur secondarily to alterations of the ground substance and fibroblasts. Although a few lipid droplets were observed in the early lesions, lipid-containing foam cells were encountered only in later ones. ACTH injections and unilateral nephrectomy augmented the early arteriosclerotic lesions. The severity of arteriosclerotic lesions appeared greater in males.

Hummel and Barnes (1938) found medial calcification in the aortas of old rats. The disease was not extensive in males and females that had received a basic diet adequate in all respects except for calorie content. The lesions in the aorta were similar to those induced by hypervitaminosis D and were characterized by loosening of medial fibers and the appearance of either fine calcific deposits along the elastic fibers or solid masses in the media.

Kittinger *et al.* (1960) studied enzyme changes accompanying arterial disease in female breeder, Sprague-Dawley rats. Extracts of arteriosclerotic aortas of these animals contained significantly less lactic dehydrogenase than did extracts of normal or slightly affected aortas. Production of reduced triphosphopyridine nucleotide (TPNH) by combined action of glucose-6-phosphate and 6-phosphogluconic dehydrogenases was significantly depressed in moderately and severely sclerosed aortas. But there were no significant changes in levels of 6-phosphogluconic dehydrogenase.

Gillman and Hathorn (1959) investigated naturally occurring aortic and coronary arteriosclerosis in breeding and nonbreeding male and female stock rats. Lesions were absent in males, and among females, were more common in breeders than in nonbreeders. The aortas were most severely affected. They showed rigidity, calcification, and even cartilage and bone formation, together with intimal and medial fibrosis, ectasia, and heavy mucopolysaccharide accumulations. The coronary arteries were not so severely damaged. These lesions occurring spontaneously in breeding females were regarded as indistinguishable from those found in arteries healing after toxic doses of calciferol. A number of changes occurring during pregnancy were suggested as etiological factors in arteriosclerosis meriting investigation.

In an electron microscopic study of the normal rat aorta, Keech (1960a) described intercellular boundaries between endothelial cells. The subendothelial layer increased in width with age, and contained blunt processes and localized whorls of fine collagen which were believed to anchor the endothelium to the internal elastic membrane. The latter contained linear streaks embedded in a matrix. The smooth muscle cells were obliquely attached to adjacent elastic laminas. It was concluded that this arrangement should be more effective in controlling aortic diameter than would radially oriented smooth muscle cells. Pease and Paule (1960) confirmed Keech's electron microscopic description of the aorta of the rat. In addition, they conceived of the aortic wall as a three-dimensional network of elastic cords interspersed between medial cells and tying together the principal elastic laminas. Muscle cells appeared attached directly to elastin by thin layers of cement substance. There was no evidence either of direct attachment of the smooth muscle cells to collagen, or of connections or fusions of collagen with elastin. The intimal connective tissue contained thin strands and tiny units of elastin associated with a mucopolysaccharide matrix. These units were regarded as active centers of elastin formation and deposition in the intima. An apparently similar origin of regenerating elastic fibers in a mucopolysaccharide matrix was observed by light microscopy in early arteriosclerotic lesions in the cat (Lindsay and Chaikoff, 1955).

Keech (1960b) examined the aortas of lathyritic rats with the electron microscope. The aortic wall of these rats thickened and displayed widened interlaminar spaces, radial orientation of smooth muscle cells, progressive loss of desmosomes, and a progressive increase in dense, finely stippled material that coated the edges of the elastic laminas and extended outward between the muscle cells. The ends of these cells were separated from the laminas. The stippled material was periodic acid-Schiff positive. An increase in subendothelial and interlaminar collagen was also observed.

Numerous reports have appeared dealing with the production of arteriosclerosis in rats by lipid administrations. Page and Brown (1952) induced hypercholesterolemia and atherogenesis in hypothyroid rats by feeding them diets rich in cholesterol and cholic acid. Although the aortas and coronary arteries were infiltrated with lipid, foam cells and proliferative reactions were absent. Wissler *et al.* (1952) found hypercholesterolemia and coronary atheromas in old rats fed high-fat diets for long periods. Hartroft *et al.* (1952) reported on the occurrence of lipid deposits in coronary arteries of rats fed choline-deficient diets. Malinow *et al.* (1954) found atheromatous lesions in rats fed vegetable oil and subjected to unilateral experimental perinephritis. Bragdon (1952b) has described the atheromatous lesions that appear in rats subjected to repeated intravenous injections of lipoproteins contained in the serum of cholesterol-fed rabbits. Bragdon and Mickelsen (1955) further described these lesions, which were first characterized by groups of foam cells in the endocardium and intima and later by masses of anisotropic crystals embedded in fibrous tissue. One such lesion was found in a coronary artery, but these vessels were usually the site of massive infiltration of lipid without tissue reactions. Similar heavy deposits of lipid in the aortic intima were not associated with tissue proliferation. Fillios *et al.* (1956) induced atheromatosis of the aorta and coronary arteries in rats by feeding them cholesterol-containing diets, sodium cholate, and thiouracil. The early vascular lesions were characterized by deposition of extracellular lipid and cholesterol in the medial and intimal ground substance, whereas the older lesions contained predominantly intracellular lipid within foam and other mesenchymal cells. In some intimal plaques, proliferation of fibroblasts and deposition of ground substance, elastic tissue, and collagen were secondary to lipid and cholesterol deposition.

According to Humphreys (1957), spontaneous arteriosclerosis of coronary vessels can be found in 60% of normal rats more than 500 days of age. The incidence and structure of the atheromatous lesions in the coronary arteries of rats fed synthetic diets containing palm-kernel oil, ground-nut oil, palm oil, or butterfat were similar. These lesions consisted of intimal fibrous plaques and were composed of collagen, swollen endothelial cells, and hyaline material; lipid in the form of fine droplets was present throughout the plaques. Wilgram (1958, 1959) also studied coronary arteriosclerosis in rats and found coronary arterial plaques containing fibrin-like material that he did not regard as atherosclerotic. Pronounced hyperlipemia and hypercholesterolemia, induced by feeding a high-fat, egg-yolk diet supplemented with cholesterol, cholate, and thiouracil, led to the development of severe coronary atherosclerosis with occlusion and myocardial infarction. O'Neal *et al.* (1961) studied atherosclerosis in the aorta of rats fed similar diets. The aortic disease was limited to the thoracic portion, and appeared as elevated yellow plaques affecting as much as 25% of the intimal surface. The lesions involving the intima and inner media consisted of foam cells distended with lipid. Cholesterol deposits were present. Overlying the internal elastic membrane, the lesions also displayed a thin layer of amorphous or finely fibrillar eosinophilic material that stained with phosphotungstic acid or periodic acid-Schiff reagents. This layer also contained lipid droplets and a few foam cells.

Hartroft and O'Neal (1962) found a high incidence of thrombosis with infarction in the hearts and kidneys of rats that had been fed a diet containing 40% butter and 5% cholesterol, sodium cholate, and thiouracil. Lesions of the vascular walls, however, were not described. Feeding of unsaturated fats (corn or cottonseed oil) protected the rats against development of ischemic infarcts. Removal of any one of the four dietary constituents decreased the incidence of infarcts and removal of any two completely protected against vascular thrombosis and infarction.

Loustalot (1960) produced gross atheromatous lesions in the aortas of rats by feeding them low- or high-protein diets containing cholesterol, cholic acid, and thiouracil. Lipid infiltration was found in the intima and extended into the deeper layers of the media; lipid-filled macrophages were present. Eades et al. (1962) showed that hypertensive rats fed an all-meat diet developed hypercholesterolemia and coronary arteriosclerosis within 16 weeks, indicating that hypertension coupled with a diet high in fat and proteins, but low in cholesterol, was related to the production of hypercholesterolemia and coronary arteriosclerosis.

Arteriosclerosis has been produced by ionizing radiation in the rat. Berdjis (1960) studied the effects of irradiation of either the whole body or the heart, kidney, or leg. The aortas displayed partial thickening, the result of medial proliferation. Early degeneration and/or calcification was not severe enough to form real arteriosclerosis. Subintimal alterations and fibrous plaques were seldom found. Elastic fibers were disassociated, fragmented, and duplicated. The general picture of aortic disease was regarded as a form of early Mönckeberg's sclerosis. Irradiated femoral arteries exhibited focal fragmentation or disassociation of elastic fibers. More pronounced sclerotic changes were observed in uterine, ovarian, spermatic, and testicular arteries. Cerebral vessels, however, appeared resistant to irradiation. Gold (1961) reported on the production of arteriosclerosis in Wistar rats fed a high-fat diet to which had been added cholic acid and cholesterol; half of the rats received a total of 2500 r (X-rays) to the thorax. Atherosclerosis in the aorta, coronary arteries, pulmonary arteries, and endocardium occurred in both groups of rats. Severe coronary disease was observed in 26% of the irradiated animals as compared with none in the nonirradiated groups; similar differences were noted in the main pulmonary arteries and endocardium of the two groups. The lesions were characterized by an infiltration of lipophages and deposits of mucopolysaccharide material in the intima, a decrease in interlaminar elastic fibrils, and increased deposition of mucopolysaccharide in the medial aortic layers. The most striking changes were found in the coronary arteries of the irradiated group. Some lumens were almost occluded by greatly thickened intima containing accumulations of mucopolysaccharide and lipophages. The internal elastic membrane was largely obliterated. Occasional aneurysmal dilatation of these vessels had occurred.

I. Cetacea (Whales, Dolphins, Porpoises)

Arteriosclerosis has not been extensively studied in this order of mammals. Race *et al.* (1959) described the heart and aorta of an adult male sperm whale measuring 44 feet in length, but found no evidence of arteriosclerosis. The aortic wall consisted of very large, interwoven bundles of elastic tissue, and was apparently devoid of muscle.

J. Carnivora

1. CANIDAE

Among carnivora, naturally occurring as well as experimentally induced arteriosclerosis has been studied most extensively in the domesticated dog.

a. *The Naturally Occurring Disease.* Köllisch (1910) was one of the first to report degenerative disease in the dog aorta. Strauch (1916) described aortic lesions, streaks, or oval plaques, mainly in the abdominal aorta near bifurcations and vascular ostea. Although rare in young dogs, most older animals were afflicted, especially after 8 years of age. Consistent splitting and fragmentation of the internal elastic membrane were followed by intimal proliferative thickening and hyalinization. Fatty degenerative lesions were seldom encountered. Krause (1922) frequently found abdominal aortic plaques in dogs 5 years of age or older; he described hyperplastic intimal plaques containing fine elastic fibrils. Nieberle (1930) demonstrated only calcific deposits in the canine arterial media. Zinserling (1932) studied arteriosclerosis in old dogs, and concluded that primary intimal sclerosis preceded lipid deposition and that alteration of the connective tissue as well as cholesterol deposition in the vascular wall was important in the pathogenesis of the canine disease.

Morehead and Little (1945) found localized intimal plaques associated with splitting and reduplication of the internal elastic membrane even in 10-day-old puppies. Medial disease was more pronounced in the aortas of older dogs. Focal loss of elastic tissue, medial necrosis with cyst formation, hyperplasia of smooth muscle cells, and localized fibrosis and calcification were features of the medial disease in the dog.

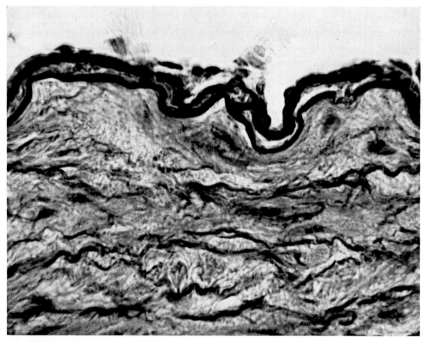

Fɪɢ. 20. Lower abdominal aorta (male dog, age 12). Magnification: 800. Weigert-van Gieson stain. The internal elastic membrane is reduplicated. Some segments show granular degeneration, beading, and fragmentation. No lipid is present at this stage (Sudan IV stain).

Lindsay *et al.* (1952a) studied aortic and coronary arteriosclerosis in dogs, most of which were over 8 years of age. The earliest evidence of aortic disease consisted of fragmentation, splitting, and reduplication of the internal elastic membrane (Fig. 20). Intimal thickening resulted from accumulations of mucoid ground substance followed by intimal fibroblasts which were first arranged irregularly (Fig. 21), then perpendicularly, and finally circumferentially (Figs. 22, 23). These plaques frequently were distinctly layered (Fig. 24). A still later development in these intimal plaques was the elaboration of collagen, reticulum, and elastic fibers which gradually replaced the mucopolysaccharide ground substance (Fig. 23). Lipids did not seem to be involved in the early aortic disease of the dog, but when they did occur, they usually involved only the deeper portions of the larger plaques.* Progressive enlargement of the intimal plaques resulted in compression, distortion, and further degeneration of the internal elastic membrane. Disease in the media

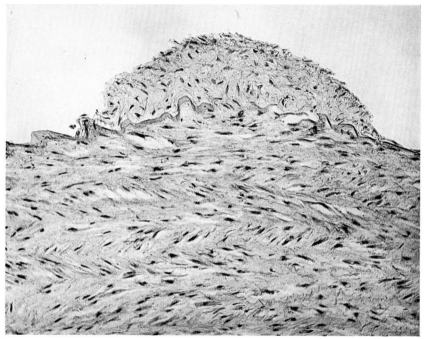

Fig. 21. Abdominal aorta (male dog, age 12). Magnification: 250. Hematoxylin-eosin stain. Small, early intimal plaque. The intimal fibroblasts have an irregular arrangement. No lipid is demonstrable by Sudan IV staining, but delicate elastic fibers are shown by Weigert-van Gieson staining. Note fragmentation of internal elastic membrane.

resembled that in the intima, and was characterized by collagenous replacement, focal degeneration, loss of elastic tissue, and focal proliferation of smooth muscle cells. Cystic deposits of acid mucopolysaccharide were also observed. Intimal fibrous thickening was demonstrated in coronary arteries, and myocardial fibrosis and acute infarction were found in several animals. Indeed, chronic myocardial failure closely resembling

---

* In old hunting dogs, however, Bevans (personal communication) found extensive lipid deposition in only moderately thickened intima.

that in man was observed in 5 dogs. In these studies of arteriosclerosis of the dog aorta (Lindsay *et al.,* 1952a) the lesions were found to be more numerous and prominent in the abdominal segment. It should be noted that Harkness *et al.* (1957) had found that the elastic content in the thoracic aortic was twice that of the collagen content, whereas twice as much collagen as elastic tissue was found in the abdominal aorta.

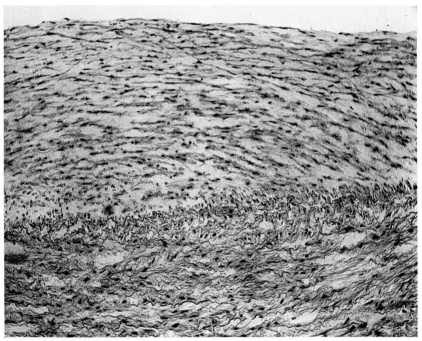

Fig. 22. Thoracic aorta (male dog, age 12). Magnification: 125. Hematoxylin-eosin stain. This plaque shows circumferential arrangement of fibroblasts. Abundant muco-polysaccharide (colloidal iron-Prussian blue stain) and pericellular elastic fibrils (Weigert-van Gieson stain) are present.

However, McGill *et al.* (1957), who studied sites of vascular vulnerability in dogs by injections of Evans blue, did not find unusual localization of the dye in sites in the aorta where arteriosclerosis is likely to develop.

Medial disease in the dog aorta has been described by Corwin and Cragg (1938). The elastic fibers of the media of the first portion of the aorta were unusually tortuous and slightly fragmented, and the media contained nodular, amorphous calcific deposits. Negligible amounts of lipid were present. The morphological evidence suggested an infectious origin rather than sclerosis due to aging. Bloom (1946) described xanthomatosis of the arterial media in the dog characterized by collections of foam cells in muscular arteries and, to a lesser degree, in elastic arteries. The foam cells, which contained unsaturated glycerides and cholesterol esters, were believed to be derived from smooth muscle cells. The lesions were further complicated by connective tissue proliferation and deposition of iron pigment.

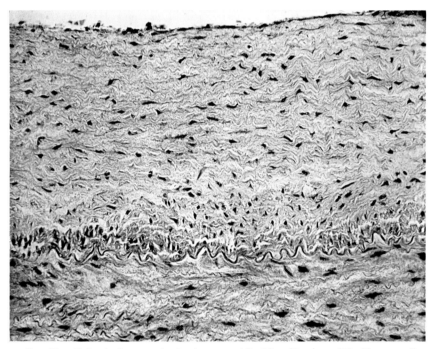

FIG. 23. Abdominal aorta (male dog, age 13). Magnification: 250. Hematoxylin-eosin stain. At this stage, the cells and fibers comprising the intimal plaque are arranged circumferentially. Considerable collagen is noted. No lipid substance is present (Sudan IV stain).

Arteriosclerosis in 3 wild canines was described by Fox (1933). A jackal showed intimal hyaline and calcified plaques, irregular thinning and calcification of the media, and multiple aneurysms of the thoracic and upper abdominal aorta. Fibrosis, calcification, and small aneurysms were also observed in the mesenteric arteries. Vastesaeger (1959a) did not find arteriosclerosis in 3 jackals (*Canis aureus*) that he examined. All of the captive wild Canidae, including wolves, foxes, and coyotes, examined by Ratcliffe *et al.* (1960) showed arteriosclerosis of the intimal fibrous type, mainly in the deep myocardial arteries.

b. *Experimentally Induced Arteriosclerosis.* Lindsay *et al.* (1952b) investigated cardiovascular disease in dogs subjected to both hypophysectomy and thyroidectomy (HT). Two basic types of lesions were observed in the aorta and coronary arteries: (1) lesions identical with those observed in normal dogs, but usually with more pronounced lipid in-

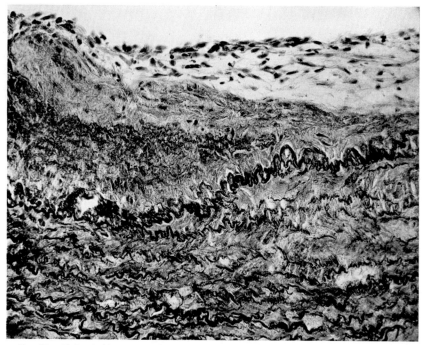

FIG. 24. Abdominal aorta (male dog, age 13). Magnification: 250. Weigert-van Gieson stain. This intimal plaque has three distinct layers. The deepest consists of condensed connective tissue and many elastic fibers. The superficial layer consists of immature connective tissue. No lipid material is demonstrable by Sudan IV staining.

filtration of the thickened intima of the aorta and believed to be secondary to hyperlipemia and hypercholesterolemia; (2) lesions in medium-sized arteries, mainly coronaries, characterized by primary deposition of lipid in the intima or media, by accumulations of lipid-containing foam cells, and by varying degrees of secondary intimal and medial mucopolysaccharide deposition and fibrosis. Refractile material, presumably cholesterol, was found in these foam cell lesions.

Arteriosclerosis resembling that seen in HT dogs has been produced by ingestion of cholesterol and thiouracil. In dogs so treated, Steiner and Kendall (1946) found cream colored, intimal plaques in the aorta that were most numerous distally. The lesions consisted of accumulations of intimal foam cell that sometimes penetrated the media. The internal elastic membrane appeared secondarily thickened, duplicated, and occasionally fragmented. Elastic fibers were found in the thickened intimal layer. Anisotropic cholesterol crystals and calcific deposits were present in some lesions. Steiner *et al.* (1949) extended these observations on cholesterol and thiouracil feeding to young dogs. The resulting arterial lesions were believed to have the same anatomical distribution as those in man, including involvement of cerebral arteries. Elevated yellow plaques in the aorta, coronary arterial narrowing, and involvement of anterior mitral valve leaflets were observed. The lesions consisted of intimal foam cell collections, and the older lesions showed extensive fibrosis with localization of foam cells in the deeper layers. Lipid infiltration also involved the medial layers of arteries. It should be emphasized that large amounts of lipids were stored in liver, spleen, and kidneys of these animals. Bevans *et al.* (1951a) studied the pathogenesis of these cholesterol-thiouracil-induced lesions in dogs and found rough correlations between severity of disease, time of exposure to the treatment, and cholesterol levels of blood. Two months after cholesterol feeding was begun, lipid accumulations were found in fibrocytes and smooth muscle cells, and by 4 months intimal proliferation had occurred. By 6 months intimal proliferation and abundant lipid were present in the media, although foam cells were limited to the intimal layer. Bevans *et al.* (1951b) also studied regression of the thiouracil-cholesterol-induced lesions in the dog. The vascular lesions diminished in number and severity during a period of stock diet feeding when the cholesterol levels had returned to normal. The slightly thickened intima contained little or no lipid, but relatively large amounts remained in the outer media and adventitia. The longer the animals were fed the stock diet, the less lipid remained in the vascular walls. The healed plaques were devoid of lipid, and beneath the plaques the media was scarred and the elastic fibers distorted. In some instances regression of plaques, particularly in the thyroid arteries, occurred despite sustained hypercholesterolemia. Davidson *et al.* (1951) found that the addition of choline to the cholesterol-thiouracil regimen in dogs did not affect serum lipid levels, degree of lipid infiltration of the liver, or severity of the arteriosclerotic disease.

Creech *et al.* (1955) implanted aortic homografts into the abdominal aortas of dogs rendered hypothyroid by administration of I[131] and fed cholesterol. A control group with autogenous aortic grafts was similarly treated. When cholesterol levels were over 1000 mg per 100 ml, the

host aorta and homograft were equally affected by cholesterol atherosclerosis. When cholesterol levels were below 1000 mg per 100 ml, the
host aortas showed little or no atherosclerosis but the homografts were
moderately to extensively involved. In animals with autogenous grafts,
the host aorta and graft were equally affected by atherosclerosis when
cholesterol levels were above 1000 mg per 100 ml, whereas when the levels
were below 1000 mg per 100 ml, the grafts were unaffected.

Haimovici *et al.* (1958) placed fresh thoracic homografts in the abdominal aortas of dogs and later fed them cholesterol and thiouracil.
In most cases the abdominal aorta of the host exhibited intimal plaques
consisting predominantly of foam cells with only minimal fibrosis,
whereas the homografts showed predominantly fibrous plaques, only a
few of which contained foam cells. It was suggested that the thoracic
origin of the homograft may have accounted for this result, indicating
a biological difference between the two aortic segments.

Milch *et al.* (1958) studied hyperlipoproteinemia and cholesterol deposition in the arteries of I^{131}-treated dogs. Tissue analysis at autopsy
revealed significantly elevated levels of cholesterol in coronary arteries,
aortas, and livers in treated male dogs as compared with control male
dogs. However, gross and microscopic examinations of the coronary
arteries and aortas of these I^{131}-treated dogs failed to demonstrate arteriosclerotic lesions.

Atherosclerosis has been induced in dogs in as short a period as 8
weeks by feeding them an "infarct-producing diet" which was high in
fat and cholesterol and contained sodium cholate, choline, and thiouracil (DiLuzio and O'Neal, 1962; Hartroft *et al.*, 1962). The arterial
lesions were characterized by lipid infiltration of the intima and inner
media, and by accumulations of foam cells with fibrosis. These investigators concluded that advanced foam cell lesions preceded experimental
arterial thrombosis in the dog.

Sabiston *et al.* (1961) produced primary lipid atherosclerosis in dogs
that were: (1) subjected to surgical coarctation of the aorta; (2) made
hypothyroid by total thyroidectomy and administration of I^{131}; and (3)
fed a high-cholesterol diet. After 18 to 20 months, all of the dogs had
atherosclerosis at some point in the arterial system, and coronary atherosclerosis was present in 8 of 10 dogs that had been subjected to aortic
coarctation. Fatty intimal lesions, which progressed to fibrosis and hyalinization, occlusion of the lumen, medial infiltration, and calcification,
were identical with those produced previously by cholesterol feeding
alone. The creation of coarctation immediately above the orifices of
the coronary arteries accentuated the production of atherosclerosis in

the segment exposed to hypertension. Coronary arteriosclerosis was less pronounced in hearts without coarctation of the aorta. It was concluded that hypertension accentuated the development of this form of experimental atherosclerosis.

Stephenson *et al.* (1962) studied dogs treated with I^{131} and fed a high-cholesterol, high-fat diet containing cholic acid and thiouracil. In as short a period as 2 months, 17 of 20 dogs developed foam cell lesions of the coronary arteries followed by reactive fibroplasia, intimal proliferation, calcification and, in some cases, intramural hemorrhage and ulceration.

Sako (1962) observed the effects of turbulent blood flow and hypertension on experimental atherosclerosis induced by cholesterol feeding, total thyroidectomy, and thiouracil administration. Severe primary lipid atheromatosis was found proximal to where surgical iliac arterial-venous fistulas had been created and above points of surgical thoracic aortic coarctation. Sako concluded that turbulence, increased blood flow, and hypertension were abetting factors in production of this form of experimental atherosclerosis. Moss *et al.* (1951) studied the effects of experimental renal hypertension on cholesterol-induced atherosclerosis and found a fair correlation between severity of lesions, duration of treatment, hypercholesterolemia, and average mean blood pressure. Moses (1954) studied atherosclerosis in dogs that resulted from cholesterol feeding and induction of chronic hypertension by injections of silica into the renal arteries. Hypertension increased the severity of aortic atherosclerosis, but marked hypercholesterolemia was associated with increased severity of aortic atherosclerosis even in normotensive dogs.

Conrad *et al.* (1956) described canine coronary and aortic lesions induced by intravenous allylamine. Early lesions displayed medial edema and deposition of periodic acid-Schiff positive material. In most instances the internal elastic membrane was swollen and exhibited exaggerated periodic acid-Schiff staining. Necrosis was observed in the severe lesions, which also gave an intense periodic acid-Schiff reaction; acid mucopolysaccharide could not be detected in these lesions, nor was lipid found in them after the animals had received injections of egg yolk suspended in saline.

Waters (1957) investigated the effect of a large, high-fat meal on the course of the acute inflammatory lesion in the coronary arteries and aortas of dogs produced by an intense episode of hypertension resulting from repeated intravenous injections of epinephrine. During the lipemic period, abundant amounts of lipid accumulated at the site of arterial injury. The vascular lesions resembled those of medial arteriolonecrosis and arteriosclerosis. Acute injury with hemorrhage had occurred, and perivascular exudate was present. No foam cells appeared, and for 2 to 3 weeks lipid remained extracellular and in droplet form.

Waters (1962) investigated the effects of short-term feeding of high-fat diets, with or without addition of cholesterol, upon coronary arteries

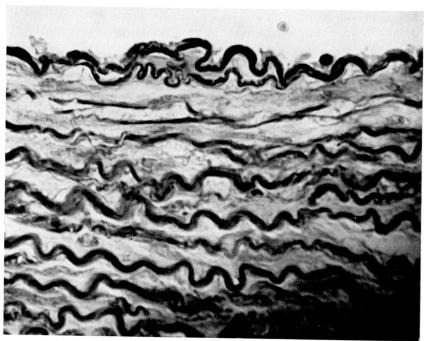

Fig. 25. Abdominal aorta (young male cat). Magnification: 800. Weigert-van Gieson stain. The internal elastic membrane is degenerating, beaded, and fragmented. The newly formed reduplicating fibers show similar degeneration. Lipid is absent (Sudan IV stain).

of dogs. Both groups of animals received coronary injury by means of intravenous allylamine. Lipid accumulated equally in the coronary arteries of both the cholesterol-fed dogs and those not fed cholesterol. In the former, the lesions progressed to fatty, foam cell granulomas, whereas in the latter, foam cell lesions did not develop.

Lindsay et al. (1962a, b) produced arteriosclerosis in the abdominal aortas of dogs by irradiating localized segments with X-rays or electrons. The arteriosclerotic lesions were similar in all respects to those that occur naturally in dogs, particularly in older animals. It was proposed that irradiation may have caused a selective injury of the internal elastic membrane and that this degenerative process was followed by development of intimal fibrosis, plaque formation, and minimal lipid infiltration. In these studies, irradiation with the doses employed apparently might have caused disruption of the internal elastic membrane without injury to other vascular layers. Senderoff *et al.* (1961) irradiated hearts

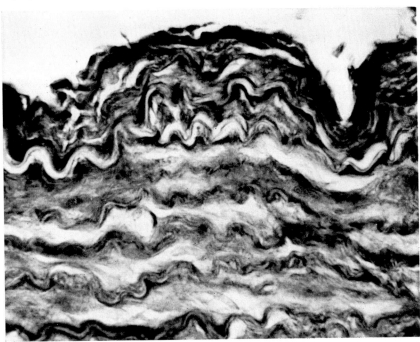

FIG. 26. Abdominal aorta (male cat, age 14). Magnification: 800. Colloidal iron-Prussian blue stain. Small intimal plaque composed of reduplicated internal elastic membrane and increased deposition of acid mucopolysaccharide. No lipid is present (Sudan IV stain).

of dogs. One group was also subjected to coronary artery ligation. Better preservation of the myocardium was observed in the irradiated dogs subjected to coronary ligation, and in those, myocardial lesions healed more rapidly. This was believed to have resulted from development of functioning intercoronary, anastamotic channels. No evidence of coronary injury by irradiation was seen on gross or microscopic examination.

2. FELIDAE

Although Fox (1933) asserted that domestic cats rarely developed arteriosclerosis, disease consisting of intimal granulations of the thoracic and abdominal aortas was observed. Lindsay and Chaikoff (1955) found considerable arteriosclerosis in 36 cats, 14 of which were 5 years of age or older. The initial lesion in the coronary arteries and aorta consisted of degeneration and fragmentation of the internal elastic membrane (Fig. 25) or inner medial elastic lamina and of deposition of an increased

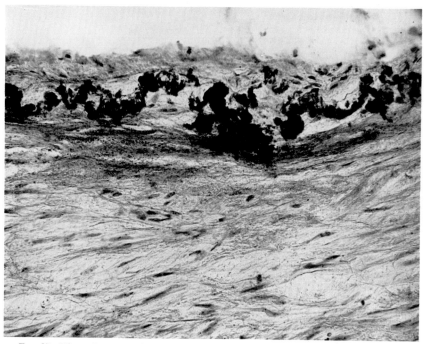

Fɪɢ. 27. Thoracic aorta (female cat, age 19). Magnification: 250. Sudan IV-hematoxylin stain. Granular, amorphous, calcific deposits are present in the slightly thickened intima. Fine lipid droplets are present in the intima and adjacent media. A few amorphous, refractile crystals were demonstrable in this lesion (polarized light).

amount of acid mucopolysaccharide (Fig. 26). In some instances fine lipid droplets were found adhering to or near the degenerating internal elastic membrane (Fig. 27). The latter was occasionally partially calcified (Fig. 27). There was evidence of considerable regeneration of the elastic tissue (Fig. 28). Some intimal mucoid deposits apparently persisted and were invaded by proliferating fibroblasts (Figs. 29, 30). Collagen, reticulum, and elastic fibers gradually replaced the mucoid ground substance as the plaques matured (Fig. 31). Lipid seemed not to be concerned in the pathogenesis of these lesions, and cholesterol could not be identified in them. Coronary arteriosclerosis was prominent in these old cats (Fig. 32-35). Olcott *et al.* (1946) described pronounced hypertrophy and hyperplasia of the smooth muscle of the media of the pulmonary arteries of cats. Since associated intimal disease was not observed, this lesion was not regarded as true arteriosclerosis.

Fox (1933) found only 8 instances of aortic disease among 184 wild

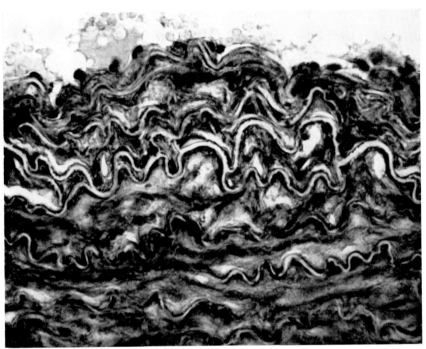

FIG. 28. Abdominal aorta (young female cat). Magnification: 800. Colloidal iron-Prussian blue stain. Considerable duplication of internal elastic fibers is present. Note bridging of gaps in degenerated fibers by new fibers. Increased amounts of acid mucopolysaccharide are present. No lipid is present at this stage (Sudan IV stain).

Felidae, and cited a report from the London Zoological Society of a tigress with arteriosclerosis and aneurysms. In these wild Felidae the disease appeared mainly in the aorta and its chief branches, and consisted of hyaline intimal thickenings, often associated with aneurysm formation. The intima between the aneurysms was slightly roughened in some cases. The intima was thickened by growth of fibrils and hyaline deposits, and the internal elastic membrane was interrupted by calcific deposits. Lipid deposition was not prominent. Fox concluded that parasitism was responsible for many cases of feline arteriosclerosis. Ratcliffe *et al.* (1960) listed the occurrence of arteriosclerosis in the coronary ar-

teries and aortas of 12 captive wild Felidae. Examples of aortic arteriosclerosis in a tiger and jaguar (Lindsay and Chaikoff, unpublished) are
shown in Figs. 36, 37.

3. OTHER CARNIVORA

Fox (1933) found minimal arterial disease in Procyonidae (raccoons)
and Ursidae (bears) that had lived in the Philadelphia Zoo. In 2 para-

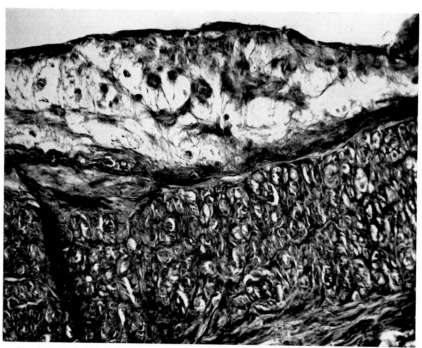

FIG. 29. Abdominal aorta (female cat, age 19). Magnification: 800. Colloidal iron-
Prussian blue stain. The intimal plaque consists of loosely arranged fibroblasts. The
stroma is rich in acid mucopolysaccharide. No lipid is present (Sudan IV stain).

doxures, he observed a saccular aneurysm in one and complete arteriosclerosis with atheroma, cartilage formation, calcium deposition, and
elastic disorganization in the other. Three animals in the skunk, otter,
badger group had arterial lesions consisting of atheromatous streaks running the length of the aorta. The innermost layer showed heavy fibrillar
thickening with elastic participation. Calcific deposits on and between
elastic fibers were associated with elastic fragmentation. Only 2 raccoons
were found to have renal arteriosclerosis. A bear showed mid-thoracic
aortic, intimal thickening consisting chiefly of frayed elastic fibers ex-

tending from the main bundles. These lesions were not regarded as true arteriosclerosis. We have observed mild thoracic and abdominal aortic arteriosclerosis (Lindsay and Chaikoff, unpublished) in old bears (Figs. 38, 39). Vastesaeger *et al.* (1959b) found coronary arteriosclerosis and thrombosis causing death of a panda (*Ailurus fulgens*). There was fi-

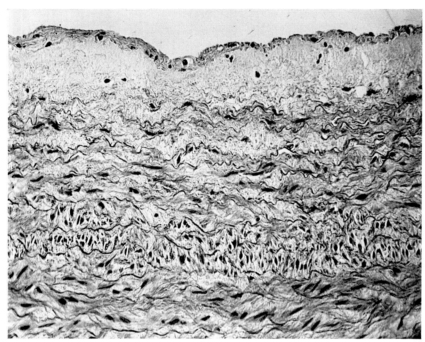

FIG. 30. Thoracic aorta (young female cat). Magnification: 250. Hematoxylin-eosin stain. The thickened intima consists of loose, fibrillary, mucoid connective tissue. The Weigert-van Gieson staining shows a few delicate elastic fibers and Sudan IV staining fine lipid droplets in the intima.

brous thickening of the coronary intima, which contained cholesterol clefts. The internal elastic membrane was stretched and interrupted. Ratcliffe *et al.* (1960) listed 9 families of Mustelidae showing coronary and aortic arteriosclerosis.

K. Pinnipedia (Seals, Sea Lions)

Arteriosclerosis was found in 2 of the 35 sea lions (Otariidae) examined by Fox (1933). In one, he described intimal fibrillar thickening, and in the other a calcific atheroma of the intima with elastic splitting and alizarin-staining muscle fibers in the underlying media. Kelley and

Jensen (1960) described lesions in the aortas of 3 mature bull sea lions. The intimal surface of the aortas contained numerous punctate elevations measuring 1 to 15 mm in diameter. As judged by the Liebermann-Burchard reaction, the cholesterol content of the sclerotic area was higher than that in adjacent normal regions. An inflammatory process

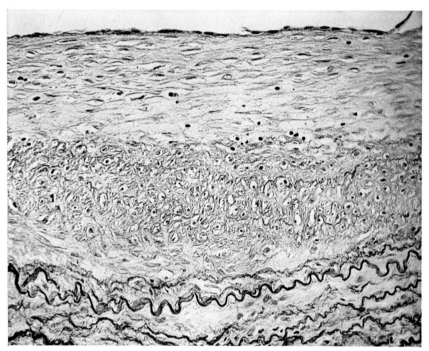

Fig. 31. Abdominal aorta (male cat, age 5). Magnification: 250. Weigert-van Gieson stain. This abdominal plaque consists of moderately dense connective tissue. Note distinct layering and fragmentation with reduplication of internal elastic membrane. Although moderate amounts of mucopolysaccharide are present (colloidal iron-Prussian blue stain), this plaque is devoid of lipid (Sudan IV stain).

in the media, involving elastic tissue destruction and infiltration with plasma cells, macrophages, and lymphocytes, was found. Subintimal fibrosis completed the resemblance of the lesion to that of human syphilis.

L. Tubulidentata (Aardvarks)

Arteriosclerosis has not been described in members of this order.

M. Proboscidea (Elephants)

Few autopsies have been reported on elephants. Galen (cited by Benedict, 1936) described a sclerotic cardiac lesion as "a bone of the heart." Fox (cited by Benedict, 1936) found pale, fibrous thickening about the left coronary arterial orifice of an elephant. Myocardial fibrosis and chronic inflammation were also observed, but the aorta appeared normal. In Fox's later studies (1933), none of the elephants examined showed arteriosclerosis.

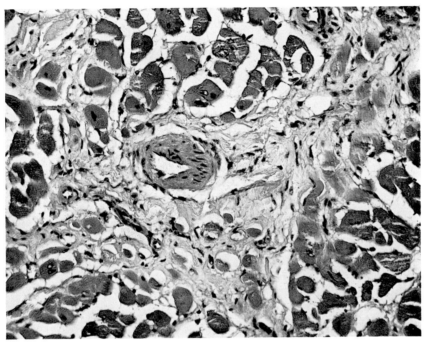

Fig. 32. Small coronary artery (male cat, age 12). Magnification: 250. Hematoxylin-eosin stain. The arterial wall is thickened and the lumen narrowed. Note myocardial fibrosis that involves the adjacent myocardium.

Lindsay *et al.* (1956) found severe generalized arteriosclerosis in a 47-year-old female Indian elephant that died of acute cardiac failure, the result of pronounced arteriosclerosis in many small coronary arteries. These myocardial as well as other small arteries revealed fragmentation and degeneration of the internal elastic membrane apparently followed by deposition of collagen and reticulum fibers. The lesions, which were identical with those observed in muscular arteries of other species, occluded many vascular lumens almost completely, and were devoid of lipid. Similar intimal disease leading to formation of intimal plaques was observed in major coronary and pulmonary arteries and in the aorta. Degeneration of the internal elastic membrane preceded the intimal deposition of mucopolysaccharides and connective tissue fibers. Medial calcification was a prominent feature of the arteriosclerotic process in the aorta and—to a lesser degree—in the major coronary arteries. This was believed to have resulted from medial elastic degeneration followed by accumulations of mucopolysaccharides and collagen. Minimal lipid

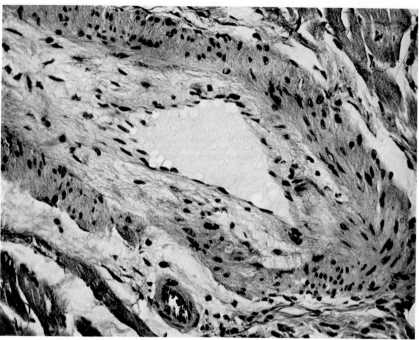

Fig. 33. Medium-size coronary artery (male cat, age 12). Magnification: 250. Hematoxylin-eosin stain. The thickened intima consists of loose, fibrillar connective tissue. Abundant mucopolysaccharide substance is demonstrable in the intima (colloidal iron-Prussian blue stain).

infiltration in the intimal and medial lesions of the large muscular and elastic arteries appeared to be clearly a secondary process and did not seem to be concerned with the early development of the vascular lesion. Cholesterol was not demonstrable. The calcific medial disease resembled aortic medial sclerosis in the human being and the medial calcific lesions commonly observed in old cows by Fox (1933).

Vastesaeger et al. (1959a) described cellular fibrous intimal thickening of the major coronary arteries of an African elephant (Loxodonta africana cyclotis). However, they did not observe significant changes in the internal elastic membranes in these sclerotic coronary arteries.

N. Hyracoidea (Hyraxes)

Arteriosclerosis has not been described in this order of mammals.

O. Sirenia or Sea Cows

Lindsay and Chaikoff (unpublished) found no evidences of arterial disease in a young male dugong.

P. Perissodactyla (Odd-Toed Ungulates: Horses, Rhinoceroses, Tapirs)

Fox (1933) stated that intimal lesions are common in the aorta of the horse and appear as granular or irregular thickenings in the cardiac region. Minimal amounts of Sudan-staining materials were present, and atheromas were not conspicuous, at least until advanced age was reached. Thoracic aortic arteriosclerosis in an old horse (Lindsay and Chaikoff, unpublished) is shown in Fig. 40. In a wild horse, Fox described low-

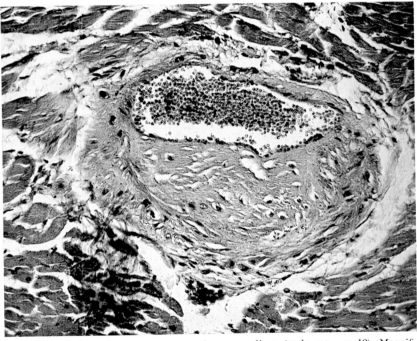

Fig. 34. Medium-size coronary artery in myocardium (male cat, age 12). Magnification: 250. Hematoxylin-eosin stain. An eccentric, fibrous intimal plaque has severely narrowed the lumen. Abundant mucopolysaccharide and a few collagen fibers are present (colloidal iron-Prussian blue stain). Several defects in the internal elastic membrane are noted (Weigert-van Gieson stain).

grade intimal thickening with fatty deposits in the thoracic aorta around the intercostal orifices.

Fox (1933) described mild intimal thickening of the thoracic aorta in a tapir. An aged Malayan tapir examined by Lindsay and Chaikoff (unpublished) showed pronounced aortic arteriosclerosis with linear cal-

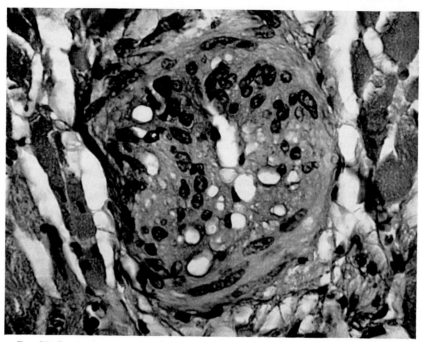

Fig. 35. Coronary artery (female cat, age 19). Magnification: 800. Hematoxylin-eosin stain. Plump fibroblasts fill the thickened intima. The vacuolated cells are devoid of lipid (Sudan IV stain).

cific deposits in the inner media (Fig. 41) closely resembling those observed in ruminants. Considerable intimal thickening, with plaque formation and lipid deposition, was found throughout the aorta (Figs. 42-45).

Q. Artiodactyla (Even-Toed Ungulates)

1. Suiformes (Pigs, Hippopotamuses)

Fox (1933) did not find arteriosclerosis in wild swine that he examined. Vastesaeger et al. (1959a) studied only one specimen, an aged warthog (*Phacochoeros aethiopicus*). The major coronary arteries of this animal showed moderate arteriosclerotic thickening; the internal elastic membrane was frequently interrupted and was not undulating.

More extensive studies have been made in domestic pigs. Gottlieb and Lalich (1954) found the incidence of aortic arteriosclerosis in 3% of 200 pigs ranging in age from 4 months to 3 years. Pale yellow, elon-

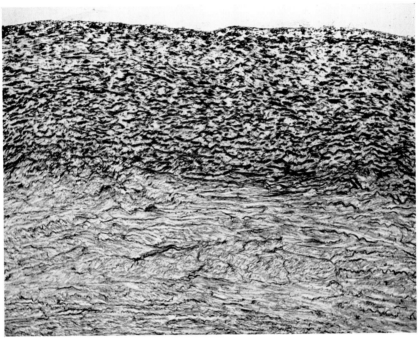

Fig. 36. Abdominal aorta (male tiger, age 20). Magnification: 125. Weigert-van Gieson stain. The widened intimal layer contains abundant, coarse, circumferential, elastic fibers and is rich in mucopolysaccharide substance (colloidal iron-Prussian blue stain). No lipid is demonstrable (Sudan IV stain).

gated intimal plaques 0.5 to 1 mm, or larger (5 to 10 mm), were aligned to the long axis of the aorta. They were most numerous in the descending arch and upper thoracic portions. An increase was noted with age, but there were no sex differences. Abdominal aortic disease was less frequent. The thoracic lesions were composed of fibrous connective tissue containing minute quantities of sudanophilic material in and around fibroblasts; lipid-containing macrophages, cholesterol, and hemorrhage were absent. In the abdominal segment there was edema, hyalinization, and disruption of elastic connective tissue fibers with medial atrophy. Calcific deposits were present in diseased portions of the media.

Peifer (1955a) observed naturally occurring arteriosclerosis in the aorta of several 5-year-old sows. Lipid streaking was prominent in the aortic arch. Fatty infiltration of the intima was accompanied by accumulations of collagenous fibers. No medial calcification was observed. Peifer (1955b) also studied arterial disease in miniature pigs fed different forms

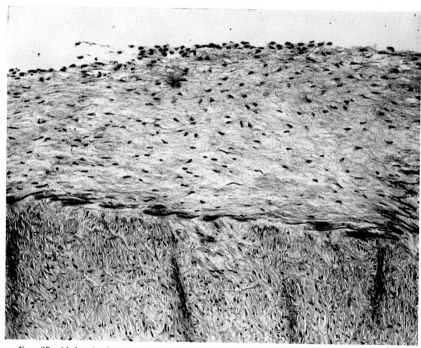

FIG. 37. Abdominal aorta (male jaguar, age 16). Magnification: 125. Hematoxylin-eosin stain. This intimal plaque consists of compact fibrous tissue with relatively few fibrocytes. Mucopolysaccharide substance is abundant (colloidal iron-Prussian blue stain), but elastic fibers are sparse in the plaque (Weigert-van Gieson stain). Lipid (Sudan IV stain) is absent.

of lipids. Although many of them had marked lesions covering the entire surfaces of the thoracic aortas, he found no intimal disease. He did, however, find lesions in the media resembling Mönckeberg's sclerosis.

Jennings et al. (1961) found extensive arteriosclerosis in a 7-year-old sow. Several intimal coronary plaques, thoracic plaques, and pearly thickening and plaque formation of the abdominal aorta represented the disease in this animal. The internal elastic membrane of the coronary arteries was reduplicated, and the plaques in these vessels consisted of fibroblasts, collagenous and elastic fibers, and mucopolysaccharides. Small amounts of lipid were present, particularly in the larger plaques, some of which were partially calcified. Very few lipid-filled macrophages were noted in these lesions, but the Schultz reaction for cholesterol was positive. In the aortic arch there was intimal swelling with granulation of collagenous and elastic fibers. Some finely divided lipid was present.

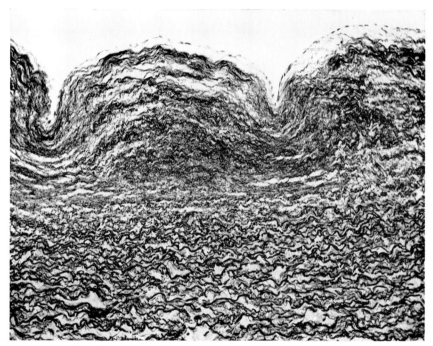

FIG. 38. Thoracic aorta (female brown bear, age 17). Magnification: 125. Weigert-van Gieson stain. The intima is considerably thickened and contains numerous elastic fibers. Only a few fine intracellular lipid droplets are demonstrable in this plaque (Sudan IV stain).

The thoracic and abdominal aortas revealed minimal intimal thickening composed of fat-filled connective tissue lying just within the internal elastic membrane. The fibrous plaques contained elastic and collagenous fibers, varying amounts of lipid, and a few smooth muscle fibers. The internal elastic membrane was fragmented. The largest plaque found contained cholesterol clefts. No fibrin was detected in any of the aortic plaques. The lesions in the femoral, renal, and cerebral arteries consisted of fibrous plaques that contained elastic fibers and mucopolysaccharides, but no lipids.

Skold and Getty (1961) examined the aortas and iliac arteries of 45 pigs of many breeds, ranging from 1 to 8 years in age. Lesions were observed in all animals, most frequently in the abdominal aorta and in the iliac arteries near the aortic bifurcation. Coronary plaques were also observed. Rough, elevated, soft intimal plaques, 2 to 15 mm in size, covered much of the abdominal aorta. The plaques and streaks stained with Sudan IV to varying degrees. The intima was thickened by foamy

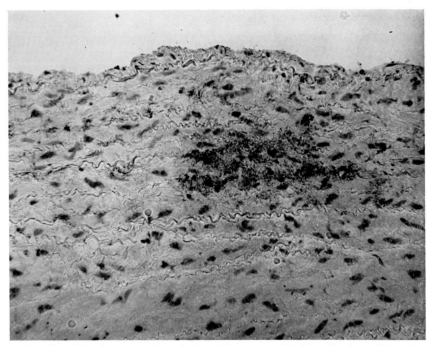

Fig. 39. Abdominal aorta (female brown bear, age 15). Magnification: 250. Sudan IV-hematoxylin stain. Extracellular lipid deposits are noted in the media. Elsewhere the slightly thickened intima also contains similar deposits.

macrophages. Alterations in ground substance resembled those observed in man. The internal elastic membrane was fragmented. In the photomicrographs shown, the lesions seem to be predominantly fibrous, and although they contained considerable amounts of lipids, foamy macrophages are not detectable. Murphy et al. (1962) described arteriosclerosis in the aortas of 140 swine. Microscopic evidences of intimal thickening were observed at the classic sites before grossly evident lesions were visible. The slightest change consisted of a subendothelial fatty streak confined to the intima; the elastic lamina was usually intact. Larger nodular lesions usually showed diffuse accumulations of fat and considerable amounts of connective tissue. In larger lesions, connective tissues were often the major constituent and lipid was detected only at the margins and deep below the fibrous cap. The early lesions were rich in mucopolysaccharides and did not always contain fat. Extensive lesions that consisted of mature connective tissue contained little mucoid material, although lipid was sometimes abundant.

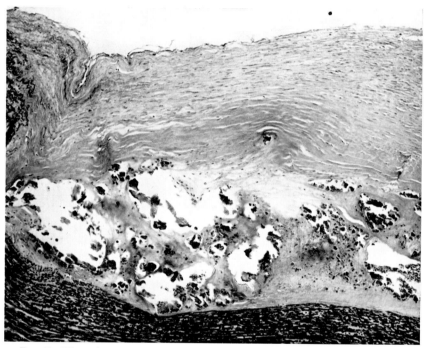

Fig. 40. Thoracic aorta (old horse). Magnification: 125. Weigert-van Gieson stain. This large fibrous intimal plaque contains extensive calcific deposits. Large and small lipid droplets are present about the calcific areas (Sudan IV stain).

Bragdon *et al.* (1957) fed corn oil or butter (40%) to boars. The addition of butter to the diet significantly elevated the blood cholesterol, but no such elevation occurred when corn oil was added. Half of the aortas examined contained lesions similar to those described by Gottlieb and Lalich (1954), but the incidence was the same in control and in fat-fed animals. Rowsell *et al.* (1958) studied arteriosclerosis in pigs fed 40% butter or 40% margarine. The aortic plaques in these animals consisted of intimal fibrous thickenings infiltrated with macrophages and lymphocytes. Fragmentation of the internal elastic membrane was observed in some. In the butter-fed animals, lipid droplets

were abundant next to the internal membrane, whereas few droplets
were found in animals fed a grower ration only. It was concluded that,
whereas margarine caused little increase in the amount of arteriosclerosis,
the high-butter diet did produce considerable increase in the disease.
It was noted that plaques tended to localize in areas where changes in

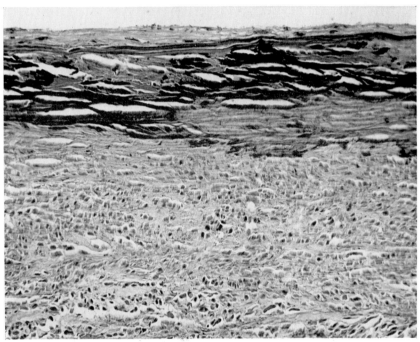

FIG. 41. Upper abdominal aorta (Malayan tapir, age 30). Magnification: 125. Hematoxylin-eosin stain. Extensive linear calcific deposits in the inner media appear first
on medial elastic fibers and eventually coalesce. Note slight intimal fibrous thickening.

blood flow occur, such as near vessel bifurcations, in the aortic valve,
near vascular orifices, and near a patent ductus arteriosus. Rowsell et al.
(1960) compared the effects of egg yolk or butter feeding on the development of atherosclerosis in swine. As judged by Sudan IV staining of
the aorta, atheromatosis was three times as severe in animals fed butter
as in the controls, whereas in animals fed egg yolk it was six times as
severe. Pearly plaques stained only peripherally or not at all, and such
plaques were found in some control animals. Two sorts of lesions were
observed microscopically. In areas of Sudan IV staining without gross
evidence of intimal thickening, extensive accumulations of lipid were
observed just beneath the endothelium. This had not provoked a cel-

lular response. The second type of lesion consisted of a fibrous plaque showing connective tissue proliferation and the presence of mucopolysaccharide substance. Lipid was found in the deeper layers or at the margins. The lipid consisted of neutral fat, phospholipids, and cholesterol, but no cholesterol clefts were found. In the larger plaques, elastic

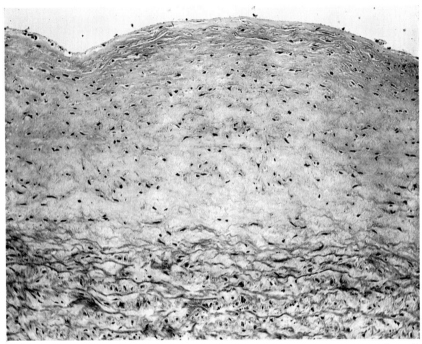

Fig. 42. Aortic arch (Malayan tapir, age 30). Magnification: 125. Hematoxylin-eosin stain. The thickened intima consists of delicate, mucoid connective tissue. Fine calcific deposits were found in several areas. Abundant mucopolysaccharide (colloidal iron-Prussian blue stain) is present, but collagen fibers (van Gieson stain) are sparse. Sudan IV staining reveals moderate amounts of finely divided lipid, mainly extracellular, but cholesterol is absent (polarized light).

fragmentation and reduplication were noted. Many plaques were definitely layered. The deeper portions appeared as mature connective tissue, and the more superficial portions consisted of immature connective tissue and mucopolysaccharide substances. Lipophages were present here. Significant increases in cholesterol and phospholipids were observed only in the egg-fed swine.

McKinney (1962) found fatty streaks in the aortas of 2 of the 5 hippopotamuses that he examined, but neither had aortic plaques. The lesions were described as resembling those of the human being in three respects: (1) subintimal fibrosis and thickening; (2) intimal sudanophilia; and (3) presence of refractile material, probably cholesterol, in the deeper intimal layer.

2. TYLOPODA (LLAMAS)

Fox (1933) found arteriosclerosis in 3 llamas. In 2, only simple calcific deposits were observed, but in the third, advanced plaques were

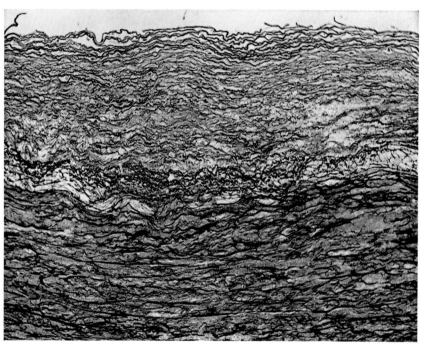

FIG. 43. Lower thoracic aorta (Malayan tapir, age 30). Magnification: 125. Weigert-van Gieson stain. The intimal plaque contains numerous, wavy elastic fibers. Mucopolysaccharide (colloidal iron-Prussian blue stain) and collagen (van Gieson stain) are present in equal amounts.

covered by an atheromatous type of intima. Rigg *et al.* (1960) has also mentioned the occurrence of arteriosclerosis in 2 llamas. An example of abdominal aortic arteriosclerosis in the llama (Lindsay and Chaikoff, unpublished) is illustrated in Fig. 46.

3. RUMINANTIA (CATTLE, SHEEP, GOATS, DEER, GIRAFFES)

Arteriosclerosis has been described in a variety of ruminants. In Bovidae, which include domestic and wild cows and buffalo, Fox (1933) found lesions characterized by calcific deposits in the inner media and plaques just beneath the intima. The musculoelastic layers contained long, narrow plates of calcified material, often associated with fragmentation of elastic laminas. Fox stated that the intima of these species becomes thick and nodular with advancing age. Although delicate fat droplets might be distributed along the collagen and elastic fibrils, atheromatous lesions were not observed. In the severest lesions the

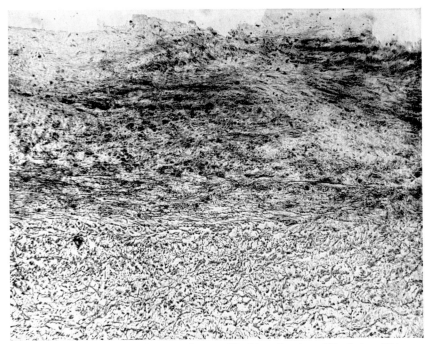

FIG. 44. Aortic arch (Malayan tapir, age 30). Magnification: 125. Sudan IV-hematoxylin stain. Fine lipid droplets are seen in connective tissue cells and in intercellular spaces, mainly in the thickened intima. Some droplets appear adherent to elastic fibers. No foam cells are present.

plaques may be overlain by intimal thickening. A common finding in elderly cows is the formation of cup-like intimal depressions with medial calcification of the Mönckeberg type. Ratcliffe *et al.* (1960) has also recorded the occurrence of aortic and coronary arteriosclerosis in Bovidae. Alibasoglu *et al.* (1962) found that 67% of relatively young cattle condemned for Johne's disease had gross arteriosclerotic lesions. Scattered, irregular, patchy, shell-like plaques were found in the abdominal aorta. Fibrotic endocardial changes, fibrosis and hyalinization of the intima, with mucoid deposition, calcification and plaque formation of the endocardium and thoracic intima, a medial calcification in the abdominal aorta, and intimal and coronary thickening were found in these cattle. Foamy and vacuolated cells and an increased fragmentation of the medial elastic fibers were accompanied by an increase in smooth

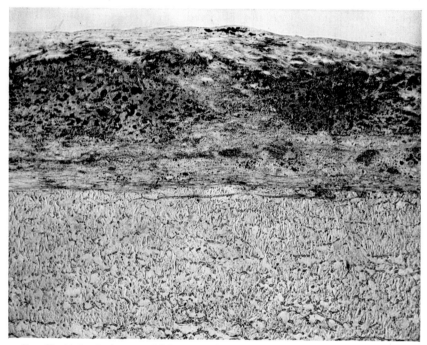

Fig. 45. Abdominal aorta (Malayan tapir, age 30). Magnification: 125. Sudan IV-hematoxylin stain. Lipid infiltration is limited to the intimal plaque and is less pronounced in the superficial layer. The dense lipid deposits noted are in macrophages. Cholesterol is absent (polarized light).

muscle bundles. Small lipid droplets in swollen endothelial cells overlying the fibrotic intima were observed. The high incidence of arterial disease in these animals was believed to be related to infection with *Mycobacterium paratuberculosis*. McKinney (1962) described both fatty streaks and fibrous plaques in 4 wild buffalo and 3 wild cows. We have observed similar aortic lesions in old domestic cows (Lindsay and Chaikoff, unpublished, Fig. 47).

Fox (1933) found only three instances of intimal thickening in deer (Cervidae). Calcification of the media beneath the intimal thickening was noted, and an axis deer (*Axis axis*) showed calcification in its coronary arteries. Vastesaeger *et al.* (1959a) found arterial disease in several species of deer. A fallow deer (*Dama dama*) showed minimal intimal fibrous thickening of the right coronary artery. The internal elastic membrane was stretched but intact. A Canadian deer (*Cervus canadensis*) also showed intimal fibrosis of a coronary artery, and the internal

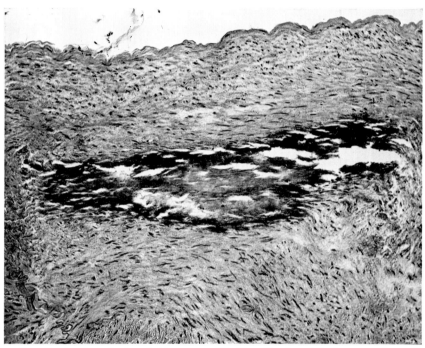

Fig. 46. Aortic arch (female llama, age 18). Magnification: 125. Hematoxylin-eosin stain. A large intimal fibrous plaque contains an extensive calcific deposit. Earlier calcification elsewhere in this plaque appears on collagen and elastic fibers. Small lipid droplets (Sudan IV stain) and a few cholesterol crystals (polarized light) are present in the deep layers of the plaque.

elastic membrane was replaced by a layer of parallel fibers. Enormous sclerotic thickening of the right coronary artery was observed in a musk deer (*Hyemoschus aquaticus*). The internal elastic membrane was frequently broken. Many histiocytes were present in the deeper layers of the thickened intima. In several deer that we have examined (Lindsay and Chaikoff, unpublished) elastic formation in intimal plaques was pronounced (Fig. 48). The wildebeeste also is subject to aortic arteriosclerosis (Lindsay and Chaikoff, unpublished, Fig. 49). Goetz and Keen (1957) did not find arteriosclerosis in an old bull giraffe.

Hulland (1960) studied arteriosclerotic changes in the visceral arteries of 67 mature sheep and 15 ovine fetuses. Even in 7-year-old sheep, few gross lesions were observed, except for prominent longitudinal folds in the thoracic aorta. However, Sudan staining revealed lipids in well defined areas adjacent to many arterial branches, and more pronounced

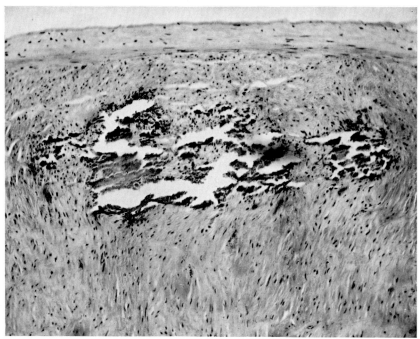

FIG. 47. Abdominal aorta (old cow). Magnification: 125. Hematoxylin-eosin stain. Large calcific deposits in the media and slight intimal fibrous thickening are noted. Lipid is absent (Sudan IV stain).

in older animals. Some fraying and reduplication of the internal elastic membrane was noted in these older animals. Intimal sclerosis varied from small plaques to complete circular fibrous bands. The intimal lesions in the older animals had become confluent, but in young animals no thickened intima was present between plaques. The latter contained collagen and mucopolysaccharide materials, but the amount of elastic tissue varied. Muscle fibers were seen penetrating the interrupted internal elastic membrane. Some plaques were laminated with more elastic tissue in the deeper portions. Sudan IV staining of sections of the aorta showed intracellular and extracellular lipid throughout the intimal plaque. Frequently droplets were concentrated on the intimal side of the internal elastic membrane or just beneath the endothelium. It was emphasized that not all plaques contained fat and that some fat was found in the inner media. Foam cells were rare.

In sheep, Jensen *et al.* (1962) found arteriosclerotic lesions occurring discontinuously in the internal spermatic artery and in the arteries of

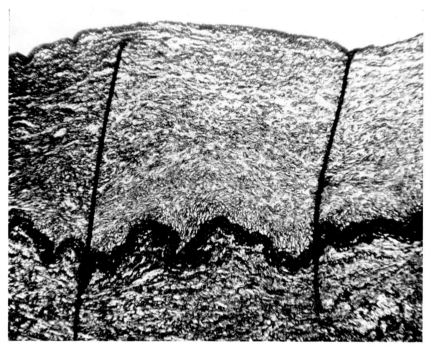

FIG. 48. Thoracic aorta (female axis deer, age 4). Magnification: 125. Weigert-van Gieson stain. The intimal plaque is rich in elastic fibers, especially adjacent to the media. Lipid is absent (Sudan IV stain).

the epididymis and testis. These lesions consisted of intimal fibroplasia with edema. The internal elastic membrane was occasionally fragmented and longitudinally split. Fox (1933) mentioned definite atheroma around the intercostal arterial orifices in 1 Barbary sheep. Aortic arteriosclerosis (Fig. 50) has also been observed in old domestic goats (Lindsay and Chaikoff, unpublished).

V. Pathogenesis of Naturally Occurring and Experimentally Induced Arteriosclerosis in Animals

In much of the work cited here, the late lesions of the naturally occurring and experimentally induced types of arteriosclerosis have been compared with the human lesion without taking into account the possibility that the developmental sequence of the lesions may differ considerably in man and animals. Unfortunately, in many studies, too little attention has been paid to the mechanism of development or pathogenesis of the lesion. There is need, moreover, to distinguish the spon-

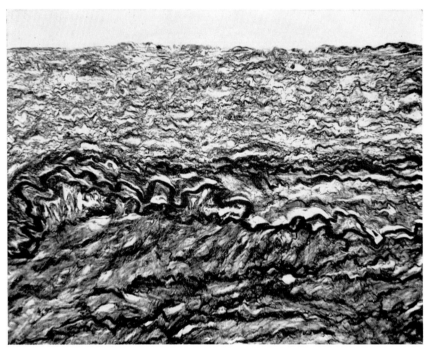

FIG. 49. Abdominal aorta (Wildebeeste). Magnification: 125. Weigert-van Gieson stain. Abundant elastic fibers are present in the intima. A few fine lipid droplets are demonstrable along deeper elastic fibers in this plaque (Sudan IV stain).

taneous from the experimentally induced lesion. For example, certain of the experimental lesions are in reality cases of naturally occurring disease that were modified by the experimental procedures. The present review, as well as studies from this laboratory, of naturally occurring and experimentally induced arteriosclerosis in many animal species demonstates that arteriosclerosis in animals consists of two basic forms: (1) a primary degenerative lesion, with or without secondary lipid infiltration, and (2) a primary, lipid-induced lesion, which may be associated with secondary fibrosis.

In most species of mammals and birds, arteriosclerosis seems to be initiated by degeneration of certain components of the vascular wall. If lipids appear during the course of the development of the arterioscle-rotic lesions, this appearance seems clearly to be a secondary phenome-non. The primary degenerative lesion is characteristic of the abdominal aorta, the coronary arteries, and other muscular arteries of the bird, whereas in the thoracic aorta of this animal, arteriosclerosis is the result

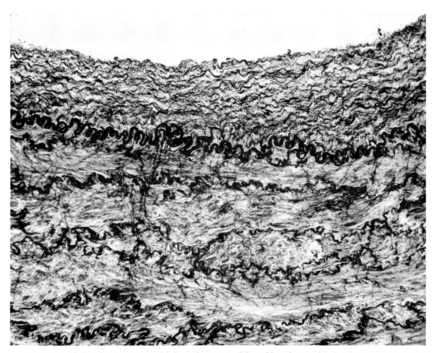

FIG. 50. Abdominal aorta (old female goat). Magnification: 125. Weigert-van Gieson stain. Diffusely thickened intima contains many wavy coarse elastic fibers. Note re-duplication of some segments of the internal elastic membrane. Lipid (Sudan IV stain) is absent.

of primary lipid deposition. Although most lesions of animal arterio-sclerosis involve primarily the intima, disease initiated mainly in the media occurs in a number of species (rats, bovines, elephants). In other species, including the dog and cat, both intimal and medial degenera-tive disease may occur together. There is considerable histological evi-dence that the basic degenerative changes leading to both intimal and medial disease are similar if not identical. Certainly some forms of me-dial arteriosclerosis in animals closely resemble medial aortic disease observed in the human being.

The earliest visual evidence of degeneration in the arterial wall appears in the internal elastic membrane or in the innermost layer of the medial elastica (Figs. 20, 25). The elastic lamina loses its uniform refractile appearance and becomes beaded and segmentally fragmented (Figs. 20, 25). Vacuoles often appear in the degenerating membrane, and these stain less intensely than do adjacent normal segments. Calcification of the degenerating membrane may also occur (Figs. 16, 27). Although a thin layer of acid mucopolysaccharide material normally envelops the internal elastic membrane, this material accumulates in greater quantities in areas adjacent to the fragmented elastic segments, particularly on the side adjacent to the endothelium (Figs. 26, 28). Vastesaeger *et al.* (1959a) have stressed the deformation of the internal elastic membrane with stretching and loss of characteristic undulation as early evidence of elastic degeneration in the arterial wall. The degenerated segments of the internal elastic membrane gradually disintegrate and disappear within the mucoid ground substance. Eventually, newly formed elastic laminas appear in the mucoid ground substance, bridging the gap that resulted from the degeneration and fragmentation (Fig. 28). The small stubs at either end of the defect seem to disappear gradually. The newly formed elastic layer must presumably be formed by some sort of molecular rearrangement of material within the ground substance, since at this stage no connective tissue or endothelial cells are in the immediate vicinity. It is possible that this regenerative phenomenon is identical with the formation of elastic substance from mucoid ground material as observed in the aorta of the rat (Pease and Paule, 1960) and in the pial arteries of the cat and monkey (Pease and Molinari, 1960). The newly formed elastic layer may become degenerated and fragmented, and still again regeneration may occur. It is of interest that in one species at least—the cat—this sort of degenerative lesion was commonly observed even in young animals and was found on the convex surface of the aortic arch and on the posterior wall of the thoracic and, particularly, the abdominal aortas (Lindsay and Chaikoff, 1955). These, of course, are the sites where mature arteriosclerotic lesions are often found in older animals. Apparently this degenerative lesion is a reaction of wear and tear, and must occur frequently throughout the vascular system. It is conceivable that arteriosclerotic lesions eventually develop only in areas subjected to repeated injuries of this sort.

As degeneration and regeneration with reduplication of the elastic laminas recur, and as acid mucopolysaccharide substance accumulates, a small plaque protruding into the vessel lumen eventually appears (Fig. 26). The source of this mucoid substance is not known, although mucopolysaccharide granules may be found in the cytoplasm of the overlying endothelial cells.

The next stage in the development of the arteriosclerotic lesion is the appearance of scattered, immature fibroblasts in the areas of mucoid accumulation (Figs. 21, 29, 30). These seem to originate both from medial connective tissue and possibly from the surface endothelium. Further growth of the intimal plaque or, in some instances, diffuse intimal thickening results from proliferation of fibroblasts. The intercellular substance of the earliest intimal plaque consists entirely of fibrillar acid mucopolysaccharides, but as the plaque enlarges and matures, delicate reticulum, collagen, and elastic fibers appear, first around individual fibroblasts, and gradually replace the fibrillar mucoid ground substance (Figs. 22, 23, 24).

These newly formed elastic fibers should be distinguished from fibers derived from the internal elastic membrane even though their histological staining reactions are similar. In the earlier, smaller plaques, the cells and fibers have an irregular arrangement which later becomes perpendicular to the endothelial surface. In the older, mature plaques, the cells and fibers generally assume a circumferential arrangement (Figs. 22, 23). Distinct layering of plaques (Figs. 24, 31) suggests an episodic development of the arteriosclerotic lesion.

In most species of animals, demonstrable lipid material cannot be found in the early degenerative lesions and in the early arteriosclerotic plaques. In most species in which lipid material is found in fibrous intimal plaques, its presence is restricted mainly to larger and presumably older mature plaques, usually in the deepest segments adjacent to or in the media. Such lipid localization is characteristic of the naturally occurring fibrous plaques of the abdominal aorta of birds (Fig. 2), dogs, cats, and other species (Figs. 18, 19, 45). The source of the lipid that enters preexisting fibrous plaques is not known, but since the lipid is likely to be found in the deeper segments, presumably it does not enter from the vascular lumen. Its appearance may result from local synthesis. It has been shown that the normal arterial wall of various animals is capable of synthesizing fatty acids and cholesterol (Chernick *et al.,* 1949; Siperstein *et al.,* 1951; Werthessen *et al.,* 1954). In some early lesions fine lipid droplets appear adjacent to and on the surface of degenerating segments of internal elastic membranes. We have observed these deposits in early lesions in the cat, rhesus monkey, other macaques (Fig. 13), chimpanzee (Figs. 18, 19), and baboon. This finding may reflect an affinity of lipid for the enveloping mucopolysaccharide, or this lipid accumulation may result from a lipoidal degeneration of the arterial elastic tissue as suggested by Adams and Tuqan (1961). Although considerable amounts of lipid may eventually appear in and near these earlier primary fibrous plaques, foam cells that have ingested lipid are rarely observed. These cells, of course, appear early and form the bulk of primary lipid lesions induced by hyperlipemia and/or hypercholesterolemia.

Although cholesterol deposition occurs frequently in human arteriosclerosis and is largely responsible for the serious sequelae of arteriosclerosis in man, cholesterol is not often demonstrable in animal arteriosclerotic lesions and its presence is almost limited to lesions found in birds and primates. Vastesaeger et al. (1959a) stressed the importance of the role of cholesterol in coronary arteriosclerosis because, in the only two cases of thrombotic coronary occlusion that they observed in chimpanzees, the intima was filled with cholesterol crystals.

It must be emphasized that, unlike the arteriosclerotic lesion in man, most later arteriosclerotic plaques in animals do not usually contain large amounts of lipid. However, the primary fibrous lesion of the abdominal aorta of the chicken, particularly when modified by experimentally induced lipemia, often does show extensive secondary accumulations of lipid, including cholesterol, and the appearance of necrosis, ulceration, and local thrombosis seems identical with the arteriosclerotic sequences so common in the human being.

In a number of animal species, medial disease overshadows intimal fibrosis and thickening. Extensive calcification of degenerating elastic tissue and the appearance of increased amounts of mucoid ground substance suggest that the medial lesion may be basically similar to that of the intima. In old dogs and cats the elastic tissue degeneration, the accumulations of mucopolysaccharide, and the eventual collagenous scarring occur in the media as well as in the intima. Medial disease with calcification and with relatively minor intimal involvement is characteristic in the rat, in most bovine species, and in the elephant. In these and other animals, identical calcific deposits in the internal elastic membrane may be observed in the absence of medial disease in some segments of the aorta (Fig. 16).

Arteriosclerosis arising primarily from deposition of lipids and followed by reactive fibrosis is not a feature of the naturally occurring disease in mammals—in sharp contrast to arteriosclerosis induced by cholesterol feeding in which deposition of lipid and cholesterol in the vascular wall is followed by fibrosis. In the thoracic aorta of the bird, however, naturally occurring arteriosclerosis is initiated by deposition of lipid material, first in the endothelial cells and eventually in connective tissue cells and macrophages which proliferate in the intimal layer. Accumulations of these cells form elevated intimal plaques, and these lipid-containing intimal cells eventually give rise to mucopolysaccharide, reticulum, and collagenous fibers which represent the secondary fibrous component of this lesion. Among mammals, mild primary lipid lesions of this sort seem to be limited to the rabbit and squirrel (Bragdon, 1952a, 1954). It is likely that the so-called milk streaks or lipid-containing lesions which occur transiently and early in life in the rabbit and also in the human being are examples of lipid deposition in an otherwise normal intima. Similar lipid infiltration has been observed in the walls of the aortas of newly hatched chicks (Nichols *et al.*, 1961). Although the lipid may persist for a number of weeks, a sclerotic reaction does not ensue. It is possible that careful examination of these early lipid lesions in mammals may reveal preexisting degenerative changes which so far have not been recognized.

VI. Etiological Factors in Animal Arteriosclerosis

It seems likely that, in animals as in humans, arteriosclerosis is related to the process of aging. In the dog, cat, primates, and other species, the incidence and severity of naturally occurring arteriosclerosis are greater in older animals and, except for the earliest degenerative lesions of the elastic tissue, seem to be absent in younger animals. In the human being, at least, degenerative changes of the elastic tissue of the skin and the lung as well as of blood vessels are clearly related to the age of the individual.

Genetic factors may be important in the development of animal arteriosclerosis, as they must be in the human disease. So far, however, genetic differences are claimed only for certain strains of domestic pigeons. Which of the factors in the vascular lesion are determined genetically in these pigeons is not at present known (Clarkson *et al.*, 1959; Prichard *et al.*, 1962).

Sex differences in incidence and severity of arteriosclerosis are not apparent in most animals so far described. Limitation of severe disease of the media to female rats and its absence in male rats may be related to frequency of pregnancies. The naturally occurring fibrous lesion in the abdominal aorta is more pronounced in male than in female birds, and the occurrence of the lipid-induced, naturally occurring arteriosclerotic lesion of the thoracic aorta is more pronounced in female than in male birds. The lipid-induced lesion seems clearly to be caused by the periodic lipemia and hypercholesterolemia associated with egg laying in the female bird (Lorenz, 1954).

Intravascular pressure is undoubtedly related to the development of arteriosclerosis in animal blood vessels. Since the pulse pressure in the abdominal aorta is greater than in the thoracic aorta, this factor may be related to the higher incidence and greater severity of arteriosclerosis in the abdominal than in the thoracic aorta even in quadrupeds. Greater pulse pressure would be expected to be associated with greater degrees of injury and fragmentation of the internal elastic membrane. Experimental arteriosclerosis of any form would be expected to be adversely affected by the added induction of hypertension.

The sites of arteriosclerosis observed in many animal species are identical with those observed in human beings. These include: the convex surface of the first portion of the aortic arch; sites about the intercostal and abdominal arterial openings; the lower portion of the abdominal aorta; areas near bifurcations; and the upper portion of the anterior descending branch of the left coronary artery. Relative immobility of certain of these segments might be expected to result in greater degrees of fragmentation and injury of the internal elastic membrane. In addition, turbulence of blood flow at certain of these sites may contribute to the injury. Although turbulence may be important in experimental arteriosclerosis associated with hyperlipemia, this factor would not seem so important in naturally occurring disease in most animal species since the amount of lipid material found in intimal lesions is relatively insignificant and since blood lipid levels in most animal species are relatively low as compared with those in human beings.

Rindfleisch (1870) was one of the first to suggest that mechanical and hemodynamic factors might be important in the pathogenesis and localization of arteriosclerotic lesions. More recently, Schwartz and Mitchell (1962) investigated the distribution of arterial plaques in the human aorta and other arteries and found that pressure differences in various parts of the aorta and in neck and iliac arteries were related to differences in the incidence of plaque formation in these vessels: fewer plaques were found where the pressures were lower. In addition, raised plaques were more frequently found at sites where turbulent blood flow was thought to occur—for example, within the mouths of coronary arteries. On the other hand, flat plaques or fatty streaks did not show this correlation with zones of turbulence, but were found more often in a fan-shaped area in the upper thoracic aorta, narrowing down to a posterior strip in the lower thoracic aorta. The fatty streaks were believed to result from shearing forces exerted by flow patterns in the aorta. Since the distribution of the fatty streaks was different from that of the raised plaques in this study, Schwartz and Mitchell (1962) regarded these two lesions as separate processes and emphasized that different mechanical and hemodynamic factors were important in the localization of the two types of injury.

Since many herbivorous animals develop significant degrees of arteriosclerosis, diet apparently has little to do with the onset of the naturally occurring disease in most animals. It is recognized, however, that more information is needed on the dietary habits of animals that develop arteriosclerosis spontaneously.

Muscular activity does not appear to be significantly related to the incidence or severity of arteriosclerosis in animals since comparable arterial disease may be found in placid animals and in those that are extremely active. No relation between exercise and degree of arteriosclerosis was demonstrated in the pigeon (Lofland and Clarkson, 1959), but such a relation was demonstrated by Orma (1957) in the cholesterol-fed chicken.

Ratcliffe *et al.* (1960) claim that the frequency of arteriosclerosis in mammals and birds in the Philadelphia Zoological Garden has increased tenfold since 1935. Increases in the variety of animals developing the disease, and changes in location and character of the arteriosclerotic lesions, as well as in the rate of their development, are pointed out. These investigators note the improvements in the nutrition and the increased population density of their zoo animals, and present the hypothesis that social pressure was responsible for increased arteriosclerosis, as has been suggested in the case of the human being.

Incorporation of intimal thrombi by fibrous tissue, with subsequent formation of plaques (Duguid, 1952), was not observed in the development of animal arteriosclerosis by Vastesaeger *et al.* (1959a) nor by us in studies of domestic and captive wild animals.

VII. The Relation of Naturally Occurring Arteriosclerosis to That Induced Experimentally in Animals

A. Arteriosclerosis Primarily of Lipid Origin

In the bird (chicken), naturally occurring disease in the thoracic aorta, observed mainly in the female, is initiated by deposition of lipid in an otherwise normal thoracic aorta. This lesion can be duplicated experimentally by diethylstilbestrol injection or by the feeding of cholesterol or other sterols. Lesions so induced are composed of foam cell plaques that eventually display varying degrees of fibrosis. These experimental procedures result in the appearance of similar foam-cell-containing plaques throughout the vascular system. In addition, excessive lipid, including cholesterol, is deposited in naturally occurring fibrous plaques of the abdominal aorta if such lesions should be present.

A similar, primarily lipid-type of arterial disease has been induced in the rabbit by cholesterol feeding. The lesion is of the foam cell type, which later—when complicated by fibrosis, degeneration, and liquefaction—may resemble human arteriosclerotic lesions. It should be recalled that this form of experimentally induced arterial disease is but one manifestation of a widespread storage of lipids in the animal body.

A similar primary lipid lesion, consisting of foam cells, may also be induced in the rhesus monkey by feedings of large amounts of cholesterol. There is no histological evidence so far that the resulting lesions represent deposition of cholesterol in preexisting fibrous intimal plaques. Identical foam cell lesions are found in the arteriosclerosis induced in cebus monkeys by cholesterol feeding. In the dog, cholesterol feeding accompanied by hypothyroidism results in the development of foam cell arterial lesions. It should be noted, however, that in the dog, particularly in older ones, not only do primary lipid lesions with accumulations of foam cells appear, but preexisting fibrous lesions may also be modified by excessive deposition of lipid and cholesterol. Experimentally induced atheromatosis in rats is a result of dietary manipulations causing hyperlipemia and hypercholesterolemia, and consists of infiltration of lipid material into vascular walls, usually without significant reactive fibrosis.

In these various species, primary lipid arteriosclerosis appears to result from infiltrations of fat and cholesterol from the lumen into the vascular wall. The latter reacts by mobilization of macrophages which ingest the lipids. Eventually necrosis and scarring, with narrowing of the media and destruction of the internal elastic membrane, may appear. Although the late lesions induced by these experimental procedures may closely resemble later human arteriosclerotic lesions, their pathogenesis seems entirely different.

B. Naturally Occurring Arteriosclerosis Modified by Lipid Deposition

The feeding of excessive amounts of lipids has been shown to result in secondary lipid deposition in preexisting, naturally occurring fibrous plaques in birds, dogs, and swine. However, the administration of cholesterol to aged female breeding rats is not accompanied by cholesterol or lipid deposition in preexisting, degenerative lesions of the media.

C. Experimental Production of Degenerative Elastic and Fibrous Arteriosclerosis

Few studies on the experimental production of the degenerative type of arteriosclerosis have been reported. Arteriosclerosis induced in the rhesus monkey by a pyridoxine-deficient diet (Rinehart and Greenberg,

1949, 1951) closely resembles the naturally occurring disease in this species. It seems likely that disturbances in protein metabolism accompanying the pyridoxine deficiency may be related to elastic tissue degeneration and abnormalities of vascular ground substance that resulted in fibrous intimal proliferation. Indeed, it has been shown that suboptimal protein intake in male birds is accompanied by a significant increase in naturally occurring fibrous arteriosclerosis in the abdominal aorta (Chaikoff *et al.*, 1961).

Injury of the vascular wall, apparently localized to the internal elastic membrane and resulting from irradiation, has been shown to induce experimental arteriosclerosis similar to, if not identical with, that of the naturally occurring disease of the dog (Lindsay *et al.*, 1962a, b). Elastic destruction associated with deposition of ground substance and profound connective tissue proliferation has also been induced by enzymic (papain) injury of the aorta in rabbits (Tsaltas, 1962). Obviously, further investigation of this important, early degenerative phase of animal arteriosclerosis is needed.

VIII. Relation of Naturally Occurring Arteriosclerosis in Animals to Human Arteriosclerosis

The findings presented here indicate that the basic pathogenesis of naturally occurring arteriosclerosis in various mammalian orders is identical with that of the disease in the human being. In the human coronary artery (Moon and Rinehart, 1952) and aorta (Taylor, 1953) elastic degeneration, mucoid deposition, and fibrosis appear to antedate lipid deposition.

In animal species, degenerative lesions and fibrosis also predominate, and lipid accumulation is clearly a secondary phenomenon. It seems highly unlikely that the pathogenesis of arteriosclerosis in the human being should differ significantly from that in other species. Lesions in primates more closely resemble the human lesions than do those of other species because of their considerable content of lipid, including cholesterol.

In avian species, the two forms of arteriosclerosis, the primary lipid lesion and the primary fibrous lesion, have not always been clearly differentiated. In many experimental studies, this fact has sometimes been ignored, and arteriosclerosis in the bird has been treated as a single process. The fibrous lesion in birds, occurring in the abdominal aorta, does, however, clearly resemble the human lesion, particularly when the former is complicated by lipid deposition resulting from cholesterol feeding or diethylstilbestrol injections. Most of the lesions involving the aorta and coronary and other arteries in cholesterol-fed birds must be regarded as part of a generalized storage disease. (The only counterpart of this phenomenon in man is found in essential hypercholesterolemia.)

The earliest gross evidence of the human disease, manifested as fatty streaks in the aorta, consists of lipid in connective tissue cells and in the intercellular spaces of the intima. The primary lipid lesion found naturally in the bird and rabbit and that which may be experimentally induced in birds, rabbits, monkeys, and dogs, appear first as a lipid infiltration of the endothelial cells and later as lipid-laden foam cells probably derived from the endothelial layer. It seems likely, however, that lipid infiltration in the intima in the human being is preceded by intimal degeneration, although this process may not always be visible or recognizable by the usual methods of examination.

The late foam cell lesions of the lipid-induced experimental disease in several species have shown fragmentation and disruption of the internal elastic membrane. This is clearly a late mechanical effect, however, and not to be mistaken for the early fragmentation of the internal elastic membrane, which seems to initiate arteriosclerosis in mammalian and, in part, in avian species.

ACKNOWLEDGMENTS

We are indebted to Dr. C. R. Schroeder, Dr. W. P. Heuschele, and Mr. B. W. Sheridan of the San Diego Zoological Gardens, San Diego, California; to Dr. A. J. Riopelle of the Yerkes Laboratories of Primate Biology, Inc., of Emory University, Orange Park, Florida; to Dr. W. Mottram and Mr. Cary Baldwin of the San Francisco Zoological Garden; and to Dr. J. W. Gilmore for furnishing us with the hearts and arteries of many of the animals referred to in this chapter. Our thanks are due to Mrs. Thelma Gotham for preparation of the histological sections and to Mr. Hal Strong of the Veterans Administration Hospital, Oakland, for assistance in preparation of the photomicrographs. The many helpful discussions with Mr. C. W. Nichols, Jr., and his assistance in assembling the bibliography are gratefully acknowledged. Our own studies on the cardiovascular systems of domestic and wild animals in captivity were aided by grants from the U. S. Public Health Service, the Life Insurance Medical Research Fund, the Alameda County Heart Association, and the Committee on Research of the School of Medicine.

REFERENCES

Adams, C. W. M., and Tuqan, N. A. (1961). *J. Pathol. Bacteriol.* **82**, 131.
Alibasoglu, M., Dunne, H. W., and Guss, S. B. (1962). *Am. J. Vet. Res.* **23**, 49.
Altschul, R., and Fedoroff, M. E. (1960). *Arch. Path.* **69**, 689.
Anitschkow, N. (1913). *Beitr. Pathol. Allgem. Pathol.* **56**, 379.
Aronson, W. (1962). *Arch. Pathol.* **74**, 509.
Benedict, F. G. (1936). *Carnegie Inst. Wash. Publ.* **474**.
Berdjis, C. C. (1960). *Strahlentherapie* **112**, 595.
Bevans, M., Davidson, J. D., and Abell, L. L. (1951a). *A.M.A. Arch. Pathol.* **51**, 278.

Bevans, M., Davidson, J. D., and Kendall, F. E. (1951b). *A.M.A. Arch. Pathol.* **51**, 228.

Bloom, F. (1946). *Am. J. Pathol.* **22**, 519.

Bragdon, J. H. (1952a). *Circulation Res.* **5**, 641.

Bragdon, J. H. (1952b). *Federation Proc.* **10**, 350.

Bragdon, J. H. (1954). *Circulation Res.* **2**, 520.

Bragdon, H., and Mickelsen, O. (1955). *Am. J. Pathol.* **31**, 965.

Bragdon, J. H., Zeller, J. H., and Stevenson, J. W. (1957). *Proc. Soc. Exptl. Biol. Med.* **95**, 282.

Buck, R. C. (1962). *Brit. J. Exptl. Pathol.* **43**, 236.

Chaikoff, I. L., Lindsay, S., Lorenz, F. W., and Entenman, C. (1948). *J. Exptl. Med.* **88**, 373.

Chaikoff, I. L., Nichols, C. W., Jr., Gaffey, W., and Lindsay, S. (1961). *J. Atherosclerosis, Res.* **1**, 461.

Chernick, S. S., Srere, P. A., and Chaikoff, I. L. (1949). *J. Biol. Chem.* **179**, 113.

Clarkson, T. B., Prichard, R. W., Netsky, M. G., and Lofland, H. B., Jr. (1959). *A.M.A. Arch. Pathol.* **68**, 143.

Conrad, L. L., Gonzalez, I. E., Joel, W., and Furman, R. H. (1956). *Circulation Res.* **4**, 263.

Corwin, W. C., and Cragg, R. W. (1938). *Am. J. Med. Sci.* **195**, 47.

Creech, O., Jordan, G. L., Jr., DeBakey, M. E., Overton, R. C., and Halpert, B. (1955). *Surg., Gynecol. Obstet.* **101**, 607.

Dauber, D. V. (1944). *A.M.A. Arch. Pathol.* **38**, 46.

Dauber, D. V., and Katz, L. N. (1942). *A.M.A. Arch. Pathol.* **34**, 937.

Dauber, D. V., and Katz, L. N. (1943). *A.M.A. Arch. Pathol.* **36**, 473.

Davidson, J. D., Meyer, W., and Kendall, F. E. (1951). *Circulation* **3**, 332.

DiLuzio, N. R., and O'Neal, R. M. (1962). *Exptl. Mol. Pathol.* **1**, 122.

Duff, G. L., McMillan, A. B., and Ritchie, A. C. (1957). *Am. J. Pathol.* **33**, 845.

Duguid, J. B. (1952). *Lancet* **ii**, 207.

Eades, C. H., Jr., Phillips, G. S., and Solberg, V. B. (1962). *Proc. Soc. Exptl. Biol. Med.* **110**, 65.

Fillios, L. C., Andrus, S. B., Mann, G. V., and Stare, F. J. (1956). *J. Exptl. Med.* **104**, 539.

Finlayson, R., and Hirchinson, V. (1961). *Nature* **192**, 369.

Fisher, H., Feigenbaum, A. S., Leveille, A. S., Weiss, H. S., and Griminger, P. (1959). *J. Nutr.* **69**, 163.

Fox, H. (1933). *In* "Arteriosclerosis" (E. V. Cowdry, ed.), pp. 153-193. Macmillan, New York.

Gey, K. F., and Pletscher, A. (1961). *Nature* **189**, 491.

Gilbert, C., and Gillman, J. (1960). *S. African J. Med. Sci.* **25**, 59.

Gillman, J., and Gilbert, C. (1957). *Exptl. Med. Surg.* **15**, 181.

Gillman, J., Gilbert, C., and Prates, M. D. (1960). *S. African J. Med. Sci.* **25**, 47.

Gillman, T., and Hathorn, M. (1959). *Nature* **183**, 1139.

Goetz, R. H., and Keen, E. N. (1957). *Angiology* **8**, 542.

Gold, H. (1961). *A.M.A. Arch. Pathol.* **71**, 268.

Gottlieb, H., and Lalich, J. J. (1954). *Am. J. Pathol.* **30**, 851.

Gresham, G. A., Howard, A. N., and King, A. J. (1962). *Brit. J. Exptl. Pathol.* **43**, 21.

Haimovici, H., Maier, N., and Strauss, L. (1958). *A.M.A. Arch. Surg.* **67**, 282.

Harkness, M. L. R., Harkness, R. D., and McDonald, D. A. (1957). *Proc. Roy. Soc.* **B146**, 541.

Hartroft, P. M., Suzuki, M., and O'Neal, R. M. (1962). *Exptl. Mol. Pathol.* **1**, 133.

Hartroft, W. S., and O'Neal, R. M.   (1962).   Am. J. Cardiol. 9, 355.
Hartroft, W. S., Ridout, J. H., Sellers, A. E., and Best, C. H.   (1952).   Proc. Soc. Exptl. Biol. Med. 81, 384.
Hass, G. M., Trueheart, R. E., and Hemmens, A.   (1960).   Am. J. Pathol. 37, 521.
Heuper, W. C.   (1942).   A.M.A. Arch. Pathol. 33, 267.
Heuper, W. C.   (1946).   Am. J. Pathol. 22, 1287.
Higginbotham, A. C., and Higginbotham, F. H.   (1958).   A.M.A. Arch. Pathol. 65, 631.
Horlick, L., and Katz, L. N.   (1949).   J. Lab. Clin. Med. 34, 1427.
Howard, A. N., Gresham, G. A., and Jennings, I. W.   (1962).   Proc. Nutr. Soc. (Engl. Scot.) 21, 20.
Hulland, T. J.   (1960).   Can. Vet. J. 1, 195.
Hummel, K. P., and Barnes, L. L.   (1938).   Am. J. Pathol. 14, 121.
Humphreys, E. M.   (1957).   Quart. J. Exptl. Physiol. 42, 96.
Jennings, M. A., Florey, H. W., Stehbens, W. E., and French, J. E.   (1961).   J. Pathol. Bacteriol. 18, 49.
Jensen, R., Flint, J. C., Brown, W. W., and Collier, J. R.   (1962).   Am. J. Vet. Res. 23, 480.
Karrer, H. E.   (1961).   J. Ultrastruct. Res. 5, 1.
Kawamura, R.   (1927).   "Neue Beiträge zur Morphologie und Physiologie der Cholesterinsteatose," p. 267. Fischer, Jena.
Keech, M. K.   (1960a).   J. Biophys. Biochem. Cytol. 7, 533.
Keech, M. K.   (1960b).   J. Biophys. Biochem. Cytol. 7, 539.
Kelly, A. L., and Jensen, D.   (1960).   Nature 186, 731.
Kittinger, G. W., Wexler, B. C., and Miller, B. F.   (1960).   Proc. Soc. Exptl. Biol. Med. 104, 616.
Köllisch, P.   (1910).   Zur pathologischen Anatomie und Aetiologie der sogenannten Atherosklerose der Arterien bei den Haustieren. Inaugural dissertation (Bern). J. L. Stich, Nürnberg.
Krause, C.   (1922).   Beitr. Pathol. Anat. Allgem. Pathol. 71, 121.
Leary, T.   (1949).   A.M.A. Arch. Pathol. 47, 1.
Lindsay, S., and Chaikoff, I. L.   (1950).   A.M.A. Arch. Pathol. 49, 434.
Lindsay, S., and Chaikoff, I. L.   (1955).   A.M.A. Arch. Pathol. 60, 29.
Lindsay, S., and Chaikoff, I. L.   (1957).   A.M.A. Arch. Pathol. 63, 460.
Lindsay, S., Chaikoff, I. L., and Gilmore, J. W.   (1952a).   A.M.A. Arch. Pathol. 53, 281.
Lindsay, S., Feinberg, H., Chaikoff, I. L., Entenman, C., and Reichert, F. L.   (1952b).   A.M.A. Arch. Pathol. 54, 573.
Lindsay, S., Nichols, C. W., Jr., and Chaikoff, I. L.   (1955).   A.M.A. Arch. Pathol. 59, 173.
Lindsay, S. Skahen, R., and Chaikoff, I. L.   (1956).   A.M.A. Arch. Pathol. 61, 207.
Lindsay, S., Kohn, H. I., Dakin, R. L., and Jew, J.   (1962a).   Circulation Res. 10, 51.
Lindsay, S., Entenman, C., Ellis, E. E., and Geraci, C. L.   (1962b).   Circulation Res. 10, 61.
Lofland, H. B., Jr., and Clarkson, T. B.   (1959).   Circulation Res. 7, 234.
Lofland, H. B., Jr., Clarkson, T. B., and Goodman, H. O.   (1961).   Circulation Res. 9, 919.
Lorenz, F. W.   (1954).   Vitamins Hormones 12, 235-275.
Loustalot, P.   (1960).   Helv. Physiol. Pharmacol. Acta 18, 343.
McGill, H. C., Jr., Geer, J. C., and Holman, R. L.   (1957).   A.M.A. Arch. Pathol. 64, 303.

McGill, H. C., Jr., Strong, J. P., Holman, R. L., and Werthessen, N. T. (1960). *Circulation Res.* **8**, 670.

McGill, H. C., Jr., Frank, M. H., and Geer, J. C. (1961). *A.M.A. Arch. Pathol.* **71**, 96.

McKinney, B. (1962). *Lancet* **ii**, 281.

Malinow, M. R., Hojman, D., and Pellegrino, A. A. (1954). *Acta Cardiol.* **9**, 480.

Malinow, M. R., Hojman, D., and Pellegrino, A. A. (1956). *A.M.A. Arch. Pathol.* **61**, 11.

Mann, G. V., Andrus, S. B., McNally, A., and Stare, F. J. (1953). *J. Exptl. Med.* **98**, 195.

Manning, G. W. (1942). *Am. Heart J.* **23**, 719.

Milch, L. J., Renzi, A. A., Weiner, N., Robinson, L. G., and Wilson, S. S. (1958). *Proc. Soc. Exptl. Biol. Med.* **97**, 56.

Moon, H. D., and Rinehart, J. F. (1952). *Circulation* **6**, 481.

Morehead, R. P., and Little, J. M. (1945). *Am. J. Pathol.* **21**, 339.

Moses, C. (1954). *Circulation Res.* **2**, 243.

Moss, W. G., Kiely, J. P., Neville, J. B., Bourque, J. E., and Wakerlin, G. E. (1951). *Circulation* **4**, 462.

Murphy, E. A., Rowsell, H. C., Downie, H. G., Robinson, G. A., and Mustard, J. F. (1962). *Can. Med. Assoc. J.* **87**, 259.

Nichols, C. W., Jr., Lindsay, S., and Chaikoff, I. L. (1955). *Proc. Soc. Exptl. Biol. Med.* **89**, 609.

Nichols, C. W., Jr., Lindsay, S., Chapman, D. D., and Chaikoff, I. L. (1960). *Circulation Res.* **8**, 16.

Nichols, C. W., Jr., Lindsay, S., and Chaikoff, I. L. (1961). *J. Atherosclerosis Res.* **1**, 133.

Nieberle, K. (1930). *Verhandl. Deut. Pathol.* **25**, 291.

Oester, Y. T., Davis, O. F., and Friedman, B. (1955). *Am. J. Pathol.* **31**, 717.

Olcott, C. T., Saxton, J. A., and Modell, W. (1946). *Am. J. Pathol.* **22**, 847.

O'Neal, R. M., Still, W. J. S., and Hartroft, W. S. (1961). *J. Pathol. Bacteriol.* **82**, 183.

Orma, E. J. (1957). *Acta Physiol. Scand.* **41** (Suppl. 142), 75.

Page, I. H., and Brown, H. B. (1952). *Circulation* **6**, 681.

Parker, F. (1958). *Am. J. Anat.* **103**, 247.

Paterson, J. C., Slinger, S. J., and Gartley, K. M. (1948). *A.M.A. Arch. Pathol.* **45**, 306.

Paterson, J. C., Mitchell, C. A., and Wallace, A. C. (1949). *A.M.A. Arch. Pathol.* **47**, 335.

Pease, D. C., and Molinari, S. (1960). *J. Ultrastruct. Res.* **3**, 447.

Pease, D. C., and Paule, W. J. (1960). *J. Ultrastruct. Res.* **3**, 469.

Peifer, J. J. (1955a). *Hormel Inst. Univ. Minn. Ann. Rept.* p. 35.

Peifer, J. J. (1955b). *Hormel Inst. Univ. Minn. Ann. Rept.* p. 37.

Prichard, R. W., Clarkson, T. B., Lofland, H. B., Jr., Goodman, H. O., Herndon, C. N., and Netsky, M. G. (1962). *J. Am. Med. Assoc.* **179**, 49.

Prior, J. T., Kurtz, D. M., and Ziegler, D. D. (1961). *Arch. Pathol.* **71**, 672.

Race, G. J., Edwards, W. L. J., Halden, E. R., Wilson, H. E., and Luibel, F. J. (1959). *Circulation* **19**, 928.

Ratcliffe, H. L., Yersimides, T. G., and Elliott, G. A. (1960). *Circulation* **21**, 730.

Rigg, K. J., Finlayson, R., Symons, C., and Hill, K. R. (1960). *Proc. Zool. Soc. Lond.* **135**, 157.

Rindfleisch, E. (1870). "Manual of Pathologic Histology," Vol. I, p. 250. New Syndenham Society, London.

Rinehart, J. F., and Greenberg, L. D. (1949). *Am. J. Pathol.* **25**, 481.

Rinehart, J. F., and Greenberg, L. D. (1951). *A.M.A. Arch. Pathol.* **51**, 12.

Rowsell, H. C., Downie, H. G., and Mustard, J. F. (1958). *Can. Med. Assoc. J.* **79**, 647.

Rowsell, H. C., Downie, H. G., and Mustard, J. F. (1960). *Can. Med. Assoc. J.* **83**, 1175.

Sabiston, D. C., Jr., Smith, G. W., Talbert, J. L., Gutelius, J., and Vasko, J. S. (1961). *Ann. Surg.* **153**, 13.

Sako, U. (1962). *J. Am. Med. Assoc.* **179**, 36.

Schwartz, C. J., and Mitchell, J. R. A. (1962). *Circulation Res.* **11**, 63.

Senderoff, E., Kaneko, M., Beck, A. R., and Baronofsky, I. D. (1961). *Am. J. Roentgenol. Radium Therapy Nucl. Med.* **86**, 740.

Siperstein, M. D., Chaikoff, I. L., and Chernick, S. S. (1951). *Science* **113**, 747.

Skold, B. H., and Getty, R. (1961). *J. Am. Vet. Med. Assoc.* **139**, 655.

Smith, C., Seitner, M. M., and Wang, H. (1951). *Anat. Record* **109**, 13.

Solowjew, A. (1932). *Centr. Allgem. Pathol. Anat.* **53**, 145.

Sperry, W. M., Jailer, J. W., and Engle, E. T. (1944). *Endocrinology* **35**, 38.

Steiner, A., and Kendall, F. E. (1946). *A.M.A. Arch. Pathol.* **42**, 433.

Steiner, A., Kendall, F. E., and Bevans, M. (1949). *Am. Heart J.* **38**, 34.

Steiner, P. E., Rasmussen, T. B., and Fisher, L. E. (1955). *A.M.A. Arch. Pathol.* **59**, 5.

Stephenson, S. E., Jr., Younger, R., and Scott, H. W., Jr. (1962). *J. Am. Med. Assoc.* **179**, 46.

Strauch, C. (1916). *Beitr. Pathol. Anat. Allgem. Pathol.* **61**, 532.

Taylor, C. B., Cox, G. E., Manalo-Estrella, P., and Southworth, J. (1962). *A.M.A. Arch. Pathol.* **74**, 16.

Taylor, H. E. (1953). *Am. J. Pathol.* **29**, 871.

Tsaltas, T. T. (1962). *Circulation* **26**, 673.

Vastesaeger, M., Gillot, P., Parmentier, R., and Mortelmans, J. (1959a). *Bull. Soc. Roy. Zool. Anvers* **14**, 1-46.

Vastesaeger, M., Gillot, P. H., and Mortelmans, J. (1959b). *Bull. Soc. Roy. Zool. Anvers* **14**, 47.

Waters, L. L. (1957). *Yale J. Biol. Med.* **30**, 101.

Waters, L. L. (1962). *Yale J. Biol. Med.* **35**, 113.

Waugh, D., Maximchuk, A. J., and Stuart, J. R. (1956). *Proc. Soc. Exptl. Biol. Med.* **93**, 197.

Weiss, H. S. (1959). *J. Gerontol.* **14**, 19.

Weiss, H. S., and Fisher, H. (1959). *Am. J. Physiol.* **197**, 1219.

Werthessen, N. T., Milch, L. J., Rodman, R. F., Smith, L. L., and Smith, E. C. (1954). *Am. J. Physiol.* **178**, 23.

Wexler, B. C., and Miller, B. F. (1958). *Science* **127**, 590.

Wexler, B. C., and Miller, B. F. (1959). *Proc. Soc. Exptl. Biol. Med.* **100**, 573.

Wexler, B. C., Brown, T. E., and Miller, B. F. (1960). *Circulation Res.* **8**, 278.

Wilens, S. L., and Sproul, E. E. (1938a). *Am. J. Pathol.* **14**, 177.

Wilens, S. L., and Sproul, E. E. (1938b). *Am. J. Pathol.* **14**, 201.

Wilgram, G. F. (1958). *Proc. Soc. Exptl. Biol. Med.* **99**, 496.

Wilgram, G. F. (1959). *J. Exptl. Med.* **109**, 293.

Wilgram, G. F., and Ingle, D. J. (1959). *A.M.A. Arch. Pathol.* **68**, 690.

Wissler, R. W., Eilert, M. L., Schroeder, M. A., and Cohen, I. (1952). *Federation Proc.* **11**, 434.

Wissler, R. W., Frazier, L. E., Hughes, R. H., and Rasmussen, R. A. (1962). *A.M.A. Arch. Pathol.* **74**, 312.

Wolffe, J. B., Diglio, V. A., Dale, A. D., McGinnis, G. E., Donnelly, D. J., Plungian, M. B., Sprowls, J., James, F., Einhorn, C., and Werkheiser, G. (1949). *Am. Heart J.* **38**, 467.

Zinserling, W. D. (1932). *Beitr. Pathol. Anat. Allgem. Pathol.* **88**, 241.

—11—

Induction of Experimental Atherosclerosis in Various Animals

W. Stanley Hartroft and Wilbur A. Thomas

I. Introduction

Less than two decades ago the rabbit and chick were the only common laboratory animals in which atherosclerosis could be produced readily at will (Katz and Stamler, 1953). The rat was generally regarded as quite resistant to the lesion and was considered an "unsuitable" animal for this purpose. But the past two decades have witnessed remarkable changes in these concepts. For example, papers concerning the experimental production of atheroma in the rat published during that time now number in the hundreds. Another significant change in the approach of investigators to the problem has been the application of sophisticated nutritional techniques. Until the last decade, many experiments involved merely adding cholesterol supplements to commercially available pellets for rabbits or "starter mash" for chicks. Semisynthetic diets with control of total caloric intake are now commonly employed by students of atheroma in their experimental forays.

The investigator who wishes to produce atheroma experimentally now has the choice of a wide range of species, rather than the few mentioned above. In addition to rabbit (Anitschkow, 1933), chicken (Katz and Pick, 1961), and dog (Steiner and Kendall, 1946), or the now popular rat (Wissler et al., 1954; Fillios et al., 1956), atheroma in some form has been produced at will by many in a variety of species including mouse (Cuthbertson et al., 1960), guinea pig (Altschul, 1950), hamsters (Goldman and Pollak, 1949), domestic pig (Reiser et al., 1959), and monkey (Mann and Andrus, 1956; Cox et al., 1958; Taylor et al., 1959, 1962). The pigeon (Lofland et al., 1961) is now providing as much useful information as the chick or cockerel, and even the duck has proven of interest (Katz and Stamler, 1953). And working in the prairies of the Canadian West, Altschul (1961) has produced experimental atherosclerosis in prairie gophers (Citellus or Arctomys richardonii, Sabine).

The methods, first developed for the rabbit and chicken, with few exceptions hinge around the production of a sustained and usually relatively severe degree of hypercholesterolemia. Ranging from simple supplementation of a normal diet with 0.5 to 5.0% cholesterol for the rabbit and chicken to more complex regimens for the rat involving not only supplements of cholesterol but also of cholic acid, thiouracil, and high levels of dietary fats, the production of hypercholesterolemia of exogenous (dietary) origin is the most firmly established approach.

Presentation of an exhaustive review of the historical aspects of experimental atherosclerosis is beyond the scope of this chapter and the reader who desires such information is referred to other sources (Katz and Stamler, 1953). We intend to present herein a list of some of the experimental animals and methods that have been used and a summary of the lessons we believe have been learned over the years from work with experimental animals that may be pertinent to the atherosclerotic problem in man. In addition we shall present a more detailed discussion of some of the observations made in our own laboratories that we believe to be relevant.

II. Terminology

The word atherosclerosis has been used in this volume thus far largely to indicate an arterial disease occurring in man which is difficult to define in any widely accepted fashion except in rather general terms. However, regardless of the difficulties in making a precise definition, it is a useful term in that it brings to the minds of practically all knowledgeable observers of human lesions the same pathological process. Almost anyone can distinguish this process, at least in its more advanced stages in the systemic circulation, from other common disease processes that occur in the arteries of man.

Unfortunately the term atherosclerosis does not have the same usefulness when applied to arterial lesions that can be produced in experimental animals. The human disease begins in childhood and develops in an irregular and variable fashion throughout a lifetime. Experimental lesions are almost always produced over a period of a few months or at most over a year or two and are almost certain to have some differences from those developing over longer periods in man even if they represent otherwise the exact counterpart of the human disease.

Also a much broader spectrum of pathological processes has been produced in the arteries of experimental animals than is commonly encountered in man, many parts of which have some features that are common to human atherosclerosis and others that are not. It is usually impossible to be certain which process is a bona fide counterpart of the human disease and which is not. Thus with experimental animals one is faced with the choice of avoiding the term atherosclerosis althogether (since it seems that one can never be sure that one has the exact human counterpart) or using it to indicate only that a process has been produced with its most prominent characteristics similar to those of human atherosclerosis. In the reports of our own work in the past we have vacillated between these two choices. However, as our thinking has evolved we have gravitated toward the second as being the most practical definition. In this chapter the term will be used only in this second sense. It will not be used to imply of itself that the exact counterpart of the human disease has been produced although in subsequent words and statements we may suggest that we hold this opinion.

III. Some of the Animals and Methods That Have Been Used for Production of Atherosclerosis Associated with Exogenous Hypercholesterolemia

A. The Rabbit

In the rabbit atherosclerosis has been produced by simple addition of cholesterol to commercial pellets or natural foods (Anitschkow, 1933). This was the first successful method to be developed and has been used in literally thousands of experiments. Advantages include the fact that lesions are produced readily within a few weeks and the ease of handling the rabbits. Critics of the lesions point out that the "foam cell" is the most prominent component, the ascending aorta is more severely involved than the abdominal, and lesions almost never proceed to ulceration, calcification, and thrombosis (all in contrast to the lesions in man). Another disadvantage often mentioned is that the rabbit is by nature a strict vegetarian with a serum cholesterol level much lower than that of man while the levels associated with arterial lesions are far in excess of those usually seen in man. The rabbit has been used also for the production of pulmonary arterial lesions by intravenous injection of blood clots (Harrison, 1948).

B. The Chicken

In the chicken also atherosclerosis has been produced by simple addition of cholesterol to commercial mash or natural foods (Katz and Pick, 1961). Among the advantages cited are the rapidity with which lesions can be produced, the fact that the chicken is a natural omnivore, the observation that at least on rare occasion lesions may calcify and even "ulcerate." Disadvantages include the nonmammalian nature of the chicken and the fact that the lesions are much less prone to ulcerate and calcify than those of man, and that thrombosis almost never occurs.

C. The Rat

Atherosclerosis has been produced in the rat by adding cholesterol, bile salts, and thiouracil to semisynthetic diets otherwise meeting normal nutritional requirements (Wissler et al., 1954; Fillios et al., 1956). Addition of large amounts of fat (such as butterfat) is also helpful particularly if thrombosis is desired. Our own work with such diets will be summarized later in the chapter. Among the work of other investigators utilizing the rat, that of Gresham and Howard at Cambridge is outstanding (Gresham and Howard, 1960; Nutrition Review, 1963; Davidson et al., 1961). These workers have studied the effects of peanut oil and butter (when fed in combination with cholesterol, bile salts, and thiouracil) on atherogenesis and have found evidence suggesting that peanut oil results in a more proliferative type of arterial lesion than does butter.

The advantages of the rat include ease of handling large numbers, the wealth of other nutritional information that is available, the fact that the morphological features of the lesions are in the opinion of the authors of this chapter more similar to those of man (at least of the early stages in man) than those of most other experimental animals, and the fact that thrombosis can be produced with relative ease. Disadvantages include the complexity of the diets that are required, the metabolic differences between man and the rat (for instance, the rat's serum cholesterol is largely esterified with arachidonic acid while in man it is with linoleic), and the fact that with currently known techniques it has not been possible to produce lesions comparable to the advanced lesions seen in man. Also the serum cholesterol levels that seem to be required are far in excess of those ordinarily present in either man or rats.

D. The Dog

By adding cholesterol and thiouracil to commercial or semisynthetic diets atherosclerosis has been produced in dogs (Steiner and Kendall, 1946). Addition of butter and bile salts is also helpful (DiLuzio and O'Neal, 1962; Hartroft *et al.*, 1962). Among the advantages of the dog are his size (facilitating sequential blood studies for instance), the amount of physiological data available, and the fact that thrombi can be induced by diet. His size is also one of the disadvantages as is the complexity of diets required and his apparent resistance to development of advanced lesions.

E. The Pigeon

Atherosclerosis has been produced in the pigeon by adding cholesterol to commercial mash for certain species (Lofland *et al.*, 1961). Advantages include ease of inducing lesions, simplicity of diet, small size, and the fact that certain species react quite differently from others. Disadvantages are the same as those with the chicken.

F. The Monkey

In the monkey atherosclerosis has been produced by adding cholesterol and saturated fatty (or unsaturated) acids to the diet (Mann *et al.*, 1953; Mann and Andrus, 1956; Cox *et al.*, 1958; Taylor *et al.*, 1959, 1962). Advantages include the "over-all" similarity of the primate to man, the apparent similarity of the lesions to the early lesions of man, and the occasional development of advanced lesions with thrombi. Disadvantages include the difficulty of handling primates, the size of the animals which limits numbers, and the length of time required to develop significant lesions.

G. The Pig

Atherosclerosis has been produced in the pig by adding cholesterol and saturated (or unsaturated) fats (or even without cholesterol) (Reiser *et al.*, 1959). Advantages claimed include the similarity of the lesions to those of man and similarity of diets required to human diets. Disadvantages include the size of the animals and the quantity of food required.

H. Other Laboratory Animals

Almost all other laboratory animals have been used with varying degrees of success but none of these would appear, on the basis of currently available information, to have any superiority over those already mentioned.

IV. Some Methods Involving Supplements Other than Cholesterol or Deficiencies of Certain Dietary Factors

Hypervitaminosis D injures many organs other than the heart and vessels by inducing metastatic calcification (Duguid, 1930). In the aorta of rats, rings of medial calcification develop. The gross appearance has been aptly designated "bamboo aorta." If the process has any counterpart at all in man, it more nearly approaches that of Monckeberg sclerosis than atheroma. But changes in the intima overlying the portions of affected media are characterized by lipid infiltration, accumulation of small numbers of lipophages, and some hyalinization in late stages. When hypervitaminosis D has been combined with supplementation of the diet with cholesterol (Wilgram and Hartroft, 1955), the amount of abnormally deposited lipid in intima and subintimal layers is correspondingly greater, and the lesion approaches that of advanced atheroma of large vessels in man somewhat more. This model has been of use for studies of basic reactions of the artery to injury. Almost certainly, however, this approach has little further to yield about etiology and pathogenesis of atheroma in man as we conceive it at present.

Deficiencies of many vitamins and essential food factors have been suspected as playing a role in the production of atheroma, if not in man at least in some of the experimental forms, including the cholesterol-induced type. These theories have led to many attempts to protect vessels of animals from the effects of cholesterol-feeding by supplements of the vitamin under study. Essential fatty acids have received considerable attention and although interrelations between dietary supplements of cholesterol and the essential fatty acid requirement of chickens and miniature pigs have been shown (Hill *et al.,* 1957), even the large amounts of essential fatty acid contained in corn oil fed at a 40% level (by weight) in the diet of rats also given cholesterol have failed to protect the vessels. The tocopherols have received similar attention and have even been used clinically (without rational justification) to treat myocardial infarction.

Pyridoxine (B_6)-deficiency was discovered by Rinehart and Greenberg (1949) to produce rather striking lesions in the aortas and particularly the coronary arteries of monkeys. Changes in the latter consisted of proliferation of intima with accumulation in and beneath of hyaline-like material showing some of the characteristics of mucopolysaccharides. Stainable lipid (including cholesterol) was absent or minimal in these lesions even in rather large ones. It should be noted however that, compared to the average American diet, Rinehart and Greenberg's monkeys were on a low fat regimen, the amount being only 2% corn oil. It is interesting to speculate whether or not significant amounts of abnormal fat might have been deposited in these lesions had the animals received a quantity of fat in their diets more closely approximating that consumed by man. It is quite likely however that monkeys could not be trained to consume such an excessive amount (40% by calories) as the average American likes to take regularly.

Almost at the same time, two completely independent lines of investigation threw dietary choline into prominence in ways which at first appeared diametrically opposed. One of us (WSH) with a collaborator encountered lesions of coronary arteries and aortas in young rats fed high fat (lard), low choline diets for even relatively brief periods. The changes in the aorta resembled the "bamboo aortas" of hypervitaminosis D grossly, but microscopically, deposition of stainable fat in both intima and media was more prominent. Moreover pathogenic studies demonstrated that the abnormal fat desposits preceded medial calcification. In the coronary arteries of these rats, intimal proliferation and lipid infiltration (including cholesterol) were unaccompanied by medial calcification and to this extent resembled those of man more than did the aortic changes. These diets did not contain any added cholesterol, and serum cholesterol levels were not elevated compared to those of choline-supplemented controls. The latter, which were pair-fed exactly the same basal diet, were entirely protected from vascular changes by the lipotropic supplement (0.85-0.2% choline chloride). The mechanism by which choline deficiency produces vascular damage in these animals is still not understood but the renal damage frequently encountered in the same rats has been postulated by some as the pathway. Lehr and Churg (1952) produced vascular damage of a similar type by inducing renal damage. Nevertheless in any group of animals so studied, a small number in which vascular lesions can be found never exhibit renal damage (by light microscopy).

Shortly after this apparent role of choline deficiency, Wissler *et al.* (1954) reported the production of atheromatous-like lesions in arteries of rats fed diets containing more choline than normal (125 mg per day). His diets also contained 62.5 mg of cholesterol per day per rat. Under these conditions, only the animals consuming the diets containing both cholesterol and choline developed lesions. Their levels of blood cholesterol were also higher than in the rats not given the additional choline. thereby reflecting the cholesterol-elevating effect of choline when exogenous cholesterolemia is also induced. Lesions in the rats of Wissler *et al.* did not exhibit medial calcification of aortas and it is likely they are similar to those produced later by Fillios *et al.* (1956) with cholesterol, sodium cholate, and thiouracil. Choline, like sodium cholate and thiouracil, here served to intensify the hypercholesterolemia. High choline levels have also been shown under certain conditions (cholesterol supplements) to increase atheroma in chickens (Stamler *et al.,* 1950) and in monkeys (Mann *et al.,* 1953). It is an interesting paradox that a deficiency and an excess of the same essential food factor under suitable conditions can produce changes at least superficially similar.

Further complicating the picture was the later publication (Buckley and Hartroft, 1954) indicating that a similar level of dietary choline (0.85%) when added to a diet containing sufficient excess vitamin D to produce vascular lesions, completely protected the aortas of the treated group and reduced changes in coronary arteries to only an occasional animal. These diets contained no added cholesterol. There are several obvious experiments that might still be done to clarify these interrelationships between dietary cholesterol, dietary choline, and hypervitaminosis D, but to the writers' knowledge nothing new of recent years has been added. Newberne and Salmon (1961) reported confirmatory evidence of the development of coronary arterial changes in choline-deficient rats.

V. Discussion of Some of Our Own Observations of Atherosclerotic Lesions in Rats Associated with Thrombogenic Diets

In a series of reports over the period 1957-1959 (Hartroft and Thomas, 1957; O'Neal *et al.*, 1959; Thomas and Hartroft, 1959; Thomas and O'Neal, 1959) we presented results of studies of a practical dietary method for producing thrombosis and myocardial infarction in rats which was developed by us jointly with the assistance of our associates. The diets used by us (one of which is presented in Table I) were modifications of

TABLE I

INGREDIENTS OF ONE THROMBOGENIC DIET FOR RATS IN PERCENTAGES BY WEIGHT

Ingredient	Percentage
Butter	40.0
Cholesterol	5.0
Propylthiouracil	0.3
Sodium cholate	2.0
Sucrose	20.5
Casein	20.0
Alphacel	6.0
Vitamin mix[a]	2.0
Choline chloride	0.2
Salt mix[b]	4.0

[a] Each kilogram of the vitamin mixture contained the following, triturated in dextrose: vitamin A concentrate, 4.5 gm (200.000 units per gram); vitamin D concentrate, 0.25 gm (400,000 units per gram); α-tocopherol, 5.0 gm; ascorbic acid, 45.0 gm; inositol, 5.0 gm; menadione, 2.25 gm; P aminobenzoic acid, 5.0 gm; niacin, 4.5 gm; riboflavin, 1.0 gm; pyridoxine hydrochloride, 1.0 gm; thiamine hydrochloride, 1.0 gm; calcium pantothenate, 3.0 gm; biotin, 0.02 gm; folic acid, 0.09 gm.

[b] This salt mixture is the Wesson modification of Osborne and Mendel Salt Mixture [*Science* **75**, 339 (1932)]. The composition in per cent by weight is as follows: calcium carbonate, 21; copper sulfate ($5H_2O$), 0.039; ferric phosphate, 1.47; manganous sulfate (anhydrous), 0.02; magnesium sulfate (anhydrous), 9; potassium aluminum sulfate, 0.009; potassium chloride, 12; potassium dihydrogen phosphate, 31; potassium iodide, 0.005; sodium chloride, 10.5; sodium fluoride, 0.057; tricalcium phosphate, 14.9.

diets previously used by others (Wissler *et al.*, 1954; Fillios *et al.*, 1956) for the production of a mild form of atherosclerosis which on rare occasions (one rat in one laboratory and two in the other) were associated with thrombosis and infarction. We had previously developed diets for rabbits that seemed to modify thrombolytic activity (Thomas *et al.*, 1956, 1957; Scott and Thomas, 1957; Rabin *et al.*, 1957) and we postulated that by combining such diets with those shown to produce mild atherosclerosis in rats, we might produce more advanced atherosclerosis and

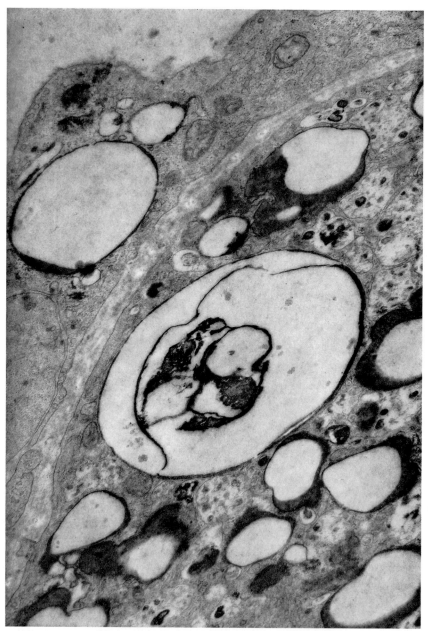

Fig. 1. A macrophage containing large amounts of osmiophilic material (a typical "foam cell") fills most of the photograph. It is in the intima of the aorta of a rat fed a diet containing butter, cholesterol, bile salts, thiouracil, and other ingredients

thrombosis. Unfortunately for the hypothesis, thrombi developed in many rats fed such diets in 3 to 5 months which was before the development of any more than the mildest stage of atherosclerosis. This observation seemed to indicate that the principal effect was on the blood itself and led to a series of studies which are still in progress on a variety of clotting characteristics in rats fed various diets for short periods (Tillman *et al.,* 1960; Scott *et al.,* 1961a, b; Thomas, 1961; Lee *et al.,* 1962, 1963a, b, c, d).

Only after our joint activities had ceased in 1959 did attention in our now separate laboratories return to any extent to the changes in the arterial walls. This bit of personal history is presented because the directions in thinking that were taken in our separate laboratories were quite different and represent respectively examples of what we believe to be two of the most important trends in experimental studies of atherosclerosis today.

In the laboratories of one of us (WSH in association with R. M. O'Neal, W. Still, and others) (O'Neal and Still, 1962; Still and O'Neal, 1962) rats were placed on a milder modification of the diet shown in Table I (thiouracil was omitted) which permitted the rats to live for longer periods of time. The rats were killed at intervals over a 12-month period on the diet and sections taken for light and electron microscopy. Atherosclerotic plaques were observed in many of the animals with thicknesses of the plaques corresponding to the very early stages of the disease in man. Although several cell types were observed in the plaques, the most significant one appeared to those of us involved in this study at St. Louis (WSH and associates) to be the "foam cell." Our observations led us to postulate that the foam cell came from the circulating blood and that it was a monocyte that had phagocytosed a large amount of lipid. We observed some foam cells that were situated partially within the intima and partially projecting into the lumen without endothelial covering. We postulated that this was the route of entry into the intima although we obviously could not be certain of the direction of movement. We found numerous foam cells in the circulating blood and the numbers corresponded in a general way to the extent of intimal disease.

(see Table I) for 14 months. The macrophage is separated from the lumen, which is in the upper left corner, by a thin cytoplasmic projection from an endothelial cell (which also contains lipid). Grossly the aorta had numerous atherosclerotic plaques, especially in the abdominal portions, which were as thick as or thicker than the remainder of the vessel wall. The number of foam cells varied considerably from plaque to plaque. In some they accounted for less than one-fourth of the total mass. In others, they were the predominant cell type. Lead hydroxide stained. Magnification: 24,000. (From Thomas *et al.,* 1963.)

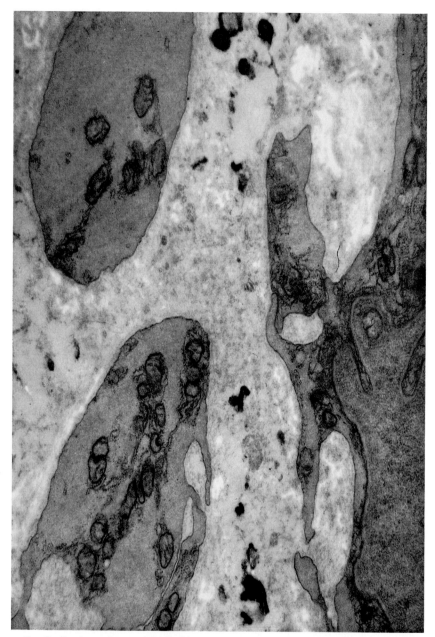

FIG. 2. Portions of several "primitive smooth muscle" cells are visible in an atherosclerotic plaque from the same rat as in Fig. I. This was the predominant cell type.
These cells are thought to be smooth muscle because they have heavy plasma mem-

On the basis of these observations we formulated the hypothesis that the atherosclerotic lesions in the rat developed as a result of macrophages migrating from the circulating blood into the arterial intima. This hypothesis seems to us to be on a sound enough basis to warrant further investigation in experimental animals and in man.

In the laboratories at Albany Medical College (WAT in association with K. T. Lee, R. F. Scott, F. Goodale, and others) studies of somewhat similar nature have been carried out but the hypotheses that have evolved and directions that are being taken are quite different. We also have fed rats for long periods on the thrombogenic diet of Table I with thiouracil omitted. In addition we have been able to get an occasional rat to live for long periods even when thiouracil was included. We too have observed foam cells but the most prominent cell type that we have seen has been a modified smooth muscle cell similar to that described by Movat *et al.,* 1958; and by Geer *et al.,* 1961 (and confirmed by us) in early human lesions. We have studied in great detail lesions from a rat (Fig. 1) that survived on the whole diet of Table I for 14 months developing plaques in the aorta that were in many places as thick or thicker than the media; illustrations from these studies are presented in the figures. Most of the changes observed in this rat have also been found in lesser degrees in rats fed for shorter periods on the same diet or for similar periods on the diet without the thiouracil (the effect of the thiouracil appearing to be principally on the quantitative and not the qualitative aspects). The lesions produced, in our opinion, correspond quite well to the early and moderately advanced atherosclerotic lesions of man (Figs. 2 and 3). The only important differences would appear to be greater medial involvement in the rat and more foam cells, but both are also present in human lesions. A detailed description and evaluation of these lesions are being presented elsewhere (Thomas *et al.,* 1963) and will not be repeated here. What we will present is the hypothesis we have drawn from our observations which is influencing the current course of our work and which represents one trend that is also being pursued in at least some other laboratories. We postulate that the diet has resulted in disturbance of the metabolism of the cells in the intima (injury) and that the response to the injury has been proliferation just as it is with most other types of intimal injury. The proliferation in the

branes, prominent pericytosis vesicles, and a cytoplasmic matrix resembling that of normal smooth muscle cells. However, their actual identity is of less interest than the fact that they are similar to cells that are prominent in early human atherosclerotic plaques. They are clearly different from the "foam cells" that have been the predominant cell type of most plaques produced in experimental animals in the past. Lead hydroxide stained. Magnification: 20,000. (From Thomas *et al.,* 1963.)

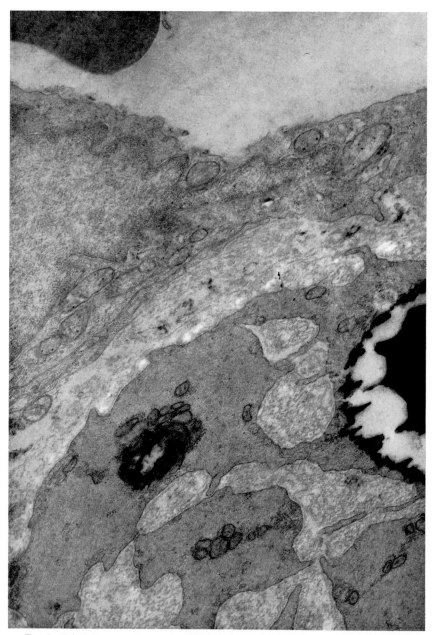

Fig. 3. Primitive smooth muscle cells are shown from another intimal plaque from the aorta of the same rat. The osmiophilic material in the smooth muscle is indistinguishable from that seen in smooth muscle cells of early human plaques. An endothelial cell separates the other cells from the lumen which is at the top. Lead hydroxide stained. Magnification: 18,000. (From Thomas et al., 1963.)

rat as in man has been largely of "modified" smooth muscle cells which are either capable themselves of producing collagen or which pass through a fibroblastic stage. Some of these cells and the endothelial cells accumulate lipid as a result of continued metabolic injury and eventually rupture with release of protein-bound lipid which accumulates in extracellular sites and is not easily removed. Macrophages enter from the circulating blood or tissue and carry out their role of scavengers just as in other situations and many of these become completely filled with lipid particles becoming the well known foam cells.

We have not as yet produced the advanced lesions of atherosclerosis in the rat with necrosis, ulceration, and thrombosis. However, the lesions observed in the early and moderately advanced stage resemble so closely those of man that it seems likely that they would progress to the advanced stage if followed over the entire life span of the rat instead of for the less than half life span that was studied even in our most prolonged experiment (14 months).

VI. Discussion of Ceroid and Other Topics

In studies of cirrhotic livers of choline-deficient rats, one of us (WSH) some years ago developed the hypothesis that whenever hemorrhage occurred into fatty tissues, polymerization of unsaturated fatty acids into the insoluble, sudanophilic pigment ceroid would almost certainly result. It appeared evident that this pigment should therefore be present in atheromatous lesions in man, and examination of coronary arteries and aortas of man proved that it was indeed present, often in large amounts (Hartroft, 1953). Because the same situation exists within thrombi (fatty acids of coagulated plasma mixed with red cells) examination of 100 occlusive thrombi in coronary arteries of man was also undertaken. Over half exhibited ceroid pigment mixed in and on platelet clumps and fibrin strands (Hartroft; unpublished), the material appearing orange to red in paraffin sections stained with oil red O. Current studies in our (WSH) laboratories in Toronto have established the presence of an intermediate form of pigment which stains with oil red O and although soluble in xylol, unlike normal fat it is insoluble in 90 and 95% ethyl alcohol. This form has been named preceroid (Hartroft, 1963) and will now be looked for in thrombi with little or no true ceroid. It is quite possible that formation of ceroid within a thrombus may well inhibit thrombolysis; in view of the present emphasis on unsaturated fats in the diet and the fact that they are the precursors of ceroid and preceroid this line of investigation will be pursued further.

Although a detailed discussion will not be included here, several provocative new lines of approach which have developed within the past year or two will be mentioned. Constantinides and his associates in British Columbia (1960) have reported the production of very striking lesions in rabbits fed cholesterol dietary supplements for brief periods alternated with others during which the animals were fed completely normal stock diets. This cyclic cholesterolemia resulted in lesions of the abdominal aorta which exhibited ulceration, calcification in the form of "egg-shelling," and the development of a truly atheromatous (atheroma-gruel) content. It is possible that the intervening periods relatively free of hypercholesterolemia permitted "healing" in the form of fibrosis and calcification. In any event, in the opinion of one of us (WSH), the resulting lesions resemble those of aortas in man more closely than any, to our knowledge, previously reported in animals.

A group in Chicago (Cohn *et al.*, 1961) showed that when chickens were permitted to nibble more or less constantly at a cholesterol-supplemented diet, they developed lower levels of cholesterol in the serum and less atherosclerosis than others fed the same amount and kind of food mixture in the form of meals where food intake was limited to a few hours a day. Similar studies have also been carried out in rats and rabbits.

No attempt has been made here to review the effects of hormonal imbalances on the development of atherosclerosis in animals (diabetes, administration of adrenal hormones, effects of sex hormones, etc.) although many reports have appeared over the years. The subject is a large one and can not be covered within a chapter in this volume.

X-irradiation of rats (Gold, 1961), implantation of wire coils to produce trauma (Friedman and Byers, 1961), and prolonged intra-aortic infusions of serotonin in dogs (Rossi *et al.*, 1961) are other interesting approaches to the production and study of arterial lesions all of which have some aspects of atheroma as seen in man. Truly, the student of atheromatosis today has a wide choice not only of species but also of methods for his purpose.

VII. Some of the Lessons Learned Over the Years from the Work of Many Investigators Concerned with Experimental Atherosclerosis

1. Arterial lesions in many respects resembling human atherosclerosis can be produced in animals by diet. The diets used successfully have usually contained large amounts of cholesterol although in all species

except the rabbit and the chicken adjuncts such as thiouracil have been found to be necessary in order to produce impressive lesions, at least in short-term experiments.

2. When an animal is fed cholesterol and then the arterial wall is damaged, lesions will be most severe at the site of damage. This phenomenon has been observed with many types of injury including such widely differing ones as trauma, bacterial infection, and medial necrosis produced by vitamin D overdosage.

3. The rapidity with which arterial lesions develop with cholesterol feeding is closely related to the levels in the blood with slow development with levels similar to those of man and more rapid development with extreme levels.

4. Species differ widely in their ability to handle cholesterol in the diet. Rats for example are highly resistant to the ill effects in contrast to rabbits which are particularly susceptible.

5. Cholesterol feeding alone apparently is not sufficient to produce the full spectrum of atherosclerotic disease with the complications that one observes in man. For example, only by using a variety of other dietary ingredients can thrombosis be produced.

6. Arterial lesions resembling human atherosclerosis can be produced by means other than dietary manipulation. For example, fibrous intimal plaques have been produced in pulmonary arteries by several investigators by intravenous injections of fibrin or whole blood clots.

7. The character of experimental arterial lesions can be influenced by hormones and by a wide variety of drugs.

8. Deficiencies of specific nutrients in the diet such as pyridoxine and (as described above) choline can influence the development of arterial lesions.

9. The roles of saturated and unsaturated fats appear to be different in the development of the spectrum of atherosclerotic disease. However, the precise mechanisms have not been entirely elucidated in experimental animals and the situation appears to be much more complex than it seemed to be a few years ago. For example, at least some evidence has been presented suggesting that diets containing butter are more "thrombogenic" than those containing corn or peanut oil but that corn and peanut oil are more "atherogenic."

VIII. Summary

It now appears that atheromatous lesions, in the sense the term has been used in this chapter, can be produced in almost all common laboratory animals and can be demonstrated as spontaneously occurring lesions in a number of wild and domesticated species (see preceding chapter). Old concepts that viewed atheroma as a unique characteristic of man or a laboratory curiosity that could be produced in only a few species have been completely demolished in the past decade. Studies in comparative pathology utilizing many different animals may provide valuable clues to both the etiology and the pathogenesis of the condition now that the tools are at hand. Those working in the field almost universally feel that important advances and new concepts are not far ahead of them.

REFERENCES

Altschul, R. (1950). *Am. Heart J.* **40**, 401.
Altschul, R. (1961). *Arch. Pathol. Anat. Physiol.* **334**, 25.
Anitschkow, N. (1933). *In* "Arteriosclerosis" (E. V. Cowdry, ed.), pp. 271-322.
Buckley, G., and Hartroft, W. S. (1954). *Am. J. Clin. Nutr.* **2**, 396.
Cohn, C., Pick, R., and Katz, L. N. (1961). *Circulation Res.* **9**, 139.
Constantinides, P., Booth, J., and Carlson, G. (1960). *Arch. Pathol.* **70**, 712.
Cox, G. E., Taylor, C. B., Cox, L. G., and Counts, M. A. (1958). *A.M.A. Arch. Pathol.* **66**, 32.
Cuthbertson, W. F., Elcoate, P. V., Ireland, D. M., Mills, D. C. B., and Shearley, P. (1960). *J. Endocrinol.* **21**, 45.
Davidson, E., Howard, A. N., and Gresham, G. A. (1961). *Brit. J. Exptl. Pathol.* **42**, 195.
DiLuzio, N. R., and O'Neal, R. M. (1962). *Exptl. Mol. Pathol.* **1**, 122.
Duguid, J. B. (1930). *J. Pathol. Bacteriol.* **33**, 697.
Fillios, L. C., Andrus, S. B., Mann, G. V., and Stare, F. J. (1956). *J. Exptl. Med.* **104**, 539.
Friedman, M., and Byers, S. O. (1961). *J. Clin. Invest.* **40**, 1139.
Geer, J. C., McGill, H. C., and Strong, J. P. (1961). *Am. J. Pathol.* **38**, 263.
Gold, H. (1961). *Arch. Pathol.* **71**, 268.
Goldman, J., and Pollak, O. J. (1949). *Am. Heart J.* **38**, 474.
Gresham, G. A., and Howard, A. N. (1960). *Brit. J. Exptl. Pathol.* **41**, 395.
Harrison, C. V. (1948). *J. Pathol. Bacteriol.* **60**, 289.
Hartroft, P. M., Suzuki, M., and O'Neal, R. M. (1962). *Exptl. Mol. Pathol.* **1**, 133.
Hartroft, W. S. (1953). *J. Gerontol.* **8**, 158.
Hartroft, W. S. (1963). *Federation Proc.* **22** (in press).
Hartroft, W. S., and Thomas, W. A. (1957). *J. Am. Med. Assoc.* **164**, 1899.
Hartroft, W. S., O'Neal, R. M., and Thomas, W. A. (1959). *Federation Proc.* **18**, Pt. II, 36.
Hill, E. G., Warmanen, E. L., Hayes, H., and Holman, R. T. (1957). *Proc. Soc. Exptl. Biol. Med.* **95**, 274.
Katz, L. N., and Pick, R. (1961). *J. Atherosclerosis Res.* **1**, 93.
Katz, L. N., and Stamler, J. (1953). "Experimental Atherosclerosis." C. C Thomas, Springfield, Illinois.
Lee, K. T., Scott, R. F., Kim, D. N., and Thomas, W. A. (1962). *Exptl. Mol. Pathol.* **1**, 151.
Lee, K. T., Kim, D. N., Milano, M., and Thomas, W. A. (1963a). *Exptl. Mol. Pathol.* (to be published).

Lee, K. T., Kim, D. N., Milano, M., and Thomas, W. A. (1963b). *Exptl. Mol. Pathol.* (to be published).

Lee, K. T., Kim, D. N., and Sherman, L. (1963c). *Exptl. Mol. Pathol.* (to be published).

Lee, K. T., Kim, D. N., and Sherman, L. (1963d). *Exptl. Mol. Pathol.* (to be published).

Lehr, D., and Churg, J. (1952). *J. Mt. Sinai Hosp. N. Y.* **19**, 106.

Lofland, H. B., Jr., Clarkson, T. B., and Goodman, H. O. (1961). *Circulation Res.* **9**, 919.

Mann, G. V., and Andrus, S. B. (1956). *J. Lab. Clin. Med.* **48**, 533.

Mann, G. V., Andrus, S. B., McNally, A., and Stare, F. J. (1953). *J. Exptl. Med.* **98**, 195.

Movat, H. Z., More, R. H., and Haust, M. D. (1958). *Am. J. Pathol.* **34**, 1023.

Newberne, P. M., and Salmon, W. P. (1961). *Federation Proc.* **20**, 90.

Nutrition Rev. (1963). **21**, 17.

O'Neal, R. M., and Still, W. J. S. (1962). *Federation Proc.* **21**, 12.

O'Neal, R. M., Thomas, W. A., and Hartroft, W. S. (1959). *Am. J. Cardiol.* **3**, 94.

Rabin, E. R., Thomas, W. A., Lee, K. T., Konikov, N., and Scott, R. F. (1957). *A.M.A. Arch. Pathol.* **64**, 75.

Reiser, R., Sorrels, M. F., and Williams, M. C. (1959). *Circulation Res.* **7**, 833.

Rienhart, J. F., and Greenberg, L. D. (1949). *Am. J. Pathol.* **25**, 481.

Rossi, P., Stevenson, M., Khaksar, P., and Bellet, S. (1961). *Circulation Res.* **9**, 436.

Scott, R. F., and Thomas, W. A. (1957). *Proc. Soc. Exptl. Biol. Med.* **96**, 24.

Scott, R. F., Alousi, K., Goodale, F., Gittelsohn, A., and Thomas, W. A. (1961a). *Arch. Pathol.* **71**, 714.

Scott, R. F., Alousi, K., and Thomas, W. A. (1961b). *Arch. Pathol.* **71**, 594.

Stamler, J., Bolene, C., Harris, R., and Katz, L. N. (1950). *Circulation* **2**, 714.

Steiner, A., and Kendall, F. E. (1946). *A.M.A. Arch. Pathol.* **42**, 433.

Still, W. J. S., and O'Neal, R. M. (1962). *Am. J. Pathol.* **40**, 21.

Taylor, C. B., Cox, G. E., Counts, M., and Yogi, N. (1959). *Am. J. Pathol.* **35**, 674.

Taylor, C. B., Cox, G. E., Manalo-Estrella, P., Southworth, J., Patton, D. E., and Cathcart, C. (1962). *Arch. Pathol.* **74**, 16.

Thomas, W. A. (1961). "Blood Platelets" (Johnson, Monto, Rebuck, and Horn, eds.), pp. 163-172. Little, Brown, Boston, Massachusetts.

Thomas, W. A., and Hartroft, W. S. (1959). *Circulation* **19**, 65.

Thomas, W. A., and O'Neal, R. M. (1959). *A.M.A. Arch. Pathol.* **68**, 461.

Thomas, W. A., O'Neal, R. M., and Lee, K. T. (1956). *A.M.A. Arch. Pathol.* **61**, 380.

Thomas, W. A., Konikov, N., O'Neal, R. M., and Lee, K. T. (1957). *A.M.A. Arch. Pathol.* **63**, 571.

Thomas, W. A., Hartroft, W. S., and O'Neal, R. M. (1959). *J. Nutr.* **69**, 325.

Thomas, W. A., Hartroft, W. S., and O'Neal, R. M. (1960). *A.M.A. Arch. Pathol.* **69**, 104.

Thomas, W. A., Jones, R., Scott, R. F., Goodale, F., Imai, H., and Morrison, E. (1963). *Exptl. Mol. Pathol.* (to be published).

Tillman, R. L., O'Neal, R. M., Thomas, W. A, and Hixon, B. B. (1960). *Circulation Res.* **8**, 423.

Wilgram, G. F., and Hartroft, W. S. (1955). *Brit. J. Exptl. Pathol.* **36**, 298.

Wissler, R. W., Eilert, M. L., Schroeder, M. A., and Cohen, L. (1954). *A.M.A. Arch. Pathol.* **57**, 333.

—12—

Enzymes of the Vascular Wall in Experimental Atherosclerosis in the Rabbit

T. Zemplényi, Z. Lojda, and O. Mrhová

I. Introduction*

A fundamental requirement of all living matter is that it must contain mechanisms to convert free energy of various chemical reactions into energy-requiring reactions of biosynthetic processes, of absorption and secretion, of mechanical or osmotic work, of active transport through membranes, and others.

There is ample evidence (also presented in other chapters of this book) to show that the arterial wall is a metabolically active living organ having its own equipment for synthesizing normal and abnormal tissue components and being capable of performing many anabolic and catabolic reactions. All such reactions are dependent upon the catalytic effects of enzymes, of enzyme systems linking energy-producing processes with energy-utilizing processes, of enzymes catalyzing basic reactions of glycolysis, of the citric acid cycle, and of other "mainstreams" of metabolism.

---

* For abbreviations used in this chapter, see page 508.

It must be stressed that the aim of investigating the enzymic structure of the arterial wall is to elucidate the relationship of the latter to spontaneous human atherosclerosis. Nevertheless, when trying to clarify general features of vascular metabolism and the nature of the regulatory factors governing this metabolism, when trying to elucidate the responses of the vascular wall to environmental changes, it is also very useful to perform investigations in animals where physiological and pathological situations can be more easily induced and relationships evaluated.

Before directing our attention to the main subject of this presentation some general notes on arterial metabolism must be made.

The oxygen consumption of arterial tissue has been repeatedly investigated. Well known are the respiration studies of Lazovskaya (1943) with rat-aorta homogenates and the studies of Briggs et al. (1949) showing that the aortas of rats are capable of oxidizing various substances of the glycolytic and citric acid cycle. The O_2 uptake of intact rat aortas was about one-tenth that of the liver.

In rabbits, Dury et al. (1957) found that the aortic arch revealed higher O_2 consumption than the other portions of the vessel. Fischer and Geller (1960) obtained similar findings and, in addition, cortisone administration, and renal hypertension (with or without cholesterol feeding) were accompanied by a significant elevation of O_2 consumption of all aortic segments. Simple cholesterol feeding of normotensive rabbits, however, resulted in a depression of O_2 consumption. Krčílek et al. (1961) reported on increased respiration utilizing a polarographic method (Šerák et al., 1961) for O_2 consumption while all the above results were obtained by the conventional Warburg technique. The results of Whereat (1961a, b) also gave similar results, showing the highest O_2 consumption (and highest lipid biosynthesis) in the aortic arch of the rabbit.

It seems to be well established that the aortic wall of the rabbit, as in other species, has a low but distinct oxygen consumption and is very much dependent on a satisfactory blood supply.

It is, however, a puzzling circumstance that the intrinsic blood supply and therefore the nourishment of the vascular system, having the important function of blood transport and distribution, is relatively poor. This applies chiefly to the inner layers of the arterial wall. Their metabolic situation is very similar to that of other organs with a low oxygen supply, such as the lens. At other places in this book more details on this subject and on arterial metabolism will be given. Nevertheless, for the purposes of this presentation it is pertinent to state that, similarly to the lens, arterial tissue reveals the phenomenon of "aerobic glycolysis."

This means that in contrast to most tissues, in the presence of oxygen there is only a slight depression of glycolysis, a relatively small decrease of pyruvate or lactate production. (In other words there is a lack of the Pasteur effect.) This seems to be important in this tissue as its rate of glycolysis is comparatively high and most of its metabolic energy is probably derived from carbohydrate. It will be, of course, important to know to what extent arterial tissue is able to utilize free fatty acids for its metabolic requirements.

Concerning the question of glycolysis, it was shown by Kirk *et al.* (1954) that the anaerobic glycolysis rates were only 30% higher in human and 27% higher in dog aortic tissue than the aerobic rate of glycolysis. The recent work of Fontaine *et al.* (1960) has given further support to the probable physiological significance of aerobic glycolysis. The latter authors found that in oxen, rabbit, and human aortas about three-quarters to four-fifths of the glucose is utilized by glycolysis and the remainder only by oxidation. Similarly to the lens (Mandel, 1956), out of 4 moles of glucose utilized, 3 give rise to lactic acid supplying only 2 moles of ATP per mole of glucose, instead of 39 moles of ATP provided by complete oxidation via the citric acid cycle. In addition, the ADP and ATP content of arterial tissue was found to be much lower than in other organs (Fontaine *et al.* 1960).

If the results of such *in vitro* studies are also applicable *in vivo,* they mean that the energy metabolism of the artery is, in comparison with other organs, very disadvantageous and "metabolic lesions" can be produced more easily than in other organs possessing a much higher rate of over-all energy metabolism connected with a better blood supply and nourishment.

II. Some General Remarks on Experimental Rabbit Atherosclerosis

The history of induction of experimental atherosclerosis had been reviewed in the book of Katz and Stamler (1953) and in the recent monograph of Myasnikow (1960) and Schettler (1961).

The detailed pathological picture of experimental rabbit athero-sclerosis is well known from the descriptions by Anitschkow (1913, 1933), Altschul (1950), Wolkoff (1929, 1930), Duff and McMillan (1951), Constantinides *et al.* (1960), and others.

Nevertheless, in the presentation of our own results on enzymes, especially from the histochemical point of view, reference will often be made to the morphological picture and, therefore, it is felt that it will be useful to summarize briefly the main morphological features of experimental rabbit atherosclerosis. Some brief comments concerning differences between human and experimetal rabbit atherosclerosis will also be given.

Grossly visible lesions are seldom to be seen before the end of the first month of cholesterol feeding. In the aorta they appear in the form of small, slightly raised, round or oval spots which are yellowish in color. The lesions are observed first of all in the aortic ring and arch. Afterward they grow large, become more prominent, their number increases, and they may also be found in the upper part of the thoracic aorta where they are localized on the posterior wall and between the ostia of the intercostal arteries. The lesions reveal a tendency to confluence so that large plaques oriented longitudinally are formed.

Toward the end of the fourth month the lesions are also seen in the caudal portion of the thoracic aorta. These lesions are usually smaller and not as severe. In rabbits on a cholesterol diet for a longer period of time irregular dilatations of the aorta and calcifications may also be found.

The lesions are best detected after the staining of the aortas with lipid soluble dyes.

The lesions can often be revealed, however, earlier under the microscope. The subendothelial ground substance becomes swollen and changes in mucopolysaccharides can be detected histochemically. Fine droplets of lipids, including cholesterol, may be demonstrated in those areas either extracellularly or in some macrophages (lipophages) which then enlarge and become typical foam cells. In endothelial cells fine lipid droplets are also found. In some initial lesions, branching, stellate, or elongated cells of the fibroblastic or muscular type laden with lipid droplets may be seen. Foam cells need not always be present. More often the fibroblastic type appears later.

As the lesions progress, the lipophages grow in size and become more numerous, and some smaller cells of monocytoid character can also be observed. In the deeper part of large lesions the cells undergo necrosis and their lipid content is released. If the cholesterol feeding lasts several months the superficial layer often reveals multiplications of fibroblasts so that a fibrocytic cap is formed. Some lesions reveal stratification, i.e., layers of fibrocytic cells, muscle cells, and foam cells alternate.

As far as the fibrillar ground substance is concerned, we observed only in the young lesions argyrophilic fibers surrounding foam cells. Collagen and elastic fibers appear in older lesions where a fibrous transformation occurs.

Some lesions are characterized by an amorphous material composed of a lipid mixture with a high content of cholesterol and covered with endothelium or with a fibrotic cap. In some lesions newly formed capillaries entering from the media can be demonstrated. Endothelium proliferation from the luminal surface also occurs in some places and may form small channels but this picture is not very common. In deeper areas of the older plaques calcareous deposits can be observed.

Concerning the changes in the media, the picture is variable. In some cases no apparent changes are seen. The internal elastic membrane is often swollen and small gaps may be found. With advancing severity of the intimal lesions, edema of the underlying media, lipid infiltration of the muscle cells, and degenerative changes in elastic membranes with degenerative fatty changes of the muscle cells and foam cells appear. In some places migration of macrophages can be found. Sometimes reorientation of the muscle cells with a picture resembling migration into the plaque can be observed. Focal necrosis of the media with calcification can also be found, but calcification may occur without apparent necrosis. Capillaries penetrating from the adventitia may be met rather often. In other places almost all elements of the media are replaced by foam cells.

The changes described in the aorta can also be seen in other arteries, especially in the coronary and pulmonary arteries, in small arteries elsewhere, and less frequently in the cerebral and renal arteries.

Constantinides *et al.* (1960) showed that rabbit cholesterol lesions could develop into changes more similar to those found in humans (with a thick collagen capsule, capillarized gruel, calcification, and secondary medial degeneration), if the animals, following a period of cholesterol feeding, were allowed to age on a normal diet for 2 years, or if they were exposed to intermittent hyperlipemia. In the latter case the same type of lesions could be observed in 10 months and in a few lesions hemorrhage, ulceration, and thrombosis were also found.

In view of the above findings of Constantinides it seems to be established that it is possible to induce in rabbits not only changes similar to fatty streaks, but also the more complicated lesions of human pathology. It is sound to compare such changes only to the advanced (chronic) lesions of human atherosclerosis. It is, however, important to realize that morphological similarity of lesions does not necessarily mean causal identity.

We wish to stress the fact that the detailed picture may differ under various experimental conditions and that even under identical conditions some variations may often occur.

All the described changes and variations must be taken into consideration if enzymic activities and their changes are described and evaluated (Lojda, 1961b).

There are also some other facts that have to be considered in this connection.

The intima of the human arteries is thicker and has a subendothelial fibrous and musculofibrous layer which grows thicker with advancing age ("physiosclerosis"). In rabbits such a distinct subendothelial layer is seen only exceptionally. Usually there is a very thin layer of amorphous ground substance between endothelium and inner elastic membrane and rarely some fibrocytes can be observed.

As the structure of the arteries is not identical the details of pathological processes are also more likely to be different. With this in mind we can summarize the differences between human and experimental rabbit atherosclerosis as follows:

a. In rabbits the arterial lesions are part of the universal cholesterol thesaurismosis. In humans this is encountered only exceptionally.

b. The distribution of the atherosclerotic changes is in rabbits slightly different from that in man. In rabbits the part of the aorta mainly affected is the arch, the ascending and upper thoracic aorta. Caudally the number and severity of the lesions decrease. In the human the most severe changes are encountered in the abdominal aorta, the proximal part being mainly affected only in syphilitic aortitis. The cerebral arteries are affected in the rabbit only rarely, whereas in the human they are rather frequently affected.

c. The microscopic appearance is also different. The fatty streaks in humans are similar in structure to the early lesions in rabbits. The older lesions of man are, however, more pleomorphic; exulceration, hemorrhage, and thrombosis—so common in humans—are only exceptionally (see Constantinides, 1961) observed in the rabbit.

Despite the above differences and evident limitations we believe that experimental rabbit atherosclerosis remains a useful model for studies concerned with the effect of increased fat intake upon the morphology and metabolism of the arterial wall and the relationships to atherosclerosis, especially in its early stages.

III. Methods Utilized in Studies of Enzymes of the Vascular Wall

Enzyme activity of the vascular wall can be assessed by biochemical and histochemical methods. In this chapter devoted to enzymes of the vascular wall in experimental rabbit atherosclerosis findings obtained by both approaches will be given.

All organs, including the arterial wall, are heterogeneous, being composed of different tissues. The cells of these tissues possess different metabolic activities. There are also various amounts of extracellular substances (ground substance, connective tissue fibers, etc.) where most of the enzyme activities studied are absent. Estimation of enzyme activities (in tissue homogenates, extracts, etc.) by biochemical techniques yields valuable quantitative data on the over-all activity of tissues, especially when due attention is given to the above aspects of extracellular material and calculations are based on the deoxyribonucleic acid (DNA) or soluble protein nitrogen content.

It is important, however, to realize, in accordance with Lehninger (1959), that variations in over-all measurements of metabolic reactions must ultimately be analyzed with respect to the part taken by individual cells.

We believe that the histochemical approach is often capable of fulfilling at least in part the above requirement and of giving valuable informations on enzyme activities at the cellular level. In addition, it enables us to study enzyme activities in tissues (e.g., organ vessels and capillaries) where biochemical techniques often meet with considerable difficulties.

This approach has, of course, its limitations as well, especially from the point of view of quantitative evaluation and the limited number of enzymes detectable by histochemical methods. In our experience careful comparative analysis of findings given by both approaches makes it possible to eliminate many of the inherent limitations of each of them and to obtain the most reliable results.

For our own experiments, we used animals and methods as follows: female albino rabbits about 5 months of age were fed, in addition to a standard laboratory diet, 1 gm of cholesterol dissolved in 10 gm of margarine daily. Control rabbits of the same strain, age, and sex were fed the standard laboratory diet. The duration of the experiment was 2 weeks (16 rabbits), 4 weeks (14 rabbits), and 10 weeks (18 rabbits); 19 rabbits of an additional series were handled in the same way as the rabbits of the 4-week series.

The animals were killed by a blow on the cervical vertebrae and blood removed by cardiac puncture for biochemical determinations.

Immediately after killing the animals the aortas were removed and carefully cleaned of periaortic tissue and practically of the whole adventitia with the exception of those parts which were destined for histological and histochemical study. After rinsing the aortas several times in ice-cold saline to remove all adherent blood, samples of 200 mg wet weight (combined from different parts of the vessel) were sliced on a freezing microtome to a thickness of 20-30 μ and afterward a 2% homogenate in ice-cold saline (adjusted to pH 7.0) was prepared using a Potter-Elvehjem glass homogenizer.

The homogenate was extracted with ice-cold saline for 2 hours, then centrifuged at 3000 rpm for 5 minutes, and the supernatant used for determinations of the activity of some enzymes.

In studies of dehydrogenase systems the preparation of aortic tissue was carried out in another way. Aorta samples of about 30 mg weight (combined from different parts of the vessel) were put into liquid nitrogen, immediately pulverized, and quantitatively transferred to test tubes. (The further steps will be given later, in connection with the individual enzymes.)

In addition to the above experimental groups, reference will also be made to previous experiments with rabbits fed during a period of 6 months and used for the determination of lipolytic (lipoproteinolytic) activity of aortas.

In this case the aortas were prepared for further work by finely mincing with scissors (Zemplényi and Grafnetter, 1958a, b).

The aortas of the other species mentioned in the following pages were prepared for enzyme activity determinations in the same way as the rabbit aortas.

The nitrogen content of the aorta extracts was determined by a conventional Kjehldal procedure. The protein content of the extracts was determined by the method described by Lowry *et al.* (1951).

Deoxyribonucleic acid determinations were carried out according to the method of Schneider (1945) and Ceriotti (1952).

Details of enzyme activity determinations will be given in Section IV of this chapter. A few words have to be said, however, concerning the techniques we used for dehydrogenase (system) activity estimations. Both the dye (neotetrazolium) reduction method and the spectrophotometric method were used, the latter only in LDH determinations.

There is general agreement that in the case of DPN-linked dehydrogenases the spectrophotometrically obtained changes in the amount of reduced or oxidized DPN are reliable measures of dehydrogenase activity. On the other hand the precise nature of the sites of tetrazolium reduction in the electron transport system is so far uncertain. As shown by Lester and Smith (1961) with beef heart mitochondrial preparations this reduction (by DPNH) is probably at or close to the site of the DPNH-linked dehydrogenase. But, according to the work of Nachlas *et al.* (1960) and especially in view of histochemical experience (Pearse, 1960; Lojda, 1961a), it seems highly probable that in cruder preparations, such as ours, more intermediate steps of the electron transport chain are involved between either DPNH (in DPN-linked dehydrogenases) or succinic dehydrogenase and the tetrazolium salt.

Our own experience with LDH determinations by both spectrophotometric and tetrazolium methods in aortas of different animal species and under the influence of vitamin D and catecholamines (Zemplényi *et al.,* 1961b; Zemplényi and Mrhová, 1962a) revealed in most instances parallel changes obtained by both techniques. Nevertheless, we believe it to be more exact to refer to dehydrogenase systems rather than to dehydrogenases when using simple tetrazolium salt methods.

Histochemical determinations of enzyme activity were performed with samples of aortas from the above experiments and, in addition, with aortas of a large number of experimental animals killed during a period of about 3 years (see Lojda and Zemplényi, 1958, 1960, 1961; Lojda and Felt, 1960; Reiniš *et al.,* 1962; Lojda, 1961b).

For histochemical studies aortas were prepared in various ways: some of them were cut transversely at various levels (ascending, arch, descending), others were cut longitudinally, being rolled on a polyethylene catheter of appropriate size. They were processed in two ways: either quickly frozen with dry ice and sectioned in the cryostat or fixed overnight in cold Baker's solution, washed in Holt's gum acacia sucrose solution, and embedded in glycerine gelatine. Afterward the blocks were cut with the freezing microtome.

With the cold microtome it was possible to obtain serial sections in which the reactions for enzymes were carried out. In addition, staining for lipids and mucopolysaccharides was also performed so that the mutual relationships between enzymes and those substances could conveniently be investigated.

Some samples were fixed in cold acetone and embedded in paraffin (Lojda, 1958b).

The heart was cut transversely in three segments which were processed alternately with all the procedures described above. The same applies to the other organs.

We used as well fixed sections for the demonstration of some enzymes because in such sections structural details are much better preserved and some enzyme activities are not too much reduced (Novikoff, 1959; Lojda, 1961a).

For enzyme activity detection we used, whenever possible, different

types of methods with different substrates and controls to exclude false
positive reactions and artifacts. The details of individual histochemical
procedures will also be given in the description of individual enzymes.

Grading of atherosclerotic lesions is very difficult. Planimetric measurement of the plaques is a very time consuming method and the
results are not much better than estimation by simple inspection. The
microscopic picture is not reflected here and, in addition, it is not quite
correct to judge the severity of the process by its extension only. Since
we could not stain our material with fat-soluble dyes (the material for
enzymic analysis must be worked up as soon as possible and the staining
could also interfere with enzymic activities), we determined the extent
of lesions only by rough estimation.

Our grading was as follows (see Fodor *et al.*, 1958):

1. Changes seen only microscopically (slight edema of the intima
with some lipids lying extracellularly between the endothelium and
the inner elastic membrane, single lipophages).

2. Changes apparent macroscopically as slight fatty streaks or spots.

3. Small single plaques in the aortic ring and/or arch and/or single
plaques in the thoracic aorta.

4. Larger plaques in the arch and ascending part of the aorta with
a tendency to confluence and single plaques in the descending part.

5. Large confluent plaques in the descending part of the aorta as
well.

IV. Enzymes of Normal and Atherosclerotic Vessels

The most convenient way to describe systematically enzymes of the
vascular wall is to follow—where possible—the well known basic metabolic cycles such as the glycolytic cycle, Krebs cycle, etc. (see Zemplényi,
1962). In this presentation, however, we decided for methodological
reasons (similarity of techniques used for enzyme activity detections), to
group the available data first of all according to the types of reactions
catalyzed (e.g., dehydrogenases, esterases, etc.). In addition to results
related to rabbit vessels, mention will also be made of findings in vessels
of other species and especially of pertinent findings of other authors in
human arteries. We hope, in this way, to make the picture more complete.

A. Dehydrogenases

Dehydrogenases are important enzymes of cell respiration. In general they catalyze the transfer of a pair of hydrogen atoms (electrons)

from appropriate substrates to other members of the electron transport chain. The passage of these electrons through a series of steps entails the stepwise liberation of energy. Dehydrogenases have, therefore, a key position in metabolic energy production.

In our own experiments we used the following techniques:

1. BIOCHEMICAL METHODS (see also Section III)

Neotetrazolium hydrochloride (NT) was used as an acceptor of electrons and the amount of diformazan formed after incubation was estimated photometrically. In all determinations the incubation vessels contained 1.5 ml of Krebs-Ringer phosphate buffer pH 7.4, 1.5 ml of the appropriate substrate (0.2 M solution of sodium lactate, succinate, malate, or α-glycerophosphate), 2 ml of 0.5% NT and the aortic powder prepared by means of liquid nitrogen as described in Section III. In LDH, MDH, and AGPDH system activity determinations 0.5 ml of DPN $(2 \times 10^{-3} \ M$ freshly prepared) and 0.5 ml of 0.1 M NaCN was also added. Following incubation (45 minutes at 38°C) and centrifugation (3000 rpm for 5 minutes) the diformazan was extracted by means of 2×5 ml redistilled acetone for 20 hours. The amount of diformazan was estimated at 470 mμ and calculations were performed on the basis of the DNA content of aliquot samples of the same aorta.

In some experiments LDH activity was also determined spectrophotometrically using a Boehringer TC-G test. In these determinations extracts of aortic homogenates were used as the sources of enzyme activities. The activity was expressed in Wroblewski units in the latter experiments, while in experiments utilizing NT the activity was expressed in μg of diformazan per 100 μg of DNA.

2. HISTOCHEMICAL METHODS

SDH activity was determined by the method of Nachlas *et al.* (1957b). In some cases phenazine methosulfate and/or menadione were added to the incubation mixture. Control tests were performed by incubating sections without succinate. DPN- and TPN-tetrazolium reductases were detected by the slightly modified method of Scarpelli *et al.* (1958) using DPNH or TPNH as substrates and NBT as electron acceptor. In some cases MTT with cobalt chelation was used. The LDH, MDH, AGPDH, BHBDH, G6PDH, ICDH, GDH, and alcohol dehydrogenase systems were detected according to Hess *et al.* (1958), but NBT was used in all cases as the electron acceptor. In addition, sometimes other tetrazolium salts were also used (see Lojda and Zemplényi, 1958, 1961; Lojda, 1961b).

The detection of all the above enzymes was performed in unfixed

cryostat sections adherent to slides. For the detection of DPN tetrazolium reductase and LDH free floating frozen sections from cold formol
fixed organs were used (see Lojda, 1961a for details). Incubations were
carried out at 37°C for 30-60 minutes.

Our results using biochemical methods are shown in text Fig. 1

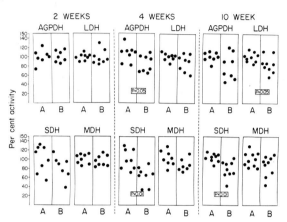

TEXT FIG. 1. The activities of some dehydrogenase systems in the aortas of
cholesterol-fat fed rabbits. A = Control rabbits. B = Cholesterol-fat fed rabbits. (For
other abbreviations see p. 508.) Average activities of aortas in control animals:
AGPDH system, 62.5 μg diformazan per 45 minutes per 100 μg DNA. LDH system,
107.5 μg diformazan per 45 minutes per 100 μg DNA. SDH system, 68.5 μg diformazan per 45 minutes per 100 μg DNA. MDH system, 53.5 μg diformazan per 45
minutes per 100 μg DNA.

which demonstrates that the activity of the AGPDH system was found
in 4 cases of the 4-week feeding experiment and in 4 cases of the 10-
week feeding experiment to be decreased as compared to the aortas of
control animals. Statistical analysis, however, revealed a borderline
significance (P < 0.05) only in the former group of animals, suggesting
that a lack of similar finding in the 10-week feeding experiment was
probably caused by the larger variation of results (45-120%). Similar
results were obtained in the determination of LDH activity. In this
case, however, statistical analysis showed a significant difference only
in the 10-week experiment. In view of the above results of borderline
significance it seems to be sound only to state that there is a *tendency*
toward decrease of activity of these enzyme systems in the aortas from
both feeding experiments of a longer duration, while the 2-week experiment did not change the activity of either system.

The study of two enzymes of the citric acid cycle revealed a significant
decrease (P < 0.01) of the aortic SDH system in both the 4-week and

the 10-week experiments. The activity of the MDH system was not changed significantly in either of the experimental series (Zemplényi *et al.*, 1962; Mrhová *et al.*, 1963a).

In normal rabbit aortas the activity of LDH system was found to be about 90% higher than the activity of the other dehydrogenase systems studied.

Estimations of LDH activity by the spectrophotometric method revealed an average activity of 1630 Wroblewski units per 100 μg of aorta extract nitrogen in the 2-week and 4-week series of control animals. No change in activity of aortas of the experimental animals in these series was found. This is in agreement with the above findings using the tetrazolium method for LDH system activity determination. Unfortunately, no data are available using this method for the 10-week experimental series.

Our histochemical findings in the aortas of normal and cholesterol-fat fed rabbits confirmed and extended our previous results (Lojda and Zemplényi, 1958, 1960, 1961; Lojda and Felt, 1960; Lojda, 1961b).

In the arterial wall of the normal rabbit all the fundamental dehydrogenase systems could be detected. Their activity was found to be confined to the muscle cells of the media and to a varying degree also to the vascular endothelium. The activity of the cellular elements in the adventitia was also variable. It was usually not so strong as the corresponding activity in the media. DPND and LDH revealed the highest activity while the activity of TPND was lower. The endothelium and the muscle cells of the media contained the following dehydrogenases (in order of decreasing activity): LDH (Fig. 1), MDH, ICDH (TPN-linked), AGPDH, G6PDH, BHBDH, and GDH. The activity of the latter was very low and it could sometimes not be distinguished from the activity of the "nothing dehydrogenase." With alcohol as the substrate we also failed to show any discernible activity. The histochemically detectable activity of SDH was found to be low in the same elements. The incubation time was shortened if the medium was supplemented with phenazine methosulfate. The highest staining intensity was observed if menadione was added to the incubation mixture. In this case the blank was also higher, showing that menadione was reduced by other substances as well.

Intracellular localization was the same regardless of the substrate used. This is due to the fact that in the case of the DPN- or TPN-linked dehydrogenases the methods used reveal the corresponding tetrazolium reductases (diaphorases) which are common for all DPN-linked and/or TPN-linked dehydrogenases (see Novikoff, 1960b; Lojda, 1961a). The

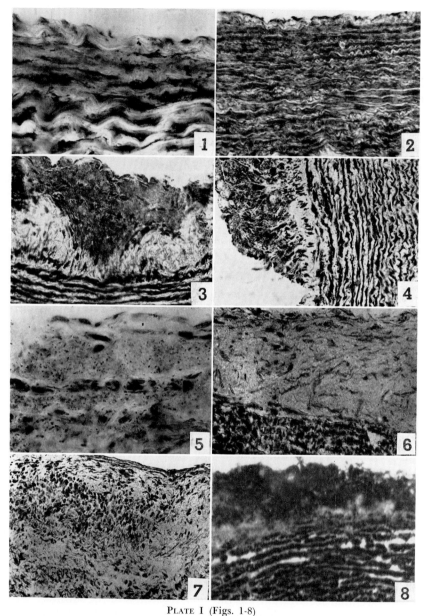

PLATE I (Figs. 1-8)

FIG. 1. LDH in normal rabbit aorta. Intima at top. Note positive reaction (black) in the endothelium and the stronger reacting muscle cells of the media. FF, NBT. Magnification: × 431.

FIGS. 2-8. LDH in atherosclerotic rabbit aortas. Note varying degree of positivity in the changed intima.

positive sites appeared as granules or short filaments resembling mitochondria.

The staining intensity of the muscle cells was found to be usually higher than or equal to the activity of the endothelium. In some cases, however, the activity of the endothelium exceeded that of the muscle cells (LDH, G6PDH, and especially ICDH in the pulmonary arteries—see Fig. 17 on Plate III). It is interesting that the staining reaction of the muscle cells of the media in the intramural intestinal arteries is higher than that of the muscle cells of the external layer of the intestine (Lojda, 1961b).

In the coronary arteries (similar to the arteries of other organs) the intensity of the reaction for dehydrogenase systems is higher than in the aorta. The corresponding reactions in the coronary arteries are, however, usually lower than in the myocardial fibers. The ratio of staining intensities of the myocardium and arterial wall shows differences with the individual dehydrogenase systems, being the highest in the case of SDH (see Figs. 14, 15, 16 on Plate II).

In the aortas of rabbits following 4-week cholesterol-fat feeding a slight decrease in staining for SDH was sometimes observed. Concerning the other dehydrogenase systems neither their activity nor their localization were at this stage apparently changed. We observed some irregularities in the staining of muscle cells and vascular endothelium

---

Fig. 2. Early stage. Intensified LDH reaction in the endothelium. FF, NBT. Magnification: × 140.

Fig. 3. Plaque with prevailing lipophages. Necrobiotic changes in the deeper parts. Strong LDH reaction in the endothelium, macrophages, and muscle cells; weaker reaction in larger lipophages; necrobiotic areas practically devoid of activity. FF, NBT. Magnification: × 140.

Fig. 4. The same as in the previous figure. (Intima to the left.) Note strong LDH reaction of muscle cells in the deeper parts of the plaques at the intimo-medial junction. Reaction in the media without apparent changes. FF, NBT. Magnification: × 126.

Fig. 5. Higher magnification of a plaque with apparent stratification. Positive LDH reaction in the endothelium and monocytoid cells. Coarse, probably artificial, formazan particles in areas occupied by larger lipophages. FF, NBT. Magnification: × 441.

Fig. 6. Late stage. Plaque with prevailing fibrocytes. In comparison with Figs. 3 and 4 the over-all LDH activity is of a lesser degree. Fibrocytes reveal a weak but distinct positive reaction. FF, NBT. Magnification: × 140.

Fig. 7. Late stage. Strong LDH reaction in the endothelium, monocytoid cells (macrophages), and muscle cells; a weaker reaction in larger lipophages and fibrocytes. FF, NBT. Magnification: × 91.

Fig. 8. Plaque with prevailing lipophages. Very strong over-all LDH activity of the plaque. A more precise localization cannot be determined. Strong reaction of muscle cells in the media. OF, NBT. Magnification: × 140.

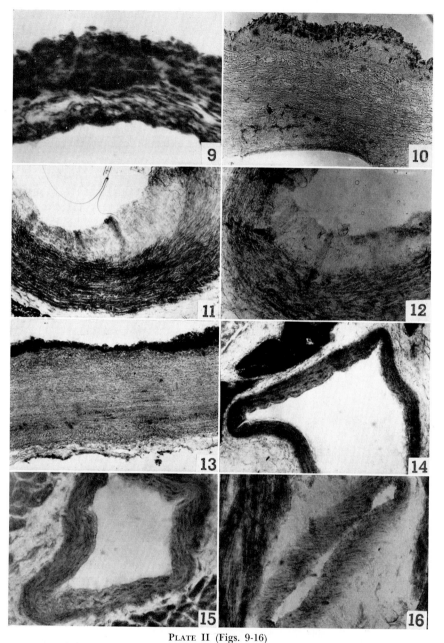

PLATE II (Figs. 9-16)

Fig. 9. LDH reaction in a plaque of the semilunar valve. Strong positivity in lipophages, somewhat weaker reaction in endothelium and fibrocytes. OF, NBT. Magnification: × 140.

but it was very difficult to evaluate them in the sections where these structures might be damaged.

With the appearance of the first lesions the changes in staining reactions become more apparent. The endothelium covering the initial lesions showed usually (but not always) a more intense reaction than the endothelium of the unaffected parts. This applies to all DPN- and TPN-linked dehydrogenases (Fig. 2 on Plate I). With succinic dehydrogenase the changes were not so marked.

The over-all intensity of the reactions in the plaques revealed very marked differences according to the cellular composition of the plaques (see Figs. 3-13 on Plates I and II). Macrophages and smaller lipophages reacted very strongly (Figs. 8 on Plate I and 9, 10, 13 on Plate II). With increasing size and increasing amount of histochemically detectable cholesterol, however, the intensity of the reaction decreased. In large foam cells with pycnotic nuclei occasional formazan particles could be seen on the surface of the lipid droplets (Fig. 5). Often no reaction could be observed at all. A very intense reaction was also encountered in some elongated cells (young fibroblasts, intermediate cells—Fig. 7) and starlike cells in which fat droplets could be demonstrated. Muscle cells also reacted very strongly (Fig. 4). In fibrocytes the degree of staining was lower (Fig. 6).

From the above findings it follows that initial plaques with predominating macrophages show a very strong over-all activity. In some small

---

FIG. 10. ICDH in an atheromatous rabbit aorta. Strong reaction in the endothelium and macrophages of the plaque. Weak staining of the muscle cells of the media. Similarly as with AGPDH in Fig. 13, the over-all activity of the plaque exceeds that of the muscle cells of the media. OF, NBT. Magnification: $\times$ 56.

FIG. 11. MDH in an atheromatous rabbit aorta. Weak reaction in the cells of the plaque, strong reaction in the muscle cells of the media. In comparison with the BHBDH (Fig. 12) the activity is higher. OF, NBT. Magnification: $\times$ 56.

FIG. 12. BHBDH in the same specimen as in the preceding figure. Almost negative reaction in the cells of the large plaque, positive reaction in muscle cells of the media. OF, NBT. Magnification: $\times$ 56.

FIG. 13. AGPDH in a smaller plaque of a rabbit aorta. Strong over-all activity of the plaque, weak reaction in the muscle cells of the media. OF, NBT. Magnification: $\times$ 56.

FIG. 14. SDH in a normal rabbit coronary artery. Positive reaction in the endothelium and muscle cells of the media. The over-all reaction is much weaker than in myocardial fibers (top left). OF, NBT. Magnification: $\times$ 140.

FIG. 15. BHBDH in a normal rabbit coronary artery. Positive reaction in the endothelium and muscle cells of the media. The staining intensity of the myocardial fibers somewhat exceeds that of the vascular wall. OF, NBT. Magnification: $\times$ 140.

FIG. 16. ICDH in a normal rabbit coronary artery. Positive reaction in the muscle cells of the media. Stronger staining in the myocardial fibers. OF, NBT. Magnification: $\times$ 140.

plaques with predominating fibrocytes the reaction is weak. In plaques with necrobiotic changes the over-all activity is low. In plaques composed of amorphous lipid masses we could not detect activity anywhere with the exception of the endothelium. Fibrous parts of older plaques were also void of a detectable reaction. Only fibrocytes showed scarce faintly positive staining.

In the underlying media the intensity of reaction was often without apparent changes but in some muscle cells it was changed (decreased or sometimes increased). In sites with calcification the reaction was lacking.

Between individual dehydrogenases differences in staining intensities could be observed in the cells of the plaques and in the muscle cells of the media, which were not always parallel to those found in the normal vascular wall. The reaction for DPND and LDH revealed the highest intensity. The intensity of the reaction for AGPDH was usually between that of MDH and BHBDH. Among the TPN-linked dehydrogenase systems the reaction for ICDH was higher than that for G6PDH. The mutual comparison of staining intensities of plaques and of the media is very instructive and can be seen in Figs. 3, 4, 6, 8, on Plate I and 10-13 on Plate II, which show clearly that the staining intensity of the cellular elements of the smaller plaques (mostly young lipophages) exceeds that of the muscle cells of the media in AGPDH (Fig. 13), ICDH (Fig. 10), and—to a lesser degree—in LDH (Fig. 8). In other dehydrogenase reactions the differences were not of such a degree. The reaction for SDH was relatively weak.

Similar changes in the reactions for dehydrogenase systems were also observed in the plaques of the larger branches of coronary arteries. In rabbits fed cholesterol for a longer period (Reiniš et al., 1962) plaques almost occluding the lumen of smaller branches and composed of larger lipophages with necrobiotic changes could be observed. The muscular elements of the media were seen in some places in such arteries. In most places they were replaced by foam cells. In the affected coronaries the endothelium revealed reactions for all dehydrogenases studied and these reactions were usually higher than the corresponding activities of the normal vessel (Figs. 19, 20, 21, 23 on Plate III). In the plaque itself a positive reaction could rarely be observed (Figs. 18, 19, 21-23 on Plate III).

The reaction in the media was variable. In the places where muscle cells were well preserved no apparent changes were encountered. At sites with degenerative changes the reaction was weakened (Fig. 20 on Plate III). (This was quite the opposite of the reaction for phosphomonoesterase II which was higher at these sites; see Section IV, B, 2, a).

The biochemical data presented here suggest that cholesterol-fat feeding in rabbits is associated with impairment of electron transport in the aortas as early as 4 weeks after starting the experiment. Changes in the activity of the SDH system seem especially to be impressive. It is interesting that at this stage of the experiment no morphological changes are to be seen in the aortas of the fed animals although the serum cholesterol levels are high (average 912 mg/100 ml) and in most instances liver steatosis is quite unequivocal.

Our findings are generally in agreement with data obtained by other authors in rat aortas (Kittinger *et al.*, 1960, 1961), and in human arteries (see Chapter 3 by Kirk).

Interestingly enough, only very few indirect biochemical data are available on succinic dehydrogenase activity of aortas and they simply show the presence of such an activity in the vessel wall without any information on changes in atherosclerotic vessels (see Kirk and Laursen, 1955; Kirk *et al.*, 1955; Maier and Haimovici, 1957). According to Malinow *et al.* (1962) gonadectomy in rats of both sexes stimulates the activity of the aortic SDH system.

From all the above studies and those described by Kirk, lacking homogeneity as they do, one gets the same impression as in our findings, that there is a decrease of some dehydrogenase activities in atherosclerotic vessels. We found such decreases in very early stages of cholesterol feeding and it is possible, in accordance with Hueper's theory (1944, 1945) that a metabolic lesion of the arterial wall, resulting from the formation of a lipid film on the intimal surface, is a prerequisite for later atheromatous changes to develop in the arteries of such animals.

Our histochemical findings were confirmed by Fouquet (1961). The histochemically detected activities of the dehydrogenases (systems) are in rough correlation with activities found biochemically, the highest activity being that of LDH.

The biochemically determined differences in the over-all activity of aortas from normal rabbits and from rabbits fed for a short period with cholesterol are too low to be observed under the microscope by the naked eye. At this stage no differences in enzyme localization could be found.

As soon as micro- and macroscopic changes (streaks and plaques) can be detected, a focal increase of staining reactions for most dehydrogenases, confined to the endothelium and young lipophages, becomes apparent. It must be underlined that the mean activity of the plaque is dependent upon its structure (see Figs. 3-13 on Plates I and II). This focal increase of activity develops in a "terrain" with decreased over-all dehydrogenase activity (see above) and, therefore, it is obviously not high enough to influence the over-all activity of the vessel wall. (As shown above the mean activity of larger plaques is decreased.)

It must be added that in our experience the changed permeability of the atherosclerotic vessel itself does not seem to be a factor if the detection of enzymes is performed in thin cold microtome sections such as ours.

Finally, it is interesting that the over-all dehydrogenase activity of the coronaries (at least in the rabbit), detected histochemically, is unequivocally higher than that of the aorta.

B. Enzymes Hydrolyzing Ester Links

These enzymes can be grouped into carboxylic esterases, phosphoesterases, sulfatases, thiolesterases, and phenolic esterases. So far only the first two groups have been extensively investigated in the vascular wall. Phenylsulfatase activity was observed by Kirk and Dyrbye (1956) to be decreased in arteriosclerotic aortas of older individuals. The histochemical findings of Fouquet (1961) indicate an enhanced sulfatase activity in atheromatous rabbit aortae.

1. Group-Specific Carboxylic Esterases

Carboxylic esterases are enzymes of comparatively low specificity. They hydrolyze a large number of different esters, though not all at the same rate. Differentiation into aliesterases (or simply *esterases,* their substrates being aliphatic esters of low molecular weight) and *lipases* is on a quantitative rather than on a qualitative basis: some of them are of a lipase character acting rapidly on triglycerides and slowly on other esters while the behavior of the others is quite the opposite.

a. Let us begin with an interesting enzyme of this group, the enzyme of the *clearing factor* or so-called *lipoprotein lipase* which seems to be associated with the removal of chylomicra from the plasma.

In our own experiments (in cooperation with D. Grafnetter) the *lipolytic (lipoproteinolytic) activity* of tissues was estimated by a method consisting of incubation of lipemic human serum, diluted 1:1 with Sörensen phosphate buffer pH 7.35, with a weighed amount of minced tissue or homogenate. In some more recent experiments activated Ediol or rat chyle (in a 3% solution of beef albumin and glucose in a final concentration of 120 mg/100 ml) were also used. Incubation was carried out for 150 minutes (in later experiments only 90 mintes) in a water bath at 37°C under steady agitation of the mixture.

The amount of free fatty acids (FFA) liberated was estimated by the method of Dole (1956) modified by using Nile blue as an indicator.

The extent of lipolysis was determined by the difference between the final and the initial concentrations of FFA in the incubation mixture. Enzyme activity was expressed either in milli-equivalents of FFA liberated per liter per gram of tissue or in μmoles of FFA released per gram of tissue (for further details see Zemplényi and Grafnetter, 1958a, b; 1959a, b).

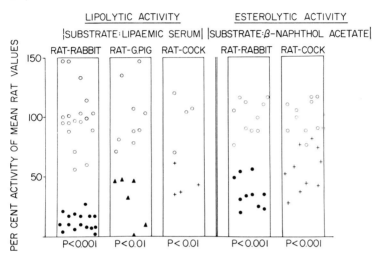

Text Fig. 2. Aortic lipolytic and esterolytic activity in various animal species. Esterolytic activity estimated in ammonia extracts of butanol acetone dried powder. (Partly reproduced from Zemplényi and Grafnetter, 1958b.)

With this technique we first investigated whether there is a difference in the lipolytic activity of the aorta of different animal species susceptible to experimental atherosclerosis, as compared with the rat which is relatively resistant (Zemplényi and Grafnetter, 1958a, b).

Text Fig. 2 presents the results of studies in which the activity of the aortas of some animal species was compared with the activity of rat aortas. Each value was obtained from a different animal. From the data it appears clear that the rat aorta has a high lipolytic activity as compared with the rabbit aorta (P < 0.001). The difference in the activity in guinea pig (P < 0.001) and cock aortas (P < 0.01) as compared with the activity of rat aortas is also unequivocal. It is important that differences in the DNA content of the aortas between these species are very small (Zemplényi *et al.*, 1961b). It is, therefore, highly improbable that the differences in lipolytic activity are caused by differences in extracellular fractions of the aortic walls.

Another problem was the relationship of lipolytic activity to the age of the animal. We compared the lipolytic activity of aortas of male rats of different age groups in which the average activity of 7-month-old rats, i.e., adult but not old rats, was taken as 100 per cent (Zemplenyi and Grafnetter, 1959b). We found that the lipolytic activity of 24-month-old rats is significantly lower than the activity of 7-month-old animals

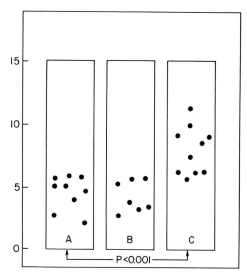

TEXT FIG. 3. Lipolytic activity of atherosclerotic rabbit aortas. A= Control animals. B = Animals with degree of atherosclerotic alterations 0-2.5. C = Animals with degree of atherosclerotic alterations 3.0-5. (Reproduced from Zemplényi and Grafnetter, 1959a.)

(P < 0.02). The decrease in activity in 12-month-old animals was of only borderline significance. The lipolytic activity of aortas of quite young rats was significantly low when compared with adult rats (P < 0.001). Estimations of the dry substance and the nitrogen content in the aortas did not reveal any differences between different age groups.

In this connection findings reported by Dury (1961) are instructive. Using our technique (but with Ediol as substrate) he showed that heparin injection of young rats resulted in increase of the lipolytic activity of aortas. In old rats no such effect could be observed.

In further experiments changes in lipolytic activity of the aortas of rabbits fed a cholesterol-fat diet for 6 months were investigated (see Section III). Text Fig. 3 shows significant differences in activity (expressed in wet weight) between controls and experimental animals with grade 3-5 atherosclerosis, while the differences compared to animals with moderate grades of atherosclerosis were not significant. Text Fig. 4

indicates the relationship between the degree of atherosclerosis and the lipolytic activity of the aorta expressed on a fat-free dry weight basis. It is obvious that there is a close linear relationship between the two values, expressed by the high value of the calculated coefficient of correlation, with the probable error smaller than 0.001. The relationship

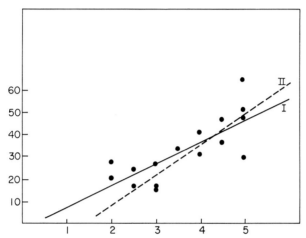

TEXT FIG. 4. Correlation of lipolytic activity of aorta (fat-free dry weight basis) with degree of atherosclerotic changes. Regression line I (for degree of atherosclerotic changes 0-5): Y = —3.48 + 9.93 X, r = 0.7842, P < 0.001. Regression line II (for degree of atherosclerotic alterations 3-5) Y = — 18.7 + 13.42 X, r = 0.7902, P < 0.01. (Reproduced from Zemplényi and Grafnetter, 1959a.)

becomes even closer after excluding mild degrees of atherosclerosis, i.e., up to 3 according to our evaluation. The results are basically equal when the lipolytic activity is calculated on a wet or dry weight basis (Zemplényi and Grafnetter, 1959a).

A few words have to be said on the enzymic properties of the lipolytic activity determined in the above way. It was shown (Grafnetter and Zemplényi, 1959, 1961, 1962) that in the presence of typical concentrations of protamine sulfate, NaCl, Ca++, Mg++ and Na glycocholate, the inhibition is practically identical when lipemic serum is incubated with myocardial tissue or with post-heparin plasma and that it is equally low in the presence of quinine sulfate and NaF. On the other hand the lipolytic activity of liver tissue is inhibited only slightly by protamine sulfate or glycocholate suggesting that in the latter case no lipoprotein lipase is involved. In the case of aortic tissue there is only partial inhibition with protamine sulfate and 1 M NaCl (Zemplényi et al., 1961a) suggesting that other esterases, less affected by these inhibitors, are also present in the aortic wall.

The latter could be proved not only qualitatively and quantitatively by our histochemical investigations (see below) but also quantitatively by biochemical techniques.

b. *The* ("nonspecific") *esterase activity* of aortas was determined as follows: 10 mg of β-naphthol acetate was dissolved in 2 ml of acetone and transferred into a swirling mixture of 20 ml veronal buffer pH 7.4 and water (final volume 100 ml) as described by Seligman *et al.* (1949). This solution served as substrate and the incubation vessels contained 2.5 ml of the freshly prepared substrate, 0.5 ml of tissue extract (see Section III), and 1.5 ml of water or of a $10^{-6} M$ solution of physostigmine in water. The incubation was carried out for 30 minutes in a water bath at 27°C. At the end of this period 1 ml (4.5 mg) of a freshly prepared cool solution of benzidine tetrazonium fluoroborate (for preparation see Lojda, 1958b) was added and shaken into each incubation vessel. An orange azo dye formed immediately and this was extracted after adding 1 ml of 40% trichloracetic acid by vigorous shaking with 10 ml of ethyl acetate. After centrifuging for 15 minutes at 1500 rpm the supernatant was measured at 490 mμ photocolorimetrically against a blank treated in the same manner but containing only the substrate mixture without aortic extract. A calibration curve for pure β-naphthol was constructed and used for the estimation of liberated naphthol. The results were expressed as μg of β-naphthol per hour per 1 mg N_2 of extract.

In some experiments a butanol-acetone powder was prepared from the aortas and an ammonia extract prepared as described by Korn (1955) was used as the source of enzyme activity. In this case the activity was expressed as μg of β-naphthol per hour per 100 mg powder.

With this technique we reinvestigated first of all the question of species differences in esterase activity (Zemplényi *et al.*, 1963b). In text Fig. 2 results of activity determinations using ammonia extracts of butanol-acetone aorta powders are shown. In these experiments calculations were carried out on a dry weight basis, all extracts being prepared from the same amount (5 mg per ml) of tissue powder. It is obvious that the esterolytic activity determined in this way is very significantly higher (P < 0.001) in the rat aorta than in either the rabbit or the chicken aorta. It must be pointed out again that there was practically no variation in the DNA content of the aortas among the above species. It is clear that findings on the esterolytic activity are quite similar to previous findings on the lipolytic activity of the aortas in these species.

Although it is highly improbable that a different degree of extraction from dried powder could be a source of error in our experiments, such a possibility was excluded in all subsequent experiments where the activity was expressed directly on the basis of the N_2 content of the aorta extract. A further error could be caused by the fact that cholinesterase activity may also be included in determinations performed in the above way, in the absence of an appropriate inhibitor (Zemplényi,

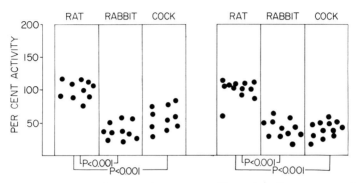

TEXT FIG. 5. Species differences in group-specific carboxylic esterase activity of aortas. The average rat aorta activity is 801 µg of β-naphthol per hour per 1 mg of nitrogen of aortic extract.

1962). Therefore, in all subsequent experiments incubations were carried out in the presence of $10^{-6}\,M$ physostigmine to minimize the interference of the latter enzyme. As seen from text Fig. 5, we obtained a pattern of activity similar to that in the previous series. We can state, therefore, that rat aorta activity estimated in different ways is always very significantly higher than aortic activity in the other species studied.

The results of the cholesterol-fat feeding experiments are collected in text Fig. 6. No significant difference between experimental and control animals could be found in either of the series. It should be mentioned that definite atherosclerotic changes were found only in aortas of animals on a cholesterol-fat diet of 10 weeks duration. The changes were, however, in most animals of a minimal degree (1–2.5 in our grading system), in one animal of medium degree (3), and in one animal of degree 4.5. Interestingly enough, the esterolytic activity of the latter rabbit aorta was the highest (323%) of the whole experimental series.

In both groups of experiments calculation of results on the protein content yielded practically identical relationships as when calculating on the nitrogen content of extracts.

Histochemically the esterases were detected by the following methods (see Lojda, 1961b):

a. Gomori's method (1952) using Tween 60 and 80.

b. Azo-coupling methods with α-naphthol acetate, naphthol AS acetate, and indoxyl acetate. For inhibition and activation the following reagents were used: E_{600} ($10^{-6} M$), eserine salicylate ($10^{-6} M$ and $10^{-3} M$), sodium chloride ($1 M$), protamine sulfate (1.5 mg per ml), sodium taurocholate ($5.10^{-3} M$), and heparin ($10^{-4} M$).

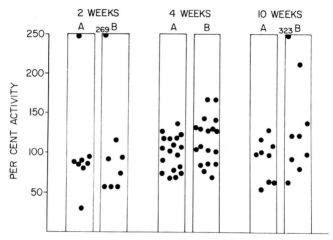

Text Fig. 6 Group-specific carboxylic esterase activities of aortas in rabbits. A = Control animals. B = Cholesterol-fat fed animals. Average activity of aortas in control rabbits 283.1 μg of β-naphthol per hour per 1 mg nitrogen of aortic extract.

c. Indoxyl methods using acetates of indoxyl and 5-bromo indoxyl as substrates.

d. Koelles' methods as modified by Gerebtzoff (1953) using iodides of acetylthiocholine and butyrylthiocholine as substrates.

When using the Gomori procedure with Tweens as substrates no regular reaction in normal rabbit arteries could be observed (only in unique cases a few places in the adventitia of rat aorta showing a positive reaction were seen). In the case of the azo-dye methods the acetate of α-naphthol was split much faster than that of naphthol AS. The activity demonstrated by azo coupling was located chiefly in the muscle cells of the aortic media. The reaction increasing radially toward the adventitia was not of the same degree along the whole aorta, but the differences were usually not great. So far we have not been able to decide whether the surfaces of elastic fibers and lamellae are involved, since a very strong positive reaction is found between the elastic lamellae following protracted incubations, and an exact localization is not possible. The reaction shown by the muscle cells of organ arteries was much weaker (Figs. 30, 31). A clear reaction could also be observed in some cells of the adventitia (fibrocytes, histiocytes). The reaction of the aortic endothelium in the rat, rabbit, and golden hamster cannot always be seen in a given section. The preparations incubated *in toto* show, however, a pronounced reaction in the endothelium. A more regular reaction could be observed in the endothelial cells of some organ vessels (especially of pulmonary arteries).

The reaction of the muscle cells of the aortic media shows considerable species differences (Lojda and Zemplényi, 1958, 1960; Zemplényi *et al.*, 1959). The strongest reaction was found in rat aortas; in rabbits the reaction was weaker and the weakest reaction could be observed in guinea pigs and golden hamsters. In chicken, macaque, and human aortas the reaction was also found to be very weak (Lojda, 1958b, 1961b).

Quantitative differences could be seen even with the naked eye, becoming very pronounced when determined photocolorimetrically after elution of the azo dye with dioxane (Lojda, 1958a). The activity in rat aortas was about five times as high as in rabbit aortas. Inhibition and activation studies were performed only with rat aortas. The enzyme activity was entirely inhibited by E_{600} and only partly by eserine salicylate. Application of taurocholate, sodium chloride, protamine sulfate, and heparin was without substantial effect.

From these results it follows that the reaction is due in part to cholinesterase and in part to nonspecific esterase. The presence of cholinesterase could also be confirmed by the use of acetylthiocholine iodide and butyrylthiocholine iodide which were both split by the muscle cells of the aortic media (Lojda, 1961a). By the use of the latter two substrates, species differences could also be detected. With both of these substrates only a weak reaction in the coronary arteries could be observed. The indoxyl methods provided a similar picture. Precise localization was obtained with 5-brome-indoxyl acetate, although the reaction was weaker than with unsubstituted indoxyl acetate.

In rabbits 2 to 4 weeks on the cholesterol-fat diet no apparent changes in the intensity and localization of staining reaction in their arteries could be observed.

The first changes could be detected with the appearance of streaks and plaques in the vessels of the animals fed 10 weeks. The endothelium covering most of the early plaques reacted more intensely than the endothelium of the unaffected portions of the vessel. The intensity of the reactions in the plaques was, of course, dependent upon their cellular composition (see Figs. 24 on Plate III and 25-29 on Plate IV). Smaller macrophages (lipophages) reacted very strongly when using the azo dye, indoxyl, or Tween 60 technique. With increasing size and increasing

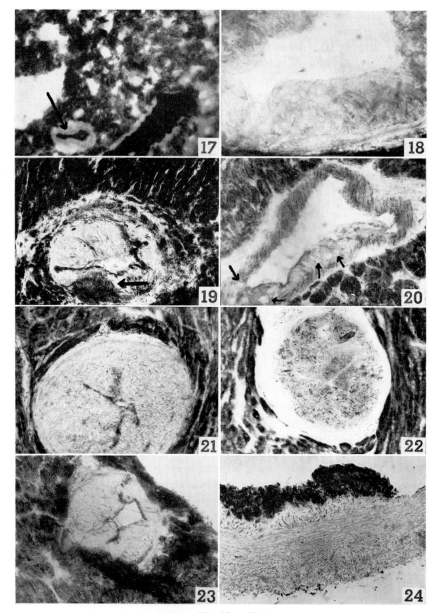

PLATE III (Figs. 17-24)

Fig. 17. ICDH in the lung of a normal rabbit. Arrow showing a small branch of the pulmonary artery. The strong activity of its endothelium much exceeds the activity in the muscle cells of the media. OF, NBT. Magnification: × 84.

Fig. 18. SDH in a larger atheromatous branch of a rabbit coronary artery. Very

amount of cholesterol, there was (similar to that observed with dehydrogenases) a drop in intensity of all staining reactions. In the deeper layers of the plaques with necrobiotic processes, esterases were obviously released from macrophages and could also be found extracellularly. A strong reaction was observed in transitional and muscle cells whereas fibrocytes showed only a lesser degree of staining (Fig. 27 on Plate IV).

Using the azo-dye methods the cytoplasm of positively reacting elements was diffusely stained along with some granular staining. The latter was detected especially when using naphthol AS-acetate as substrate. So far it is not possible to decide to what extent the diffuse cytoplasmic staining is due to the solubility of the azo dyes in fat.

In larger plaques some stratification could be observed, loci of higher activity alternating with those of lesser or no activity (Fig. 28). In plaques where a fibrous transformation took place the reaction was very weak or it could not be detected at all. Positively reacting macrophages could sometimes be found in the media. Muscle cells in the media in the vicinity of the plaque revealed a variable degree of staining, being increased or decreased but in most instances unchanged. At sites with calcification of the media positive staining reaction was absent.

---

weak staining in the elements of the plaque, somewhat stronger staining of the media-muscle cells. Strongly reacting myocardial fibers (bottom of the figure). OF, NBT. Magnification: × 140.

Fig. 19. SDH in an atheromatous smaller branch of a rabbit coronary artery. Strong positive reaction in the endothelium covering the plaque, weaker staining of the residual muscle cells of the media. No activity of the plaque itself, consisting of an amorphous mass mainly of lipid nature. Strong staining reaction of smaller lipophages (arrow). OF, NBT. Magnification: × 140.

Fig. 20. G6PDH in a larger branch of a rabbit coronary artery revealing changes mainly in the media. Arrows show foci of foam cells with almost negative reaction as compared with the distinct staining of the muscle cells of the media and the preserved endothelium. Very strong staining of the myocardial fibres. OF, NBT. Magnification: × 140.

Fig. 21. G6PDH in a small atheromatous branch of a rabbit coronary artery. Strong reaction in the endothelium and myocardial fibers. No reaction in the plaque itself. OF, NBT. Magnification: × 140.

Fig. 22. AGPDH in a small atheromatous branch of a rabbit coronary artery. Plaques occluding the lumen. No reaction in the changed vessel wall. Positive reaction in the myocardial fibers. OF, NBT. Magnification: × 140.

Fig. 23. ICDH in a small atheromatous branch of a rabbit coronary artery. Positive reaction in the endothelium, in the residual muscle cells of the media, and in myocardial fibers. OF, NBT. Magnification: × 140.

Fig. 24. Nonspecific esterase in an atheromatous rabbit aorta. Very strong positive reaction in the endothelium, macrophages, and lipophages (upper part of the plaque) and in muscle cells (deeper part of the plaque). The reaction of the muscle cells of the media is much weaker. OF, α-naphthol acetate, OD. Magnification: × 56.

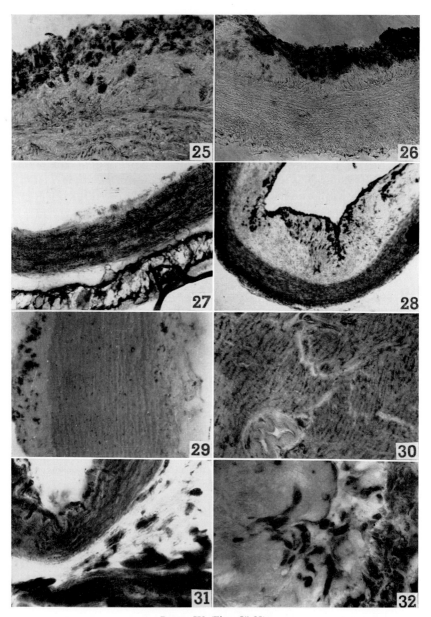

PLATE IV (Figs. 25-32)

FIG. 25. Nonspecific esterase in an atheromatous rabbit aorta (at higher magnification). Strong positive reaction in the upper part of the plaque confined to the endothelium and macrophages (lipophages). No reaction in deeper parts of the

In plaques of other arteries, including the coronaries, practically the same changes of esterase activity as those found in the aortas could be observed (Fig. 32).

There are several reports on the lipolytic and esterolytic activity of the arterial wall and the pertinent literature has been recently summarized (Zemplényi, 1962; Lojda, 1961b).

Tween-esterase was demonstrated in plaques of rabbit aortas by McMillan *et al.* (1954) and in some plaques by Narpozzi (1957). Wegmann and Fouquet (1961) and Fouquet (1961) using azo-dye methods with β-naphthol acetate observed marked changes in atherosclerotic rabbit aortas in early and late stages of chronic cholesterol feeding. Enhanced esterase activity in human atherosclerotic plaques was reported by Gomori (1946), Tischendorf and Curri (1959), Müller and Neumann (1959), Deribas *et al.* (1960), and Levonen *et al.* (1960).

The lipolytic activity of aortas of various species was investigated by Korn (1955), Gore and Larkey (1960), Dury (1961), Patelski and Szendzikowski (1961), Szendzikowski and Patelski (1961), and Gerö *et al.*

---

plaque. Weak reaction in the muscle cells of the media. FF, α-naphthol acetate, OD. Magnification: × 140.

Fɪɢ. 26. Nonspecific esterase in an atheromatous rabbit aorta. Strong positivity in the plaque macrophages (lipophages) and in the endothelium. The actually weak reaction of the muscle cells of the media cannot be seen in the picture. FF, naphthol AS-acetate, OD. Magnification: × 56.

Fɪɢ. 27. Nonspecific esterase in a small fibrotic plaque of the upper segment of the abdominal rabbit aorta. Note almost negative reaction of the plaque and the much higher staining of the muscle cells of the media. Very strong reaction in adipose tissue. OF, α-naphthol acetate, HF. Magnification: × 56.

Fɪɢ. 28. Nonspecific esterase in a later stage of rabbit aorta atheromatosis. Strong positivity in the endothelium and smaller lipophages. Somewhat weaker reaction in the muscle cells of the media. Very weak reaction in the fibrocytes of the plaque. FF, 5-bromoindoxyl acetate. Magnification: × 56.

Fɪɢ. 29. "Tween esterase" in a medium-sized plaque of a rabbit aorta. Positive reaction in lipophages. FF, Tween-60. Magnification: × 84.

Fɪɢ. 30. Nonspecific esterase in the myocardium of a normal rabbit. Positive reaction in the endothelium of smaller arteries and capillaries. Positively reacting pericytes. FF, naphthol AS-acetate, OD. Magnification: × 56.

Fɪɢ. 31. Nonspecific esterase in a larger branch of a rabbit coronary artery. Positive reaction in the endothelium. Somewhat weaker staining of the muscle cells in the media. Positively reacting fibrocytes and histiocytes in the interstitium. Stronger positive reaction in myocardial fibers. OF, α-naphthol acetate, HF. Magnification: × 315.

Fɪɢ. 32. Nonspecific esterase in a large atheromatous branch of a rabbit coronary artery. Positive reaction in the endothelium covering the plaque, in monocytoid cells, and in the muscle cells of the media (on the right of the picture). FF, α-naphthol acetate, HF. Magnification: × 441.

(1961). Evidence for a possible relationship between lipoprotein lipase and elastase has been recently reviewed by Hall (1961).

Our own findings on the lipolytic and esterolytic activities in the various species investigated, indicate the possible significance of these enzymes in regard to susceptibility of atherosclerosis. Findings in the aortas of old animals lend further support to such a possibility. In this relation the lesser degree of histochemically demonstrable esterase activity of the coronary arteries seems also to be interesting, although the precise relationship between lipolytic and esterolytic activities is so far not settled.

The histochemical results clearly show the presence not only of nonspecific esterase but also of cholinesterase in the arterial wall. This is in agreement with previous biochemical data of Thompson and Tickner (1953) and with our own findings (Zemplényi, 1962).

Results on the lipolytic activity of aortas in atherosclerotic rabbits were interpreted as signs of functional adaptation of the latter to chronic feeding of cholesterol and fat (Zemplényi and Grafnetter, 1959a). Only in aortas with high degrees of atherosclerosis could an increase of lipolytic activity be observed while aortas with lesser degrees of lesions revealed no change in activity. Determinations of the esterolytic activity of aortic extracts gave much the same results in early stages of atherosclerotic changes.

On the other hand, the histochemical evidence (Lojda and Zemplényi, 1958, 1960, 1961) clearly showed that the over-all activity even of early plaques surpassed the activity of the media (Figs. 24, 26). As with the other enzymes investigated, there was a close relationship between the degree of staining reactions and the cellular composition of the plaques.

We assume that the difference in the above results can easily be explained by the small amount of plaques in the early stages of atherosclerosis, their increased activity not being large enough to influence the high over-all activity of the arterial wall. In addition, one cannot exclude the possibility of a simultaneous decrease in mean activity of the media, not observable by the naked eye.

2. Phosphoesterases (Phosphatases)

These represent a large group of enzymes that act on a variety of phosphate esters. In the vascular tissue we are dealing particularly with phosphomonoesterases hydrolyzing monoesters of phosphoric acid.

a. *Nonspecific Phosphomonoesterases.* The best known representative of this group is the nonspecific ("group specific") phosphomonoesterase I, called also alkaline phosphatase, and phosphomonoesterase II, known usually as acid phosphatase.

In our own experiments (Zemplényi and Mrhová, 1963; Zemplényi *et al.*, 1962, 1963a) for the determination of phosphomonoesterase I activity the slightly modified method of Kaplan and Nahara (1953a), utilizing 0.005 *M* disodium phenylphosphate in a borate buffer of pH 9.8 as substrate, was applied. In contradistinction to the original method

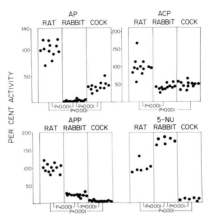

Text Fig. 7. Species differences in the activity of phosphomonoesterase I (AP), II (ACP), adenylpyrophosphatase (APP) and 5'-nucleotidase (5-NU) of aortas. Average rat aorta activities for AP 13.1 and for ACP 0.99 μmoles of phenol liberated per hour per 1 mg N$_2$ of aortic extract. For APP 23.7 and for 5-NU 5.77 μg of phosphate liberated per 30 minutes per 100 μg of nitrogen of aortic extract.

designed for estimations in blood serum, we used 1 ml of undiluted aortic extract (see Section III) as the source of enzyme activity and a different diazo reagent (0.25% paranitroaniline, water, and 0.2% NaNO$_2$ in a ratio of 1:2:1, freshly prepared). The amount of phenol liberated was determined spectrophotometrically at 445 mμ using a standard curve prepared with increasing concentrations of phenol solutions. A more detailed description is given elsewhere (Zemplényi *et al.*, 1963a).

The activity was expressed in μmoles of phenol per hour per 1 mg N$_2$ of extract.

In determinations of phosphomonoesterase II activity the method of Kaplan and Nahara (1953b) using 0.005 *M* disodium phenylphosphate in a 0.05 *M* acetate buffer of pH 5.0 was utilized. The same deviations from the original method as described above with the determination of phosphomonoesterase I activity were made, and the activity expressed in the same way.

Before turning to our main topic, it is again interesting to compare the activity of these enzymes in some animal species. As seen from text Fig. 7 there was a very significant difference in the activity of phosphomonoesterase I, rat aortas having the highest and rabbit aortas the lowest activity, while the activity of cock aortas was higher than that of the rabbit, but very significantly lower than the activity of rat aortas. The average rat aorta activity expressed in μmoles of phenol per hour per mg of N_2 (13.1) is about 36 times as high as the average rabbit aorta

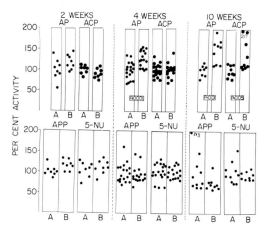

TEXT FIG. 8. The activity of AP, ACP, APP, and 5-NU in rabbit aortas. A = Control rabbits. B = Cholesterol-fat fed rabbits. Abbreviations as in Text Fig. 7. Average activities of aortas of control animals for AP 0.25, for ACP 0.86, for APP 6.2 and for 5-NU 10.7. (Values expressed in units as in Fig. 7.)

activity (0.36) and 3.5 times as high as the average cock aorta activity (3.78).

As seen from the same figure, the activity of phosphomonoesterase II in rat aortas in respect to this enzyme was very significantly higher than the activity in the other species, although the differences are not as striking as for phosphomonoesterase I.

It is also interesting to compare the phosphomonoesterase I and II activity within the same species. In this small series of experiments there was only a slightly higher activity of the latter enzyme in rabbit aortas. The data of text Fig. 8 indicate, however, that in a much larger group of rabbits the activity of phosphomonoesterase II is about 3.5 times as high as that of phosphomonoesterase I. On the other hand, in the cock aorta the average activity (3.78) of phosphomonoesterase I is about 8 times as high as the activity of phosphomonoesterase II and in the rat aorta the ratio is 13.1:0.99 (Zemplényi and Mrhová, 1963).

It is fair to add, however, that these relative figures might be a bit distorted in favor of phosphomonoesterase I by the differences in the methods used in determinations of the activities of these enzymes.

Our findings in cholesterol-fat fed rabbits are summarized in text Fig. 8. We could not detect any changes in activity of phosphomono-esterase I at a time 2 weeks after cholesterol-fat feeding. In both ex-perimental series of 4-weeks duration, however, there was a significant increase in the activity of the aortas of fed animals with a probable error of less than 0.001. The increase in the enzyme activity in the aortas of fed animals from the 10-week experiment is also unequivocal.

In contradistinction to the activity of the previous enzyme, only in the experimental series of 10-weeks duration could a slight increase of phosphomonoesterase II activity be detected with a borderline signifi-cance of 0.05.

Histochemically phosphomonoesterase I was detected using both Gomori's method (1952) and the azo-coupling method with α-naphthol phosphate, naphthol-AS-phosphate, and naphthol-AS-MX-phosphate as substrates. As coupling agents the diazo-fluoroborate of 5-chloro-2-tolui-dine, 4-benzamido-2.5-dimethoxyaniline, and fast red violet LB Salt were used. The sections were incubated for 0.5-4 hours.

Control tests were performed by incubating heat-inactivated sections with the substrate, and also normal sections in a medium which did not contain the substrate.

Phosphomonoesterase II was detected by Gomori's method (1952) and by the azo-coupling method, using the same substrates as for alka-line phosphatase, at pH 5.0 and pH 5.9. As coupling agents various diazonium salts including freshly prepared hexazotized fuchsin were used (Beneš *et al.,* 1961). Control tests were performed as with the previous enzyme.

In normal rabbit aortas phosphomonoesterase I was detectable in some sections only, and then exclusively in the adventitia. Its activity was low. It was impossible to decide in all cases to which structural component it was bound. We were able to demonstrate it in some cases on the collagen fibers and in others in the endothelium of some of the *vasa vasorum* (Figs. 34 and 35 on Plate V).

Concerning the intensity of the reactions, species differences could also be demonstrated histochemically (Lojda, 1961b). The activity in the various species (in order of decreasing degree) was as follows: rat, guinea pig, cock, golden hamster, rabbit, human.

In the rabbit coronary arteries the reaction was almost negative. Only in the vascular endothelium of some arterioles and some capillaries could a weak positive reaction be observed. On the other hand, the endothelium in the branches of pulmonary arteries showed a high degree of positivity (Fig. 33 on Plate V).

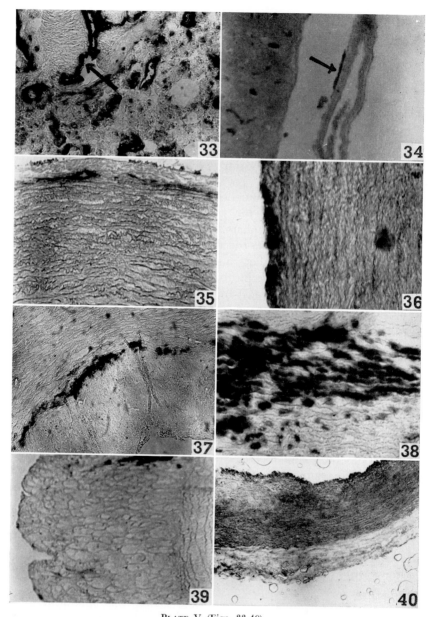

PLATE V (Figs. 33-40)

FIG. 33. AP in the lung of a normal rabbit. Arrow pointing to the strongly reacting endothelium of a branch of the pulmonary artery. PA, α-naphthol phosphate,
OT. Magnification: × 140.

In the aortas of the 2- and 4-weeks cholesterol-fat fed rabbits no changes in intensity or localization of staining reactions could be observed.

Simultaneously with the appearance of plaques, changes of activity took place. Activity was detectable in certain loci of the affected intima. This activity was difficult to locate more precisely in frozen sections after the azo-coupling reaction (Fig. 36 on Plate V). In paraffin-embedded sections, following acetone fixation, it could be observed that the activity was not equal in all areas; there existed plaques completely lacking in activity as well as plaques showing activity. In the latter, the enzyme was located mainly in the endothelium of newly formed capillaries and in the cellular membranes of some macrophages (Fig. 32 on Plate IV) and in calcified foci (Fig. 37 on Plate V). We failed to demonstrate any activity of the endothelium covering the plaques, even after *in toto* incubation. At some sites of the media a remarkably high activity, accompanying calcification, could be detected (Fig. 38 on Plate V). In this relation it is interesting that in atheromatous aortas of cockerels a higher overall activity in the plaques (including the covering endothelium) could be observed (Lojda, 1961b). In human atherosclerotic aortas the picture was very variable.

In normal rabbit aortas phosphomonoesterase II gives a weak but distinct positive reaction in the endothelium and muscle cells by Gomori's method. No significant differences were observed between various parts of the aorta. The azo-coupling method with α-naphthol

FIG. 34. AP in a cerebral artery of a normal rabbit. Positively reacting *vasa vasorum* (arrow) and capillaries. PA, α-naphthol phosphate, OT. Magnification: × 105.

FIG. 35. AP in an atheromatous rabbit aorta. On the boundary between the adventitia and media, positively reacting *vasa vasorum*. The plaque cannot be seen in the picture. PA, α-naphthol phosphate, OT. Magnification: × 140.

FIG. 36. AP in a small plaque of an atheromatous rabbit aorta. Plaque (on the left) shows a very intense reaction, a more precise localization cannot be unequivocally determined. FF, α-naphthol phosphate, DA. Magnification: × 105.

FIG. 37. AP in an atheromatous rabbit aorta. A very intense reaction in the area of calcification of the plaque at the boundary between intima and media. PA, naphthol AS-phosphate, OT. Magnification: × 140.

FIG. 38. AP in an atheromatous rabbit aorta. Positive reaction in the media at sites with calcification. PA, α-naphthol phosphate, OT. Magnification: × 140.

FIG. 39. AP in a large plaque of an atheromatous rabbit aorta. Positively reacting endothelium of newly formed capillaries. PA, α-naphthol phosphate, OT. Magnification: × 140.

FIG. 40. ACP in an atheromatous rabbit aorta. Early stage. The endothelium and the cellular elements of the small plaque reveal a stronger activity than the muscle cells of the media. OF, α-naphthol phosphate, HF. Magnification: × 56.

phosphate also detected the enzyme at the same sites. When using naphthol-AS-MX-phosphate in frozen sections, the activity in the muscle cells of the media was very low and the activity of the endothelium almost negligible. A distinct reaction could, on the other hand, be observed in the endothelium incubated in the *in toto* preparation.

In the coronary arteries the reaction was found to be weaker.

Concerning the intensities of staining reactions in various species practically the same differences as with phosphomonoesterase I were found (Lojda, 1961b).

Changes in the activity of this enzyme in the aortas were noted with the appearance of streaks and plaques, i.e., in our 10-weeks experimental series. As described previously (Lojda and Zemplényi, 1958, 1960, 1961) a high activity was detectable in the plaque elements particularly in the cytoplasm of young macrophages (lipophages) by all methods used (Figs. 40, 41, 43, 45, 46). The endothelium covering the smaller plaques and their nearest surroundings had a higher activity than the endothelium covering the unaffected areas. In larger lipophages the staining reactions were found to be decreased in intensity and some of them did not react at all. Fibroblasts usually revealed a weak staining reaction. As with the other enzymes the over-all staining intensity of the plaques depended upon their cellular composition. In plaques with necrobiotic changes as well as in plaques where a fibrous transformation took place no activity could be found.

The activity in the media was in general similar to the activity in normal aortas in those places where the appearance of the media was normal. At the sites with edema, the phosphomonoesterase II reaction was in some sections stronger, but in other sections it was weaker. At some sites of the media positively reacting macrophages could be demonstrated. In the areas where calcification appeared, a weak positive reaction could be detected. The muscle cells surrounding calcified foci revealed enhanced activity which was localized in small plasmatic granules.

In atheromatous coronary arteries (Figs. 42-44 on Plate VI) the pattern was generally similar to that seen in affected aortas. In rabbits fed for a longer period of time, the smaller coronary branches with severe lesions revealed a high activity in the endothelium and a weaker one in the muscle cells (Fig. 44).

In atheromatous chicken vessels practically the same results were obtained (Lojda, 1961b).

Before trying to discuss the interpretation of our findings on the activity of phophomonoesterase I and II we feel that it would be useful to present results on the activity of other enzymes concerned with phosphorus metabolism.

b. *5'-Nucleotidase and Adenylpyrophosphatase (Adenosinetriphosphatase)*. 5'-Nucleotidase is a specific phosphomonoesterase acting on 5'-nucleotides such as adenosine-5'-monophosphate (AMP). Adenylpyrophosphatase belongs, however, to the group of polyphosphatases which actually split polyphosphatic and not ester links. The reason why we included the latter enzyme activity under this heading was that it is more convenient to describe them together since very similar methods were used for their determination.

Concerning our biochemical determinations using aortic extracts at pH 9.0 it is reasonable to refer to aortic-adenylpyrophosphatase activity according to the definition given by Baló *et al.* (1948-1949) and by Banga and Nowotny (1951). On the other hand in histochemical determinations where desmoenzymes are first of all dealt with, it is hard to decide whether the former enzyme or adenosinetriphosphatase or both are actually detected. So far we have not attempted to differentiate them and we refer in our histochemical results to adenosinetriphosphatase activity.

For determination of 5'-nucleotidase activity the slightly modified procedure of Ahmed and Reis (1958) was used. Each test tube contained 1.2 ml of 0.05 M veronal-HCl buffer at pH 7.5, 0.2 ml of 0.003 M MgCl$_2$, and 0.2 ml of 0.01 M adenosine-5'-monophosphate. After equilibration in a water bath at 38°C for 5 minutes, 0.4 ml of aortic extract was added and the sample incubated for 30 minutes. Enzyme activity was stopped by adding 4 ml of 5% trichloracetic acid. After 5 minutes the sample was filtered through a Schleicher and Schnell filter No. 589 and a 5-ml aliquot of the filtrate was used for estimation of free phosphate by the method of Fiske and Subbarow (see King and Allot, 1947). A blank containing the same constituents but without incubation was run with each sample. The results were expressed as μg phosphate per 30 minutes per 100 μg of N$_2$ of extract.

Adenylpyrophosphatase activity was estimated essentially in the same way as the activity of 5'-nucleotidase, the difference being that 1.4 ml of a veronal-acetate buffer of pH 9.0 and 0.2 ml of 0.0075 M ATP (adenosine-5'-triphosphate) as substrate was used. The amount of aorta extract added was only 0.2 ml in each test or blank respectively. The results were expressed in μg phosphate per 30 minutes per 100 μg N$_2$ of extract.

Concerning species differences the data collected in text Fig. 7 show that rat aortas reveal again a very significantly higher adenylpyrophosphatase activity than the other species. But, interestingly enough, cock

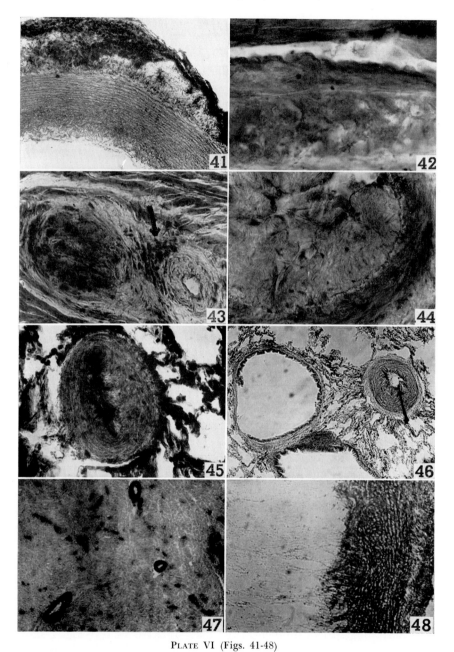

PLATE VI (Figs. 41-48)

FIG. 41. ACP in a large plaque of an atheromatous rabbit aorta. Strong positive
reaction in the macrophages (lipophages) of the plaque and in the muscle cells of the

aorta has a significantly lower activity than rabbit aorta, a finding quite the opposite of that with phosphomonoesterase I activity.

The determination of 5′-nucleotidase activity revealed the most surprising results. With this enzyme, as shown in text Fig. 7 the activity of rabbit aortas was very significantly higher and the activity of cock aortas very significantly lower than the activity of rat aortas. (The average activities in μg phosphate per 30 minutes per 100 μg N_2 are 10.09, 0.52, and 5.77 for rabbit, cock, and rat aortas respectively.)

A comparison of the activities of the latter enzymes within the same species shows that there is practically no difference in phosphate production between adenylpyrophosphatase and 5′-nucleotidase in cock aortas (0.47:0.52). On the other hand in rabbit aortas the ratio is 5.32:10.09 and in rat aortas 23.71:5.77.

In aortas of cholesterol-fat fed rabbits (text Fig. 8) no significant difference could be detected between experimental and control animals in the activity of either of these enzymes.

Histochemically both 5′-nucleotidase and ATPase activities were

---

deep part of the plaque. The muscle cells of the media reveal a weaker positivity. FF, α-naphthol phosphate, HF. Magnification: × 56.

Fig. 42. ACP in an affected branch of a rabbit coronary artery. Positive reaction in the endothelium. Somewhat weaker staining in the damaged muscle cells of the media. The boundary between intima and media appearing as a white line. FF, α-naphthol phosphate, HF. Magnification: × 440.

Fig. 43. ACP in atheromatous branches of a rabbit coronary artery. In the occluded artery (on the left) strongly reacting lipophages. Positively reacting endothelium of the artery on the right. Arrow pointing to a group of strongly reacting smaller lipophages in the interstitium. FF, α-naphthol phosphate, HF. Magnification: × 140.

Fig. 44. ACP in an atheromatous branch of a rabbit coronary artery. Positively reacting endothelium and muscle cells of the media. The amorphous mass in the plaque consisting mainly of cholesterol (needles) is without any distinct staining reaction. FF, α-naphthol phosphate, HF. Magnification: × 440.

Fig. 45. ACP in an atheromatous branch of a rabbit lung artery. Positive reaction in the endothelium and macrophages. Weaker staining of muscle cells. FF, α-naphthol phosphate, OD. Magnification: × 140.

Fig. 46. ACP in a branch of rabbit lung artery with early changes. Strong reaction of the endothelium (arrow), a weaker one in the muscle cells. FF, Gomori reaction. Magnification: × 56.

Fig. 47. ATPase in the myocardium of a normal rabbit. Strong positive reaction in the endothelium of small arteries and capillaries and in the muscle cells of the media. The myocardial fibers reveal a weak positivity. OF, Padykula and Herman reaction. Magnification: × 56.

Fig. 48. ATPase in an atheromatous rabbit aorta. Plaque to the left. Positive reaction of the muscle cells of the media. No reaction in the plaque itself. PA, Padykula and Herman reaction. Magnification: × 140.

detected according to the methods of Wachstein and Meisel (1957), and ATPase also according to Padykula and Herman (1955).

The presence of ATPase was ascertained in the endothelium and in the muscle cells of the normal arterial media (Fig. 47 on Plate VI). The reaction in muscle cells was relatively intense and in the cryostat sections it could be detected after 15 minutes. When using in the incubation medium AMP instead of ATP a positive reaction in the endothelium and muscle cells could only be demonstrated after a prolonged incubation period. When followed continuously the reaction appeared first in the adventitia, similar to the case of phosphomonoesterase I. The localization is thus at the transition between the results given by ATP and glycerophosphate as substrates. With Wachstein and Meisel's method the ATPase reaction is also shown by some cellular membranes of the muscle cells.

In atheromatous rabbit aortas a weak or almost negative reaction was observed in the cells of the plaques (Fig. 48) and in some cases the reaction in the media was weaker than the corresponding reaction in the intact media.

There are many reports in the literature on phosphoesterases and polyphosphatases of the arterial wall and these are discussed in Chapter 13 by Sandler and Bourne.

Malinow *et al.* (1959) pointed out the high alkaline phosphatase activity of cerebral arteries as compared with the aortas of many species and stressed the fact that cerebral lesions are not seen in rabbits even when they are fed cholesterol. These authors also found a much higher activity in the aortas of rats than in chicken or rabbit aortas. Our findings, both biochemical and histochemical, confirmed these species differences but in addition we found a similar difference—although not to such a degree—in the activities of acid phosphatase and adenylpyrophosphatase activities as well.

The significance of such differences is very difficult to evaluate as there is very little known of the physiological significance of the above enzymes. They could reflect in some way the higher general level of metabolic activity of the arteries of the rat, a species highly resistant to induction of experimental atherosclerosis by simple procedures. The activity of 5'-nucleotidase does not follow such a pattern, however, its activity being significantly higher in the chicken than in the rat aorta.

In normal aortas there is a good correlation between the biochemically and histochemically estimated activities of phosphomonoesterase II, 5'-nucleotidase, and the ATP-splitting enzyme. With phosphomonoesterase I, however, some discrepancy exists between findings obtained by these methods. In the latter case the activity is localized according to histochemical evidence, in the adventitia, even in unfixed cryostat sections. On the other hand for biochemical determinations samples of aortas practically devoid of adventitia have been used, and a definite, although low, activity in rabbit and cock aortas and a high activity in rat aortas, could always be detected. So far it is unsettled to what extent these different findings are caused by the presence of *vasa vasorum* in the external part of the media, or to the lower sensitivity of the histochemical methods, or simply to partial or complete loss of extractable enzymes during the histochemical procedure.

The most puzzling of our biochemical findings is the unequivocal increase in phosphomonoesterase I activity as early as 4 weeks following the cholesterol-fat feeding.

We must point out that we have little definite knowledge of the significance of this enzyme. Our histochemical results show, apart from other findings, a distinct phosphomonoesterase I activity in the media and intima at sites of calcification, and therefore the question arises on the relationship between the increase of this activity and the early calcification in atherosclerosis, as reported for human aortas by Blumenthal *et al.* (1950). Most present-day theories of calcification, however, deny any causal relationship between calcification and phosphomonoesterase I activity (see Glimcher, 1959). In this connection there is some interest in our negative finding of changes in 5′-nucleotidase activity, this enzyme being supposed by some authors (Reis, 1951) to be an important factor in the regulation of tissue calcification.

Another much disputed function, ascribed to phosphomonoesterase I, is in the formation of collagen fibers (for review see Gould, 1960). It is possible that such a causal relationship may exist in some tissues and not in others. As a matter of fact Schlief *et al.* (1954) found an increase in the activity of this enzyme in human atherosclerotic vessels where increased fiber formation could be detected. Nevertheless, in the case of aortic tissue the real existence of such a relationship between collagen fiber formation and the activity of phosphomonoesterase I has so far not been proved.

Paterson *et al.* (1957) assume that the presence of this enzyme in human atherosclerotic lesions is an evidence of an early vascularization of the affected intima. Our evidence in the rabbit aortas, however, shows a distinct activity in the macrophages and calcified loci apart from positively reacting capillaries.

In contradistinction to our findings Fouquet (1961) could not prove the presence of either phosphomonoesterase I or phosphomonoesterase II in rabbit aortas.

Similarly, as with the previous enzyme, the significance of phospho-monoesterase II is so far unclear. Our data demonstrate both histo-chemically and biochemically an enhanced activity simultaneously with the formation of plaques, its localization being in the macrophages (lipophages) and endothelium. These findings together with the dem-onstration of an increased activity in damaged muscle cells surrounding calcified foci seem to be interesting in connection with the views ex-pressed by Novikoff (1960a, 1961a, b) on the significance of lysosomal enzymes, playing important roles in pinocytosis, phagocytosis, lytic proc-esses, and so on.

Concerning adenylpyrophosphatase or ATPase and 5'-nucleotidase activities we could not detect either biochemically or histochemically any unequivocal changes in early stages of experimental atherosclerosis. Fouquet (1961) investigated the ATPase activity of rabbit aortas at different pH levels. No activity at pH 6.3, a weak activity in the intima at pH 7.4, and a strong activity even of muscle cells in the media at pH 8.5 and pH 9.4 were reported. In cholesterol-fed rabbits there was an enhanced activity after 16 days of feeding while after 30 days the enhanced activity tended to decrease.

In evaluating the latter results it is, however, important to realize that quantitative estimation of over-all enzyme activities, based upon staining reactions performed on unprotected cryostat sections only, may lead to erroneous conclusions (see Section III). These are due mainly to *hardly* controllable tissue damage under such conditions.

C. Other Enzymes

1. Glycogen Phosphorylase

Wegmann and Fouquet (1961) and Fouquet (1961) using the histo-chemical method of Guha and Wegmann (1960), observed an irregular positive reaction in the muscle cells of the media of rabbit aortas, a finding similar to the observations made previously by Takeuchi (1958). No changes were reported in aortas of rabbits fed 16 days on a cholesterol diet.

2. Phosphoglucoisomerase

The activity of phosphoglucoisomerase in aortic extracts was deter-mined in our experiments only in rabbits fed 4 and 10 weeks respectively. The method of Roe as modified by Slein (1955) was used for activity measurements. As seen from text Fig. 9 no significant difference could be detected between fed and control animals in either of the experi-mental series.

It is interesting that Brandstrup *et al.* (1957) found a definite decrease of the activity of this enzyme in atherosclerotic human aortas and Kirk *et al.* (1958) were able to detect a significant decrease in atherosclerotic segments of coronary arteries. The results were, however, expressed on a wet weight basis only.

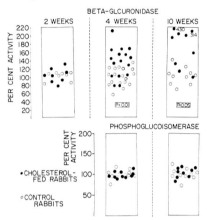

Text Fig. 9. The β-glucuronidase and phosphoglucoisomerase activity of rabbit aortas. ○ = Control rabbits. ● = Cholesterol-fat fed rabbits. Average β-glucuronidase activity of aortas in control animals 110.5 μg phenolphthalein per 100 μg nitrogen per 18 hours. Average phosphoglucoisomerase activity 139 arbitrary units per 1 mg of N_2 of aorta extracts. (Unit defined as the optical density change of 0.001 per minute measured at 540 mμ and using cuvettes of 10-mm diameter.)

3. β-Glucuronidase

This enzyme seems to have intimate though not clarified connections with the metabolism of connective tissue, especially its ground substance. We used for estimation of the activity of the aortic extracts the method of Talallay *et al.* (1946) with slight modifications of Dyrbye and Kirk (1956). Histochemical detection was carried out by the method of Fishman and Baker (1956), using 8-hydroxyquinoline glucuronide as substrate and by a modified azo-coupling method using the same substrate and freshly prepared hexazotized fuchsin as coupling agent.

As shown in text Fig. 9 we could not detect any changes in activity of this enzyme after 2 weeks of cholesterol-fat feeding. In the experimental series of both 4- and 10-weeks duration there was an increase of activity in the aortas of fed animals, this increase being of a somewhat lower degree in the 10-weeks experiment. Practically the same relationships were obtained when calculating results either on the protein or on the nitrogen content basis of the extracts (Mrhová *et al.*, 1963b).

Histochemically activity was found in the muscle cells of the media and also in the endothelium. Differences in activity resembled the differences found in phosphomonoesterase II activity, the reaction of the rat aortas being more intense than that of the rabbit aortas (Lojda, 1961b). So far we have been able to study histochemically the activity pattern only in later stages of experimental atherosclerosis. There was a focal increase in activity in some plaques especially at sites with an accumulation of alcian blue stainable mucopolysaccharides.

The physiological importance of β-glucuronidase is thus far not clear. It is known that many aromatic compounds are excreted in the urine as derivatives of D-glucuronic acid, this being an important mechanism for detoxification. β-Glucuronidases attack most β-glucuronides, for example estriol-β-glucuronides. It seems to be well established that some degradation products of hyaluronic acid can be further split by a β-glucuronidase. On the other hand the relationship of this enzyme to the synthesis of the above substances is still not clarified.

Let us assume for a moment that the change in β-glucuronidase activity is actually a reflection of a changed catabolism or anabolism, or both, of the connective tissue elements. If so, our findings of an increase of activity in the aortas of rabbits fed only 4 weeks, and without any morphological changes, could be interpreted to mean that even in cholesterol-fed animals changes in the ground substance are a prerequisite for the development of later atheromatous changes of the arterial wall.

In this connection it is interesting that there is a significant increase ($P < 0.001$) of glucosamine levels of the serum (in mg/100 ml) of experimental rabbits (47.8 ± 4.8) in comparison with control animals (34.8 ± 5.2). This is in agreement with the findings of Gerö et al. (1962).

In human atherosclerotic vessels Dyrbye and Kirk (1956) also found a tendency for the enzyme activity to be increased.

4. Aminopeptidase

The activity of this enzyme using L-leucyl-β-naphthylamine hydrochloride was studied biochemically in human arteries by Green et al. (1955) and Kirk (1960). No differences were observed between arteriosclerotic and normal segments of the same vessel. The histochemical findings of Levonen et al. (1960) indicate a moderate activity in the earliest plaques and sometimes in the media.

We investigated the activity of this enzyme histochemically by the method of Nachlas et al. (1957a). In the endothelium and muscle cells of the aortas of normal rabbits there was in unfixed sections sometimes a slight activity. In the coronary arteries no activity could be observed under the same conditions. In guinea pig aortas the staining reaction was always more intense than in the rabbit or rat aortas (Lojda, 1961b).

In early plaques of atherosclerotic rabbit aortas we observed a somewhat higher activity but a more accurate localization was not possible due to diffusion of both the enzyme and the liberated β-naphthylamine. The endothelium covering the plaques or in their neighborhood revealed a more intense staining reaction but this finding was not as unequivocal as with some other enzymes studied, e.g., phosphomonoesterase II or nonspecific esterase (Lojda and Zemplényi, 1961).

The above data are consistent with the assumption of an enhanced protein metabolism in early atherosclerotic lesions.

5. CATHEPSIN

Kritsman and Bavina (1955) investigated the activity of this enzyme in the aortas in experimental rabbit atherosclerosis using denaturated hemoglobin as substrate. The extent of activity was measured by the amount of free tyrosine. Both the total proteolysis and autolysis were found increased in comparison with normal animals, while proteosynthesis (measured with C^{14}-labeled material) was decreased.

Kirk (1962) in a recent paper carried out similar determinations on samples of human aortas and pulmonary and coronary arteries. He observed a higher total proteolytic activity for arteriosclerotic tissue portions than for normal tissue and the same applied for cathepsin activity, i.e., the difference between total proteolysis and autolysis.

Cathepsin, similar to phosphomonoesterase II (see above) seems to be connected with lysosomes and its higher activity may reflect a higher proportion of damaged cells, phagocytic cells, or dead cells in the tissue.

6. TRANSAMINASES

The activity and charateristics of various transaminases in extracts of rabbit arteries have been recently studied by Chattopadhyay (1961).

In our own investigations in cooperation with Graftnetter (so far unpublished) we estimated in aortic extracts the activity of glutamic oxalacetic transaminase by the method of Reitman and Frankel (1957). The activity of cock aortas was significantly higher ($P < 0.001$) than the activity of rat or rabbit aortas. The average activities of cock, rat, and rabbit aortas were 51.5, 29.3, and 25.4 units per 100 μg N_2 of aorta extract respectively.

No changes of activity could be detected, however, in early stages of experimental atherosclerosis.

7. Monoamine Oxidase

Thompson and Tickner (1951) demonstrated the activity of this enzyme in the aorta, pulmonary artery, and muscular arteries of rabbit, rat, and guinea pig and in small muscular branches of the human popliteal artery. In the larger arteries there was in general a higher activity than in the muscular arteries.

Spinks (1952) observed a significant decrease in the activity of this enzyme in aortas of rabbits fed dried thyroid for 14 days. It was suggested that actions of thyroid hormone on the blood pressure could be due to reduction in the activity of blood vessel amine oxidase.

8. Cytochrome Oxidase

Maier and Haimovici (1957) observed an activity of this enzyme of approximately equal magnitude in dog and rabbit aortas, and a lower activity in human aortas.

We studied the activity of this enzyme only histochemically, using the method described by Nachlas *et al.* (1958) and Burstone (1959). It was impossible to detect any activity of the arterial wall in the absence of exogenous cytochrome C (Lojda, 1961b). After adding the latter substance, there was a distinct activity in the muscle cells of the media and in the endothelium of normal rabbit aortas. In the coronary arteries the staining intensity at the same sites was somewhat higher.

Thus far we have not followed the activity of this enzyme in atherosclerotic rabbit aortas.

We feel this chapter would be incomplete without mentioning that many other enzymes have been studied in normal and diseased arteries of species other than the rabbit and especially in human vessels. A separate chapter of this book deals with the latter subject and it suffices to mention at this point that owing to the work of Kirk and collaborators and of others, we have detailed knowledge of the activities of hexokinase, phosphoglucomutase, aldolase, enolase, aconitase, fumarase, adenylate kinase, ribose-5-phosphate isomerase, purine nucleoside phosphorylase, glyoxalase I, diaphorase, cytochrome C reductase, and carbonic anhydrase of normal, and also to some extent of diseased human arteries.

Such studies are extremely valuable for investigation of the relationship between arterial wall metabolism and atherosclerosis. Nevertheless they also have limitations, as it will probably always be difficult to ascertain whether these *static* differences in activity between normal and atherosclerotic arteries in man are the result or the cause of vascular lesions. For this reason we have been applying in our own investigations, apart from studies in human vessels, the more *dynamic* approach of experimental models in animals.

V. Concluding Remarks

There is no doubt that the arterial wall is an organ with a distinct metabolism of its own, with a particular form of nourishment of its own, and with specific functions related to the transport of blood with pulsatile movements and to the distribution of blood. In no consideration of the pathogenesis of atherosclerosis can such important facts be neglected. Whatever the origin of this disease, the participation of the arterial wall in the formation of pathological changes is, in our opinion, one of the important factors (if not *the* most important factor) and metabolic disturbances of the arterial tissue itself must be suspected and intensively looked for. The study of the enzymic structure of the vessel wall under normal and various pathological conditions represents one of the promising approaches to the clarification of metabolic problems of this kind.

So far the observations on changes of enzyme activities of the arteries in experimental rabbit atherosclerosis are scanty and it would be too early to make a synthesis of the findings accumulated. In the preceding pages, we have discussed results obtained in connection with individual enzymes and we intend to underline a few points which seem to emerge from the data presented.

Accumulation of lipids is an outstanding feature in most types of atherosclerosis. The question of whether it is a primary event or whether it is a secondary phenomenon following changes in connective tissue, vascular injury, or even vascular thrombosis, is so far not settled. There is no doubt, however, that factors of a local character play an important role in the pathogenesis of atherosclerosis, a fact underlined also in the classic papers of Anitschkow (1933).

The studies of enzymes reported in this presentation show that there is a very early local response of the arterial wall to an increase of fat and cholesterol intake (at least in the rabbit). The over-all activity of some dehydrogenase systems, especially of succinate dehydrogenase, tends to decrease while the over-all activity of other enzymes, such as phosphomonoesterase I and β-glucuronidase show an enhanced activity at stages where no apparent morphological changes can be observed. The activities of the other enzymes studied, including the esterolytic activity, do not reveal any changes at this stage of the feeding experiments.

With the appearance of streaks and plaques there is a focal increase in the activity of many enzymes and the picture varies very much according the cellular pattern of the lesion. This is described in detail in Section IV.

The changes in enzyme activities observed before the appearance of morphological changes and before the signs of accumulation of lipid material lend support to the importance of local factors, especially ground substance changes, even in cholesterol-fed animals. Much more work is, of course, needed before a definite answer can be expected to the above complicated problems.

It is also important to keep in mind that the detection of a certain enzyme activity in a tissue proves only that it may work but not that it really does work *in vivo*. Nevertheless, the knowledge of such "potentialities" is an important step toward the understanding of the functioning of all living matter.

Finally it must be realized that the arterial wall is, of course, dependent upon the plasma for nourishment; plasma constituents are the building-stones in anabolic processes, regulatory humoral impulses (in addition to nervous impulses) reach the artery also in this way, and catabolic products are drained by blood and lymph channels as well. Problems of the metabolism of the vessel wall and problems of the transport and metabolism of blood constituents are, therefore, very intimately interrelated.

Acknowledgments

The authors wish to express their appreciation for statistical calculations carried out by Mrs. B. Buriánová and Mr. M. Bartoníček, and for technical assistance given by Miss J. Dvořáková, Mrs. J. Hájková, Mrs. I. Knížková, Mrs. M. Krabcová, Mrs. E. Procházková and Mrs. J. Vecková. The authors also wish to thank Dr. A. G. E. Pearse for samples of MTT, Dr. A. M. Seligman for samples of NBT, Dr. Z. Pádr for supply of NT, Dr. J. Škoda for samples of DPNH and NT, C. F. Boehringer u. Soehne, Ltd., Mannheim, for samples of TC-G Boehringer test.

Finally we thank the editors or publishers of *Brit. J. Exptl. Pathol., Časopis Lékařů Českých, Česk. Morfol., Experientia,* and *J. Atherosclerosis Res.* for permission to reproduce certain figures. Microphotographs 8 and 9 were reproduced from Lojda and Felt (1960), with the kind permission of *Experientia, Birkhäuser Verlag,* Basel. Microphotographs 17, 29, and 34 were reproduced from Lojda (1961a) with the kind permission of the editor of *Česk. Morfol.* Microphotographs 35, 36, 38, and 39 were reproduced from Lojda and Zemplényi (1961) with the kind permission of Elsevier Publishing Co.

Abbreviations

The following abbreviations are used throughout this chapter including the figure legends:

AMP   adenosine-5'-monophosphate
ATP   adenosine-5'-triphosphate

DPN   diphosphopyridine nucleotide
DPNH   reduced diphosphopyridine nucleotide
TPN   triphosphopyridine nucleotide
TPNH   reduced triphosphopyridine nucleotide
DPND   "DPN-diaphorase"
TPND   "TPN-diaphorase"
DNA   deoxyribonucleic acid
SDH   succinate dehydrogenase (system)
LDH   lactate dehydrogenase (system)
MDH   malate dehydrogenase (system)
AGPDH   α-glycerophosphate dehydrogenase (system)
G6PDH   glucose 6-phosphate dehydrogenase (system)
BHBDH   β-hydroxybutyrate dehydrogenase (system)
ATPase   adenosine triphosphatase
AP   phosphomonoesterase I
ACP   phosphomonoesterase II
APP   adenylpyrophosphatase
5 NU   5′-nucleotidase
NBT   2,2′-di-p-nitrophenyl-5,5′-diphenyl-3,3′-(3,3′-dimethoxy-4,4′-biphenylene)dite-
           trazolium chloride (Nitro BT)
INT   2-(p-iodophenyl)-3-(p-nitrophenyl)-5-phenyltetrazolium chloride
MTT   3-(4,5-dimethylthiazolyl-2)-2,5-diphenyltetrazolium bromide
NT   2,2′-diphenyl-3,3′-(4,4′-biphenylene)-5,5′-diphenylditetrazolium chloride (Neo-
           tetrazolium)
BT   2,2′-diphenyl-3,3′-(3,3′-dimethoxy-4,4′-biphenylene)-5,5-diphenylditetrazolium
           chloride
FFA   free fatty acids
FF   frozen section after cold formol calcium fixation
OF   cold microtome section from unfixed tissue
PA   paraffine section after cold acetone fixation
OD   tetrazonium fluoroborate of o-dianisidine
OT   diazonium fluoroborate of 5-chloro-2-toluidine
DA   diazonium fluoroborate of 4-benzamido-2,5-dimethoxyaniline
HF   freshly prepared hexazotized fuchsin

REFERENCES

Ahmed, Z., and Reis, T. L. (1958). *Biochem. J.* **69**, 386.
Altschul, R. (1950). "Selected Studies on Arteriosclerosis." C. C Thomas, Spring-field, Illinois.
Anitschkow, N. (1913). *Beitr. Pathol. Anat. Allgem. Pathol.* **56**, 379.
Anitschkow, N. (1933). *In* "Arteriosclerosis" (E. V. Cowdry, ed.), p. 271. Macmillan, New York.
Baló, T., Banga, I., and Josepovits, G. (1948-1949). *Z. Vitamin- Hormone- Ferment-forsch.* **2**, 1.
Banga, I., and Nowotny, A. (1951). *Acta Physiol. Acad. Sci. Hung.* **2**, 317.
Beneš, K., Lojda, Z., and Hořavka, B. (1961). *Histochemie* **2**, 313.
Blumenthal, H. T., Lansing, A. I., and Gray, S. H. (1950). *Am. J. Pathol.* **26**, 989.
Brandstrup, N., Kirk, J. E., and Bruni, C. (1957). *J. Gerontol.* **12**, 166.
Briggs, F. N., Chernick, S., and Chaikoff, I. L. (1949). *J. Biol. Chem.* **179**, 103.

Burstone, M. (1959). *J. Histochem. Cytochem.* **7**, 112.
Ceriotti, C. (1952). *J. Biol. Chem.* **198**, 297.
Chattopadhyay, D. P. (1961). *Nature* **192**, 660.
Constantinides, P. (1961). *J. Atherosclerosis Res.* **1**, 374.
Constantinides, P., Booth, T., and Carlson, G. (1960). *Arch. Pathol.* **70**, 712.
Deribas, V. I., Fuks, B. B., and Schischkin, G. S. (1960). *Dokl. Akad. Nauk SSSR* **134**, 443.
Dole, V. B. (1956). *J. Clin. Invest.* **35**, 150.
Duff, G. L., and McMillan, G. C. (1951). *Am. J. Med.* **11**, 92.
Dury, A. (1961). *J. Gerontol.* **16**, 114.
Dury, A., Leigly, F., and Dury, M. (1957). *Sci. Studies St. Bonaventura Univ.* **19**, 37.
Dyrbye, M., and Kirk, T. E. (1956). *J. Geront.* **11**, 33.
Fischer, E. R., and Geller, T. H. (1960). *Circulation Res.* **8**, 820.
Fishman, W. H., and Baker, J. R. (1956). *J. Histochem. Cytochem.* **4**, 570.
Fodor, J., Zemplényi, T., Lojda, Z., and Felt, V. (1958). *Časopis Lékařů Českých* **97**, 316.
Fontaine, R., Mandel, P., Pantesco, V., and Kempf, E. (1960). *Strasbourg Med.* **9**, 605.
Fouquet, J. P. (1961). *Ann. Histochim.* **6**, 153.
Gerebtzoff, M. A. (1953). *Acta Anat.* **19**, 366.
Gerö, S., Gergely, T., Dévényi, T., Virag, S., Székely, T., and Jakab, L. (1961). *Proc. 4th Intern. Congr. Angiology Prague 1961; see* (1963) "Metabolismus Parietis Vasorum" (B. Prusík, Z. Reiniš, and O. Riedl, eds.), p. 34. SZN, Prague.
Gerö, S., Gergely, J., Farkas, K., Dévényi, T., Koscár, L., Jakab, L., Székely, J., and Vikás, S. (1962). *J. Atherosclerosis Res.* **2**, 276.
Glimcher, M. J. (1959). *In* "Connective Tissue, Thrombosis and Atherosclerosis" (I. H. Page, ed.), p. 140. Academic Press, New York.
Gomori, G. (1946). *A.M.A. Arch. Pathol.* **41**, 121.
Gomori, G. (1952). "Microscopic Histochemistry. Principles and Practice." Univ. Chicago Press, Chicago, Illinois.
Gore, I., and Larkey, B. J. (1960). *J. Lab. Clin. Med.* **56**, 839.
Gould, B. S. (1960). *Vitamins Hormones* **18**, 89.
Grafnetter, D., and Zemplényi, T. (1959). *Z. Physiol. Chem.* **316**, 218.
Grafnetter, D., and Zemplényi, T. (1961). *Cor et Vasa* **3**, 63.
Grafnetter, D., and Zemplényi, T. (1962). *Experientia* **18**, 85.
Green, M. N., Tsou, K.-C., Bressler, R., and Seligman, A. M. (1955). *Arch. Biochem. Biophys.* **57**, 458.
Guha, S., and Wegmann, R. (1960). *Bull. Soc. Chim. Biol.* **42**, 115.
Hall, D. A. (1961). *J. Atherosclerosis Res.* **1**, 173.
Hess, R., Scarpelli, D. G., and Pearse, A. G. E. (1958). *J. Biophys. Biochem. Cytol.* **4**, 753.
Hueper, W. C. (1944). *A.M.A. Arch. Pathol.* **38**, 162, 245, 350.
Hueper, W. C. (1945). *A.M.A. Arch. Pathol.* **39**, 51, 117, 187.
Kaplan, A., and Nahara, A. (1953a). *J. Lab. Clin. Med.* **41**, 819.
Kaplan, A., and Nahara, A. (1953b). *J. Lab. Clin. Med.* **41**, 825.
Katz, L. N., and Stamler, J. (1953). "Experimental Atherosclerosis." C. C Thomas, Springfield, Illinois.
King, E. J., and Allot, E. N. (1947). *In* "Recent Advances in Clinical Pathology" (S. C. Dyke, ed.), p. 222. Churchill, London.
Kirk, J. E. (1960). *J. Gerontol.* **15**, 136.

Kirk, J. E. (1962). *J. Gerontol.* **17**, 158.

Kirk, J. E., and Dyrbye, M. (1956). *J. Gerontol.* **11**, 129.

Kirk, J. E., and Laursen, T. J. S. (1955). *J. Gerontol.* **10**, 8.

Kirk, J. E., Effersøe, P. G., and Chiang, S. P. (1954). *J. Gerontol.* **9**, 10.

Kirk, J. E., Laursen, T. J. S., and Schaus, R. (1955). *J. Gerontol.* **10**, 178.

Kirk, J. E., Matzke, J. R., Brandstrup, N., and Wang, I. (1958). *J. Gerontol.* **13**, 24.

Kittinger, G. W., Wexler, B. C., and Miller, B. F. (1960). *Proc. Soc. Exptl. Biol. Med.* **104**, 616.

Kittinger, G. W., Wexler, B. C., and Miller, B. F. (1961). *Proc. 4th Intern. Congr. Angiology Prague 1961;* see (1963) "Metabolismus Parietis Vasorum" (B. Prusík, Z. Reiniš, and O. Riedl, eds.), p. 60. SZN, Prague.

Krčílek, A., Janoušek, V., and Šerák, L. (1961). *Proc. 4th Intern. Congr. Angiology Prague 1961;* see (1963) "Metabolismus Parietis Vasorum" (B. Prusík, Z. Reiniš, and O. Riedl, eds.), p. 50. SZN, Prague.

Kritsman, M. G., and Bavina, M. V. (1955). *In* "Atheroscleroz" (N. N. Anitschkow, ed.), p. 127. Medgiz, Moscow.

Korn, E. D. (1955). *J. Biol. Chem.* **215**, 15.

Lazovskaya, L. N. (1943). *Biokhimiya* **8**, 171.

Lehninger, A. L. (1959). *In* "The Arterial Wall" (A. L. Lansing, ed.), p. 220. Williams & Wilkins, Baltimore, Maryland.

Lester, L. R., and Smith, A. L. (1961). *Biochim. Biophys. Acta* **47**, 475.

Levonen, E., Raekallio, J., and Uotila, U. (1960). *Nature* **188**, 677.

Lojda, Z. (1958a). *Acta Histochem.* **5**, 236.

Lojda, Z. (1958b). "Azocoupling Reactions in Histochemical Detection of Enzymes." SZN, Prague (in Czech.).

Lojda, Z. (1961a). *Česk. Morfol.* **9**, 179 (in Czech.).

Lojda, Z. (1961b). *Proc. 4th Intern. Congr. Angiology Prague 1961;* see (1962) *Česk. Morfol.* **10**, 46.

Lojda, Z., and Felt, V. (1960). *Experientia* **16**, 514.

Lojda, Z., and Zemplényi, T. (1958). Paper delivered at the 1st Congress of the Italian Society for Histochemistry, Messina, 1958; see (1959). *Monit. Zool. Ital.* **67** (Suppl. 291).

Lojda, Z., and Zemplényi, T. (1960). *In* "Modern Problems of Cardiology" (I. I. Speranskij, ed.), p. 261. Moscow.

Lojda, Z., and Zemplényi, T. (1961). *J. Atherosclerosis Res.* **1**, 101.

Lowry, O. H., Rosebrough, N. J., Farr, A. L., and Randall, R. J. (1951). *J. Biol. Chem.* **193**, 265.

McMillan, G. C., Klatzo, I., and Duff, G. L. (1954). *Lab. Invest.* **3**, 451.

Maier, N., and Haimovici, H. (1957). *Proc. Soc. Exptl. Biol. Med.* **95**, 425.

Malinow, M. R., Fernandes, M. A., Gimeno, A. L., and Bur, G. E. (1959). *Nature* **183**, 1262.

Malinow, M. R., Moguilevsky, J. A., and Lacuara, J. L. (1962). *Circulation Res.* **10**, 624.

Mandel, P. (1956). *Exposes Ann. Biochem. Med.* **18**, 187.

Mrhová, O., Zemplényi, T., and Lojda, Z. (1963a). *Quart. J. Exptl. Physiol.* **48**, 61.

Mrhová, O., Zemplényi, T., and Lojda, Z. (1963b). *J. Atherosclerosis Res.* **3**, 44.

Müller, E., and Neumann, W. (1959). *Frankfurter Z. Pathol.* **70**, 174.

Myasnikow, A. L. (1960). "Ateroscleroz." Medgiz, Moscow.

Nachlas, M. M., Crawford, D. T., and Seligman, A. M. (1957a). *J. Histochem. Cytochem.* **5**, 264.

Nachlas, M. M., Tsou, K. C., De Souza, E., Cheng, C. S., and Seligman, A. M. (1957b). *J. Histochem. Cytochem.* **5**, 420.

Nachlas, M. M., Crawford, D. T., Goldstein, T. P., and Seligman, A. M. (1958). *J. Histochem. Cytochem.* **6**, 445.

Nachlas, M. M., Margulies, S. I., and Seligman, A. M. (1960). *J. Biol. Chem.* **235**, 2739.

Narpozzi, A. (1957). *Boll. Soc. Ital. Biol. Sper.* **33**, 467.

Novikoff, A. B. (1959). *J. Histochem. Cytochem.* **7**, 301.

Novikoff, A. B. (1960). *In* "Developing Cell Systems and their Control" (D. Rudnick, ed.), p. 167. Ronald, New York.

Novikoff, A. B. (1960b). *J. Histochem. Cytochem.* **8**, 345.

Novikoff, A. B. (1961a). *In* "Analytical Cytology" (R. E. Mellors, ed.), p. 69. Mc-Graw-Hill, New York.

Novikoff, A. B. (1961b). *In* "The Cell" (J. Brachet and A. E. Mirsky, eds.), Vol. II, p. 423. Academic Press, New York.

Padykula, H. A., and Herman, E. (1955). *J. Histochem. Cytochem.* **3**, 161.

Patelski, J., and Szendzikowski, S. (1961). *Proc. 4th Intern. Congr. Angiology Prague 1961;* see (1963) "Metabolismus Parietis Vasorum" (B. Prusík, Z. Reiniš, and O. Riedl, eds.), p. 55. SZN, Prague.

Paterson, J. C., Mills, J., and Moffatt, T. M. (1957). *A.M.A. Arch. Pathol.* **64**, 129.

Pearse, A. G. E. (1960). "Histochemistry, Theoretical and Applied." Churchill, London.

Reiniš, Z., Wenke, M., Lojda, Z., Šulc, K., Kubát, K., and Vanĕček, R. (1963). *Vnitřní Lékař.* (in press).

Reis, J. L. (1951). *Biochem. J.* **48**, 548.

Reitman, S., and Frankel, S. (1957). *Am. J. Clin. Pathol.* **28**, 56.

Scarpelli, D. G., Hess, R., and Pearse, A. G. E. (1958). *J. Biophys. Biochem. Cytol.* **4**, 747.

Schettler, G. (1961). "Arteriosklerose." Thieme, Stuttgart.

Schlief, H., Schmidt, C. G., and Hillenbrand, H. J. (1954). *Z. Ges. Exptl. Med.* **122**, 497.

Schneider, W. C. (1945). *J. Biol. Chem.* **161**, 293.

Seligman, A. M., Nachlas, M. M., and Mollomo, M. C. (1949). *Am. J. Physiol.* **159**, 337.

Šerák, L., Krčílek, A., and Janoušek, V. (1961). *Proc. 4th Intern. Congr. Angiology Prague 1961;* see (1963) "Metabolismus Parietis Vasorum" (B. Prusík, Z. Reiniš, and O. Riedl, eds.), p. 483. SZN, Prague.

Slein, M. W. (1955). *In* "Methods in Enzymology" (S. P. Colowick and N. O. Kaplan, eds.), Vol. I, p. 304. Academic Press, New York.

Spinks, A. (1952). *J. Physiol. (London)* **117**, 35.

Szendzikowski, S., and Patelski, J. (1961). *Proc. 4th Intern. Congr. Angiology Prague 1961;* see (1963) "Metabolismus Parietis Vasorum" (B. Prusík, Z. Reiniš, and O. Riedl, eds.), p. 202. SZN, Prague.

Takeuchi, T. (1958). *J. Histochem. Cytochem.* **6**, 208.

Talallay, P., Huggins, C., and Fishman, W. H. (1946). *J. Biol. Chem.* **166**, 757.

Thompson, R. H. S., and Tickner, A. (1951). *J. Physiol. (London)* **115**, 34.

Thompson, R. H. S., and Tickner, A. (1953). *J. Physiol. (London)* **121**, 623.

Tischendorf, F., and Curri, S. B. (1959). *Acta Histochem.* **8**, 158.

Wachstein, M., and Meisel, E. (1957). *Am. J. Clin. Pathol.* **27**, 13.

Wegmann, R., and Fouquet, J. P. (1961). *Ann. Histochim.* **6**, 61.

Whereat, A. F. (1961a). *Circulation* **9**, 571.
Whereat, A. F. (1961b). *Circulation* **24**, 1070.
Wolkoff, K. (1929). *Beitr. Anat. Pathol. Allgem. Pathol.* **82**, 555.
Wolkoff, K. (1930). *Beitr. Anat. Pathol. Allgem. Pathol.* **85**, 386.
Zemplényi, T. (1962). *J. Atherosclerosis Res.* **2**, 2.
Zemplényi, T., and Grafnetter, D. (1958a). *Brit. J. Exptl. Pathol.* **39**, 99.
Zemplényi, T., and Grafnetter, D. (1958b). *Časopis Lékařů Českých* **98**, 97.
Zemplényi, T., and Grafnetter, D. (1959a). *Brit. J. Exptl. Pathol.* **40**, 312.
Zemplényi, T., and Grafnetter, D. (1959b). *Gerontologia* **3**, 55.
Zemplényi, T., and Mrhová, O. (1962). *Česk. Fysiol.* **11**, 226.
Zemplényi, T., and Mrhová, O. (1963). *Brit. J. Exptl. Pathol.* **44**, 278.
Zemplényi, T., Lojda, Z., and Grafnetter, D. (1959). *Circulation Res.* **7**, 286.
Zemplényi, T., Grafnetter, D., and Lojda, Z. (1961a). *In* "Enzymes of Lipid Metabolism" (P. Desnuelle, ed.), p. 203. Pergamon, New York.
Zemplényi, T., Mrhová, O., Grafnetter, D., and Lojda, Z. (1961b). *Proc. 4th Intern. Congr. Angiology Prague 1961;* see (1963) "Metabolismus Parietis Vasorum" (B. Prusík, Z. Reiniš, and O. Riedl, eds.), p. 63. SZN, Prague.
Zemplényi, T., Mrhová, O., and Lojda, Z. (1962). Paper delivered at the Czechoslovak Cardiological Society, Prague, 1962.
Zemplényi, T., Mrhová, O., and Lojda, Z. (1963a). *J. Atherosclerosis Res.* **3**, 50.
Zemplényi, T., Knížková, I., Lojda, Z., and Mrhová, O. (1963b). *Cor et Vasa* **5**, 107.

—13—

Histochemistry of Atherosclerosis in the Rat, Dog, and Man

MAURICE SANDLER AND GEOFFREY H. BOURNE

I. Introduction

The vascular system functions to carry nutrients to, and to remove metabolites from, the tissues of the body. The arterial system while carrying out its function as a pipeline for the body must at the same time perform all the normal functions of living tissue in general such as the repair of injury and the maintenance of its own homeostasis. In addition, special requirements must be met by the arterial organs as they are under tension due to the pressure of blood that is constantly traversing them. Diseases of the arterial system have been implicated as the underlying cause for such apparently unrelated clinical entities as myocardial infarction, cerebral vascular accidents, and dry gangrene of the lower extremities (see Chapter 2 by McGill *et al.*).

The aorta has been shown to possess many enzyme systems that are present in other systems of the body. Specifically, aortic tissue has the capability of oxidative phosphorylation, glycolysis, synthesis of complex substances such as phospholipids, cholesterol, long-chain fatty acids, and of course, the enzymes necessary for these functions. Up until the late 1950's, relatively few papers had appeared concerning the histochemical distribution of enzymes in the aorta. This was due, in part, to the relative lack of interest on the part of histochemists in the aorta and to the apparent lack of reproducibility of the results. While the biochemical studies such as those discussed by Dr. Kirk in Chapter 3 of this volume are extremely important, the problem of where individual enzymes are located within the vascular wall and perhaps even more important, within the cells of the vascular wall is information which is essential for us to have. It is well known that the concentration of a given enzyme may vary tremendously from cell to cell in a given tissue. Because of this importance of the histochemical localization of enzymes we have in our laboratory for some time been studying the distribution of several enzymes in the human aorta with atherosclerosis, the rat aorta in experimental atherosclerosis, and more recently in the dog aorta in experimentally produced atherosclerosis. In addition, a great deal of work in the histochemical study of experimental atherosclerosis in the rabbit has been done in Czechoslovakia by Zemplényi and Lojda and their colleagues (see Chapter 12 by Zemplényi *et al.*). The reader upon perusing this chapter will soon find that there is a paucity in the amount of information which we have at the present time had made available to us through the use of histochemical techniques. In view of the fact that the biochemistry of the aorta has been discussed by Dr. Kirk in a rather thorough manner in his chapter (Chapter 3 in this volume) we will not discuss biochemical studies in any detail except to show to what extent results of biochemical studies and histochemical studies corroborate or do not corroborate each other where both types of studies have been done.

II. Oxidative Enzymes

Cytochrome oxidase was studied in the dog aorta by Sandler (1962) and no activity was seen. When the enzyme was studied by Lojda (1962) it was not detected in any of the animals which he studied, including the human, rat, and rabbit aorta, unless exogenous cytochrome C was added to the incubation medium. This is in contradistinction to biochemical studies as summarized by Kirk in Chapter 3. Studying succinic dehydrogenase (Sandler, 1962), using sodium succinate as a substrate and Nitro BT as a coupling agent, in the dog aorta a slight activity can be seen in the endothelial cells and in the cells in the inner third of the media with a considerable activity being present in the outer two-thirds of the media and in the adventitia and vasa vasorum. The localization appears to be mitochondrial. Similar studies in the human, rat, and rabbit aorta have been reported by Lojda (1962). Probably the earliest studies of dehydrogenase activity were done by Fried and Zweifach (1955) in which the authors utilize neotetrazolium as a coupling agent. They found dehydrogenase activity in the media and the endothelium of rat mesenteric and carotid arteries utilizing the intermediary metabolites mannose, glucose, succinate, and hexoses. DPN and TPN diaphorase were studied in the aortas of human, rat, and rabbit by Lojda (1962). This author utilized Nitro BT as a coupling agent to study these enzymes and found that DPN diaphorase was present to a greater extent than was TPN diaphorase. The activity was present mainly in the smooth muscle cells of the media, appearing in the endothelium and adventitia only after prolonged incubation. In addition, these authors studied lactic, isocitric, malic, α-glycerphosphate, β-hydroxybutyric, glucose-6-phosphate and glutamic dehydrogenases. In the majority of instances they reported that the muscle cells of the media were stronger reacting than the endothelium with very little activity present in the adventitia. They found no alcohol dehydrogenase present. The technique which these authors used was the utilization of Nitro BT as an electron acceptor as indicated previously. The intracellular localization, using Nitro BT, is in all instances the same and appears to be mitochondrial. The reason for this is owing to the technique. In the histochemical visualization of the enzyme activity the last step requires that the intrinsic DPN or TPN dehydrogenases be coupled to the tetrazolium acceptor (in most instances this is Nitro BT). Because of this, one would expect the localization for this enzyme to be the same. For this reason, one cannot place much emphasis on the intracellular localization at the present time. No studies have been recorded utilizing exogenous diaphorase so as to alter the distribution to that of the original dehydrogenase. No histochemical studies are available to date concerning the changes which occur in oxidative enzymes in human atherosclerosis. Experimental studies in the rabbit have been performed by Lojda and his co-workers and are reported in detail in Chapter 12 of this volume.

III. Enzymes Hydrolyzing Ester Links

A. Carboxylic Esterases

Carboxylic esterases may be separated on the basis of rates of reaction. The first group, or simple esterases, act more rapidly on simple esters of low molecular weight compounds and the second consists of lipases which act rapidly on triglycerides and slowly on other esters. The originator of the first technique for esterases, Gomori (1939), reported lipase activity to be absent in the aortas of several species but to be present in the aortas of pregnant rats. He utilized Tween 60 or Tween 40 as the substrate. In this same paper he reported that esterase activity was increased in plaques in human atherosclerosis. Using α-naphthol acetate, naphthol AS acetate, indoxal acetate, Tween 60 or Tween 80 as substrates, simple esterase has been studied in the aortas of rats, rabbits, guinea pigs, and hamsters by Lojda and Zemplényi and their co-workers and are discussed in detail elsewhere (Chapter 12) in this book. Some important findings though should be discussed. The inhibition of lipolytic activity has been reported by Gerö *et al.* (1961) using mucopolysaccharides which were extracted from the human aorta in biochemical studies. But no changes of esterolytic activity have been reported in histochemical studies in the rat. Levonen *et al.* (1960), utilizing naphthol AS acetate as the substrate stated that esterase activity appeared in human atheroma in connection with foam cells. The activity was most intense in the innermost layer of the intima and in the region of the internal elastic membrane. When the whole of the aorta was involved in the atherosclerotic process, distinct esterase activity could be seen localized throughout the media. The possible significance of the changes in esterase and lipolytic activity have been discussed in detail elsewhere in this book and will not be repeated here.

B. Choline Esterase

Choline esterase has been described in the muscle cells of the media of the aorta of the various species by Lojda (1962) using acetylthiocholine iodide and butyrylthiocholine iodide as substrates. This author could not detect any distinct reaction of the coronary arteries of any of the species studied. However, from this paper it is very difficult to determine exactly what species were studied; the only species specifically referred to were the rabbit and rat.

C. Nonspecific Alkaline Phosphatases

The importance of the intermediary metabolism of phosphorus in the transfer and storage of energy in cells is well recognized and it is reasonable to assume that it has as an important place in arterial tissue as elsewhere in the body. The ability to demonstrate the intermediary metabolism of phosphorus in cells histochemically is limited to the demonstration of phosphatase activity. Alkaline phosphatase was first demonstrated by Gomori (1939) to be present in the adventitia of medium sized arteries. Newman *et al.* (1950) showed the enzyme alkaline phosphatase to be cytoplasmic in localization in blood vessels and to be present within the capillaries rather than in the larger vessels. Kirk and Praetorius (1950) reported the presence of phosphatase, using disodium phenylphosphate as the substrate, in homogenates of the human aorta. They found two peaks of activity, one at pH 5.75 which we call an acid phosphatase that had a large amount of activity, and another peak at pH 9.5 which we call an alkaline phosphatase which had only a slight amount of activity. It is interesting that Balo *et al.* (1948) were unable to find any alkaline phosphatase activity when they used the substrate sodium-β-glycerophosphate and reported its increase in tissue culture when estradiol was included in the media. From the information derived from histochemical studies the apparent discrepancies in the above results might be accounted for by the fact that there is no histochemically demonstrable alkaline phosphatase in the human aorta except in the adventitia and vasa vasorum (Woerner, 1959; Sandler and Bourne, 1960a, b). It has been shown by Patterson *et al.* (1957) that this enzyme was present in the capillaries which were revascularizing the plaques present in human atherosclerotic aortas. It would appear that the alkaline phosphatase that was demonstrated by Kielly and Meyerhof (1950) and Malinow (1960) may well have been due to the activity of the vasa vasorum in the adventitia and those vasa vasorum which are known to penetrate into the outer third of the media. Sandler and Bourne have shown that alkaline phosphatase, using the Gomori type procedure, is not present in the media or intima in the aortas of the dog, rat, cat (Sandler and Bourne, 1960a, b), monkey (Sandler and Bourne, 1960), or human (Sandler and Bourne, 1962). Lojda *et al.* (1963) reported that the enzyme was not present in any degree in normal rat aorta but that it was present in the media of vitamin-D-fed rats in those areas of the media which had not yet become calcified.

D. Acid Phosphatase

Acid phosphatase has been studied in the human aorta by Levonen *et al.* (1960). These authors found the enzyme to be absent in the normal human aorta but present to a large extent in the atheromatous plaques. Lojda and Zemplényi (1961) found the enzyme to be present in the endothelium and in the cytoplasm of the muscle cells of the media in the human aorta. There is a marked increase in activity of atheromatous aortas especially in the proliferating endothelium and in the macrophages in the plaques. In the fibrous plaques of the rat aorta only a low order of activity is observed, and the above studies in the human atheroma were parallel to the observations in the rat. It is interesting that Schlief *et al.* (1954) studying acid phosphatases at a pH of 4.9, observed an increase of acid phosphatase activity in thromboangitis but an apparent decrease of activity in atherosclerosis. In a later paper Kirk (1959), studying acid phosphatase activity using *p*-nitrophenyl phosphate as a substrate, showed that in the aortas of children there was a lower activity than in adult aortas and observed no change in activity in atherosclerotic aortas. However, in the atherosclerotic coronary arteries there was an increase in activity. What this may mean is that in the biochemical studies, which Kirk performed on the aorta measuring the total amount of acid phosphatase over the whole aorta, were unable to measure the small difference (which could be measured histochemically) in the amount of activity between the various portions of the same vessel. This serves to emphasize the advantage of using histochemical methods in studying tissue metabolism in connection with biochemical studies.

E. 5-Nucleotidase

5-Nucleotidase is an enzyme which acts on adenosine-5-monophosphate (AMP) as well as other 5′-nucleotides and may be an important factor in the regulation of tissue phosphate and adenylate concentrations and possibly in the regulation of tissue calcification as well. The histochemical demonstration of 5-nucleotidase in arterial tissue was first described in human and rat coronary arteries by Newman *et al.* (1950). It was shown to be present in the media of the human aorta by Lupton *et al.* (1952) who studied this enzyme using a modified Gomori type procedure. These authors found 5-nucleotidase to be present in the cytoplasm of the media in the human aorta. The results of these authors have been confirmed since, both histochemically (Sandler and Bourne, 1960a, b) and biochemically by Kirk (1959). Kirk observed that in homogenates of human aortas and pulmonary arteries there was an increase of 5-nucleotidase activity with age. This was also reported by Lupton histochemically. In the atherosclerotic portions of coronary arteries Kirk found no significant change but in the atherosclerotic aortas he found a slight decrease in activity.

It is interesting that Sandler and Bourne (1960a) showed a gradient of activity for 5-nucleotidase in the normal aortas of cats and rats; the highest activity was present in the thoracic portions of the aorta with the enzyme decreased in quantity toward the descending aorta, disappeared in the abdominal portion of the cat aorta, and decreased in activity in the abdominal portion of the rat aorta. They did not find such a gradient in the monkey or human aorta (Sandler and Bourne, 1960b). In the human aorta with atherosclerosis, 5-nucleotidase activity was found to be decreased in the atheroma. This decrease was in the individual cells within the plaque, comparing the activity of these cells to the amount of activity present in the surrounding relatively normal smooth muscle cells.

Here again one can point to the importance of carrying out histochemical studies in addition to biochemical ones so as to be able to differentiate different parts of the same piece of tissue in terms of differences in amount of enzymic activity. It is interesting that in the dog aorta Higginbotham *et al.* (1963) found that there was no histochemically demonstrable 5-nucleotidase activity present in the smooth muscle cells of the media or endothelium.

F. DPNase and TPNase

In studying the enzymes which release inorganic phosphate from the co-dehydrogenases tri- and diphosphopyridine nucleotide (which will be called TPNase and DPNase for convenience) Sandler and Bourne (1960b) observed the following: In the young aortas free of obvious atheroma, there was very little enzymic dephosphorylation of TPN, on the other hand, DPNase activity was intense and evenly distributed throughout the entire intima media. In the older aortas with atheroma, there was a general increase in TPNase activity spread over the entire wall, not only in the normal parts but in the atheromatous portions as well. The DPNase activity was not changed in these aortas. In addition, no differences were found between the normal and atheromatous aortas for the enzyme glucose-6-phosphatase which had a distribution similar to that for alkaline phosphatase.

G. Adenosine Triphosphate

Banga and Nowotny (1951) reported a decrease in ATPase activity
in arteriosclerotic arteries studied biochemically. This decrease was greatest when measured in the presence of magnesium ions at a pH of 7.0 as
compared to a pH of 9.0—a finding which suggests the presence of at
least two ATPases in arteries. More recently Kirk (1959) has shown that
there was a "decrease in the mean adenylpyrophosphatase activity in
arteriosclerotic areas of human aortas when compared to the normal
portions of the same vessel." He obtained similar results in the coronary
arteries of these same individuals and confirmed the presence of at least
two ATPases in the human aorta. The histochemical localization of
ATPase in arterial tissue was first reported in coronary arteries by
Newman *et al.* (1950). It was shown to be present in the media of the
human aorta by Antonini and Weber (1951) and its localization there
has since been confirmed by Sandler and Bourne (1960a, b). Sandler and
Bourne (1960a) reported a gradient of ATPase activity decreasing along
the length of the aorta in the cat and rat aortas. They reported (Sandler
and Bourne, 1960b) in the human aorta a decrease in the ATPase activity
in atheromatous areas. They also found areas in the aorta that were
normal appearing histologically in which the ATPase activity was decreased. It had been shown that synthetic diets free of essential fatty
acids could be used to produce experimental atheroma in the rat
(Thomas and Hartroft, 1959). We believed that it would be interesting
to obtain information as to whether preatheromatous areas devoid of
enzyme activity would develop in these animals on an essential fatty
acid deficient diet. The results of these studies will be discussed below.

H. Amino Peptidase

Levonen *et al.* (1960) studied amino peptidase activity using the substrate L-leucyl-β-naphthylamide. This enzyme was first found in aortas
with occasional atheroma in which moderate activity could be seen only
in the earliest plaques, mainly in the thickening intima. In severely
affected human aorta many sites of activity were present even in the
media. The importance of amino peptidase activity has previously been
much speculated upon by several authors. However, at this time it would
only be confusing to say anything about it concerning the reason for its
increase in human atheroma except that it is the only histochemical
method we have at the present time for estimating or at least for giving
us some information concerning the protein metabolism of arterial tissue.
Lojda and Zemplényi (1961) studied this enzyme histochemically in rab-

bit aortas in unfixed sections. It was present in the endothelium and in the muscle cells. In the endothelium covering atheromatous plaques they found an increase in activity of this enzyme.

I. β-Glucuronidase

This enzyme has been studied histochemically in the aorta by Lojda (1962). However, in view of the criticism of the technique by Janigan and Pearse (1962) in which they demonstrated that the amount of activity demonstrable by the available techniques is completely unrelated to the amount of enzyme activity, we can say that this enzyme remains to be studied histochemically.

IV. Enzyme Changes Demonstrable Histochemically in the Rat in Experimental Atherosclerosis

The animals used in this study were discarded female breeder rats, obtained from the Holtzman Rat Company, Madison, Wisconsin. The animals were maintained in an air-conditioned room, fed and watered daily for the duration of the experiment. The animals included in the study remained apparently free from disease. They were fed a commercial diet, purchased from the Rockland Company, until placed on the experimental diet. Control animals were maintained on the commercial diet. The experimental diet, listed in Table I was a modification of one used by Thomas and Hartroft (1959), and is "fat-free" and "essential fatty acid free."

Food was provided in the animal cages daily *ad libitum* in the form of a paste made by adding a small amount of water to the diet mixture. All animals were weighed weekly to make certain that they maintained a normal rate of growth.

A histochemical technique for the demonstration of phosphatases

TABLE I

EXPERIMENTAL DIET

Ingredient	Amount (%)
1. Casein	20
2. Sucrose	60
3. Salt mixture	4
4. Vitamin fortification mixture	2
5. Choline chloride	0.2
6. Alpha Cel (bulk filler)	8.8
7. Cholesterol	5

was designed independently by Gomori (1941) and Takamatsu (1939). A variation of the technique described by Gomori (1941) is the one which has been used for the demonstration of specific and nonspecific phosphatases in this work. The technique depends on the deposition of calcium phosphate at the site of enzyme activity. The sections were incubated with the phosphate ester in the presence of calcium ions at a pH of 9 or higher. After the sections are incubated in the buffered Ca++ solution containing the substrate, and when necessary, a suitable activator, there then remains the visualization of the calcium phosphate precipitate. The technique, as originally employed by Gomori, utilized the Von Kossa silver stain, but Gomori (1941) used the following system which produced a cobalt sulfide precipitate at the site of the calcium phosphate precipitate. The calcium is first replaced by cobalt and then the section is placed in an ammonium sulfide solution and the phosphate is replaced by the sulfur. This technique is the one preferred by Gomori (1941), Bourne (1943), and Pearse (1960).

A. Results

For the sake of convenience in describing the results the term alkaline phosphatase will be used for the enzyme hydrolyzing sodium-β-glycerophosphate, ATPase for that hydrolyzing adenosine triphosphate, AMP-ase for that hydrolyzing adenosine monophosphate, etc. It must be remembered however, that in actual fact, all that is being shown definitely by the technique is the site of production of inorganic phosphate.

B. Alkaline Phosphatase

When the substrate sodium-β-glycerophosphate was used the reaction was present only in the adventitia and vasa vasorum. The amount of the enzyme and its localization was not different in the animals on the diet from that in the controls.

C. Pyridoxal Phosphate Phosphatase

The enzyme dephosphorylating pyridoxal phosphate was studied in the rat because of the role that phosphorylated derivatives of pyridoxine appear to play as cofactors in certain enzyme reactions such as the conversion of linoleic acid to arachidonic acid. The fact that pyridoxine deficiency had been used to produce atherosclerosis experimentally also makes the study of this system interesting. No change in enzymic activity was seen in experimental atherosclerosis in the rat and the distribution was found to be similar to that of nonspecific alkaline phosphatase.

D. DPNase and TPNase

The dephosphorylation of the codehydrogenases DPN and TPN were also studied in experimental atherosclerosis in the rat.

DPN was present in all three layers of the aorta and it did not differ in experimental animals from the controls. The reaction was similar in appearance to that observed for 5-nucleotidase to be described presently.

TPNase was present in greatest quantity in the adventitia with some reaction present in the media and less in the intima. In the rat, when compared to the previous studies by Sandler and Bourne (1960a), there was no change in experimental atheroma. This points out something known to all workers with experimental animals in this field, that is: that there is a species difference in the metabolism and reactivity to various stimuli of the vascular tree. Owing to this and perhaps other unknown factors the exact development and sequelae of classic human atherosclerosis has not been reproduced in experimental animals.

E. Dephosphorylation of Glycolytic Intermediates

The localization observed when hexose diphosphate, glucose-6-phosphate, and fructose-6-phosphate were used as substrates was very much like that of alkaline phosphatase. Because of this no significance can be attributed to these results except to lend importance to the results obtained with other specific phosphate esters.

F. Riboflavin-5-Phosphatase

Riboflavin-5-phosphate was studied to see how it would be dephosphorylated because of its importance in the electron transport system and to compare it to the codehydrogenases tri- and diphosphopyridine nucleotide. Here again the reaction was similar to that obtained with alkaline phosphatase and it served mainly to emphasize the specificity of the DPNase and TPNase reactions (Sandler and Bourne, 1962).

G. 5-Nucleotidase

The sites of activity observed when adenosine monophosphate was used as a substrate were as follows: the reaction was present in all three layers of the aorta; the reaction was strong but uneven, giving a somewhat spotty appearance along the length of the aorta. There did not appear to be any difference in the reaction observed in the experimental animals as compared with that in the controls. Lojda (1961), in rabbits, found 5-nucleotidase activity in the endothelium of smooth muscle cells in the media. In atheromatous rabbit a weak reaction was observed in the cells of the plaque and in some instances the reaction in the media was weaker than in intact aortas. To demonstrate still another species difference, in the chicken atheromatous aorta this same author demonstrated a strong reactivity in the endothelium covering the plaque.

H. Adenosine Diphosphatase

When adenosine diphosphate was used as a substrate, the reaction was extremely sporadic, being located mainly in the intima and media. The reaction tended to decrease in intensity along the length of the aorta, being strongest in the thoracic portion and weakest in the abdominal portions. There was no observable difference between the experimental animals and the controls.

I. Adenosine Triphosphatase

In the normal rat aorta the reaction was strong and uniform, decreasing in intensity from the thoracic portions to the abdominal portions. The reaction was located mainly in the media and intima with some reactivity in the vasa vasorum. In the aortas of animals maintained 4 weeks on the experimental diet, there could be seen areas or spots of decreased enzymic activity. This reduction in activity is especially interesting in view of the fact that these aortas showed no histological differences when compared with the controls in either the hematoxylin and eosin preparations or those prepared by the Verhoeff and Van Gieson techniques. Neither was there any evidence of lipid deposition in the light microscope in the preparations stained with Sudan black B. However, after 12 weeks on the diet these aortas developed typical atheroma with intimal hypertrophy as seen in the hematoxylin and eosin, and Verhoeff and Van Gieson preparations and deposition of lipid as seen in Sudan black B preparations. In other words, we have in this instance a change in enzymic activity evident in one-third of the time it takes for histologically evident atherosclerotic changes to occur. When this series of experiments was repeated in young rats (3 months of age) obtained from the same source, the results were essentially the same with the exception that it took approximately twice as long, 9 weeks for the enzyme and 25 weeks for the histological changes to become evident.

V. Histochemistry of Enzyme Changes in Experimental Atherosclerosis in the Dog

Since lesions resembling human atherosclerosis have been reported to occur spontaneously in dogs (Detweiler *et al.,* 1961) and since it is possible to produce some of the lesions in these animals by administering thiouracil and a cholesterol-oil-rich diet (Higginbotham and Higginbotham, 1960; Steiner *et al.*, 1949), a study was undertaken of ATPase and 5-nucleotidase in pure bred normal dogs and in genetically similar ones subjected to experimental atherogenic procedures. The two experimental dogs included in the preliminary experiments (Higginbotham *et al.*, 1963) were started at 6 months of age on 0.5 mg of thiouracil daily, and an *ad libitum* diet of dog chow fortified with 3% cholesterol, 5% oil, and approximately three egg yolks daily. They were maintained on this regimen for 12 months at which time they were sacrificed and studied for the enzymes discussed below.

A gradient of ATPase activity was found in the normal dog aortas, both in the circumference of the vessels and along their length. In the root of the aorta, some portions showed a fairly uniform activity throughout the wall of the vessel, while the remainder of the circumference showed a variable decrease in activity in the intima and subintimal portions of the vessels. In longitudinal sections of the aorta, the decreased activity in the intima and inner media persisted to about the middle of the descending thoracic aorta. Activity then appeared to be uniform throughout the width of the wall, but somewhat decreased when compared with the activity in the middle and outer media of the ascending aorta and arch. In the abdominal aorta the activity was reduced when compared with that of the thoracic aorta, being strongest in the outer third of the media. The endothelium showed strong and uniform activity along the whole of the aorta. These findings agree with results obtained in cat and rat aortas (Sandler and Bourne, 1960a).

The over-all ATPase activity in the aortas of the cholesterol-fed dogs was generally decreased when compared with the normal. The reaction was quite irregular, particularly in the abdominal aorta where foci of intense activity appeared throughout the relatively inactive media. Only in the outer third of the media and in the adventitia did the reaction appear as great as in the control. In areas of intimal thickening and of fragmentation and disruption of the elastic elements, a consistent local decrease in activity was noted. One of the experimental animals had a dissecting lesion in the media of the ascending aorta, which had become endothelialized. Little or no activity was demonstrable in this lesion, with the exception of a strongly positive reaction in the new endothelium.

No 5-nucleotidase activity was noted after 5 hours of incubation in any of the aortas, except for a small area in the medial dissection described above. Apparently a species difference exists in the activity of this enzyme since a great deal of activity was noted in the aortas of man (Sandler and Bourne, 1960b), monkey (Sandler and Bourne, 1960), cat, and rat (Sandler and Bourne, 1960a).

Lojda (1962), studying histochemically ATPase activity in rabbit aortas, found the activity present mainly in the endothelium and the muscle cells of the media. In atheromatous aortas in the rat he confirmed the presence of a weak reaction in the cells of the plaque and that in some cases the reaction in the media is weaker than in intact aortas, confirming in the rabbit our experiments in the rat and dog.

VI. Discussion of Experimental Findings

Evidence has thus been presented that a loss of ATPase activity from the aortic wall precedes the development of fatty infiltration in atheroma in the rat and dog and that the same sequence may occur in human aorta.

We should now consider what metabolic significance could be contributed to this finding and what bearing it could have on the accumulation of lipid substance in the formation of atheroma. First of all, the question as to where the various types of lipoidal substances that are present in the atheroma come from must be considered. It has been shown that most of the lipid deposited in the plaque is a product of the aortic tissue itself and is synthesized there (Zilversmit *et al.*, 1961). The cholesterol of the atheroma, however, appears to be mostly from the plasma although some of it is undoubtedly synthesized in the aorta. However, it is probably largely esterified by the aortic tissue itself.

Recent observations with the electron microscope (Greer *et al.*, 1961) indicate that the lipid in the aorta first appears in the smooth muscle cells. Transitional cells between the smooth muscle cell and the foam cell were observed, indicating that these cells are of smooth muscle cell origin and not what would normally be considered as macrophages. This is of special interest in view of the fact that the enzyme changes we observed take place in the smooth muscle cells.

The atheroma contains fatty acids and fats mainly of the longer chain variety; there appear to be two separate mechanisms for the synthesis of fatty acids; for short-chain fatty acids the reversal of β-oxidation is well known. On the other hand, recent work has shown that in the synthesis of long-chain fatty acids there is another system at work involving the formation of malonyl coenzyme A (CoA), a step requiring ATP. The malonyl coenzyme A then combines with fatty aldehyde to add two more carbons on the fatty acid chain. It has in fact been shown that the rate of formation of fatty acids from malonyl CoA in any given tissue is many times faster than from acetyl CoA. Here we see a specific requirement for ATP for the step which may be rate-limiting in the synthesis of a lipoidal component of atheroma, and it must be stated that if the control of the availability of ATP is deranged then an overabundance of long-chain fatty acids will be formed and will cause the typical picture of atheroma.

A role for essential fatty acids in the development of atheroma has been suggested by Sinclair (1956). Evidence has been cited that with essential fatty acid deficiency there is a change in the metabolism of an individual which causes an increase in atheroma formation. The mechanism of action might well be in a defect in the production of this very same ATPase we have been studying. That some ATPases have a phospholipid as an active part of the enzyme molecule has been shown by Kielley and Meyerhof (1950), and it might be postulated that with a deficiency of essential fatty acids there is a deficiency of certain types of phospholipids, and because of this, a deficiency of ATPase in such critical regions as the aorta. Recently, Borst and Loos (1959) reported the direct stimulation of a mitochondrial ATPase by unsaturated long-chain fatty acids with a maximum stimulation at a pH of 9.0.

A similar situation exists in the synthesis of cholesterol with regard to the requirement for ATP for steps that may be rate-limiting. However, since the origin of most of the cholesterol in the atheroma seems to be the plasma, it would not be necessary to emphasize this role here (Sandler and Bourne, 1960b).

It must be understood that the above thought concerning the function of this ATPase we have been studying is at the very best a naive speculation. In all probability the ATPase we have been describing is not an ATPase at all but is a phosphotransferase. This is not hard to understand when one considers that all of the metabolic reactions that utilize adenosine triphosphate as a source of energy, when studied in isolated systems, in the absence of the specific substrate upon which they act, may act as an ATPase. It is only because at the present time we lack a means of measuring this other possible function (which may be the primary function *in vivo*) histochemically that we are forced to speculate as loosely as we have above as to the meaning of the derangement in ATP metabolism we have described. We are however, making some progress in the characterization of this enzyme through the use of specific activators and inhibitors in the histochemical demonstration of this enzyme. Studies in our laboratory indicate that the enzyme is heat-stable, resistant to alcohol, not dependent on magnesium, and is not inhibited by *p*-chloromercuribenzoic acid (Sandler, 1962). In addition the enzyme is being investigated by means of a histochemical technique (Sandler and Bourne, 1961) applied to starch-gel after electrophoresis of homogenates of rat aorta in an attempt to keep track of this enzyme during purification and then determine what other metabolic properties are present with this fraction. In this manner using combined histochemical and biochemical techniques, we may expect to gain further information concerning the metabolic derangements occurring in the arterial wall leading to and/or occurring with and subsequent to atheroma formation.

VII. Summary

Histochemical studies of the aortas of various animals have demonstrated little activity for cytochrome oxidase and a variable succinic dehydrogenase activity according to the layers of the aorta being studied. In general the outer half of the wall of the vessel shows more activity than the inner half. The muscle of the media contains dehydrogenases and on the whole is more active for DPN diaphorase than for TPN diaphorase. Lipase is not common in the normal aorta. Cholinesterase has been recorded in the muscle cells of the media. Simple esterase distribution is also discussed in this chapter.

Alkaline glycerophosphatase activity is low in most of the aortic wall although it is present in fair activity in the adventitia and vasa vasorum.

In the case of other phosphatases, however, there is a good deal of species variation both in the degree of reactivity of the layers of the aortic wall and in the response given by the wall at different levels of the aorta.

It has been shown that in the human aorta there is a decrease of 5-nucleotidase and ATPase activity in human atheromatous plaques and that these enzymes are also decreased in areas which show no histological signs of plaque formation and which possibly represent pre-atheromatous spots. In human atheromatous aortas there is also an over-all increase in TPNase activity compared with that of young normal aortas. No significant changes were found in other phosphatases. Decrease of ATPase activity was also noted in the aortas of dogs afflicted with experimental atheromas and such a decrease precedes atheroma formation.

In rats similarly affected, spotty loss of ATPase activity is found in the aortas to precede deposition of lipid in these regions. This decrease of enzyme activity takes place after 4 weeks on the experimental diet and precedes by 8 weeks the first signs of accumulation of lipid. The atheroma-producing diet in this case is a fat- (and fatty acid) free, high-cholesterol diet found by previous experimenters to produce characteristic atherosclerotic lesions.

It is possible that the deficiency of unsaturated fatty acids in the diet of these animals is responsible for the failure of adequate synthesis of ATPase, the absence of which is responsible for the derangement of the normal metabolism of the aorta resulting in the accumulation of fatty material to form an atheromatous plaque.

ACKNOWLEDGMENT

In the course of this work there were many persons for whose help and suggestions the authors are grateful. We are especially indebted to Mrs. Sara Langly, Miss Susan Drury, Miss Maria Atonopolo, and Mr. John Rieser for their technical assistance. Our thanks also to Miss Jane Maddox for her patience in the typing of the drafts and final copies of the manuscript.

This work was supported in the main by USPHS Grant H4553, with additional support from the Georgia Heart Association, National Science Foundation, and the Muscular Dystrophy Association.

The authors wish to express their gratitude to Dr. A. C. Higginbotham, Department of Anatomy, West Virginia Medical Center, for supplying some of the specimens of dog aorta and for permitting us the use of unpublished work.

During the course of a portion of this work, Dr. Sandler was USPHS Post-Doctoral Trainee in Anatomy (USPHS 2G505).

REFERENCES

Antonini, F. M., and Weber, G. (1951). *Arch. "de Vechi" Anat. Patol. Med. Clin.* **16**, 985.

Balo, J., Banga, I., and Josepovite, G. (1948). *Z. Vitamin-Hormon-Fermentforsch.* **2**, 1.

Banga, I., and Nowotny, A. (1951). *Acta Physiol. Acad. Sci. Hung.* **2**, 327.

Borst, P., and Loos, J. A. (1959). *Rec. Trav. Chim.* **78**, 874.

Bourne, G. (1943). *Quart. J. Exptl. Physiol.* **32**, 1-20.

Detweiler, D. K., Patterson, D. F., Hubben, K., and Botts, R. P. (1961). *Am. J. Public Health* **51**, 228.

Fried, G. H., and Zweifach, B. W. (1955). *Anat. Record* **121**, 1.

Gerö, J. G., Devenyi, T., Virag, S., Szekely, J., and Jakab, L. (1961). Paper delivered at the 4th International Congress of Angiology, Prague, Czechoslovakia, September 4-9, 1961.

Gomori, G. (1939). *Proc. Soc. Exptl. Biol. Med.* **42**, 23.

Gomori, G. (1941). *J. Cellular Comp. Physiol.* **17**, 71-84.

Gomori, G. (1946). *A.M.A. Arch. Pathol.* **41**, 121.

Greer, J. C., McGill, H. C., Jr., and Strong, J. P. (1961). *Am. J. Pathol.* **38**, 263.

Higginbotham, A. C., and Higginbotham, F. H. (1960). *Anat. Record* **136**, 210.

Higginbotham, F. H., Sandler, M., Higginbotham, A. C., and Bourne, G. H. (1963). Unpublished data.

Janigan, D., and Pearse, A. G. E. (1962). *J. Histochem. Cytochem.* **10**, 6.

Kielley, W. W., and Meyerhof, O. (1950). *J. Biol. Chem.* **183**, 391.

Kirk, J. E. (1959). *J. Gerontol.* **14**, 181.

Kirk, J. E., and Praetorius, E. (1950). *Science* **111**, 334.

Levonen, E., Raekallio, J., and Uotila, U. (1960). *Nature* **188**, 677.

Lojda, Z. (1961). Paper delivered at the 5th International Congress of Angiology at Prague, Czechoslovakia, September 4-9, 1961.

Lojda, Z. (1962). *Cesk. Morfol.* **10**, 1.

Lojda, Z., and Zemplényi, T. (1961). *J. Atherosclerosis Res.* **1**, 101.

Lojda, Z. Zemplényi, T., and Grafnetter, D. (1963). *Cor et Vasa* (in press).

Lupton, E. S., Miller, J. L., Slatkin, M. H., and Brodley, M. (1952). *Am. J. Syphilis Gonorrhea Venereal Diseases* **36**, 559.

Malinow, M. R. (1960). *Circulation Res.* **8**, 506.

Newman, W., Feigin, I., Wolf, A., and Kabat, E. A. (1950). *Am. J. Pathol.* **26**, 257.

Patterson, J. C., Mills, J., and Moffatt, T. M. (1957). *A.M.A. Arch. Pathol.* **64**, 129.

Pearse, A. G. E. (1960). *In* "Histochemistry Theoretical and Applied." Little, Brown, Boston, Massachusetts.

Sandler, M. (1962). Unpublished observations.

Sandler, M., and Bourne, G. H. (1960). Unpublished observations.

Sandler, M., and Bourne, G. H. (1960a). *J. Gerontol.* **15**, 32.

Sandler, M., and Bourne, G. H. (1960b). *Circulation Res.* **8**, 1274.

Sandler, M., and Bourne, G. H. (1961). *Exptl. Cell Res.* **24**, 174.

Sandler, M., and Bourne, G. H. (1962). *Nature* **193**, 4821.

Schlief, H., Schmidt, C. G., and Hillenbrand, H. J. (1954). *Z. Ges. Exptl. Med.* **122**, 497.

Sinclair, H. M. (1956). *Lancet* **i**, 381.

Steiner, A., Kendall, F. E., and Bevans, M. (1949). *Am. Heart J.* **38**, 34.

Takamatsu, H. (1939). *Trans. Soc. Pathol. Japon.* **29**, 429.

Thomas, W. A., and Hartroft, W. S. (1959). *J. Nutr.* **69**, 4.

Woerner, C. A. (1959). *In* "The Arterial Wall" (A. I. Lansing, ed.), pp. 1-14. Williams & Wilkins, Baltimore, Maryland.

Zilversmit, D. B., Sweeley, C. C., and Newman, H. A. I. (1961). *Circulation Res.* **9**, 235.

Author Index

Numbers in italics refer to pages on which the complete references are listed.

A

Abell, L. L., 395, *430*
Abraham, S., 330, *345*
Achaya, K. T., 303, 305, 333, *343*, *346*
Acker, M. S., *298*
Ackerman, R. F., 233, *259*, 340, 342, *346*, *347*
Adams, C. M., 287, *293*
Adams, C. W. M., 425, *432*
Adelson, S. F., 271, 276, *298*
Aftergood, L., 305, *343*
Agmon, J., 275, 276, *294*, *298*, *299*
Ahmed, Z., *114*, 497, *509*
Ahrens, E. H., Jr., 284, *292*, *298*, 305, *343*
Albers, H. J., 303, 304, 309, *343*
Albrechtsen, C. K., 98, *114*
Albrink, M. J., 284, *292*, *298*
Alderberg, D., 245, 289, *297*, *360*
Alex, M., 140, 155, 159, *163*
Alfin-Slater, R. B., 303, 305, 333, 343, *346*
Alibasoglu, M., 417, *432*
Alivirta, P., 280, *298*
Allalouf, D., 275, 276, *298*, *299*
Allot, E. N., 497, *510*
Almy, T. P., 245, *262*
Alousi, K., 449, *457*
Altschul, R., 3, 11, 13, 14, 15, 20, *36*, 382, *432*, 440, *456*, 461, *509*
Altshuler, C. H., 139, *162*
Anastasopoulos, G., 289, *294*
Andelman, S. L., 234, 244, *262*
Anderson, D. V., 143, *162*
Anderson, J. T., 240, *262*, 268, 271, 276, 278, 279, 280, 281, 282, 286, 289, *292*, *294*, *295*, *296*
Anderson, P., 283, *293*
Andrus, S. B., 367, 387, *433*, *435*, 440, 442, 443, 446, 447, *456*, *457*
Angevine, D. M., 139, *162*
Anitschkow, N., 198, *227*, 350, *432*, 440, 442, *456*, 461, 507, *509*
Antonini, F. M., 92, 94, *114*, 522, *531*

B

Antonis, A., 280, 284, *292*
Apostolakis, M., 303, 336, *343*
Archer, M., 270, *295*
Armstrong, E. C., 269, *297*, *299*
Aronson, W., 361, *432*
Arteaga, A., 280, *294*
Asboe-Hansen, G., 240, *259*
Aschoff, L., 126, *162*, 272, 293
Asher, G., 275, *293*
Ashikawa, J. K., 304, *346*
Astrup, T., 98, *114*, *115*, 289, *297*
Atkinson, D. I., 338, *347*
Auda, B. M., 333, *345*
Axelrod, A. E., 125, *164*
Azarnoff, D. C., 91, *114*

B

Baczko, A., 240, *259*
Baker, J. R., 503, *510*
Baldwin, D., 21, *38*
Baló, J., 92, *114*, 497, *509*, 519, *531*
Banga, I., 92, 94, *114*, 497, *509*, 519, 522, *531*
Bansi, H. W., 272, 273, *293*
Bardwil, W. A., 83, *117*
Barford, R. A., 314, 317, 319, 320, 322, 324, 325, 326, *344*, *345*
Barker, N., 225, *229*
Barker, S. A., 124, *165*
Barker, S. B., 77, *114*
Barnes, B. O., 274, 282, *293*
Barnes, L. L., 385, *434*
Baronofsky, I. D., 399, *436*
Barr, D. P., 244, 245, *259*, *261*
Barron, E. J., 312, *345*
Barrow, J. G., 287, 288, *293*
Barry, P., 233, *260*
Bartley, W., 314, 316, 317, *344*
Bassiouni, M., 142, *162*
Bavina, M. V., 90, *114*, *116*, 505, *511*
Beadenkopf, W. G., 41, *64*
Beaumont, J. L., *298*

533

Subject Index

A

Acid mucopolysaccharides, 142-143

Acid mucopolysaccharides of connective tissue, 122

Acid phosphatase activity of human arterial tissue, 92

Aconitase activity of human arterial tissue, 84-85

Adenosinetriphosphatase activity of human arterial tissue, 92

Adenylpyrophosphatase activity of human arterial tissue, 92

AGPDH in a plaque from rabbit aorta, 475

AGPDH in rabbit coronary artery, 487

Aldolase activity of human arterial tissue, 79

Anatomical aspects of aortic metabolism, 72-73

Aorta, histochemistry, 127-131
  appearance in a 40-year-old person, 129
  appearance of elastic fibers in the tunica media, 128
  appearance of fibrous plaque, 130
  atherosclerotic intima, 130-131
    appearance of lipoidal plaque of the luminal intima, 131
    primary fibrous plaques, 130-131
    secondary fibrous plaques, 130, 131
  calcium salts, 132-135
    appearance of fibrous plaque with calcification, 133
    appearance of medial aortic calcification, 133
  lipid, 135-141
    appearance of lipid in the tunica intima, 136
    cholesterol crystals, 135
    "foam cells," 135
  macroscopically normal intima, 128
  metachromasia, 129
  stage of fibrosis, 129-130
  stage of proliferation, 129
  media, 127-128
    collagenous fibrils, 128
    elastic fibers, 128
    elastic membranes, 127

ground substance, increase with age, 127
  smooth muscle, 128

Aorta, physiochemical and chemical studies of ground substance and collagen, 141-158
  age variations in the calcium and lipid concentrations in intima, 156
  age variations in the calcium and lipid concentrations in media, 156
  calcium and lipid contents, 155-158
  collagen analyses, 148
  elastin content in percentage of tissue weight, 159
  hexosamine and sulfate contents, 147
  hexosamine content in intimal and medial aortic tissue, 150
  hexosamine, estersulfate, and hydroxyproline contents, 147-155
  hydroxyproline content in intimal and medial aortic tissue, 150
  isolation of mucopolysaccharides, 141-147
  molecular weights of hyaluronate isolated from human aortas, 145
  mucopolysaccharide fractions expressed in percentages of dry, defatted tissue weight, 146

Aortic atherosclerosis, 54-60
  correlation with coronary artery lesions, 56-57
  histology and electron microscopy, 57-60
    fatty streaks, 57-60
    fatty streaks, electron microscopic appearance, 58
    fatty streaks, histologic appearance, 58
    fibrous plaques, 60
    intracellular lipid inclusions, 59-60
    musculoelastic intimal thickening, 57
  incidence by age, race, and sex in New Orleans, 55
  natural history of gross lesions, 54
    fibrous plaques, 54
    prevalence, 54
    racial comparison, 54-55
    topographical distribution, 54